May, 2002.
To Winnie & Branch.
With love,
Allie (Bury).

The Military Nurses of Canada

Recollections of Canadian Military Nurses

E.A. Landells, Editor

published with the assistance of

Co-Publishing
a division of Addison Graphics Ltd.

White Rock, BC, Canada V4B 3Z5

Canadian Cataloguing in Publication Data

The National Library of Canada has Catalogued this publication as follows:

Main entry under title:

The military nurses of Canada
Includes bibliographical references and index.
ISBN 0–9699561–0–X

1. Military nursing – Canada – Anecdotes. I. Landells, E.A., 1922-II Title.UH 495.C3M44 1995 355.3`45`082 C95-900390-8

Distribution Address:
Co-Publishing
1430 Johnston Road
White Rock, BC, Canada V4B 3Z5

Co-Publishing is a division of Addison Graphics Ltd.

Cover Design: A collage of photographs from *Canada's Nursing Sisters* by G.W.L. Nicholson, published by Samuel Stevens, Hakkert & Co., Toronto, 1975

Printed and Bound in Canada by Addison Graphics Ltd.

TABLE OF CONTENTS

ACKNOWLEDGEMENTS

This project could not have been accomplished without the assistance of the many sincere and helpful individuals who contributed not only their stories but also their unfailing support. Completing this book has been one of the happiest experiences of my life. Following are some of the many to whom I am indebted:

Alberta Association of Registered Nurses including Archivist Lorraine Mychajluno; British Columbia History of Nursing Professional Practice Group; Dr. Shirley M. Stinson, Faculty of Nursing, University of Alberta; the Nursing Sisters Association of Canada, British Columbia Unit; the Nursing Sisters Association of Canada, Toronto Unit; the Ministry of Defence, London, England; Colonel Marielle Gagné, Directorate of Health Care Personnel, National Defence Headquarters, Ottawa; Colonel Helen Ott, CFMS, retired; Lt. Colonel Harriet Sloan, CFMS, retired; Lieut. Commander S.T. Richards, RCN, retired; all the nurses who contributed their stories and photographs and assisted in so many ways to provide information and support; Alexandra Bury, who was instrumental in contacting numerous nurses and urging them to complete their stories for publication; Gerry Gerow, Dorothy Karr, Doug Lunn, and Pat Truant, copy editor and word processor. Information in the brief history at the beginning of each unit of this book was the result of my research of the War Diaries at the National Archives of Canada at Ottawa. The weeks I spent at the Archives became an interesting and pleasant task largely due to the helpful staff.

Special mention must be given to Master Warrant Officer Gordon Phillips, RCAF retired, for his untiring efforts as editor. He patiently shared his technical and administrative expertise and knowledge of military history throughout the many months required to complete this book.

FOREWORD

Edith Landells has tackled a monumental job in attempting to present the stories of nursing sisters.

The early nurses were adventurous for their time, some with very strong convictions, doing something daring in "enlisting." All of these women gave leadership in casualty care, sustaining patients with skilled knowledgeable care and comforting them with tender loving care.

Peacetime Nursing Sisters carried on, maintaining the health of service personnel, and in some cases their families, with steadily diminishing resources and ever increasing demands as technology and positive health measures advanced. Seldom did their resources (personnel, equipment, etc.) keep up with the increasing tasks assigned to the Canadian Armed Forces across Canada and around the world. nursing sisters trained professional and non-professional personnel, and they themselves adapted and evolved into assuming full officers responsibilities beyond their specialties, showing strong loyalty to their profession, to their fellow service personnel and to their country.

Edith Landells has given recognition to these military nursing officers and has attempted to accord them the respect they deserve.

I am proud to have served with some of them albeit in peacetime only.

Helen F. Ott
(Captain RCN retired)

FOREWORD

Canada's Nursing Sisters by Colonel G.W.L. Nicholson, published in 1975 records the official history of the military nursing service from The North West Rebellion to Korea. Now, thanks to the tireless dedication of Edith Landells, their story, based on personal remembrances, is continued in *The Military Nurses of Canada*. The sisters speak of endless convoys of wounded, the long hours under canvas, no lights or running water, the heat and the cold, the rain and the mud. They tell of the compassion of the wounded men for one another. They record with gratitude the blessings of penicillin, supplies of blood and plasma, and the rapid evacuation from North West Europe by the RCAF in their flying ambulances,the *Dakotas*. Their own often threatened safety is of no consequence. Always they speak of "their boys."

The sisters of the RCN recall that their sailor patients not only suffered grievous wounds but were often soaked in oil and exposed to the rigours of the North Atlantic.

Airmen, survivors of crashes, faced painful months of reconstructive surgery to dreadful burns of heads, faces and hands. Their care required all the ingenuity, support and patience the RCAF sisters could muster.

June Newton Plummer, No. 15 CGH, speaks for all nursing sisters when in her narrative she says, *"My military experience would be incomplete without paying tribute to the wonderful, brave and grateful patients we were privileged to have in our care."*

That care is continued today with the same selfless compassion, by the nursing officers of the CFMS in Bosnia, Somalia and Rwanda.

It is fitting that this book should be published in 1994-1995, the year dedicated to "Canada Remembers."

Thank you, Edith Landells, for continuing our story.

Hallie Sloan, President
Nursing Sister Association of Canada
1994 - 1996

INTRODUCTION

On going to the National Archives in Ottawa and reading comments about nursing sisters in the War Diaries, I feel obliged to attempt an explanation. Nurses were not trained in army protocol; they did not know King's Regulations (Canada) which soldiers and male officers knew by heart.

There were some problems between enlisted men, male officers and nursing sisters which probably arose from the lack of training provided to the nurses. They were unaware, to some extent, of army protocol. They weren't given the opportunity to learn rules and regulations. Nurses were not always mobilized at the same time as the rest of the unit. It was often a well trained cohesive unit by the time they joined.

This changed with time. Nursing officers now go to Chilliwack, British Columbia, for Basic Officers Orientation.

In May 1942, Canadian nursing sisters became the first nurses in an Allied country to receive official officer status with an equivalent power of command.*

There must be some gain from writing this book other than recording anecdotes of time and place. The point of the book is not to make us out as heroes of war, but simply to show the determination and dedication of this group of ordinary human beings. Sincerity was so apparent in the narratives I received that text was retained in the original form.

* WOMEN IN THE WAR EFFORT,
H. Andrea Brown and Diane Shaffelburg, Copyright 1986, Board of Education for the City of North York resource booklet for Remembrance Day. Produced by: Women's Studies Curriculum and Staff Development Services, North York Schools.

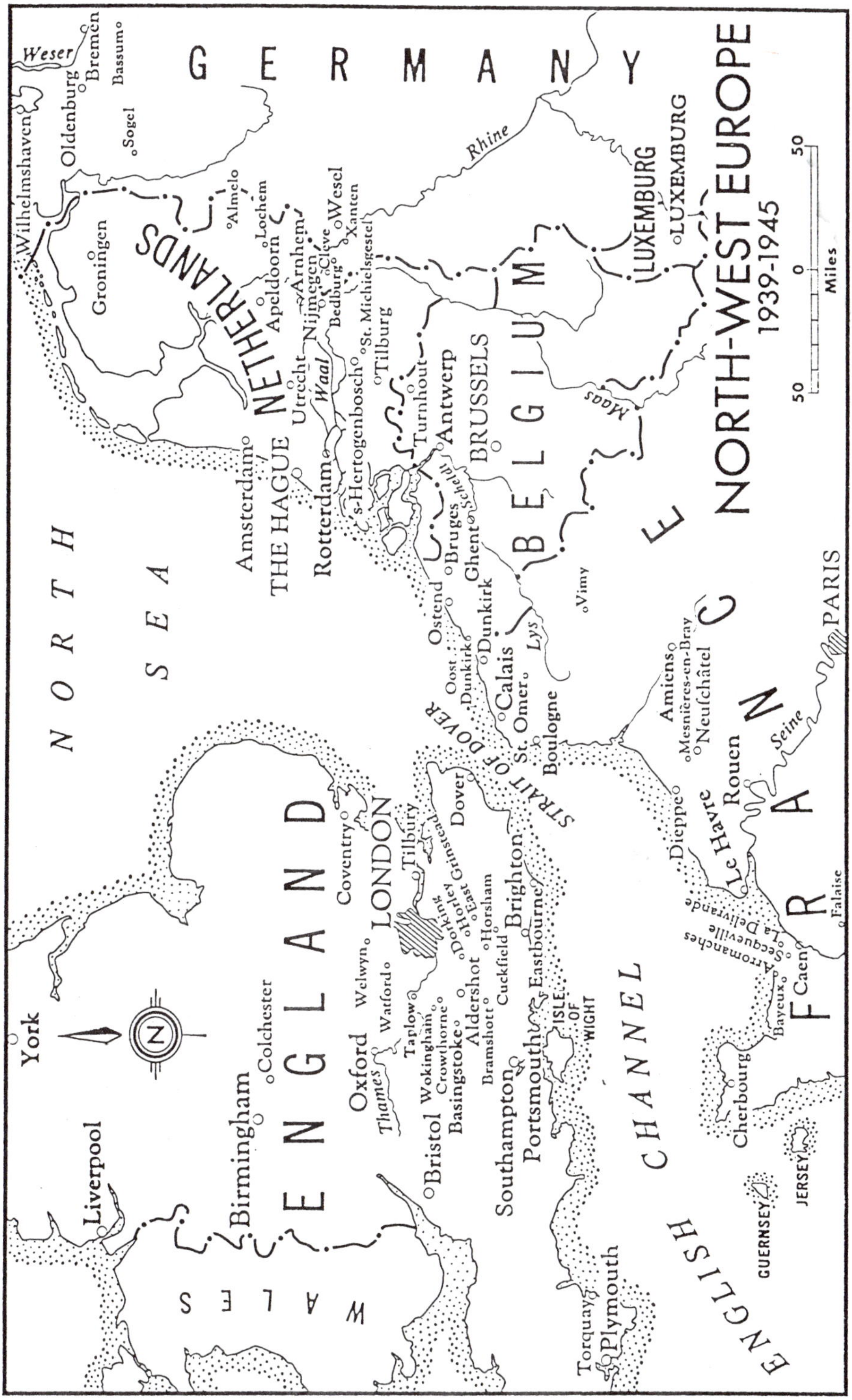
NORTH-WEST EUROPE
1939-1945
Miles
50
0
50
GERMANY
NETHERLANDS
BELGIUM
LUXEMBURG
FRANCE
ENGLAND
WALES
NORTH SEA
ENGLISH CHANNEL
STRAIT OF DOVER
ISLE OF WIGHT
GUERNSEY
JERSEY
Weser
Rhine
Waal
Maas
Scheldt
Lys
Seine
Thames
Wilhelmshaven
Oldenburg
Bremen
Bassum
Sogel
Groningen
Almelo
Lochem
Wesel
Xanten
Apeldoorn
Arnhem
Cleve
Nijmegen
Bedburg
St. Michielsgestel
Tilburg
Utrecht
Amsterdam
THE HAGUE
Rotterdam
s-Hertogenbosch
Turnhout
Antwerp
BRUSSELS
Bruges
Ghent
Ostend
Oost Dunkirk
Dunkirk
Calais
St. Omer
Boulogne
Vimy
LUXEMBURG
Amiens
Mesnières-en-Bray
Neufchâtel
PARIS
Dieppe
Rouen
Le Havre
Falaise
La Délivrande
Sequeville
Arromanches
Caen
Bayeux
Cherbourg
York
Liverpool
Birmingham
Colchester
Coventry
LONDON
Tilbury
Welwyn
Watford
Oxford
Taplow
Wokingham
Crowthorne
Basingstoke
Aldershot
Bramshott
Bristol
Dorking
Horley
East Grinstead
Horsham
Cuckfield
Dover
Brighton
Eastbourne
Southampton
Portsmouth
Torquay
Plymouth

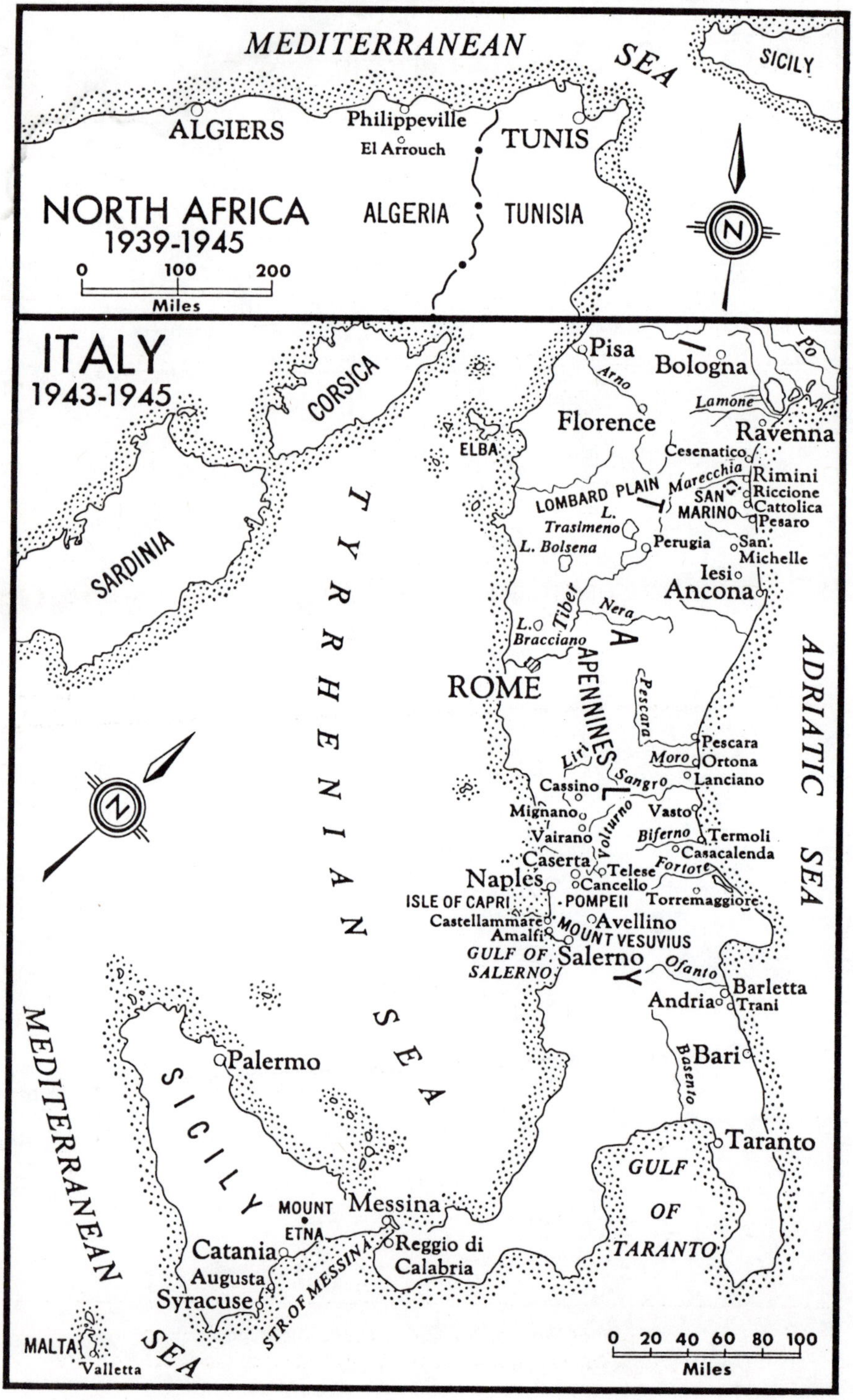
MEDITERRANEAN SEA
SICILY
ALGIERS
Philippeville
El Arrouch
TUNIS
NORTH AFRICA
1939-1945
ALGERIA
TUNISIA
0 100 200
Miles
N
ITALY
1943-1945
CORSICA
SARDINIA
ELBA
Pisa
Arno
Bologna
Po
Lamone
Florence
Ravenna
Cesenatico
Marecchia
Rimini
Riccione
Cattolica
Pesaro
LOMBARD PLAIN
SAN MARINO
L. Trasimeno
L. Bolsena
Perugia
San Michelle
Iesi
Ancona
TYRRHENIAN SEA
Nera
Tiber
L. Bracciano
ROME
APENNINES
ITALY
Pescara
ADRIATIC SEA
Pescara
Moro
Ortona
Liri
Sangro
Lanciano
Cassino
Mignano
Vasto
Volturno
Vairano
Biferno
Termoli
Casacalenda
Caserta
Telese
Fortore
Naples
Cancello
ISLE OF CAPRI
POMPEII
Torremaggiore
Castellammare
MOUNT VESUVIUS
Avellino
Amalfi
GULF OF SALERNO
Salerno
Ofanto
Barletta
Andria
Trani
Basento
Bari
Palermo
SICILY
Taranto
GULF OF TARANTO
MOUNT ETNA
Messina
Reggio di Calabria
Catania
Augusta
Syracuse
STR. OF MESSINA
MEDITERRANEAN SEA
MALTA
Valletta
0 20 40 60 80 100
Miles

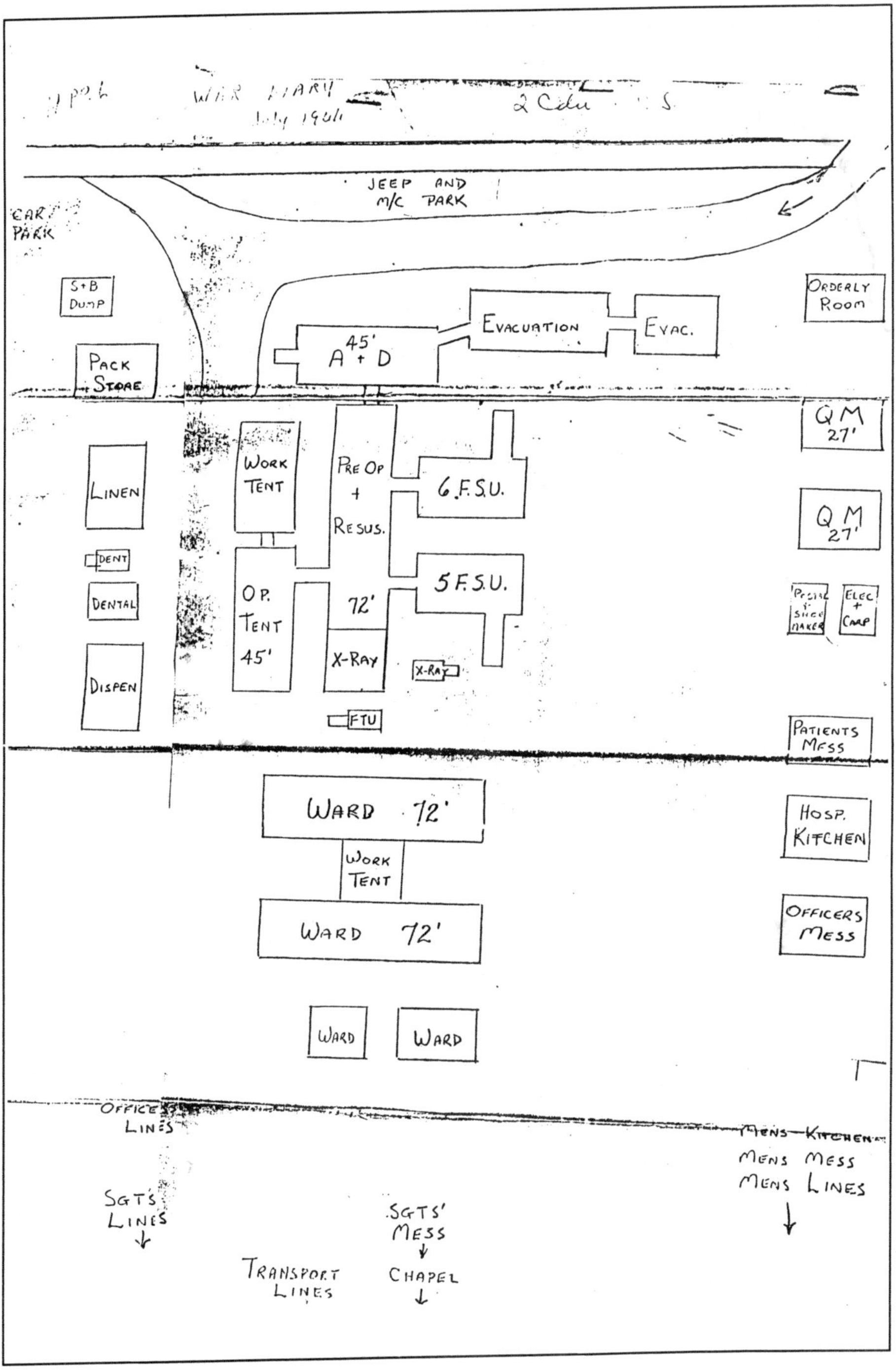

Physical Plan of No. 2 Casualty Clearing Station
Courtesy of War Diaries at National Archives of Canada, Ottawa

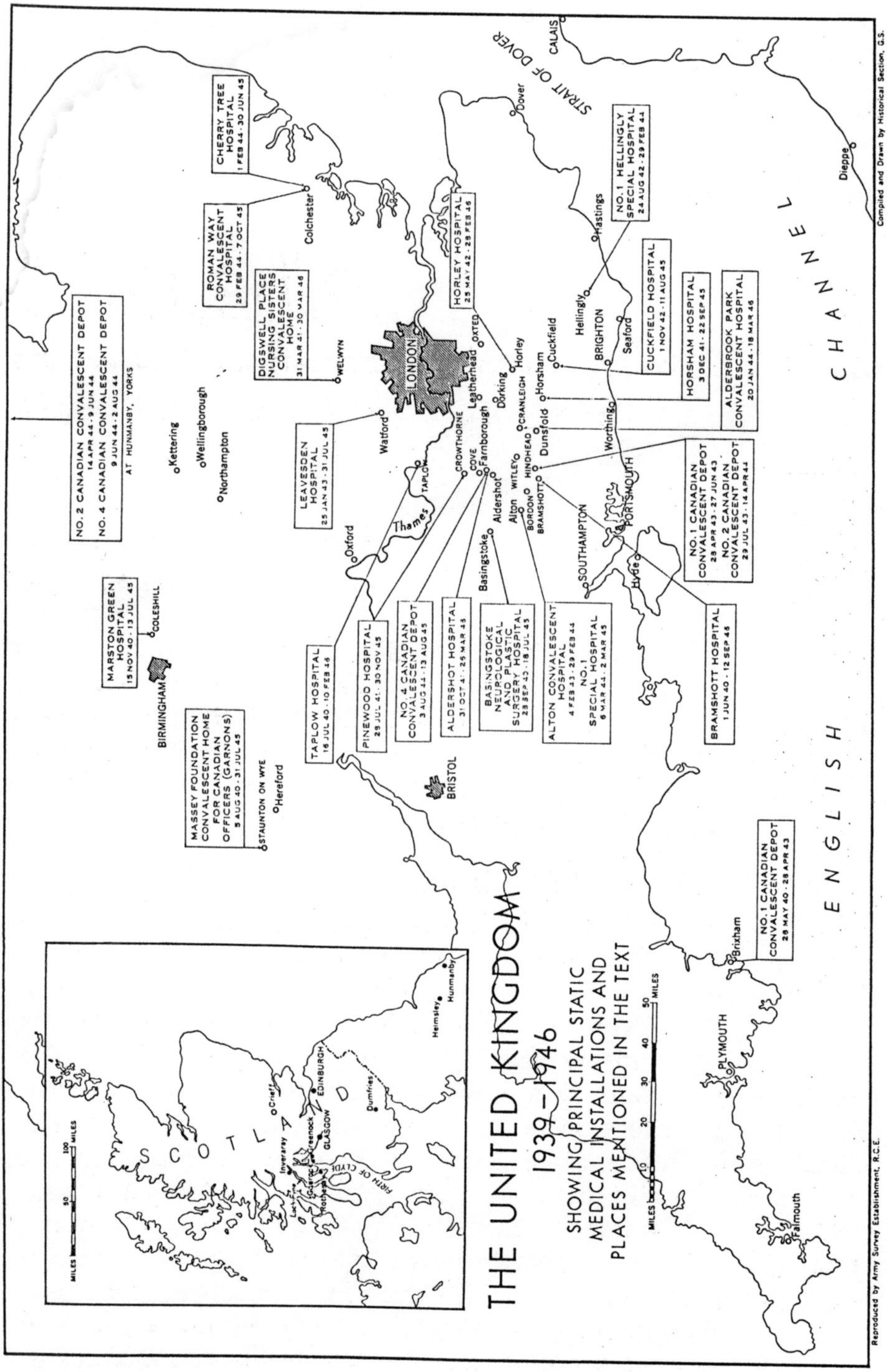

THE UNITED KINGDOM
1939–1946
SHOWING PRINCIPAL STATIC MEDICAL INSTALLATIONS AND PLACES MENTIONED IN THE TEXT
NO. 2 CANADIAN CONVALESCENT DEPOT 14 APR 44 - 9 JUN 44
NO. 4 CANADIAN CONVALESCENT DEPOT 9 JUN 44 - 2 AUG 44
AT HUNMANBY, YORKS
ROMAN WAY CONVALESCENT HOSPITAL 29 FEB 44 - 7 OCT 45
CHERRY TREE HOSPITAL 1 FEB 44 - 30 JUN 45
DIGSWELL PLACE NURSING SISTERS CONVALESCENT HOME 31 MAR 41 - 30 MAR 46
LEAVESDEN HOSPITAL 25 JAN 43 - 31 JUL 45
HORLEY HOSPITAL 25 MAY 42 - 28 FEB 46
NO. 1 HELLINGLY SPECIAL HOSPITAL 24 AUG 42 - 29 FEB 44
CUCKFIELD HOSPITAL 1 NOV 42 - 11 AUG 45
HORSHAM HOSPITAL 3 DEC 41 - 22 SEP 45
ALDERBROOK PARK CONVALESCENT HOSPITAL 20 JAN 44 - 18 MAR 46
NO. 1 CANADIAN CONVALESCENT DEPOT 28 APR 43 - 27 JUN 43
NO. 2 CANADIAN CONVALESCENT DEPOT 29 JUL 43 - 14 APR 44
MARSTON GREEN HOSPITAL 15 NOV 40 - 13 JUL 45
MASSEY FOUNDATION CONVALESCENT HOME FOR CANADIAN OFFICERS (GARNONS) 5 AUG 40 - 31 JUL 45
TAPLOW HOSPITAL 16 JUL 40 - 10 FEB 46
PINEWOOD HOSPITAL 25 JUL 41 - 30 NOV 45
NO. 4 CANADIAN CONVALESCENT DEPOT 3 AUG 44 - 13 AUG 45
ALDERSHOT HOSPITAL 31 OCT 41 - 25 MAR 45
BASINGSTOKE NEUROLOGICAL AND PLASTIC SURGERY HOSPITAL 23 SEP 40 - 18 JUL 45
ALTON CONVALESCENT HOSPITAL 4 FEB 43 - 29 FEB 44
NO. 1 SPECIAL HOSPITAL 6 MAR 44 - 2 MAR 45
BRAMSHOTT HOSPITAL 1 JUN 40 - 12 SEP 45
NO. 1 CANADIAN CONVALESCENT DEPOT 28 MAY 40 - 28 APR 43
Colchester
WELWYN
Kettering
Wellingborough
Northampton
Watford
LONDON
OXTED
Horley
Leatherhead
Dorking
Crowthorne
Cove
Farnborough
Taplow
Thames
Oxford
Aldershot
Alton
Witley
Hindhead
Cranleigh
Dunsfold
Horsham
Cuckfield
Hellingly
Hastings
Dover
BRIGHTON
Seaford
Worthing
PORTSMOUTH
SOUTHAMPTON
Bordon
Bramshott
Basingstoke
Ryde
Coleshill
BIRMINGHAM
Staunton on Wye
Hereford
BRISTOL
Brixham
PLYMOUTH
Falmouth
STRAIT OF DOVER
CALAIS
Dieppe
ENGLISH CHANNEL
SCOTLAND
EDINBURGH
GLASGOW
Greenock
Inveraray
Crieff
Dumfries
Helmsley
Hunmanby
FIRTH OF CLYDE
MILES 0 10 20 30 40 50 MILES
Compiled and Drawn by Historical Section, G.S.
Reproduced by Army Survey Establishment, R.C.E.

Chapter 1

THE HISTORY OF MILITARY NURSING IN CANADA

The North West Rebellion
South African War
World War I
World War II

By Carolyn (MacIntyre) Jones

Carolyn Jones is a 1969 graduate of Grace Hospital School of Nursing in Winnipeg with a Bachelor of Science degree in nursing from the University of Victoria in 1991. She is a civilian nurse from a military family with a high degree of interest in military nursing. Carolyn is a part-time clinical instructor at Okanagan University College in Kelowna, B.C.

THE HISTORY OF MILITARY NURSING IN CANADA

Military nursing in Canada gained its first recognition at the time of the North West Rebellion in 1885. This was long after the true beginning of military nursing but it is the time when official recognition was given by the awarding of campaign medals, a distinction that had previously been given only to soldiers. The true pioneers in military nursing were the devoted nuns of various religious orders who cared for the casualties of battle, regardless of their race, creed, colour, or religion. During the British and French battles of 1759, sisters of the Augustine and Ursuline orders "immediately took the harassing duty of nursing the sick and wounded in overcrowded wards and with hardly any proper hospital appliances."[1] The French tradition for nursing sisters belonging to various orders to serve in military as well as civilian hospitals seems to have started the practice of designating female nurses trained and commissioned to serve under military command as "nursing sisters."[2] These devoted sisters, robed in white with black gauze veils, portrayed an image of gentleness and strength. In *The History of Emily Montague* (1759), the high regard for these nursing sisters is evident. "The nuns, who are all of the noblesse, are many of them handsome, and all genteel, lively and well bred; they have an air of the world and their conversation is easy, spirited and polite."[3] About one hundred years later, it is the example of the Sisters of Charity, nursing in French military hospitals during the Crimean War that promoted the British decision to ask Florence Nightingale to organize and lead female nurses to the Crimean theatre. Florence Nightingale, credited with being the founder of military nursing, played a valuable role in the raising of the standard of education and character among nurses. These changes impacted on nurses in Canada and the United States, as hospital training schools used the Nightingale School of Nursing as their model.

THE NORTH WEST REBELLION

The North West Rebellion, a fourteen-week campaign in the spring of 1885, fought by the Canadian Militia against Louis Riel and his Metis followers, was the incentive for the organization of a Canadian Militia medical and surgical department. The newly appointed surgeon-general was Lt. Col. Darby Bergin, a prominent surgeon and member of parliament for Cornwall and commanding officer of the 59th Stormont and Glengarry Battalion of Infantry.

Dr. Bergin was responsible for two completely equipped field hospitals being sent by rail from Montreal to Swift Current. Surgeons were appointed and recommendations made to the minister of militia and defence regarding the organization of a corps of nurses. However, this organization was not done before the more than fifty casualties at Fish Creek were taken to a temporary hospital at the village of Saskatoon. Here, the lack of skilled nursing became evident and the volunteer help offered by local women was not sufficient. Help came from Winnipeg, when the head nurse of the Winnipeg General Hospital, Loretta Miller, arrived in Saskatoon on May 12. She immediately took charge of the patients in the hospital, and two days later received thirty-seven wounded from the Battle of Batoche. On May 23, four more nurses from Winnipeg arrived at the Saskatoon Field Hospital to assist with the some eighty sick and wounded, including

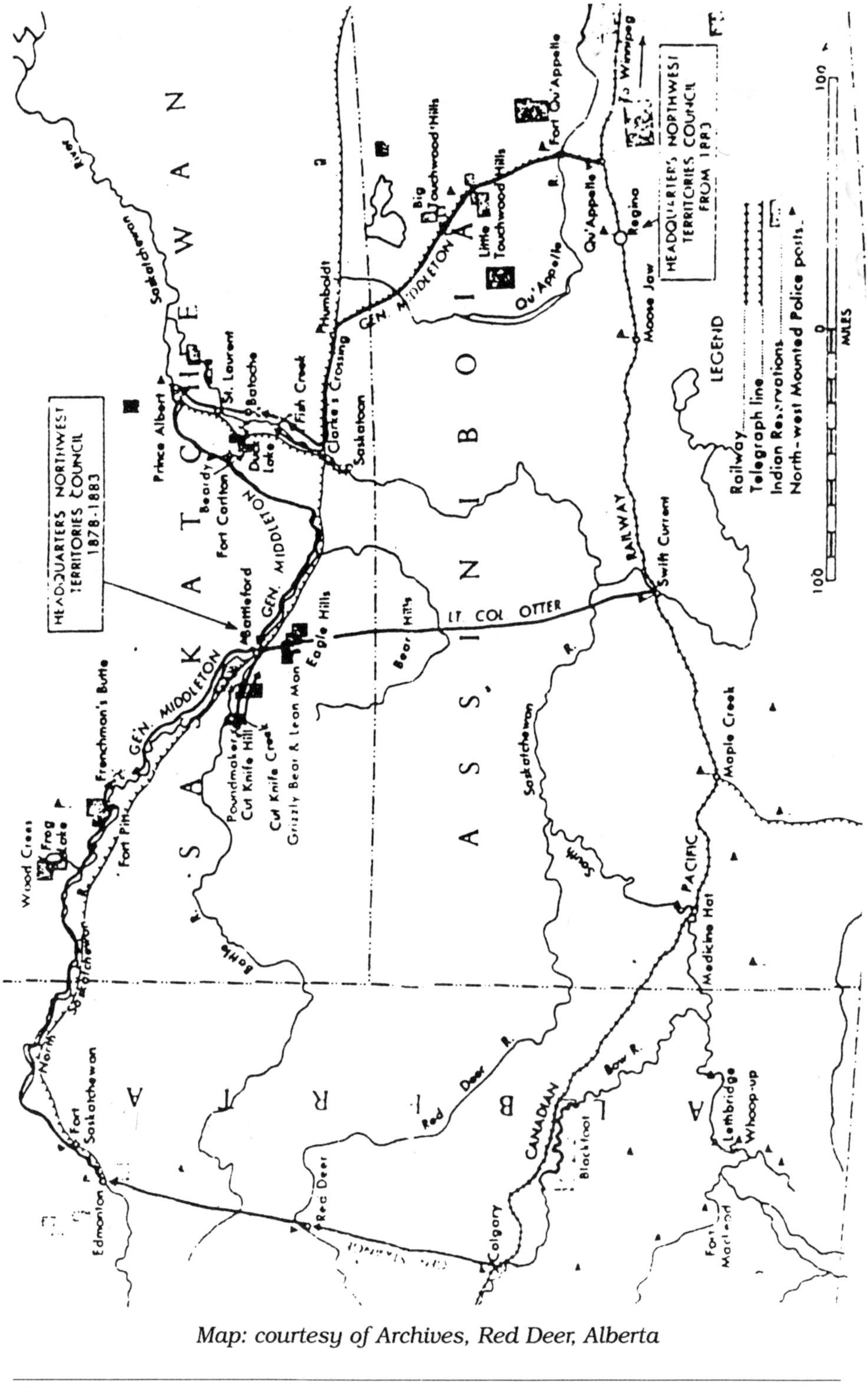

Map: courtesy of Archives, Red Deer, Alberta

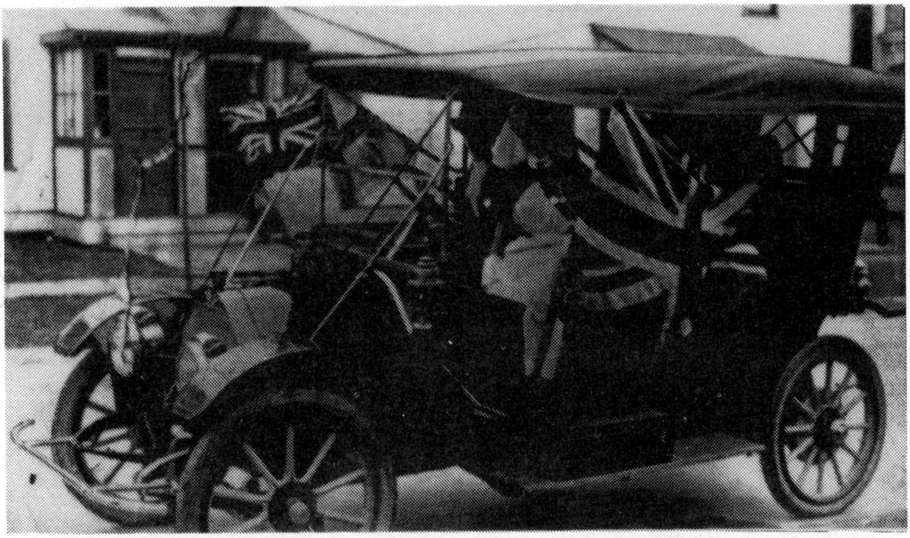

Phoebe (Parsons) Howard, born 1855 in Elora, Ontario – died after1937 (year unknown) at Winnipeg. She was the last surviving member of the group of nurses who served in the Riel Rebellion.
This photo was taken at a Decoration Parade, Winnipeg, Manitoba, 12 May 1911.
More information is available at the Provincial Archives, Winnipeg.
Photo loaned by her niece Eileen (Elliot) Radoslav
*Mrs. Howard gave her reminiscences to Lillian Gibbons of The Winnipeg Tribune, 13 April 1935.**
*Her story is also described in Canada's Nursing Sisters.***
*"More than half a century later the last surviving member of the group of nurses, Miss Parsons (who later became Mrs. H.C. Howard) recalled in an interview the tiring journey across the prairie from the railway line at Moose Jaw. The two nights on the trail they spent sleeplessly in tents, waging their own private war against sandflies and mosquitoes. Fortunately there were none of these pests at Saskatoon, where Nurse Parsons slept in a tent on a mattress on the ground. She wore no uniform - 'just a plain print dress with a small apron and a Red Cross band on her arm.' In intervals between tending their patients, many of whom were in tents set up near hospital buildings, the nurses kept themselves busy making bandages by tearing up clean pieces of old linen furnished by the women of Winnipeg."***

Gibbon, J.M. and M. Mathewson, Three Centuries of Canadian Nursing. pp.201-202.
***Nicholson, G.W.L. Canada's Nursing Sisters. p.22.*

Indian and Metis casualties.[4] When a base hospital was established in Moose Jaw, and patients transferred from Saskatoon and Swift Current, a request was sent to Ottawa for six more nurses. In charge of this corps of nurses was Sister Hannah Grier Coome, the mother superior of the Sisterhood of St. John the Divine, the first Canadian religious order in the Anglican Church.

Travel was not easy or convenient and it is recorded that during the lake voyage from Owen Sound to Port Arthur, the mother superior, having experienced difficulty in dealing with her long hair in the confined space of her cabin, and realizing the problem of managing it "in a battlefield hospital in the wilderness," cut off the long black tresses and threw them overboard, an example which the other sisters followed.[5] These seven nursing sisters completed their tour of duty in four weeks' time, and were shown a great deal of appreciation and thanks for their skilled nursing and valuable assistance.

In the meantime the hospital at Saskatoon was being closed and the remaining casualties were being sent to Winnipeg, using the one thousand mile water route of the Saskatchewan River and Lake Winnipeg. It was felt that this route would be easier on the wounded than travel on the rough trails to Moose Jaw. The five nurses from the Winnipeg General Hospital and the male medical staff accompanied the seventeen patients. The arduous journey took eleven days and was managed with great skill and care. Each of the twelve nursing sisters, along with every member of the militia force that had been on active service, was awarded the campaign medal "North West Canada, 1885." It was the first time in Canada that female nurses had been recognized as forming part of a military force in the field.[6]

SOUTH AFRICAN WAR

At the outbreak of the South African War in 1899, Canada had no organized military nursing service. This was not accomplished until 1901. However, from the large number of volunteers who applied, four nursing sisters were selected to accompany the one thousand volunteers making up the 2nd Battalion, Royal Canadian Regiment. The nursing sisters were headed by Miss Georgina Pope, a native of Prince Edward Island and graduate of Bellevue Hospital Training School in New York. Miss Pope's work in South Africa was recognized in 1903 when she was awarded the Royal Red Cross for conspicuous service in the field; the first Canadian to win this high distinction. In 1908, Nursing Sister Pope became the first matron of the Canadian Army Medical Corps, a position she held until 1914.[7]

These four nursing sisters who had the distinction of being the first Canadian military nurses to serve overseas left Canada in October 1899. In February 1900, four additional nursing sisters were sent to South Africa with a second contingent. Included in this group was 27-year-old Margaret Macdonald from Nova Scotia, whose long and distinguished career in military nursing was just beginning. She was a graduate of Mount Saint Vincent College, Halifax, and New York City Hospital Training School, Blackwell's Island, New York. Her nursing experience included service in a military hospital for American veterans who had been wounded in Cuba during the Spanish-American War, and on the hospital ship, *Relief*. She served two terms in South Africa and was at the 600-bed No. 18 Stationary Hospital in Harrismith until peace was signed in Vereenigung in 1902. She continued to gain military hospital experience, and in 1914 was sent to England to be in charge of over 100 nurses with the first Canadian Armada. In a short time, she became the matron-in-chief of the Canadian nursing sisters in France during the Great War of 1914-18.[8]

Miss Pope, writing from the large base hospital No. 1 General, at Wynberg, describes a little of the Army sister's life during the South African War.

"*We nursed in huts, and found the work at times very heavy, often times having our dinner between nine and ten P.M. We received our first convoy of wounded a few days after the Battles of Maggersfontein and Modder River, when the beds were filled with the men of the Highland Brigade. We remained at Wynberg for nearly a month, when No. 3 General Hospital of 600 beds was pitched under canvas at Rondebosch, a few miles away. Here we arrived on Christmas Day, and remained almost six months, having at times very active service; sometimes covered with sand during a 'Cape South-Easter'; at others delayed with a fore-runner of the coming rainy season, and at all times in terror of scorpions and snakes as bed-fellows.*"[9]

The following tribute paid to nursing sisters of the South African War was given by a British nursing sister during a talk to an International Congress of Nurses, and sums up the difficulties of this nursing experience and the hardiness of the nurses.

"I hear of Army sisters and Reserves who behaved badly, neglect patients and care for nothing but amusing themselves, but I have not met them. All I have seen, and I have seen many, have appeared to me to be, each in her own degree, quiet, earnest, painstaking women, saying little or nothing of their own discomforts, and most anxious to do all they possibly can for the sick under great drawbacks, not the least of which that they are strangers to one another, in a strange land, seven thousand miles away from home and hospital. I do not believe that, given all the circumstances, the numbers, the heat, the freedom, the poor food bringing its sensation of lethargy and weariness, the constant illness, the many deaths... I do not believe, I say, that any other profession could have borne it as we have done."

It was during the South African War that the Nursing Service was organized as an integral part of the Army Medical Corps and Canadian nurses were granted the rank, pay, and allowance of Lieutenant in the Army.[10]

WORLD WAR I

In 1914 there were only five nursing sisters in the Permanent Army Medical Corps and fifty-seven on the Reserve List.[11] This number grew to over three thousand during the four years of the war. The Overseas Military Forces of Canada utilized the services of 2504 of these nursing sisters and it is about some of their experiences that the following is written.

In 1914, Margaret Macdonald, Matron of the Nursing Service of the Permanent Army Medical Corps, was given the task of mobilizing one hundred nursing sisters for the two general hospitals which were to accompany the first contingent of 2300 troops to England. These nurses were chosen from the thousands of Canadian nurses who had volunteered for service overseas. The additional training received by these nurses was only a week, although they received lectures on such topics as the ethics of Army nursing, discipline, camp sanitation and military routine during the two week Atlantic crossing.[12] The Canadian nurses were welcomed with generous hospitality when they were assigned to English Emergency Stations in Boulogne, Canadian camps on Salisbury Plain, British hospitals, or No. 2 Canadian Stationary Hospital in France. This hospital was housed in Le Touquet Golf Hotel, a seaside resort area at the mouth of the River Canche, twenty-five miles from Boulogne. Thirty-four nursing sisters, under the leadership of Matron Ridley, assisted in changing this recreational hotel into a 320-bed capacity semi-modern hospital. Later, it would have a 615-bed capacity. The first patients, British soldiers, suffered mainly from trench feet, frostbite, or minor gunshot wounds. Sister M.B. Clint, author of *Our Bit, Memoirs of War Service by a Canadian Nursing Sister*, writes the following:

"It is a source of gratification that we had the honour of nursing some of the 'Old Contemptibles,' men of that deathless band which held the enemy hordes at bay beyond a thin khaki line. Our charts bore the names of nearly all the famous regiments of the British Army – the remnants of the first Expeditionary Force. The old British Tommies were the most grateful patients, and many wrote us later that they would never forget the kindness of the Canadians, the different 'atmosphere' from any hospital they had known, the eagerness and good nature of our orderlies."[13] Miss Clint also writes of the 327 Canadian casualties admitted on April 26, following the heavy fighting at Ypres. In an atmosphere of filth and pain, nursing sisters washed, fed, dressed wounds, and made patients as comfortable as possible. Assisting at operations was also a nursing duty, and Canadian nurses were known for their skill at administering anaesthesia.

In March of 1915, the No. 2 Canadian General Hospital had set up a tent hospital of 1040 beds on the high cliff outside Le Treport. Matron Rayside along with fifty-seven nursing sisters served here, caring for high numbers of casualties from the Battles of Ypres and Festubert. No. 2 General was responsible for introducing an improved system for registering admissions and enabling patients to be received, diagnosed, and allocated to wards with a minimum of delay.[14]

Meanwhile, in the Eastern Mediterranean, five Canadian Army medical corps units, along with nursing sisters, were working under horrendous conditions to care for the numerous Allied sick and wounded. Camp conditions on the Island of Lemnos were unhygienic. Sanitary provisions were primitive, and food and water supplies scarce. The heat was scorching and flies were abundant. Dressing changes required the assistance of a helper to fan vigorously to keep the flies away from open wounds.

Nursing Sister Cline wrote, *"The delirious were tormented by swarms of insects in a temperature of 100 degrees.*[15] *Many of the soldiers suffered from amoebic dysentery, a condition that soon spread to medical officers, sisters and orderlies, and resulted in the death of Matron Jessie Jattard of No. 3 and one of her nursing sisters.*[16] *With the passing of summer, the problems of heat, insects and gastro-intestinal infections were over, but a blizzard in late November left casualties as great as any battle. In the Sulva Valley, more than two hundred men were drowned or frozen to death as icy torrential rains flooded trenches.*[17] *More than twelve thousand of the sixteen thousand casualties evacuated in nine days were due to the weather.*

"Amputation of toes and feet due to frostbite and gangrene was a common operation.

"No. 4 (University of Toronto) General Hospital was the first Canadian medical unit to serve in Macedonia. The tented hospital that was set up in Salonika in early November 1915 was soon followed by nursing staff and one thousand patients. A diversion for the nurses here was the presence of French airmen at a nearby aerodrome. A New Year's greeting, thrown from one of their low-flying planes was creatively addressed to 'the Nursing Sisters whose silhouettes among their tents have added poetry to our flight'." [18]

The bed capacity of No. 4 General increased by five hundred, from the original one thousand, due to a continual rise in the number of malaria cases. Although hospital staff took quinine as a precaution, malaria took its toll, necessitating the return of groups of nurses to England. The hardships endured by Canadian nursing sisters in the Eastern Mediterranean were many, and these nurses are deserving of a special place in history.

As the war progressed, the function of Casualty Clearing Stations (CCS) changed from accommodating patients for a few hours until transfer to a general hospital to an area of treatment for life-threatening injuries. Canadian nurses aspired to be one of the dozen or more nursing sisters in a CCS and to work with some of Canada's most experienced surgeons. In times of heavy fighting, surgical teams consisting of a surgeon, a nursing sister, an anaesthetist (who might be a nursing sister with special training) and an orderly, were drawn from clearing stations in a quiet part of the line. Sometimes as many as five surgical teams worked in the tented or hut operating rooms following a major battle. The type of nurse selected for this work was spoken highly of by a surgeon who served with one of these teams. "*They deserve a great deal of praise for the very cheerful way in which they put up with the long fatiguing hours they were called upon to serve in the operating rooms and tents of the CCSs. Their steady nerves and calm demeanour were evident during the operations, even when the enemy planes were soaring overhead; the shrieking of dropping bombs, the bursting of shells from our own Archies did not seem to rattle them in any way. Their kindness and thoughtfulness in calling on the patients was a great source of hope and encouragement to many a poor fellow sorely wounded.*"[19]

In the spring of 1918, in a breach of the Geneva Convention, Germans attacked hospitals and hospital ships. During the first of one of these air raids, the nursing sisters' quarters attached to No. 1 Canadian General Hospital was completely demolished. Nursing Sister Katharine Macdonald was killed instantly and two other sisters died of their injuries a few days later. The bombing resulted in sixty-six deaths and seventy-three wounded. Remaining devoted to their duty, nurses assisted surgeons throughout the night with cases needing urgent surgery. For their heroic service during the air raids, Nursing Sisters Helene Hanson and Beatrice McNair became the first Canadian nurses in the war to be awarded the Military Medal.[20] Further hospital bombings resulted in the deaths of four more nursing sisters and the torpedo destruction of the hospital ship *Llandovery Castle*, on June 27, 1918, 116 miles off the coast of Ireland, resulting in the loss of the entire contingent of fourteen nursing sisters headed by Matron Margaret Fraser.[21] Two hundred and thirty-four lives were lost in this disaster and twenty-four survivors were rescued from the water. A sergeant, who had taken charge of the lifeboat carrying the nursing sisters, praised the fortitude of the fourteen sisters who "*unflinchingly and calmly, as steady and collected as if on parade... faced the ordeal of certain death... a matter of minutes – as our lifeboat neared the mad whirlpool of waters where all human power was helpless.*"[22]

As a tribute to the forty-seven Canadian nursing sisters who lost their lives in the Great War, a strikingly beautiful memorial was placed in the Hall of Fame of Canada's Parliament Buildings. The monument honours three centuries of Canadian nursing history by depicting the heroism and martyrdom of early religious sisters who came to Canada from France during l'ancien regime, and the heroic courage and self-sacrificing loyalty of nurses who offered their services and lives for the great cause of freedom during the Great War. The inscription on this memorial reads: *"Erected by the nurses of Canada in remembrance of their sisters who gave their lives in the Great War 1914-18 and to perpetuate a noble tradition in the relations of the old world and the new.*

"Led by the spirit of humanity across the seas women by her tender ministrations to those in need has given to the world the example of an heroic service embracing three centuries of Canadian History."[23]

WORLD WAR II

The nurses who were among the first to be sent overseas during the Second World War were better prepared than those of World War I. In order to be a member of the Nursing Service, the nurses had to be British subjects, between the ages of twenty-one and thirty-six, unmarried or widows without children, graduates of a recognized school of nursing and registered in their province of practice. Within the Army, the sisters received a special course of instruction and had to qualify before an examining board in military law and in the new responsibilities of active service. A physical training course was also required. With regard to rank, a circular issued by the Royal Canadian Army Medical Corps stated: "All members of the Nursing Service are commissioned officers. They are enlisted as second lieutenants and remain in this rank for six months after enlistment. They attend an officers' training school in Army procedure at special centres in each district, and if recommended, become full lieutenants. The matron of a small unit holds the rank of captain, and of a large unit – major.[24]

The first contingent of one hundred and twenty-nine Canadian nursing sisters under the leadership of Matron Agnes Neill (later to become matron-in-chief) left for England in June 1940, nine months after the outbreak of war.[25] No. 5 and No. 15 Canadian General Hospitals had been established about six months prior to the nurses' arrival. No. 5 General was assigned to Taplow, west of London, where a new hospital had been built on the three hundred-acre Cliveden estate of Lord and Lady Astor. The hospital was well equipped by the Canadian Red Cross Society. No. 15 General was established at Bramshott Chase, south of Taplow. It was here that Canadian Army casualties of the frequent motorcycle accidents were treated. Neurosurgery and plastic surgery became the needed specialties of No. 1 Canadian Neurological Hospital owing to the head and face injuries and burns suffered by soldiers and civilians. Sisters found the nursing of young paraplegic soldiers especially difficult.

The nursing sisters in the Canadian general hospitals in Britain had opportunities to improve their professional standing. They took courses at various civilian hospitals in or near London and learned about the changes and innovations happening in burn therapy, plastic surgery, blood transfusion and intravenous therapy.

On August 19, 1942, the day of the Dieppe raid, hundreds of casualties were sent to the Canadian general hospitals across the channel. Many of these casualties were from the 2nd Canadian Division. At one of these hospitals, ninety-five operations were performed in nineteen and one-half hours, with the staff stopping only momentarily for food.[26] Nursing sisters of No. 7 General would later recall patients that had touched them deeply – "*the young Frenchman who had lost both arms, and who would cry in the night because his twin brother had been taken prisoner in the raid. I used to go to his bed, prop him up against my shoulder, and hold a cigarette for him while he smoked it.*"[27]

The Canadian hospitals in England admitted six hundred Dieppe casualties. Divisional Commander, Major-General J.H. Roberts visited each institution where the wounded were being treated and in communication to Major-General Luton wrote the following: "*On all sides, there was nothing but the highest praise for the kindly care meted out to them by your medical staff and nursing sisters. It has been a remarkable feat of surgical skill and careful nursing that so many have by now recovered, and others are well on their way to convalescence.*"[28]

In July of 1943, Canadian nursing sisters began to experience the challenges of nursing under battle conditions. The Canadian involvement in the Allied invasion of Italy meant the provision of Canadian military hospitals. Canadian General Hospital No. 5 went to Sicily. Matron Agnes Macleod of Edmonton and fifty-five nursing sisters, on their arrival, were described as a "*group of grimy, tin-hatted girls, perspiring in the terrific heat and burdened with cumbersome equipment.*"[29] In addition to the heat, these nurses also had to endure the noise of night raids overhead, dysentery, bedbugs, mosquitoes, and the threat of malaria. Restrictions on moving malarial patients from Sicily often meant exceeding the hospital's normal bed capacity and placing patients on the balconies, in the corridors, and even on the roof.[30]

In addition to the nursing sisters in the five general hospitals at various locations on the Italian peninsula, nursing sisters were also with the two major mobile medical units of the 1st Canadian Corps (No's. 4 and 5 Casualty Clearing Stations) as they followed the forward troops to the Romagna Plain. In February 1944, No. 4 Field Surgical Unit made history by being the first to use the new miracle drug penicillin in treating a compound fracture of the femur. The unit was also the first to employ a nursing sister in its operating theater in the forward area. The war diary recorded: "*Lt. (N/S) Jean Hackland now on full time duty with the unit... She should be of great help in developing good operating technique, not to mention being good for morale.*"[31]

For many nurses, being close enough to the forward troops to be within range of the enemy's guns was a desirable position. One nursing sister of No. 1 F.S.U. wrote: "*To me personally, it was the most challenging, inspiring, and soul-satisfying work I have ever done.*"[32] These mobile units were compact and able to move quickly. They dealt with seriously wounded men who required immediate surgery. In a report to Canadian Military Headquarters, the consultant surgeon wrote the following: "*Too much praise cannot be given to these sisters who work unceasingly, often times with little sleep, and giving their best at all times, not only in post-operative care but in assisting the surgeons of the Field Surgical Units.*"[33]

Later, when a reorganization of the medical services within the 1st Canadian Corps took place, sixteen additional nursing sisters were assigned to demanding duties in these mobile units, demonstrating that the value of having nurses serving close to battle areas was recognized.

The preparation for an invasion of Normandy included planning for casualties of about 10% of the 70,000 British-Canadian personnel that were scheduled to go ashore on D-Day, June 6, 1944. On June 8, the wounded began arriving at Canadian hospitals in England, being directed from field dressing stations in France. Army nursing sisters did not cross into Normandy until July 9; however, two RCAF nursing sisters with a mobile field hospital had become the first Canadian servicewomen to land in France. A nursing sister with the first Casualty Clearing Station in France wrote about their work under canvas, caring for Canadian wounded from the Caen sector.

"*We are well forward and hear a lot of noise, jerry planes, terrific ack-ack. A red-hot tracer bullet came whizzing by my tent door yesterday. Kind of made me gulp and get down on the floor. Shelling seems close at times. We set up tents that morning and we opened at noon and have been busy up to our necks in work. We work sixteen hours out of the twenty-four. All our work is surgery. You haven't time to think or be frightened of anything going on around you. When you are off duty, you just put your tin hat over your face and go to sleep. The surgeons have been wonderful and our share has not been small. One wished for one hundred hands and ten pairs of feet and many more hours in every day."*[34]

The Allied offensive move into northern Belgium late in the year meant threats from V-bombs and the possibility of a German attack across the River Maas. By the time the Rhineland battles ended in early March 1945, more than twenty thousand casualties of all types had been evacuated through the medical services. In July 1945, the disbandment of all medical units in North-West Europe had begun.

By the end of the war, the RCAMC had some 3656 nursing sisters on strength; two-thirds of these were overseas. They had staffed one hundred major hospital units, treated over 60,000 patients, and won 386 awards.[35] Their service in war, like those of military nurses in the past, had been one of compassion.

1. Gibbon, Mathewson, 1947 p. 50
2. Nicholson, 1975, p.5
3. Gibbon, Mathewson, 1947
4. Nicholson, p.22
5. Nicholson, p.24
6. Nicholson, p.26
7. Nicholson, p.44
8. Gibbon, Mathewson, p.290
9. Gibbon, Mathewson, 1947, pp.290-291
10. Feasby pp. 1-4
11. Feasby p. 3
12. Nicholson, p.53
13. Gibbon & Mathewson, p.298
14. Nicholson, p.64
15. Gibbon & Mathewson, p.302
16. Nicholson, p.69
17. Nicholson, p.71
18. Nicholson, p.75
19. Nicholson, p.81
20. Nicholson, p.93
21. Nicholson, p.95
22. Nicholson, p.95
23. Gibbon & Mathewson, p.310
24. Gibbon & Mathewson, p.455
25. Nicholson, p.118
26. Nicholson, p.129
27. Nicholson, p.130
28. Nicholson, p.130
29. Gibbon & Mathewson, p.465
30. Nicholson, p137
31. Nicholson, p.143
32. Nicholson, p.145
33. Nicholson, p.145
33. Nicholson, p.146
34. Gibbon & Mathewson, p. 470
35. Nicholson p. 208

Chapter 2

CANADIAN ARMY MEDICAL CORPS

Ina Isabelle Grenville
Madeleine (Morrison) Jaffray
Roberta (MacAdam) Price
Margaret Jane (Landells) Roebuck
Marjorie (Young) Sanders
Edna (Gray) Williams

CANADA'S NURSING SISTERS 1914-1918

by Pamela Brunt

> The following article was provided by: Friends of the Canadian War Museum, *Fact Sheet No. 1.* Original research by Pamela Brunt, Lt. RCN retired. She retired in 1991 having served as a navy nurse from 1967-1991 and in her last two and a half years of service served at the Directorate of History doing research for the RCN History. She is now retired and does still take an interest in military history.

Although female nurses had been employed by the military during the North West Rebellion of 1885, the Canadian Army Nursing Service was only officially organized in 1901. On the outbreak of the First World War in August 1914, only five nursing sisters were serving in the Permanent Force, with a further eighty as part-time members of the Militia.

When the order to mobilize was received by the matron of the Canadian Army Medical Corps, Margaret Macdonald, in September 1914, a frenzy of recruiting and selection took place to meet the requirements of the Canadian Expeditionary Force.

Less than a month later Matron Macdonald and one hundred nurses landed at Plymouth, England. Initially these nurses were billeted at St. Thomas Hospital in London, but in November thirty-four of them, under Matron Ridley, were posted to France for duty in No. 2 Stationary Hospital. The remainder of the nurses stayed in England to work in other military hospitals.

On November 4, 1914, Margaret Macdonald was appointed matron-in-chief and granted the rank of major. This gave her the distinction of being the first woman in the British Empire to be granted this rank. It should also be mentioned that the Canadian nursing sisters were the only ones to hold military rank and be under military control, unlike those serving with other armies.

A second group of twenty Canadian nurses was sent to France in November 1914. They were attached to British stationary hospitals. Nurses from both these groups became eligible for the 1914 Star, for which very few Canadians qualified.

As the war progressed more nurses were recruited and sent overseas to staff the growing number of medical facilities being set up by the Canadian Army, both in England and France.

No. 1 Stationary Hospital, accompanied by No. 1 Canadian Casualty Clearing Station, had been sent to France in February and these were followed by No. 2 Canadian General Hospital in March. In May 1915, No. 1 Canadian General Hospital was ordered to France. This hospital remained three years at Etaples, until it was forced to move to a safer spot at Trouville, due to repeated serial bombings which claimed the lives of staff and patients alike.

In August 1915, nursing sisters were sent to Africa to work in conditions that were considered to be the worst of any in the war. The Canadian nurses were part of No. 1, No. 3, and No. 5 (later to become No. 7) Stationary Hospitals. No. 5 Hospital was set up on the outskirts of Cairo and No. 1 and No. 3 were sent to the Greek island of Lemnos.

In April 1916, No. 3 Stationary Hospital was transferred from Lemnos to Boulogne, France. By this time there were nine units of the Canadian Army Medical Corps in France and Belgium in which nursing sisters were employed. In addition to those mentioned above, No. 4 Stationary (which became No. 8 General), No. 1, No. 2 and No. 3 Casualty Clearing Stations were now in operation.

By the end of the war in 1918 a total of 16 Canadian General Hospitals, 10 Stationary Hospitals and 4 Casualty Clearing Stations had been set up and staffed with Canadian nursing sisters. A total of 3141 nursing sisters were enrolled in the Canadian Army Medical Corps during the First World War, of which 2504 served overseas. By this time the nurses had been nicknamed "bluebirds" as they work bright blue cotton uniforms for hospital duty.

During the First World War Canadian nursing sisters served in Britain, France, Greece, Malta and Egypt, while the Nursing Service operated as an integral part of the Military medical services. Nursing sister casualties included: six killed, six wounded, 15 drowned by enemy action (the result of the sinking of the hospital ship *Llandovery Castle*), and 18 dead from disease. They received 328 decorations, 169 were mentioned in dispatches, and 76 were brought to the notice of the Secretary of State for War.

Perhaps their greatest accomplishment was the undying gratitude of the thousands they saved and the realization that military nurses were capable of playing a significant role in future conflicts.

Further Reading:

McPhail, A., *Official History of the Canadian Forces in the Great War 1914-19.* The Medical Services. Ottawa: DND; 1925

Nicholson, G.W.L., *Canada's Nursing Sisters.* Toronto: Hakkert & Company, 1975

Ina Isabelle Grenville

Graduated from: Mack Training School for Nurses at St. Catharines, Ontario. Year: 1912

Submitted by her nephew John J. Savigny, Kingston, Ontario

Military History:

Service: CAMC

Rank: Lt. N/S

Served: World War One

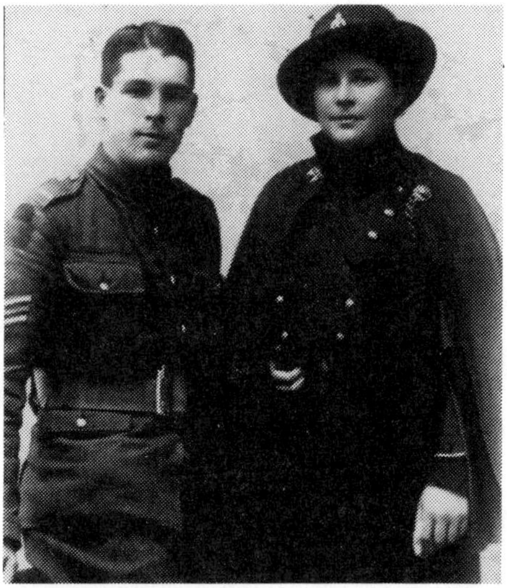

Nursing sister Ina Isabelle Grenville with her brother, Sgt. Roy Grenville Loaned by: John J. Savigny, nephew

Ina Grenville was not the only member of her family to serve overseas. Her younger brother, Roy, and her father were on active duty with the Canadian Army. Her father joined in 1916 at the age of 53.

Ina Grenville of Thorold, Ont., was among the first ten Canadian nurses to go overseas in April 1915. She was a member of St. John's Ambulance Corps Division and went directly to Gallipolli. Ina was stationed at Malta where she cared for Australian troops.

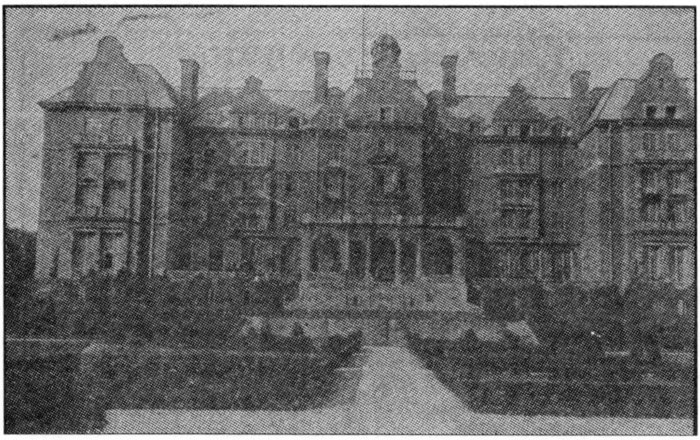

Buxton Hospital, England

She transferred to the British Red Cross and served under fire on several fronts in France before being brought into the Canadian Army Medical Corps. Ina served in England at Orpington and Buxton Hospitals.

In 1919 she returned to Canada and was on the staff of St. Andrew's Military Hospital at Toronto until it closed. Her next duty was at Christie Street Hospital.

Ina was one of the first nurses appointed to the provincial department of health staff in 1920 when a nursing service was being organized in Northern Ontario. Miss Grenville died in 1934.

Madeleine (Morrison) Jaffray

Submitted by Mary MacDonald, White Rock, B.C.

Graduated from: Clifton Springs Sanatorium Clinic in New York and the Boston Dispensary

Military History:

Service: CAMC

Rank: Lieutenant in the Canadian Army, attached to the French Red Cross

Served: World War One

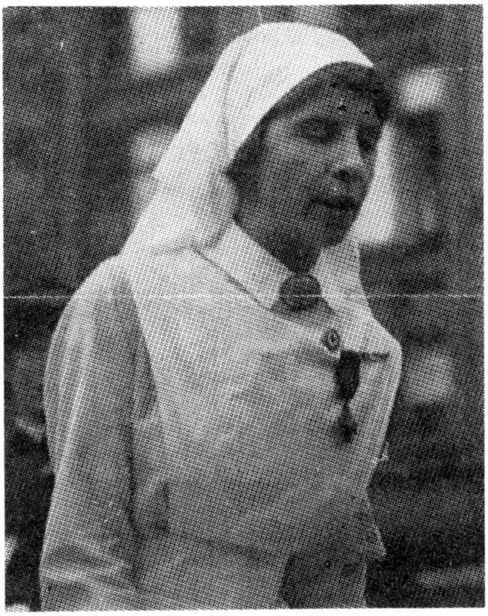

Nursing Sister Madeleine (Morrison) Jaffray, CAMC.
loaned by Mary MacDonald, White Rock

A nursing graduate of Clifton Springs Sanatorium Clinic in New York and the Boston Dispersary, she was a lieutenant in the Canadian Army, attached to the French Red Cross from 1915 to 1917.

Working in a hospital post five miles from the front lines during an air raid at Adinkerke, Belgium, Mrs. Morrison lost her left foot.

She was the first Canadian woman to be awarded the Croix de Guerre by France for valour in Belgium. She was also honoured with the Insignia in Bronze, for meritorious service, and the French medal Desepidemis for Service.

Mrs. Morrison worked with the Victorian Order of Nurses in Edmonton. She was the first woman active member of the War Amputees of Canada. She was also an honourary life member of the Nursing Sisters of America and the National Council of Women.*

* *FRAGMENT MAGAZINE,* 1972, Fall Issue p.34.

Roberta (MacAdam) Price

Submitted by Mary MacDonald, White Rock, B.C.

Graduated from: Home Economics at MacDonald College, Guelph, Ontario

Military History:

Service: CAMC

Rank: Lieutenant Dietitian

Served: World War One

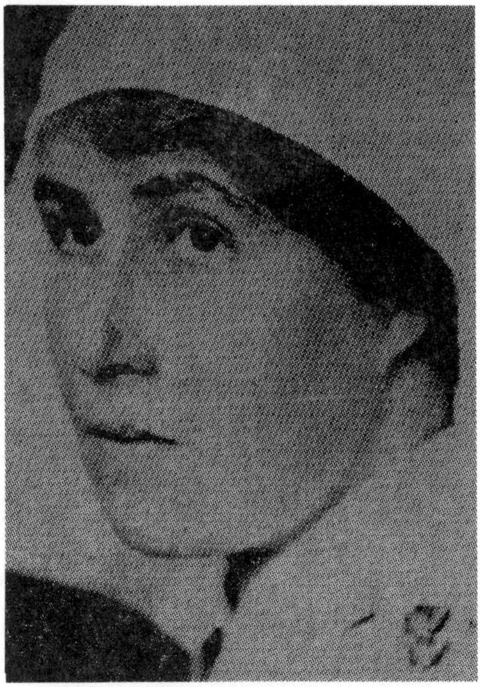

Nursing Sister Roberta MacAdam, CAMC. Loaned by Mary MacDonald, White Rock

Roberta MacAdam came to Edmonton in 1911 and joined the Alberta Department of Agriculture to pioneer for women in the extension service.

When war broke out she went overseas as dietitian for the Canadian Army Military Hospital Services with the rank of lieutenant and was granted the right to officially wear the uniform of a nurse.

She was elected as MLA (Member of the Legislative Assembly) in August 1917, when serving overseas. Her support came from soldiers and nurses all serving overseas, at that time. Her campaigning came from one small printed sheet. Miss MacAdam did not take her seat in the legislature until returning from overseas duty many months later. She was Canada's only woman to represent the Armed Services in the legislature. She served one term in legislative office but did not seek re-election. She returned to her former profession of dietitian and in 1920 married Harvey Price in Peace River.

The Nursing Sisters' Association of Canada, Edmonton Unit, planned a portrait of Roberta MacAdam to hang in the Alberta legislative gallery and sponsored a fund to pay for it. Individuals and organizations donated funds to have her portrait painted and today it hangs in the Alberta legislature.*

* THE EDMONTON JOURNAL, Wednesday, November 30, 1966. p.26

Margaret Jane (Landells) Roebuck

Written by her niece, Edith Landells

Military History:

Service: CAMC

Rank: Lt. N/S

Served: 1916 to 1919

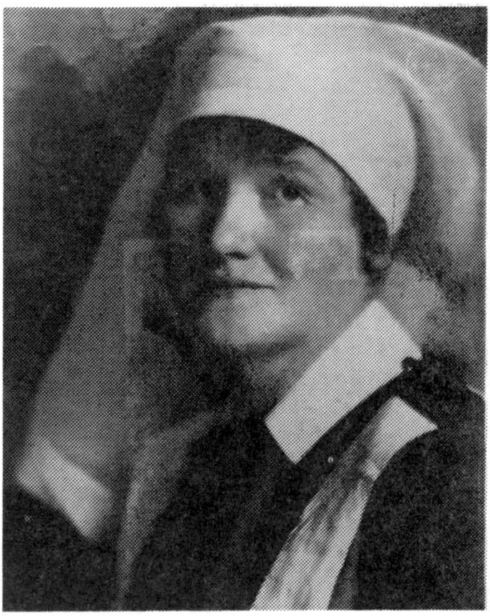

Margaret Jane Landells, No. 1 Stationery Hospital, CAMC. Loaned by Elizabeth Foxton MacInnes, 1943 graduate of Neepawa General Hospital, Manitoba and Donald MacInnes

Margaret Jane Landells enlisted in CAMC, Canadian Expeditionary Force and was appointed to commissioned rank in the Canadian Army Medical Corps CEF on the 26th day of June, 1916.

She served in Canada, England and Salonica with the CAMC and was struck off strength on the 16th day of February 1920 by reason of general demobilization. She was awarded the British War Medal and the Victory Medal.

She went overseas 21 July 1916 and was posted to No. 1 Canadian Stationary Hospital for duty in Salonica, Greece. She left Southampton on HS *Oxfordshire* for Port Said. From there she embarked on *Alexandra* for Salonica in August. Her recollections of Greece are

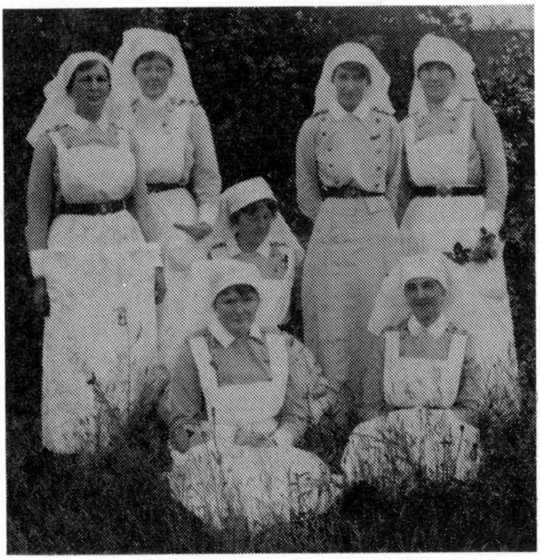

Front row left:
N/S Margaret Jane Landells, CAMC,
No. 1 Stationary Hospital

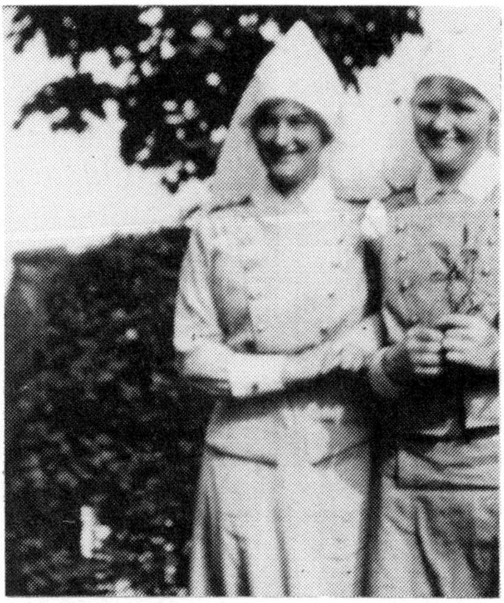

R: N/S Margaret Jane Landells
loaned by Jean (Landells) Butler

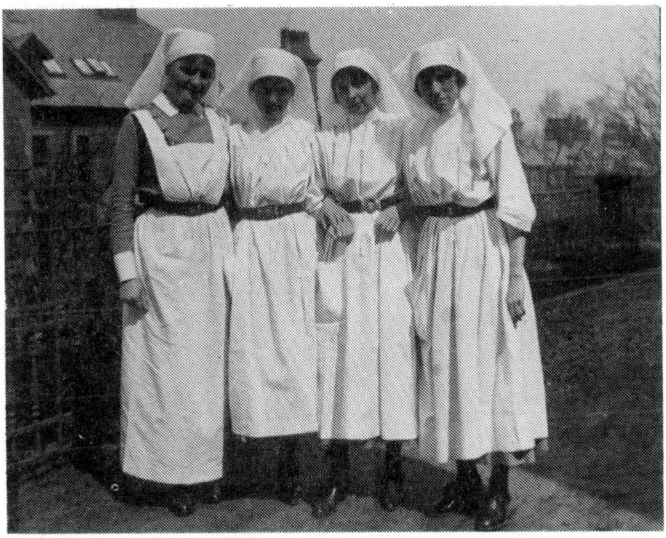

L: N/S Margaret Jane Landells
loaned by Norma (MacInnes) Wournell

of excessive heat in summer and severe cold in winter.

In March of 1917 she was invalided to the hospital in Uxbridge, England and from there to the Canadian Convalescent Hospital also at Uxbridge.

She served at Ramsgate, Basingstoke and at No. 12 CGH Bramshott until her return to Canada in July of 1919 on the SS *Orduna.*

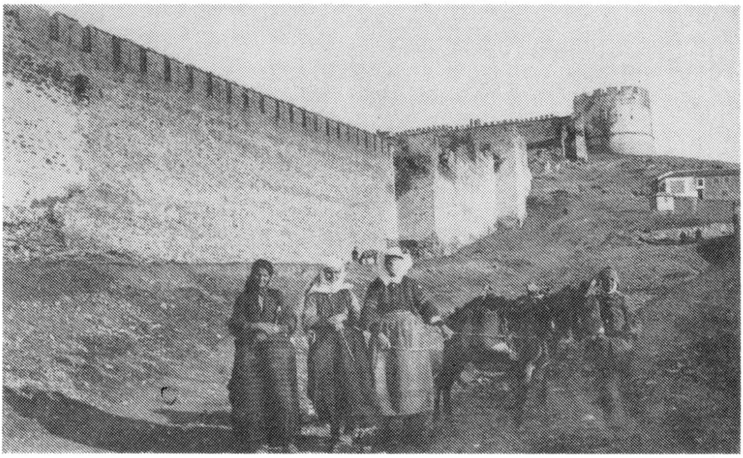

Salonica, Greece
M.J. Landells was stationed here
with No. 1 Stationary Hospital
loaned by Norma (MacInnes) Wournell

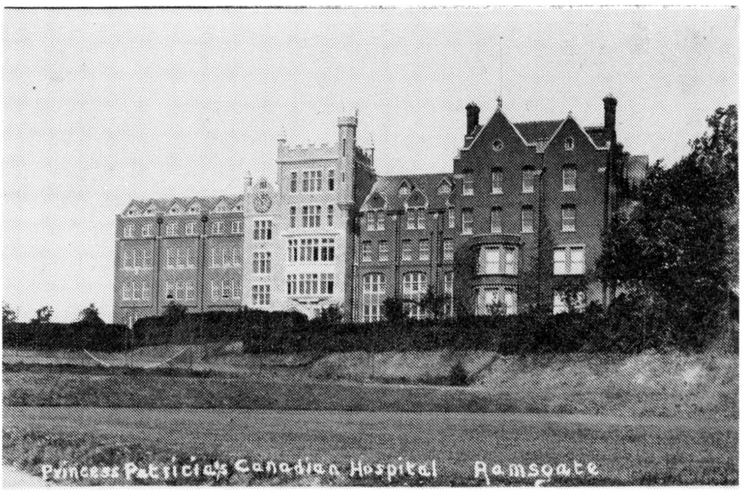

Princess Patricia's Canadian Hospital,
Ramsgate, England

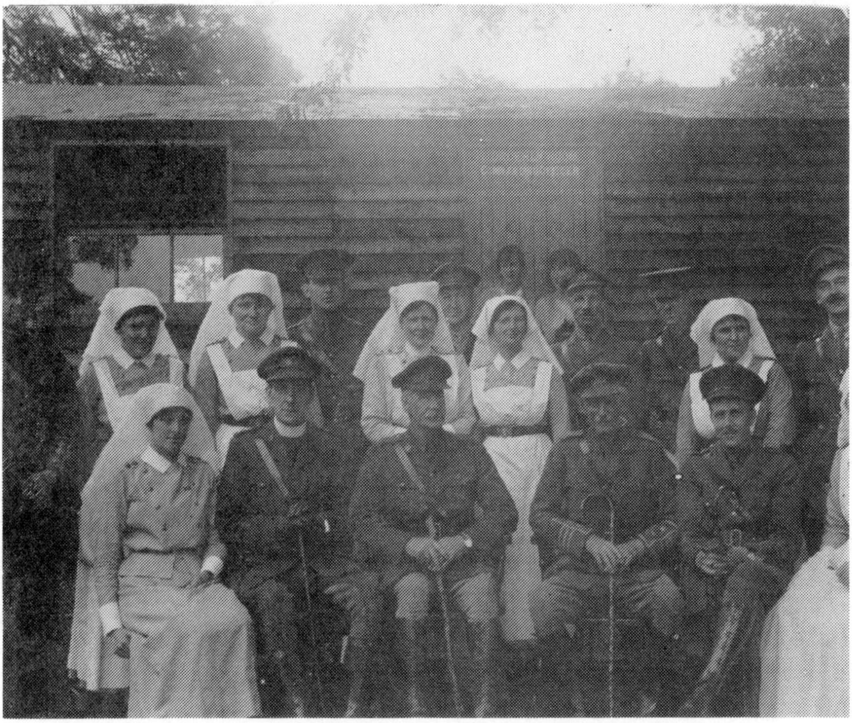

Medical staff at Uxbridge Army Hospital in England, May 1919
N/S M.J. Landells - back row, second from left
loaned by Marion (Roebuck) Walline

Marjorie (Young) Sanders

Graduated from: Toronto General Hospital School of Nursing

Military History:

Service: CAMC

Rank: Lt. N/S

Served: 1917 to 1919

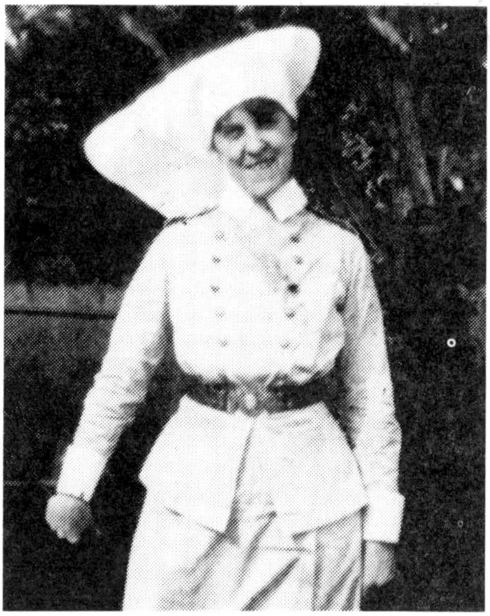

N/S Marjory (Young) Sanders at Christie St. Hospital 1917. This is the photo I gave my husband (then fiance) before he went overseas.

I decided to join the Canadian Army Medical Corps before I even graduated from nursing school, my fiance was in the Army, I knew him in high school.

I was stationed at Christie Street Military Hospital in Toronto and I was glad to be in the Army. We made a contribution, we helped to restore so many to normal health. Nurses were valuable to the Army, we gave a different outlook to military patients, we braced them up and lifted their spirits; they depended on you so much.

There were many nurses at Christie Street Hospital; we did everything but scrub the floors. There were orderlies to help lift and turn the patients. We were at Hart House when we got our first uniforms. Our capes were lined with crimson; some didn't like the bright red. The government had provided samples and the colour of the lining was changed to navy blue. Our uniform was blue with brass buttons.

I was very sorry that I didn't get overseas. We really felt we made a difference. I was discharged 16 August 1919 and was married 23 August 1919.

Edna (Gray) Williams

Graduated from: St. Joseph's Hospital School of Nursing Victoria, B.C. Year: 1916

Military History:

Service: CAMC and QAIMNS

Rank: Lt. N/S

Served: January 1917 to 1918

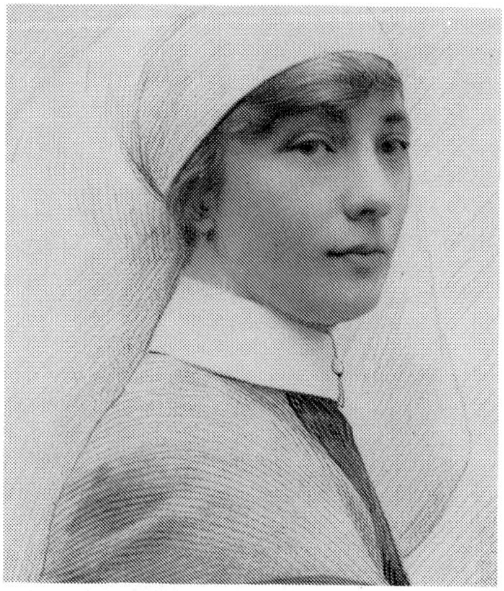

Nursing Sister Edna (Gray) Williams who responded to request for Canadian nurses to serve with QAIMNS.
Loaned by daughter Vera Bailey

Active Militia of Canada: Recommendation for Appointment to CAMC HQ of Ottawa, January 30, 1917.

Date of appointment to QAIMNS: Feb. 1, 1917 and proceeded overseas on the SS *Letitia* for service with the QAIMNS March 27, 1917.

Served in Belgium and France beginning April 1917.

I wanted to be in the Army because I was curious; I wanted to see what it was like.

Our government asked for 200 Canadian nurses to serve with the British Army overseas and I was one of 25 nurses who went from B.C. We were with the Queen Alexandra's Nursing Service. We got our uniform in England; it was grey.

Most of the time we lived in tents in France; we took care of wounded soldiers right off the battlefield. It was a very busy time, I worked in the operating room and on the wards. We worked 12 hours, from 7 to 7. Before I returned to Canada I had three days' leave.

Chapter 3

CASUALTY CLEARING STATIONS

NO. 2 CASUALTY CLEARING STATION

Lily Clegg
Constance (Bond) Young

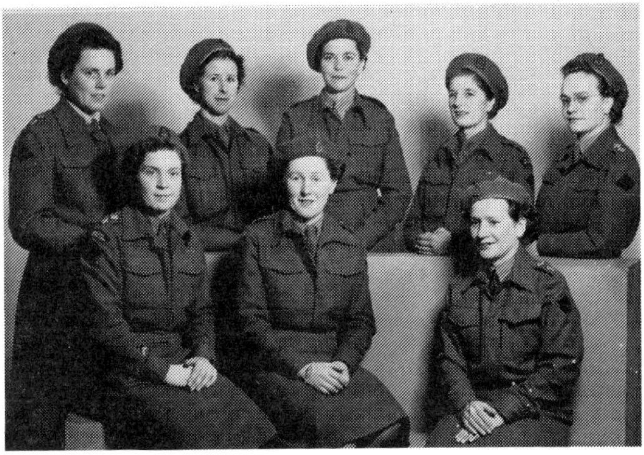

No. 2 CCS, Tilburg, Holland, December 1944
BACK ROW: L-R: Connie Bond; Bea Curtis; Matron Dorothy Ballantine; Rene Boughton; Mary Bell.
FRONT ROW: L-R:
Doris Boddy; Wilma Frey; Lily Clegg.

On 1 July 1940 No. 2 Casualty Clearing Station mobilized at Toronto and located at Camp Borden Military Hospital with Lt. Col. Harvie as OC.

The unit, including nursing sisters, reached Halifax 6 October 1941 and boarded *Warwick Castle* arriving at Liverpool, 17 October 1941.

By 29 July 1942 Matron Paterson and nursing sisters, in battle dress, practised moving in the field.

The unit arrived in France 12 July 1944 and set up under canvas 17 July at Sequeville-en-Bessin with No. 3 CCS nearby. The nursing sisters rejoined their unit from No. 77 British General Hospital.

After extremely active periods, and several moves, the unit crossed the German border at Bedburg March 1945. After a short stay they returned to Holland near Nijmegen.

The unit remained in Europe until its disbandment 12 November 1945.

Lily Clegg

Graduated from: St. Michael's Hospital School of Nursing
Toronto, Ontario. Year: 1932

Other: Registered Record Librarian

Military History:

Service: RCAMC

Rank: Lt. N/S

Served: 3 June 1940
to 3 October 1945

I nursed as a deputy sister in Paddington Hospital, SCC, London, England, 3 March 1938 to 22 August 1939. My father served in the 1914-1918 war so it was natural for me to join the Army.

I joined No. 2 Canadian Casualty Clearing Station, 1940. No. 2 CCS served in Camp Borden, Camp Sussex, October 31, 1941. Stationed in Surrey, Sussex and Kent, England

We landed in Courseulles, France 11 July 1944. No. 2 CCS served as a 100-bed hospital. We first set up at Sequeville and followed the 3rd Division to St. Germain, France; Ghent, Belgium; Bedburg, Germany; Tilburg, Holland. In May 1944 I returned to England on the point system. I found the work rewarding and remain satisfied that No. 2 CCS had done excellent work.

Connie (Bond) Young

Graduated from: St. Michael's Hospital School of Nursing Toronto, Ontario. Year: 1932

Military History:

Service: RCAMC

Rank: Lt. N/S

Served: 3 June 1940 to 10 September 1945

As I wanted to use my nursing experience to help win the war, I enlisted in Toronto 3 June 1940. By November along with medical officers, NCOs and the men of 2 CCS, I was assigned to Camp Borden Military Hospital in the first group of nurses to staff the military hospital at that camp. With Grace Paterson as matron, eight nurses were chosen to staff No. 2 CCS to go overseas with the 2nd Canadian Division. It was this group that proceeded to Camp Borden, namely Nursing Sisters Grace Paterson, Mary Bell, Lily Clegg, Lorraine Thompson, (who married and was replaced by Beatrice Curtis), Peggy Lister, Doris Boddy, Helen Lane and Connie Bond.

April 1941, No. 2 CCS transferred to Camp Sussex, N.B. Military Hospital and by 9 October we sailed from Halifax, N.S., with the 2nd Division. We disembarked at Liverpool, England, a week later. No. 2 served as a CCS at Cranleigh, Surrey until April 1944. This was a beautiful country estate loaned for the duration to the Canadian Army by Solomon Jowell, a wealthy diamond merchant who had moved his family to New York. Here we served as a general hospital for the area troops and were trained and prepared for future action. We received "walking wounded" from the Dieppe Raid.

April 1944:

We moved under canvas for short period then settled in Sussex at Elham near Folkestone.

10 July 1944:

No. 2 CCS embarked from Southampton and landed at Courseulles, France, on a landing barge at Mulberry Beach with No. 3 CCS. For six weeks we were under canvas, the forward CCS with Operation Veritable. Our location was outside Caen, eight hour duty. We were constantly under fire, and wore steel helmets on duty and off.

25 July 1944:

St. Germain, beyond Caen, still under fire. Opened a Canadian cemetery here, consecrated by our padres.

25 August 1944:

First chance to go back to General Hospital at Bayeux for rest period. Recalled after several hours to unit.

27 August 1944:

Unit on the move to Brionne in Normandy. Set up in apple orchard, better than the mud at Caen. Received casualties the same day. FSU and FTU and additional staff of nurses were sent to handle rush of casualties. 12-hour duty.

5 September 1944:

On the move again, closed the hospital at Brionne.

15 September 1944:

Long journey across the Seine, through Elbeuf, Rouen, Abbeville, Montreuil, all night journey to Steenvoorde near the Belgian border. The enemy was really on the run, the carnage and destruction was indescribable.

24 September 1944:

Settled at Ghent in the new wing of their hospital. Good to be in a building and English-speaking Belgian nurses joined our staff. Very busy here.

6 October 1944:

Evacuated all patients possible to receive casualties following 3rd Division new attack. Half the casualties were German POWs. They were given the same care as our men, except they did not receive penicillin – the reason, our supply was limited.

21 October 1944:

Matron-in-Chief, Agnes Neill and Principal Matron Shaffner arrived on tour of the Medical Units in the Theatre of War.

23 November 1944:

No. 2 CCS moved to Tilburg in Holland and set up in a school, nurses were billeted at first with civilians, then later acquired another school for residence.

25 December 1944:

Christmas in Holland. The Dutch sisters sang Christmas carols in English at midnight mass for our benefit.

26 December 1944:

Warning of German paratroopers, all night vigil at hospital, but false alarm.

February 1945:

Moved to Nijmegen, Holland, to a Jesuit seminary. From here we moved across the Rhine to Bedburg, Germany, a mental hospital set up, a short stay there, then back to Sherongberg, Holland, enemy on the run.

In early April rotation leave started for return home, five originals of 2 CCS, Lily Clegg, Beatrice Curtis, Mary Bell, Doris Boddy and Connie Bond spent V.E. Day in London. No. 2 CCS had moved to Appledoorn where they celebrated V.E. Day.

NO. 3 CASUALTY CLEARING STATION

No. 3 Casualty Clearing Station mobilized at Winnipeg, February 1942. Their job was to operate a military hospital accommodating 200 beds.

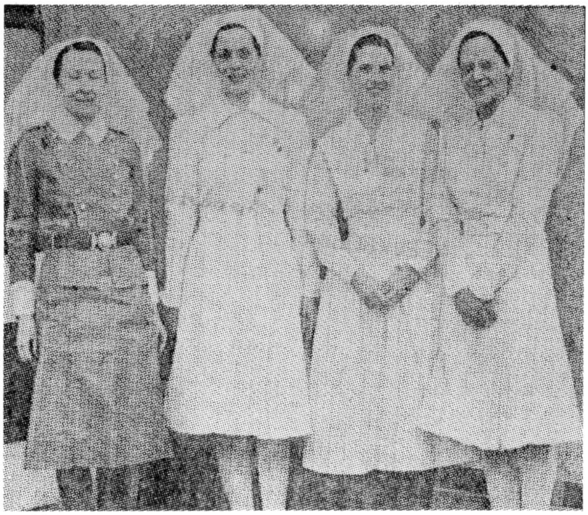

These nurses are looking forward to serving with No. 3 CCS: L-R: Nursing Sister in charge Evelyn McTavish, a graduate of McKellar Hospital, Fort William, Ont., N/S Jean Galbraith, Yorkton, Sask., a graduate of Misericordia Hospital, Winnipeg; N/S Elizabeth Hodge, a graduate of Winnipeg General Hospital, Winnipeg; N/S Sarah Horning, Binscarth, Man., a graduate of Misericordia Hospital, Winnipeg.
Other nursing sisters slated for this unit are Winona Brown, Elma Copeland, Eva Toews and Madeley Crichton, all of Winnipeg.
No. 3 Casualty Clearing Station of the RCAMC was mobilized in Winnipeg for active service. Nursing sisters who will serve with the unit are: Evelyn McTavish, Jean Galbraith, Elizabeth Hodge, Sarah Horning, Winona Brown, Elma Copeland, Eva Toews and Madley Crichton.
Courtesy: National Archives of Canada, Ottawa

Because of its size, compactness and mobility, this hospital could be moved quickly to the point of action and removed by the same means. A Casualty Clearing Station is the first point at which major operations take place and casualties are prepared for transport to a general or base hospital.

On 21 July1943 the unit boarded the *Queen Elizabeth* at Halifax and arrived in Gourock, Scotland 27 July.

They sailed for Juno Beach, 9 July 1944 and first set up their tents near Sequeville-en-Bessin while the battle at

Caen raged on. They occupied forward positions, never far behind the advancing troops; the rush of casualties was intense. By early 1945 No. 3 CCS along with No. 6 CCS was just outside Nijmegen, Holland. The large number of casualties was distributed among the various units in the area. By April the flow of casualties gradually decreased.

On 8 December 1945 all personnel were struck off strength and so ended the history of No. 3 Canadian CCS with the Canadian Army overseas.

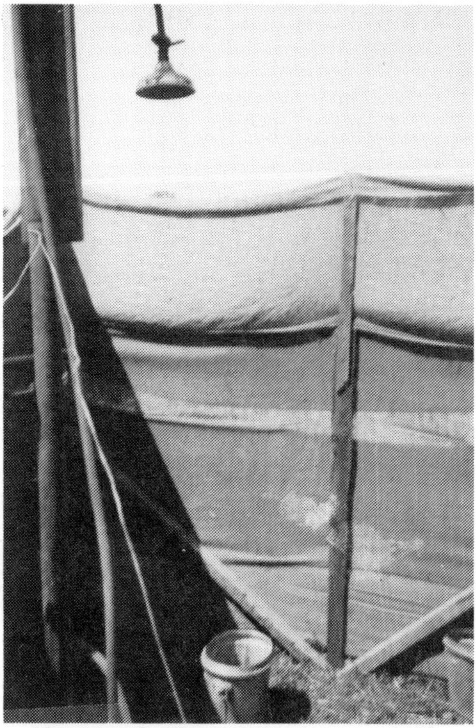

Showers for the nursing sisters at the 3rd Casualty Clearing at Caen France, July 1944.
loaned by Dolly (Vincent) Watkins

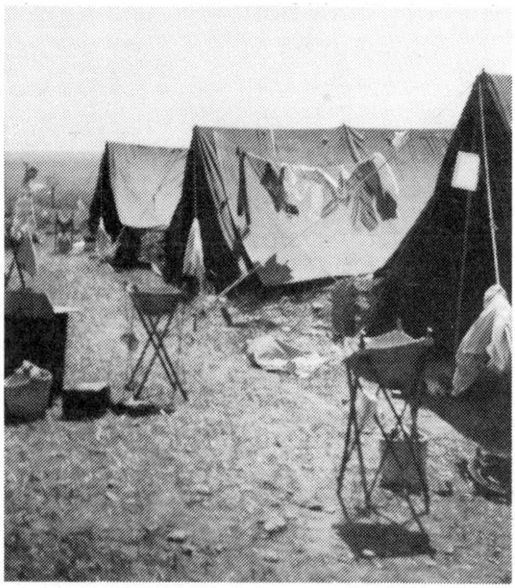

Nursing sisters' tents at No. 3CCS Caen, France July, 1944
loaned by Dolly (Vincent) Watkins

NO. 4 CASUALTY CLEARING STATION

Lillian Bibby
Margaret Brown
Maxine (Fuller) Slemon

No. 4 Casualty Clearing Station Mobilized at Edmonton in September of 1939. They embarked on the SS *Empress of Britain* January 28, 1940, and arrived in Scotland February 8, 1940. The nursing sisters joined their unit September 11, 1940, for duty in the U.K.

On October 28, 1943 they boarded the SS *Argentina* and were in the convoy when it was bombed in the Mediterranean.

February 28, 1945 No. 4 CCS departed Italy for northwest Europe. July 1, 1945, the unit disbanded.

From news clipping Nursing Sister's Association, Edmonton Unit, Archives Collection News Clipping:

Agnes McLeod entered the University of Alberta School of Nursing and graduated in 1927 with the first class. She then taught at Archer Memorial School of Nursing at Lamont, then taught at the University Hospital and later attended Columbia Teachers' College where she obtained a Masters degree.

She returned to Canada and was an instructor at Vancouver General Hospital School of Nursing. Then she returned to the University of Alberta to become the first director of the university's Graduate School of Nursing.

Miss Agnes McLeod was appointed matron of No. 4 CCS and went overseas with the unit. Shortly after, in England, she was made matron of the Neurological Unit at Basingstoke. Later she was transferred to No. 5 CGH and was with that unit when it followed the Army into Italy.

Shortly before D-Day she returned to England to become matron of No. 2 CGH which was moved to Normandy 9 August 1944. Later she returned to Italy to become senior matron of the RCAMC Nursing Services there.

Lillian Bibby

Graduated from: Calgary General Hospital School of Nursing.
Year: 1933

Military History:

Service: RCAMC

Rank: Lieutenant N/S

Served: August 1940 to June 1945, with No. 4 CCS, in England, Sicily, Italy and Europe

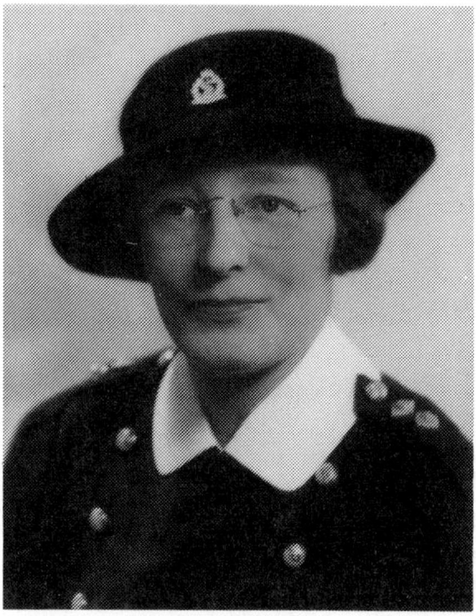

No. 4 CCS
Lillian E. Bibby

I joined the Royal Canadian Army Medical Corps in September 1940 because of a circular the Canadian Red Cross sent out after my graduation.

I served with No. 4 CCS in England, Italy and Sicily. The last few months in Europe I was attached to No. 5 Cdn. General Hospital. I returned to Canada in May 1945 and was discharged November 1945.

In February 1946 I joined the Col. Belcher Hospital staff as charge nurse. Except for a six-month course learning about OPLC supervision and management.

I remained at the Col. Belcher Hospital until retirement in May 1970.

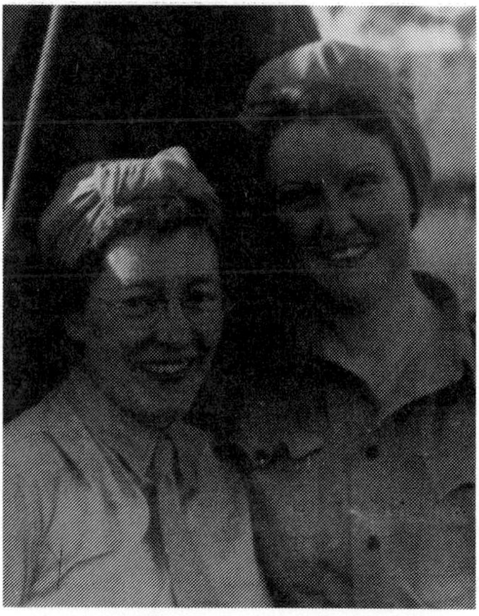

Italy, 1944 - in the field. Khaki triangles on head worn at work, chiefly under canvas.

Margaret C. Brown

Graduated from: Misericordia Hospital School of Nursing, Edmonton. Year: 1932

Military History:

Service: RCAMC

Rank: Lieutenant N/S

Served: May 22, 1940 to September 27, 1946

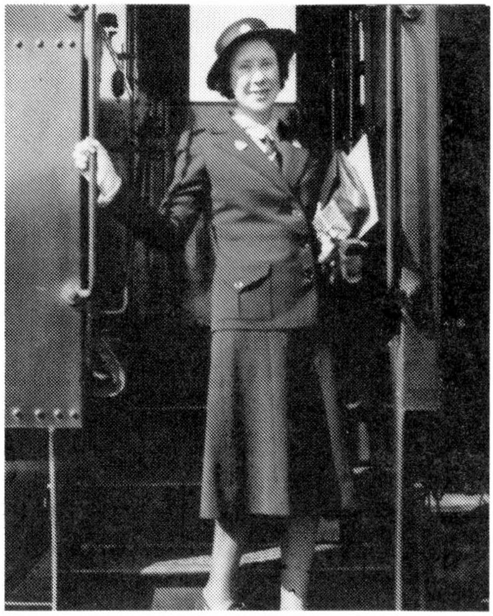

No. 4 CCS
M.C. Brown leaving Edmonton
July 18, 1940

I chose to join the Army because of patriotism mixed with a little adventure. I received both serving with No. 4 CCS from Alberta in the south of England, August 1940 to 1943.

Through blackout and blitz, night after night, falling over tent ropes or into the muddy trenches, one had to have a sense of humour for there was no glamour.

Next step, Sicily, with No. 4 CGH for a few months, then to Italy until April 1945, during which time I really knew what wartime surgery was all about as I was with the surgical team from Rome, north to firing line at Monument Hill. During those days and nights working under canvas and dim light while hearing gunfire was stressful but gave great satisfaction.

Next step, a short time in Belgium, then to England and home in June 1945 and oh, oh, ice cream and white bread and butter, but most of all, a bathtub of hot water.

On returning to Canada, I served at Currie Barracks Hospital, Calgary until September 1946 when my discharge from the Services came through.

I then worked at the Col. Belcher Hospital, Calgary until March of 1967 when it was time to retire and enjoy life.

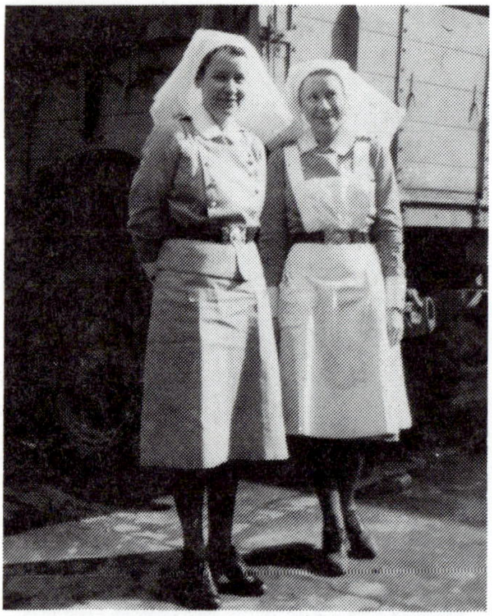

L-R: Agnes McLeod, M.C. Brown,
Dorking, England

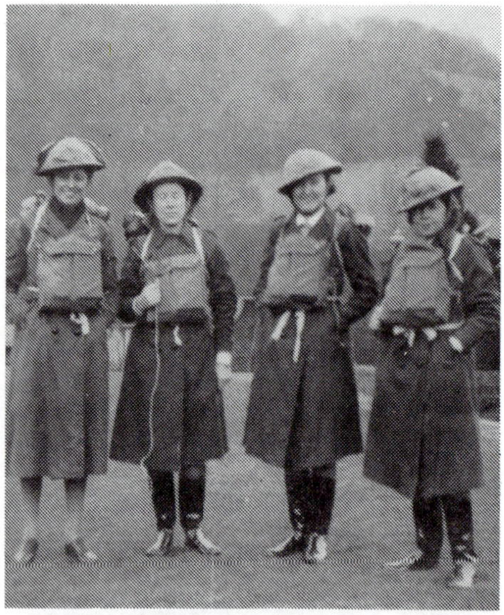

Gas Training, 1940 England, 4CCS
Margaret C. Brown 2nd from left.

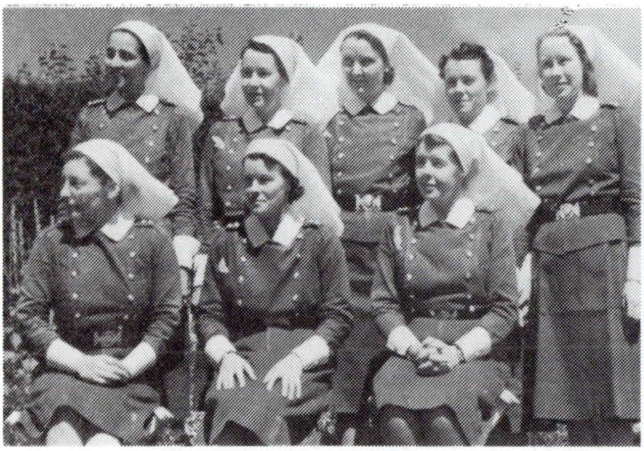

No. 4 CCS, Ashtead Park
TOP ROW L - R:
Lt. N/S Queena May Esdale,
Capt. A. McLeod, Lts.(N/S) Maxine Fuller,
M. Hodson, Margaret Brown
SITTING LEFT - RIGHT:
Lts. N/S Lillian Bibby, Robinson, M. Logan

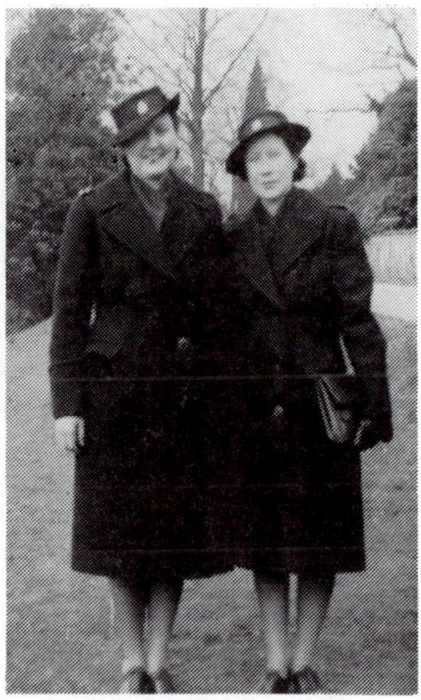

L-R: Maxine Fuller,
M.C.Brown

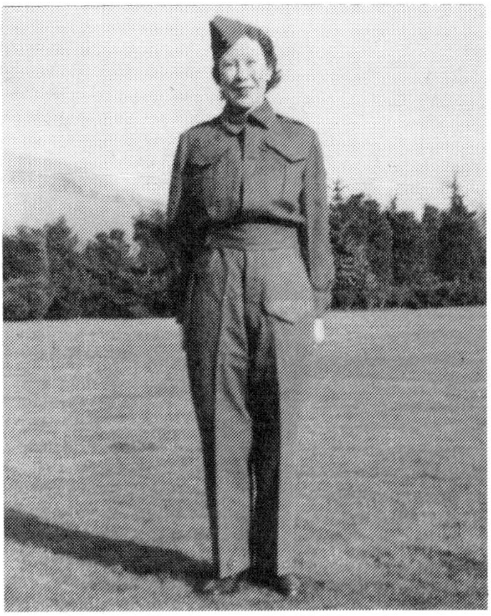

Battle dress, M.C.Brown

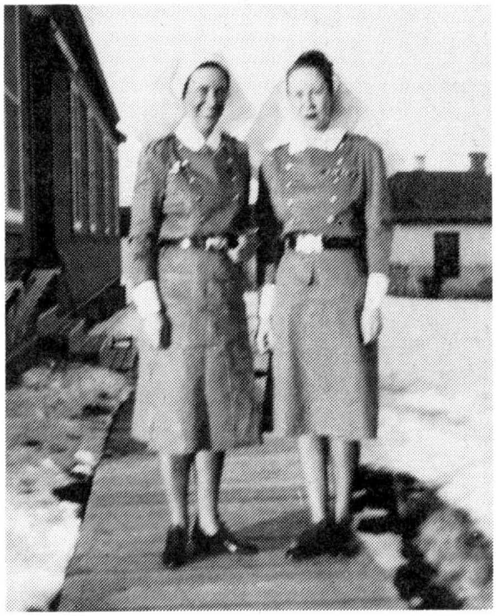

L-R; R. King, M.C.Brown, Dorking, England

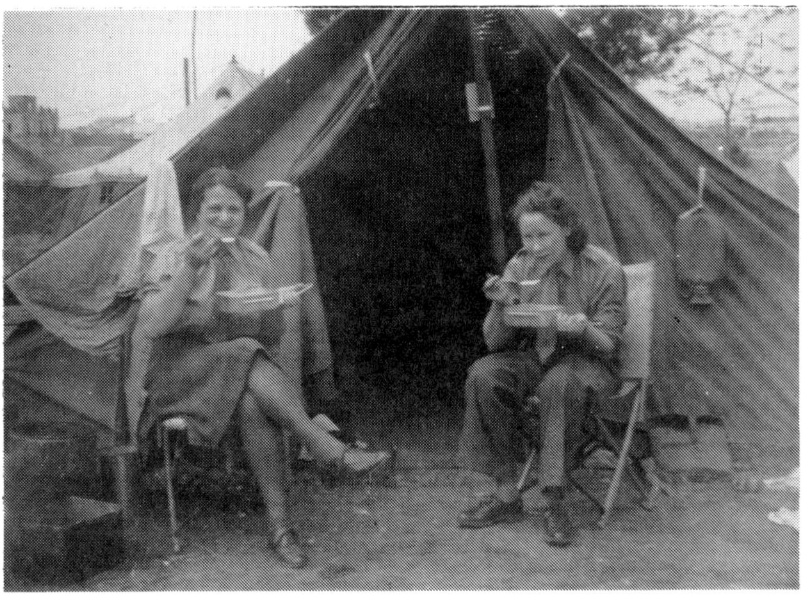

L-R: K.P. Smart, Margaret C. Brown
Moving Day 1944, Andria, Italy, No. 5 Cdn. Gen. Hosp.

Maxine D. (Fuller) Slemon

Graduated from: Royal Alexandra Hospital School of Nursing, Edmonton. Year: 1936

Military History:

Service: RCAMC

Rank: 1st Lieutenant N/S

Served: 1940 to 1945

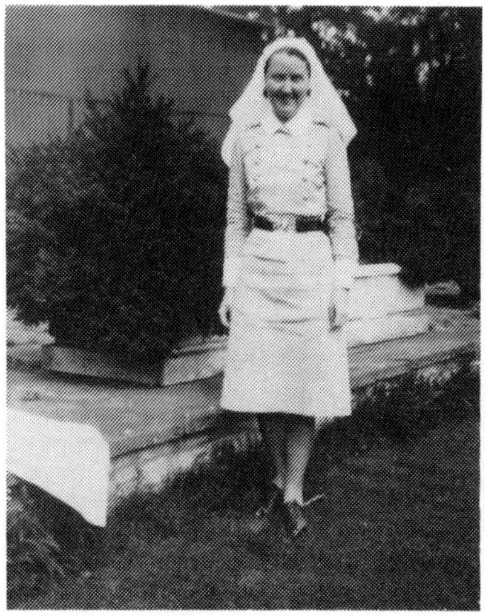

No. 4 CCS Maxine D. (Fuller) Slemon 1940-45

I wished to support the war effort and travel so I joined the Army in 1940 and was called up in August of that year. We worked for a short time in Edmonton and then the call came to go overseas. We proceeded to Calgary to join the rest of our unit and went then to Halifax and England.

As a mobile unit, No. 4 CCS, we moved to various locations in southern England, located sometimes in buildings, sometimes under canvas.

In 1943 we embarked for Sicily and then to Italy and followed the troops north.

I was married in Italy, returned to England and then to Canada where I was demobilized.

NO. 5 CASUALTY CLEARING STATION

Evelyn Pepper

No. 5 Canadian Casualty Clearing Station mobilized at Ottawa 2 September 1939.

Nursing sisters became part of the unit 1 May 1940 with Mima MacLaren as senior nurse.

On 17 June 1941 the unit boarded the SS *Andes* at Halifax and sailed four days later as part of a convoy that reached Scotland 30 June 1941. The unit functioned as an active CCS at Ford Manor.

In November of 1942 the unit moved to the field for five months of intensive training near Newdigate.

At the end of October 1943 they boarded the SS *Argentina* and arrived in Italy 8 November. They were constantly moving and were often within a few miles of the front lines tending the wounds of Canadian soldiers as well as caring for the numerous medical problems including a high incidence of malaria.

Evacuation of wounded soldiers was made difficult because of the rough terrain and narrow roads, another reason for medical personnel to be close to the front lines.

As the Italian campaign drew to a close No. 5 CCS left Italy and arrived in Holland at the end of March 1945.

Their final assignment was at Almelo, Holland, where the unit disbanded 2 September 1945.

Evelyn Pepper, RRC, CSt.J., RN

Graduated from: Ottawa Civic Hospital School of Nursing.
Year: 1928

Military History:

Served: RCAMC

Rank: Major

Served: World War II

Aspiring to be a doctor, in 1929 I applied to the Dean of Medicine, McGill University, Montreal, who granted me an interview. After discussing my goal and testing my wits for what seemed an interminable time, he rose from his desk, placed his hand on my shoulder, and said *"Go home young lady, go home, there is no place for women in medicine."* Thus ended my hope of becoming a doctor.

Early in the 1930 Depression, commonly known as "The Dirty Thirties," the radiologist of the OCH offered me a position on his staff and I was pleased to accept. Nine years later I resigned as charge nurse of the X-ray department when I enlisted as a 2nd Lieutenant with No. 5 CCS, RCAMC, on June 1st, 1940.

A matron and seven nursing sisters comprised the nursing staff of our unit. We served in Petawawa Military Hospital for over a year attending sick and injured soldiers and learning

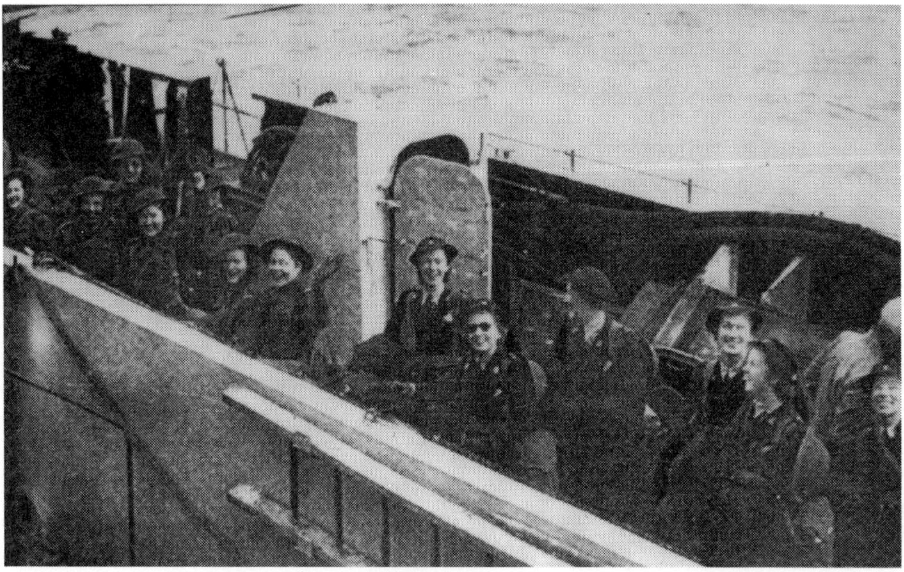

5 CCS
L-R:
Seven Canadian nursing sisters of No. 4 Cdn. Casualty Clearing Station and six Canadian nursing sisters of No. 5 Cdn. CCS: Capt. (Matron) Dorothy Macham , Lieut. Nursing Sisters Dorothy Dent, Evelyn Pepper, Ida Burkholder, H.M. Gardiner, Elizabeth Cleland

From the decks of the landing craft which had participated in the invasion of Sicily and Italy, nursing sisters and troops of the 1st Corps wait in Augusta harbour for orders to go ashore.

Courtesy: History of Canadian Army Overseas 1939-45, Whitcomb Gilmore Co., Montreal.

Army rules and regulations while teaching the other ranks their role as nursing orderlies.

On June 1st, 1941, our unit sailed from Halifax on the SS *Andes* for service abroad. We landed in Scotland and were whisked by train to London. Enroute we were happy to see how calm and seemingly unperturbed the people in the countryside were. But we noted a very opposite attitude as we ran through the populated and devastated areas. We were housed overnight in a V.A.D. Club on Cavendish Square. As we drove into the Square we had noticed a large monument bound by a chain of military warnings. We were instructed by our hostess, Mrs. Howes, not to open the blackout curtains, remain indoors and hurry to the basement in the event of an air raid. When we inquired about the cordon around the monument, our hostess calmly explained that there was an enemy bomb there which the authorities had not had time to remove.

Our next stop was Digswell Place, the beautiful estate of Col. and Mrs. Kenneth Maitland, located at Welwyn, Hertfordshire, about thirty miles from London. Their young children were safely in Canada and the parents provided their estate as a holiday house or convalescent home for Canadian nursing sisters for the duration of the war. Mrs. Gertrude Gilson, nicknamed "Squire," her maiden name, was the house-mother at Digswell Place. "Squire," a charming lady full of vigour, humour and constant kindness, had been a nursing sister during WW I, one of four Canadian nursing sisters stationed in Petrograd during the Russian Revolution. As one of the others wrote in her diary, February 24th 1917, "It is not often that one can watch the death of a monarchy and the birth of a new republic." Twenty-four years later "Squire" Gilson RRC, RN, was serving her country again.

All who stayed at Digswell Place recall how the colonel and his wife Jean, although both had wartime duties, planned that either or both would have dinner with the nursing sisters whenever possible. Their presence was always a joy to everyone as was the presence of their two Great Danes resting quietly in front of the fireplace. It was always a perfect setting for good conversation, music and the good dinner prepared and served by the friendly house-staff, one of whom, every morning, would serve us "breakfast in bed" while the other cleaned the rooms downstairs without having us under her feet.

One of my first purchases in England was a corselette. I paid for it and stood quietly waiting for it to be wrapped. "Aren't you going to wrap it?" I finally inquired. "Well, I can put a string around it," she replied. From then on I usually wrote home for such a thing unless it was small and could be tucked into my gas mask.

On July 23rd, 1941 we rejoined our unit at Ford Manor, some distance from East Grinstead, where we reopened a 150-bed hospital and engaged in intensive training for many months. Our new home was a mansion once owned, we were told, by the Earl of Buccleugh, a brother of the present Queen Mother. It was a lovely stone home with vast grounds, gorgeous gardens – 24 gardeners in peacetime – but the coldest and most awkward place in which to work. Two reasons accounted for this situation. First, no fuel was available for the multiple fireplaces.

Second, an overabundance of small rooms and few large rooms, all connected by hallways and stairways, was tiring and confusing. Nevertheless, we enjoyed our experience while there.

Shortly after our arrival we met two sisters, Jean and Meg Hadden, who lived in Dormanslad, a town adjacent to Ford Manor. They very kindly invited four of us to their home one evening. As we had to walk, we decided to take a shortcut. When they asked us if we had found the walk long we told them we had cut across a huge field. They exclaimed "You must NEVER do that again. There is a bull in that field and he's nasty. You must go home by the main road." So we took the long road. Enroute we had to pass several ominous looking camouflaged guns, all pointing skyward. This frightened us somewhat so we hastened our steps and clicked our heels harder on the pavement, to boost our confidence, as we passed up the long dark lane to the manor. Suddenly out of the darkness a voice called "Halt! Who goes there?" We all replied "Canadian Nursing Sisters." "Advance to be recognized," the voice said. As we moved forward one tremulous voice called, "Oh, you wouldn't know us. We have just arrived!"

When a scheme called "Tiger" was activated by Corps Headquarters to test our efficiency in receiving, treating and evacuating casualties we knew we were "in training."

Hundreds of faked casualties were brought to Ford Manor by train or ambulance while others were walking wounded. Each man wore a tag stating his type of wound. They were taken immediately to the triage area where two doctors made the decision as to his priority for admission and care. Detailed records were kept by each section of our unit involved in the exercise. Action taken and in what amount of time were two important factors.

For instance, a doctor, an anaesthetist and a nurse worked for eight hours in the operating room estimating "supplies needed." Following an examination of the wound the doctor would say "I will need such and such." He gave orders for everything he anticipated he would require for that particular case and then went on to the next casualty awaiting surgery. The anaesthetist and nurse did likewise. All was recorded for a period of eight hours which was the length of the exercise. A study of all reports revealed deficiencies in all sections and the corrective action to be taken. This was attained during further exercises.

As nursing sisters our intense military training started at our next location, Newdigate Place. We all wore battle dress. We did not operate a hospital. Daily training included physical exercises and long marches. The instructor was neither amused nor impressed by our high-stepping to avoid the ever present lovely flowers that lay in our path. *"WOMEN,"* he would exclaim in disgust. Hardening activities included erecting and dismantling our tents; going to the firing range where we had to fire heavy guns called .303s which gave one a bang on the shoulder when you pulled the trigger; map reading and revolver practice were also on the agenda. Getting an Army vehicle licence required that you could drive every type of vehicle in the car park which held ambulances, passion wagons – much like a Brinks truck, Jeeps, motorcycles and trucks. This training was optional and some nursing sisters preferred not to participate.

We took part in several war schemes. Some were short, others lasted two weeks or more. As nurses, we unpacked and repacked the supplies allocated for our work areas. They were always well marked and in place waiting to be used. When we were finished using them, we would repack them and they were returned to stores. We became used to moving from place to place and doing our job well despite weather conditions and short notice. We never knew when the next move would take place but we always had to be ready. Others were in charge. We did as we were instructed. Pitching tents and driving trucks was not our job. Nor was the firing of arms our job. But we were prepared to do these things if the need arose. Every scheme demonstrated how, when and where our service fitted into the master plan. All schemes were interesting, exciting and very realistic. We were being prepared for what lay ahead. Our muscles told us so.

On October 25th, 1943 our unit sailed in convoy for a "destination unknown." On November 6th the convoy was attacked off the coast of Gibraltar by enemy submarines and aircraft. Two ships were hit: one, an ammunition ship, blew up. SS *Santa Elena*, the second ship, was carrying 1900 fighting personnel and the complete staff and supplies of No. 14 Canadian General Hospital. Matron Blanche Herman and thirty of her nursing staff were, to our horror, reported missing.

When our ship, the SS *Argentina* sailed safely into Augusta Harbour, Sicily, we heard the wonderful news that Matron Herman and her nursing sisters were all safe, having been picked up from life boats by two American destroyers. The SS *Santa Elena* sank off the coast of North Africa. All medical supplies and stores went down with the ship and the nursing sisters lost all their personal belongings.

We were taken directly by car to No. 5 CGH. at Catania. We were in Sicily for just a short time during which we worked mostly at the No. 2 British Field Hospital in Messina where we attended British casualties from the Italian campaign and "Desert Rats" from North Africa.

The quartermaster of No. 5 CGH. approached Matron Macham a day or so after our arrival and explained to her that he was short of drivers and needed one of her nursing sisters to be his driver for the next two days. "Ev Pepper has her licence and I need her service," he said. Without hesitation I was assigned the task. The car I drove was a small Fiat to which they attached a truck. Elizabeth Cleland was the one who offered to come with us to sit in the truck with the sandwiches and coffee and any supplies we collected enroute. We drove from one supply depot to the next. The quartermaster knew what he was looking for and we helped him at every stop. When we stopped for lunch or tea we picked the fresh fruit nearby for dessert. There was so much on that lush island. It was a very interesting experience for us and a fascinating drive. We were not only on duty, we were seeing Palermo, Syracuse and other parts of Sicily as well.

Few of the roads in Sicily and Italy had guard-rails in those days. If you were on the outside driving along a mountainside you could see a great depth of open space. It was quite intimidating and at times the palms of my hands were moist. We were stopped, on our second day, as we approached a mountainous area. A big gun was being winched around a curve on the road ahead. We had to sit and wait until the gun was driven safely down the mountain. Meanwhile, I started the engine once and it responded well but the second time it wouldn't start. The QM said *"You are the driver lass, so you fix it."* I got out and was greatly relieved when I saw what repair was needed. Taking the foil out of my package of cigarettes, I attached two loose wires and got the car started.

During this time delay, two young German prisoners had been watching us from behind a barbed-wire fence. They clapped their hands when the car started but quickly disappeared. We were still waiting for our signal to proceed up the mountain when they reappeared with their arms full of luscious tangerines. I gave them each a cigarette and watched the enjoyment it gave them. The prisoners were so young. That was late in 1943.

I recall wondering if the Germans were beginning to show signs of their losses.

When we arrived back at the hospital laden with the needed medical supplies from the depots and an abundance of fresh fruit, Elizabeth and I decided that a part of our training at Newdigate Park had come into proper focus during our two-day expedition.

On January 14th, 1944, we were flown to Bari, Italy, five of us in a Lancaster plane. There was an iron lung stabilized in the centre, enroute probably to one of our hospitals. The co-pilot suggested we could come forward one at a time and fly the plane. It was so intriguing; one could look down through the plexiglass and see a convoy going through the Gulf of Toranto. When it was my turn, the plane was flying over water and all I had to do was watch the horizon. But as soon as we flew over land, I wanted to level with every green space below. I soon found that at the slightest touch on the control stick, the plane reacted instantly. Flying over land was much more difficult, I decided, than cruising over water.

The first location for No. 5 CCS on the mainland was an unbelievably dirty town on the Adriatic side of Italy called Corato. A sewerage system had never been built. Fortunately, the nurses were housed outside the town where the air was fresher and limited water was available. Soon after our arrival, while walking to the school where our unit had set up, some ladies asked us who we were. Leafing through our dictionaries we found "nutrice – to nurse." They seemed pleased. Later in the week we were asked what in the world we had told the villagers we were. She laughed when we told her and said "Nutrice" meant wet nurse. From then on, at her suggestion, we answered "Sona Infermere," meaning "I am a nurse."

Orders to proceed closer to the front line came in about a month's time. Lanciano was to be our destination. We moved in convoy. Tents were set up for the officers and other ranks. The nurses slept in the ambulances. The tobacco factory which we were supposed to occupy was in such disrepair from recent bombings it was ten days or so before we admitted our first casualties there.

Meanwhile the nursing sisters worked with No. 13 Canadian Field Dressing Station which was set up in an apartment building. The operating rooms were very busy. Shrapnel was falling. We soon saw what awful wounds these penetrating shell fragments caused. During one operation a noise was heard on the ceiling. The scrub nurse looked up and said, "There must be mice up there." She was told, "That's not mice. That's shrapnel." The benefit of having nursing sisters working with their team was highly proclaimed by the doctors of No. 13 FDS, and worked exceedingly well later in the campaign. As I look back I think it brought impetus to change.

An apartment opposite to No. 13 FDS was occupied by an Indian Unit. Every morning we would see the men come out in colourful trunks and wash their hair at the large water tank standing in the driveway. Someone saw us and said "You girls had better not be looking at those Indians. First thing you know they are going to be over here to visit you." We assured him we were only interested in their "hairdo," how they rolled it up and tucked it under their turbans.

As the weather improved the casualties increased and the operating teams were very busy. In a few days we were on the move again to Casacalenda, about ten miles away, where eighty beds were set up in a school. Fifteen days later we were on the move again to Telese where we were located in the Hotel Albergo Grande. Casualties were cared for on the first two floors and the nursing sisters occupied the third floor. This location was by far the best we had encountered for casualty care since arriving in Italy.

Later in April we moved into a highly camouflaged area where many medical units were concentrated. Ordinarily, being a medical unit, the Geneva Red Cross Agreement would give you a certain amount of safety. But on this occasion no evidence was in sight. We were told we were on a "rest period," the first since our arrival in Sicily in November 1943. Heavy traffic on the Naples to Cassino highway and the absence of a Red Cross flag in the area aroused our suspicion, however, that an advance attack was in the offing and we would be moving forward. One day an officer pulled into our field. The driver unrolled a large map on the side of the truck. We sat on the ground watching and listening as the officer described some of the planned action. This had never happened before and we were grateful that we were drawn into the picture but sure that he only told us what it was safe to tell. Our suspicion was confirmed. The "rest-period" was another form of camouflage and we would soon be in action again. The following day two church services were conducted by the senior Protestant and Roman Catholic chaplains from the

1st Canadian Corps. All units in the concentration area participated.

A morning or so later I lay on my cot and watched formations of planes passing overhead. The sun was rising and they were just silver specks in the air – hundreds of them. When we heard the distant bombing we knew the attack had started.

At this time, Matron Dorothy Macham was recalled to England to assume other duties. We regretted this very much but off she went carrying her usual happy smile and our very best wishes.

In a few days we were attending to the most serious casualties, Priority 1 and Priority 2, from our attack on the Hitler Line. Priority 3s were sent further down the line to a General Hospital. No. 4 CCS was open about six miles away and the motor ambulance brought one hundred cases to each unit alternately.

This system was maintained throughout the campaign. Our present location was a town called Pignataro. In the first two days we admitted 162 casualties and lost only one patient.

When our unit moved forward again, two of us were left behind with seventeen patients who were too ill to be moved. We were told that a doctor would join us as soon as possible. He arrived the next day, very dirty from a dusty, long and sweaty drive and went to a nearby stream to wash. He came back with a horribly gashed foot. We attended to his injury and evacuated the poor chap immediately.

Dorothy Dent and I had four orderlies, a cook and an ambulance driver to work with us. We had to make our plans. The other ranks worked twelve-hour shifts. Dorothy came on duty before midnight and we reviewed each case. Then I retired and returned about 7 A.M. This gave us an overlap each night and morning to assess all patients and determine which ones should be prepared and sent by ambulance to No. 3 CGH that morning. Our first objective was to get the most serious cases back to base hospital quickly and in as good condition as possible. Dorothy and an orderly accompanied them providing care enroute. They caught some rest on the return trip and later at camp.

We were working in a plowed field and all but two of the beds were low cots. Much of our nursing was done on our knees. The effort by the other ranks to help these boys recover was exceedingly good, generously given and always with cheer and a smile. Our patients were superb, very quiet and as cooperative as possible depending on the nature and extent of their wounds. Most had had surgery, some were in casts, all were in need of continuous observation and support. All were safe and resting fairly well. The look on their faces was rewarding.

The night the unit had moved forward, one tent had been left behind in the olive grove where all the nursing sisters had been housed. At first I could not sleep because olives kept dropping off the trees onto the canvas and I felt sure someone was outside. The cook realized I had not slept very much and gallantly said "Don't worry, Sister, I'll put my pup tent next to your tent; you'll sleep tonight." Frenchie, the cook, slept in his pup tent. He snored so loudly, I could not sleep in mine. That evening the lone tent was given an new home nearer the treatment area.

On rejoining our unit we asked about a uniform worn by Allied soldiers seen in the Cassino area. It was long, like a robe, made of grey-green material covering the soldier from head to foot. We were told these men were the gallant Poles who had contributed so magnificently in the recent attack. As they climbed the hills their uniform blended in with the rocks and brush of the area, adding to their success.

By mid-July the unit had returned to Telese. No place in this war-torn country could have been nicer for the wedding of Sister Helen Gardiner to Major John Hornibrook, 1st Survey Regiment, than the Grande Albergo Hotel. N/S Elizabeth Crothers was her bridesmaid and Major Larry Brown, M.D. gave the bride away. Captain Saddler was best man and Captain Eagles our, CE padre, performed the ceremony. A delightful reception was held at the First Survey Regiment Officers' Mess. The nursing sisters and Major Brown were original members of No. 5 CCS, an Ottawa-Kingston unit. This happy event was our first big social occasion of the year.

The next move was my own. I was on night duty when Matron Elva Honey woke me up at mid-day and told me I had been promoted to A/M Captain No. 1 CGH. I was sad to leave but quietly moved on. One always did as one was told. Unless you were of senior rank or working alone, as two of us had been recently, you were never a participant in the decision making.

In the first week of August we left our location in a cloud of dust which lasted most of the day. I remember the incident well because I developed an infected thumb and had to suck it all day. Nine hours later we were settled in the Canadian Officers' Club in Rome where we were to remain until further orders. It wasn't difficult to spend several days in that great city. There was so much to see and historical sites to visit. Many of us were present during an audience with His Holiness, the Pope.

Early in the morning of August 18th we said good-bye to Matron Nancy Kennedy-Reid. She was returning to the U.K. to become principal matron of a 1200-bed hospital. The nursing sisters gave her a lovely tortoise-shell vanity case, a token of their high regard and very best wishes. A newsy letter received by her replacement, PM Helen Hewton, brought word that four of the "Woofs," women of over forty, who had been returned to the U.K. were working again with her at her new posting, No. 23 CGH.

One of my first duties as a/matron No. 1 CGH was to proceed with three nursing sisters, as an advance party, in the preparation of our new location at Jesi. Two days later the remainder of the nursing sisters joined us and hundreds of beds were made in quick order. By 1800 hours on August 22nd we had completed our task and ready as a team to receive 600 patients. On opening day over 400 patients were evacuated to us from field medical units. These nursing sisters who had recently arrived adapted themselves to the situation like old timers. The unit functioned as a Casualty Clearing Station from then on. Records show that from the opening day until the end of September, of the 7119 casualties admitted, over 2094 were operated on, 1202 requiring major surgery.

No. 1 Canadian Motor Ambulance corps was bombed one night. Two boys were killed and twenty-two wounded. When these casualties were brought to us we were deeply saddened. We had come to know most of them. Since this action started they had been constantly bringing the wounded to us.

On August 30th our Canadian boys pierced the Gothic Line. Everyone was cheering.

As the battle raged on in September, more and more casualties were received. We were approaching a nursing crisis situation. As No. 1 CGH was acting as a pool for the advanced medical units, all the attached nursing sisters had been sent forward as needed. A large percentage of our admissions required surgery and treatment over and above what they had received in the forward area. P/Matron Hewton had sent an urgent message to Senior P/Matron Herman that more nurses were urgently needed. The increasing number of post-operatives was taxing our nursing staff almost to the breaking point.

The situation was solved by the attachment, for various periods of time, of two British field surgical units and surgical teams from No. 15 CGH and No. 5 CCS supplementing our own staff. Working in shifts, the operating rooms were kept functioning twenty-four hours a day and the pressure on the bedside nurses was eased. It had been a very difficult and exhausting month. Everyone involved deserved high praise.

On September 26 we received great news. Rimini had fallen.

Italians told us it had been a typical month of October, cold and bleak. Rain had hampered our activity. To the delight of some, but not all, the return sailing of nursing sisters to the U.K. had been temporarily cancelled.

Cardinal Villeneuve of Quebec visited the wards bringing happiness and comfort to all.

Two weddings took place in the nursing sisters mess during October. P/A Frances Hughes was married on October 4th to Lieut. Donald Cleveland. P/A Helen Porter was married on the 28th to Capt. Robert Metcalfe. The mess lends itself beautifully for such happy occasions.

On November 6th I joined No. 3 CGH as a/capt. matron replacing Capt. Matron M.I. Roach who had been posted to No. 1 CGH. I was sorry I had missed the vicious storm that had occurred earlier. It would have been fun to see "the high rubber boots brought out to float the nurses through the mud to the hospital."

The next day our hospital was inspected by the newly appointed GOC 8th Army. This gentleman was a treat to meet. He drove his own car. Before he arrived it was rumoured that he did not like operating rooms but he liked cooking. The culinary and most other departments were visited including the wards and Red Cross Room where he chatted with many of our patients.

A short account of the 1st Div. HQ party is deserved. It was such fun. Fourteen nursing sisters from 5 CCS and 3 CGH were guests of Commanding Officer Col. Ross. An Italian artist drew caricatures of each guest on a reserved section of each dinner menu. It was then added to a "Rogues Gallery" on the wall. Everyone enjoyed the lovely goose dinner and other entertainment as the evening went laughingly on.

No. 3 CGH remained in its same location on the Adriatic. The hospital was closed to visitors. We were acting as a clearing station for all acute throat cases in the area. The incidence of diphtheria remained high and we had evacuated 89 positive cases to base hospital. Proven malaria cases were lower than expected, reflecting our learned precautions on preventing mosquito bites through the use of mosquito netting, repellents, and exposure of as little skin as possible, especially after the sun went down.

As more penicillin was being used in the treatment of our 800-plus battle casualties, an extra nurse was added to the night staff to administer the drug throughout the hospital, thus enabling the sister in each surgical block more time for much-needed bedside care.

This had been a busy month relieved only by the joy of Christmas. Prizes were offered for the most attractive ward on each floor. Every patient in the winning wards received generous gifts of cigarettes and Canadian chocolate bars from the Red Cross girls. More than one hundred patients sat at long tables in our broad hallways for Christmas dinner. It was interesting to see the less fortunate cases being helped to get comfortably seated by their ward buddies. The snow-white table cloth laden with colourful decorations of jellies, red apples, nuts and candies interspersed with candles and greens provided a homey atmosphere. One chap remarked that it was the first time in three years he had sat at a table for Christmas dinner.

January '45 was a quiet and somewhat puzzling month. Rumours were occurring until all proposals of moving south had been cancelled. It appeared certain we were to remain where we were for the winter.

Senior/P. Matron Agnes MacLeod, recently returned to Italy, visited our unit a second time late in January. Such collaboration with headquarters where units were so far apart was very reassuring to all in charge positions and her staff.

"Before the Allied assault across the Rhine began in late March, No. 3 Canadian General Hospital, first of the Canadian hospitals to arrive from Italy, had opened at Tilburg in Holland on March 15, 1945, to be followed by No. 1 Canadian General Hospital and No. 4 Canadian Casualty Clearing Station."

This statement taken from Colonel G.W.L. Nicholson's book, *Canada's Nursing Sisters*, brought back experiences in which I was involved, especially the secret movement of the First Canadian Division from Italy to another theatre of war. As matron of No. 3 CGH, I had been called to a meeting of the unit's officers and told that we would soon be on the move; destination was not mentioned. The nursing sisters were to travel by ambulance to Naples, by ship to Marseilles and by air to a Canadian

Hospital on the coast of France. I received orders which I was to follow implicitly. All unit insignia, including shoulder patches, were to be removed from our uniforms. We were to feign ignorance of having had any overseas army experience. In other words, we were to act as though we were new recruits. We would be billeted at an American Hospital in Marseilles but at no time were we to visit or work in the hospital nor go into the city. We were, in fact, confined to barracks!

After working strenuously for well over a year, most of us with forward surgical mobile units, we welcomed this respite from nursing duty. We had access to good books, took walks in the compound, talked a lot, ate extremely well and slept like tops. Speaking of food, we never seemed to stop eating. Went to the mess dining room three times each day and always left the table with some goodies tucked away in our battle dress jacket for afternoon tea or a late night snack. A German prisoner of war kept our large barrack-room quarters clean and cosy. There was a big stove in the centre of the room and every evening he came and lit a wood fire. Later on, when there was a good bed of glowing coals, we'd whip the stove lids off, place several metal coathangers over the open area and toast the best sandwiches, made from the wide selection of goodies spirited from the mess hall. It was great fun. We were a friendly group though some had not been with No. 3 CGH for very long, including myself.

Several days after our arrival we were notified to report for duty in the hospital the next morning. I immediately asked to see the commanding officer of the hospital and told him what my orders were. He would not listen nor change his mind. So I quietly explained to him that I would have to refuse his order. I was told to do as he ordered or face disciplinary action. I was shocked! If Canadians were seen in the hospital or Marseilles the move of the Corps would have been in jeopardy. I had been instructed that if I encountered any difficulty which I could not resolve amicably, I was to contact a certain officer in movement control. This I did and that evening a Canadian medical officer came roaring into the compound on a motorcycle. To shorten the story – we did not report for duty the next morning.

We left Marseilles the following day and flew to Brussels. Enroute the soft pink clouds were unbelievable. I felt one could have bounced in them. The officer who met us said we were to fly the following day for a nine-day leave in the U.K. No. 2 CGH in Ghent was where we stayed that night and several saw old friends again.

Our accommodation in London the next night was exceptionally good. Most were placed in Grosvenor House. It was a joy to feel hot water coming through the taps and that doors did have knobs. Early in the morning a V-1 or V-2 dropped near Hyde Park where the Grosvenor stands. The explosion was terrible. Several of us got over from the other hotel as quickly as we could. Fortunately, none of the nurses in Grosvenor House were injured. But one told me that when the bomb exploded she dashed from the bath to the bedroom and found her bed covered with splintered glass.

Later that morning everyone went their own way; some to Scotland or Ireland while others preferred to remain in London or nearby. We came together again in Brussels and moved on to a large building in Tilburg, Holland, which had every facility required for medical care including 200 bright rooms. It was a Roman Catholic Children's School previously occupied by the 88 British Gen. Hospital. Everyone was happy to be back with the unit. After a good holiday we were keen to get on with the task at hand.

My stay with No. 3 CGH, however, was short lived. I was posted to No. 1 CGH the next morning.

Word had been received that No. 1 Canadian Mobile Neuro-Surgical Unit and No. 6 British Maxillo-Facial Team would be attached to our unit, the former for the duration of the Campaign. We looked forward to working with these specially-trained Canadian and British nursing sisters.

When the First Canadian Corps struck north against Arnhem to clear western Holland, No. 1 CGH was ready. The first battle casualties began arriving on March 27th in fairly large numbers. More wards were being opened as the casualty flow increased. On April 1st No. 1 Canadian Mobile Neuro-Surgical Unit and No. 6 British Maxillo-Facial Team were working by nightfall. We were receiving a great many casualties but evacuating them, providing their injury was not too serious, to nearby units, thus providing more rapid turnover of cases. In four days all wards, nevertheless, were working to capacity. No matter how frequent our evacuations were, the wards were quickly filled again. We conserved on linen by just turning the sheets and pillowcases unless they were soiled. Also, open beds, made folded to the bottom, were an asset.

In a few days we evacuated our first ambulance train. I was

very grateful when I saw this happen. Being in a mobile unit in Sicily and Italy the patients were taken by motor ambulance to the train – if there was a train. Col. Wooton, an engineer, who was a patient at the time in Nijmegen, was very interested and extremely pleased. To me it meant continuation of casualty care enroute. Casualties requiring penicillin left with a bright yellow tag tied through the top button hole of their pyjamas. On the wards a patient on penicillin had a similar yellow card prominently shown on his chart. The same technique was carried out when the patient was moved by air. All were attended to by trained personnel.

It always amazed me that battle casualties were so quiet, so uncomplaining, despite the extent of their injury. We admired "our boys" tremendously and would have liked to have given them more individual attention but it just was not possible under the stress of battle. One had to adapt the principle of "doing her best for the most."

About April 9th there was an influx of ex-POWs, including Russians, Poles, Yugoslavs and Italians; it was a pitiful sight to see. Most were suffering from malnutrition and/or tuberculosis. Some had lost their will to survive and psychological help was needed and given by all of us including our doctors and padres. Many suffering from malnutrition were naturally ravenous for food and very angry when they received only small portions as directed by the doctor and dietician. These patients were on the third floor where isolation techniques were also the rule. One day I was approaching one Russian's bed when he suddenly sat up straight and spat at me. Fortunately I was gowned. An interpreter was finally found and there were smiles from then on. We lost one of these ex-POWs despite our combined effort. This soldier really willed himself to die. It was a dark day for me because, as a care giver, I thought our team was invincible.

The number of prisoners of war admitted increased as the days of battle wore on. They were all Germans but there was considerable difference in their ages and their attitudes. The elderly prisoners were quite appreciative of the care they were receiving. Perhaps this was so because they were old, weary of war and suddenly felt safe in our hands. There were many more young German prisoners, arrogant youngsters just out of school. They had been given guns and ordered to use them. This they considered as a great honour. Their injury seemed to act as the barometer of their attitude. The worse it was, the more cooperative they were. Some cried because they were sick and in pain or because they were lonely.

Over a period of years most nursing sisters had experienced young casualties of all nationalities, crying for "Mum." She was always there to talk, give him a smile, a pat on the shoulder or squeeze his hand.

In November '44, word had been received that the large-scale plan of returning nursing sisters to Canada on a "date of enlistment" scheme would soon start. The news created mixed feelings among the nursing sisters. Some felt that because they had voluntarily offered their service, they should be given the option of completing their commitment. Others were more than pleased to return home. We had been informed about it individually and in groups. It had been widely discussed by all concerned. But it seemed odd that it should happen at the height of what we now felt was our final campaign.

The first nine replacement Canadian nursing sisters arrived from England on April 20th. The plan had begun! No. 1 CGH was to be used as a staging unit for nursing sisters coming to the Continent or going home. New faces appeared daily and the friendly spirit in the nurses' mess was cheerfully extended to the newcomers. The "let-down" feelings were soon replaced by joyful talk about "going home." The plan was working.

Early in April, Major (PM) D. Riches of CMHQ, London, accompanied Major (Senior PM) M.M. MacLaren on a tour of the forward medical units. I reminded Mima how we had driven around the block four times gathering up our courage to cross the bridge at Porter's Island in Ottawa, leading to our enlistment in June, 1940.

Life was changing quickly. We were so excited and happy about the good news we were receiving, but overwhelmed with joy by the arrival of so many Canadians from freed German prison camps and hospitals. Our welfare officer brought a young Canadian woman, who had married a Dutch businessman prior to the war, into our hospital. She and a Russian lady prisoner had escaped when their prison was damaged. Being in German territory and unable to speak the language, she was advised by her companion not to talk at any time. She had been playing dumb for a few months and was almost demented. She and her husband had been caught aiding Allied airmen to escape to England after being shot down. They were never in the same prison and incarcerated for over three years.

The lady was from Wolfville, N.S. Her married name was Mona Leonhardt. What tales these folks told us. No more imaginative books need be written. She worked in a factory scraping glue off boxes, which she thought had been Red Cross parcels. Occasionally she would come across a piece of bright coloured paper, place it on her workbench, and look at it for real enjoyment. They saved any crumbs they found in the boxes, saved them until night and then ate them together.

It was decided to bring her over to our mess to convalesce and have female company. Two of our nursing sisters were pleased to share their room with our new Canadian friend. The nurses did all kinds of nice things for her. We all had a wonderful time giving her things to wear or having her hair done. The dietician looked after all ex-POW's meals and a doctor saw her regularly every day on his rounds. We all realized early on that she needed a great deal of psychological help, proper diet and planned exercise in the fresh air.

Weeks later a doctor took her to see her home to find out how she would react. She was not allowed to remain. After a few more weeks, two nursing sisters and I took her home to stay. With the CO's permission we took a good quantity and assortment of rations with us to boost their larder.

Food was scarce in Holland, and expensive; many people were eating the tulip bulbs from their garden. We stayed overnight and saw where they had hidden the airmen they had helped to escape. When the headboard of the bed in their master bedroom was moved to one side, access to a crawl space to their sloping roof was revealed. It was in this space that flyers hid awaiting the next step in their planned escape.

In the morning her closest friend cycled over in torrential rain carrying a newspaper-wrapped parcel. In it were Mona's jewels, in their case, which her friend had thoughtfully buried for safekeeping over three years ago. The war had ended just five miles from their lovely home which was boasting sheaves of welcoming wisteria.

We left Mrs. Leonhardt and her devoted housekeeper, who had remained in the house to protect it from vandalism, waiting in great anticipation of Mr. Leonhardt's safe arrival home. It had been another type of "war experience" for we three nurses.

Below in quotations are parts of a letter written to my sisters on May 6, 1945.

"*On the evening of May 4th, 1945, it was announced that the*

Germans in Holland in Northwest Europe had surrendered. It rather startles one to think that the grim horrors of war and spectacular happenings of the past five years are over. As for the peace that will soon be ours, I trust the world deserves it and can handle it better than ever before. Everyone was overjoyed, simply speechless and the town of Nijmegen went simply mad with joy. Tracer bullets and flares were shooting up everywhere. Bonfires burned on the streets as the Dutch cast their blackouts into flaming heaps.

"I was with one of our officers attending a men's party. We had suddenly heard the townspeople screaming and becoming pretty hysterical. Then a band played the Dutch National Anthem followed by "O Canada." Some chap jumped up on a table and told us what had been announced. The crowd went wild again. With tears and cheers the Dutch people were simply dragging Canadian soldiers into their homes, feeding them and giving them native wine which they obviously enjoyed very much. Our group came back to the hospital around 11 o'clock. We got three loaves of bread, a can of butter and a fresh hot roast of lamb from the hospital kitchen and had a party.

"That night every nursing sister enjoyed her first night's sleep without a blackout, some for many a year. The world seemed startlingly bright the next morning. Jove, the news is good. It is almost beyond belief.

"Exultation among the nursing staff was slightly delayed. Some of us could not believe that the message was entirely correct. It seemed somewhat premature. The dedicated group of doctors and nurses were very busy. Casualties, though less, were still coming to the hospital. All departments were still open."

Ancillary staff were still doing their extra bit. A physiotherapist was acting as a scribe for a doctor trying to keep up on the documentation that must accompany every casualty passing through our hands. The Red Cross officers provided much-needed items to ex-POWs as well as some luxuries they had not even seen since their imprisonment. In retrospect, involved as we had been for so long in casualty care situations, we were probably in mild shock. Our thinking cleared rapidly on May 7th when a "cease fire" affecting all troops in Europe was issued and VE Day was announced by Prime Minister Winston Churchill on May 8th, 1945. The long stream of battle casualties had finally ended.

As we celebrated that night, a tremendous sense of relief and quiet thankfulness stirred in our hearts.

The war in Europe was over.

No. 1 CGH remained busy for some months caring for the sick and injured in the Nijmegen area. The hospital was also actively involved in the comings and goings of nursing sisters affected by the "date of enlistment scheme" and the closure of hospitals. On December 5th, 1945, a delightful Christmas party, ordered, I believe, by the assistant director of Medical Services of the Canadian Forces in the Netherlands, took place for two hundred war orphans between the ages of three to ten being cared for in the area. It was the only Canadian Hospital still open. In mid-January it was turned over to the British. Most of us returned home on the *Queen Elizabeth* along with about 13,000 other Canadians, in early February 1946.

No. 6 CASUALTY CLEARING STATION

Edna (Crawford) Howard
Arleeta King
Margaret (Smith) Sparling

No.6 Casualty Clearing Station mobilized at Westmount Barracks, Montreal 1 July 1941.

On 20 March 1942 they embarked on the SS *Capetown Castle* at Halifax. By mid April they had set up at Pinewood in the U.K.

In July, 1944 the unit arrived at Courselles sur Mer in France. They followed the Allies as they progressed from France to Belgium to Holland, receiving casualties until the hostilities ceased. No. 6 CCS was at Almelo, Holland on VE Day.

They were located at Amersfoort, Holland when the unit officially ceased to exist as of 26 December 1945.

Edna (Crawford) Howard

Graduated from: Moncton Hospital School of Nursing.
Year: 1942

Military History:

Service: RCAMC

Rank: Lt. N/S

Served: March 1944 to April 1946

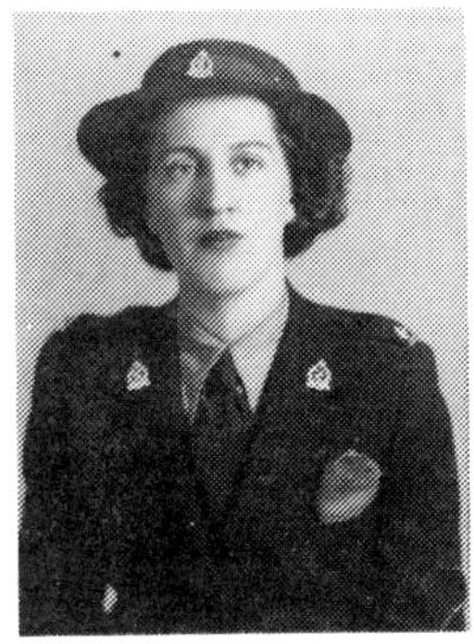

Lt N/S
Edna Crawford, Sussex 1944

It is hard to believe at present, but patriotism was in vogue when I joined the Army.

Three years of training, the usual routine day after day and finally, hard to believe, it is finished or just begun – the life for which I had worked so hard to achieve – years of working, saving, of doing without and, yes, of dreaming for. And here it was – Graduation Night. What a night! The sparkling white of nurses' uniforms, beautiful red roses, family; and wholeheartedly I dedicated myself to the nursing profession. I came back to my training school anxious to get to work. The thrill of being a White Nurse. I was anxious to really do my best and learn all I could to help others.

It was war-time, 1942; my hands and feet flew, but things were changing. My brother was in uniform. I was at home when his civilian clothes came home. My Mum and Dad were really upset. I was home on leave and was about to tell them I was joining the Army. However, I decided to wait – I tried to persuade myself I was needed where I was, but began to feel guilty when many of my friends joined up and were coming to visit us from Sussex. I became more anxious than ever to join up. One evening, we went to see *"So Proudly We Hail,"* and as we left the darkened theatre my mind was made up – I could ignore my conscience no longer. So November 9th, 1943, I was on nights, and in the cool gray dawn, I slipped a letter to MD No. 7 in the mailbox. I stood for some time, slowly returning to make morning rounds. What next. For the next 2-3 months, I constantly argued with myself. My family didn't want me to go. The doctors and superintendent needed nurses, and I was doing a job I loved – combination of charge nurse and giving nursing care.

However, in March of 1944, the mail brought the letter that changed my life. We were called in for medicals – Hayes, Godfrey, Brown, Barnes and I. Medicals cleared. We were posted to Sussex for basic training. Some disappointments – Sussex had plenty of nurses. Life was not rushed and it seemed so useless while Moncton Hospital was crying for help.

One day after another, and we're home on embarkation leave. We were going to be sent overseas as reinforcements for what was being called the Big Push coming up in June.

It was my first visit home in uniform and my sister sensed I was different, but I waved good-bye to Mum and Dad saying I'd see them next month, no need to worry them yet. Lots of time if things worked out.

We proceeded to Aldershot Transit Camp spending my 25th birthday lining up to bathrooms, meals, quarter master stores, and soon we were gathered in a quiet room and told we'd be leaving soon. It seemed like a dream. It was all happening so fast – the dark and quiet Troop Train to Halifax. Boarding the ship to take us across the Atlantic – seemed like it was all happening to someone else.

The trip was wonderful – clear, shiny days; but on the skyline was our convoy of ships. We learned later we were part of one of the largest convoys – preparing for the Great Day. What I didn't know that day was that my future husband had landed in Scotland too. Strange!

The trip was passing and then June 6th, 1944. Flash – Our boys had landed on Normandy beaches. Immediately our ship was at prayer. More precautions were being taken. We slept in our clothes, etc. Three more days and on June 9th, we were sailing into Scotland. The grass was so green - made me think of Canada. A busy day of waiting, standing. The long night from Greenock to London. Cold too. The Institute ladies, along the way serving sweet tea and "Naafi Tea" and Spam sandwiches – welcoming us with warm smiles. We got to London, wrinkled and dusty. Our matron-in-chief met us at the station and sent us to Bramshott. We arrived there but no one was expecting us, so back to the Lorries and off to No. 2 General at Hazelmere. They were receiving D-Day casualties. I wondered abut my brother. Monday morning we were off to the wards to work. The buzz bombs were flying over and the sirens were sounding, keeping everyone on the alert. It was a far cry from the home that I had left such a short time ago. Surprised to find the nurses immaculate in blues, white veils, etc. We were lined up to be sent to our wards. My friend Jeanie Barnes had worked on "Obs" for two years and was excited over being off that type of work. Down the list the matron went and we heard her say, Sister Barnes to obstetrics. Jeanie's face was something to see. She had crossed the ocean to get away from "women and babies." Ironic!

We were told not to unpack as we would be going overseas soon. Once more, we began our trips to QM stores preparing for work at the front. We were sent off to Whitby on the North Sea. A beautiful spot – bright, sunny days – we spent training, drilling, exercising; our poor bruised bodies really rebelled at all the punishment. We really needed the extra push from the pal behind us to get us up the third flight of stairs where we were billeted. We watched the planes go out and counted them coming back. This for the month of July and then we were gathered in a quiet room and given our orders for proceeding to France.

I began to realize what little nursing experience I had compared to the nurses I was with – some had five to six years. I was anxious to get to France as I knew my brother was over there. I hoped to meet him. On August 3rd we set out at Dover in rain, all day train ride through the battered cities and towns. Another cold, damp night, buzz bombs, etc. Ready to move. A lorry ride to C-22 where our Third Div. boys had waited to go to Normandy. We were under canvas. Church parade Sunday. For four more days, we slept, ate and waited – cut off from the world, no mail, no radio, no papers, etc.

Finally, August 7th up in a pearly dawn, lovely old English garden – seemed so peaceful and yet to near to war. Off to Southampton where our hospital ship waited to take us to France. As we waited to cross, we saw them bring the casualties on. It will be years before I will forget the look on those boys' faces. England looked good to them in comparison with the hell they had left. My eyes were filled with tears. We sailed along, landing at Courseulles on the French coast. It was hard to believe that only eight weeks ago the enemy was in control. The long, dusty, hot lorry ride to Bayeux, and there long rows of tents No. 10 General Hospital with 1,200 patients. It was work, working with POWs. We had thoughts of them almost as monsters, and now to find them as patients – they are very like our own boys. Worried over wives, children. Brave in suffering. It was wearisome. The sky shone brightly at night with ack ack fire.

I was sent up to 3 CCS to help out. Everything so strange – no linen – dirt, dust, flies, working 8 hours on, 8 hours off – seemed like a nightmare. How horrified I was when the charge sister told me not to bother the MO to sign a death certificate as we'd have several deaths by morning. I was so shocked! I was lost one night getting back to my tent; the flares lighted up and I got there safely. I hated being alone in the tents – the other two nurses worked 12-8. But on duty, it was smile, smile, cheer up the boys – never mind your fears. They don't know the meaning of fear... So just kept on working doing the best we could, carrying on in story book style, not as soldiers but as weary, tired – and many of them sick nurses, have carried on.

Then a promise of 12 whole hours off duty. I tumbled into my cot vowing I would sleep every precious minute from 8 A.M. to 8 P.M. At 2 P.M. I was wakened and told to be ready to move with three other nurses by 4 P.M. I struggled up, feeling cheated of my lovely sleep. But was too busy to feel sorry for myself, I had my bedroll to do. Boots to lace, etc. We arrived at 9 FDS to find 30 very ill – too ill to move – patients waiting. Just the tent up. We ate out in the open, and were told our tent would be ready by end of shift. They were in dug outs like the boys, and as three of us came off duty and went into a tent, a male voice said, *"Welcome Ladies."* It was our OC; however, we found our own dug-out and were soon settled in, near Carpiquet Airport and also close to Caen. The boys fixed up a primitive shower and we even had an iron.

It was here the OC requested that no one wave at him when he was in his office (using the latrine). There were rumours of moving but I was sent back to my own unit in Bayeux. We were busy but I loved the work, although I hated the dark, mud, wind and rain. A four-day leave at Deauville – that pleasure spot of peace times, now one riotous, mad house. It was all so strange. Boys trying to snatch some pleasure in an unbearable situation, girls trying to accommodate them. It was all too much for me. I was glad to return to Bayeux and my work sloshing through mud, darkness and oh so weary of it all.

No mail – then an order to be ready to go to Antwerp. A mad dash to pack, leaving Facey and Dot behind but Barnes was along, too, and ten other nurses. 4:30 A.M. we were off to Brussels, 14 of us in a Lorry, with luggage and only one stop all day. We arrived at the Atlantic Hotel. A bathtub, hot water. We all got cleaned up. We left for Antwerp and 8 CGH. The cold of the apartments – no heat – buzz bombs falling. The look on the boys' faces while they waited for the engines to cut out. They'd been through so much. Very shortly we were ordered to be ready to go to 6 CCS at Braachat, not far from Antwerp. The nurses there received us with open arms. I was so weary. It all looked impossible – what a night. Uppy and Katy – so busy and so much to learn all at once. But at the end of a week, we were functioning like old pros.

Another quick move to Nijmegen. We drove steadily all day through forlorn and forsaken Holland – broken bridges, the thunder of guns, the sky bright with artillery fire. Finally at A.M. a building – we piled out of the lorry – stiff, sore and cold (it was November 9th) – to find our cots set up and the cooks had hot chocolate, bread and butter ready.

On duty, and I drew nights again. Admissions all night long. How often I worked with tears in my eyes thinking of my brother. One evening on duty I looked up and he was standing before me. He looked so well, and was stationed nearby. We were very busy as we had Major Eaton's and Major Mustard's as well as the 6 CCS patients. Encouraging helping, soothing, kidding, never giving up. Those dark December days when the wail of the bagpipes were heard daily piping the boys to their last resting place. The spirit of the boys we had – so glad to be alive.

They gave us the strength and courage we needed, certain things remain in my mind. One big chap (Major Moffatt) – a leg gone, the other badly fractured – begging me to promise him he'd be okay – that he wasn't going to die. Gladys needed him too much. Calling me small fry as he clung desperately to my hand. Slipping off to sleep after 1/2 gr. of Morphia. Saying I know I'll be okay if you stay with me – and he was gone. Blessed sleep. I left his side with tears in my eyes. If his wife had only known that she was his last thought.

The big Irish lad who said, "Not so much of me to bathe today Sister." I pulled down the sheets and both legs were off at the knees.

Thus: December, January, and February went by. Days of hard work, Discouraging at times but always with the feeling that we were making life easier for some. We had a leave in Gent – an uneasy leave. Buzz bombs were still dropping. We were anxious not to miss the so-called Big Push. Due at any time, we were alerted for 5 A.M. I heard the first planes come over and we had a busy time ahead. Casualties poured in until evening when the thunder of the guns rolled away. The tracer bullets and ack-ack made the sky look like Fairyland. And by next morning, we were on the move. Spring had come. I was over at the Annex with the walking wounded. A hundred men – the CO called me, "The maid with a million men!"

A 72-hour leave to Paris – we went by train all night and arrived in Paris at daybreak. Stayed at the Metropole Hotel. What an exciting 72 hours. Facey and I were buddies, and she made every minute count, strolling the Champs Elysees – the Rue de Rivoli. Facey went to the opera to see Faust and Notre Dame, the Palace of Versailles, the Eiffel Tower, and finally to the Folies- Bergeres. Paris lighted again. Back to 6 CCS again. The tension was lifting and we were winning – April slipped away and then a leave to London. All the hurry and rush – strolling in Westminster Abbey, viewing Buckingham Palace, the King in his gardens, the day at Windsor Castle. Flying over the countries so lately occupied. What happiness.

Came back to pack again – no secrecy this time. Holland is free. We packed up from the place we had spent six months and we moved to Almelo to find patients already waiting. It was Sisters' Hospital, and had hot and cold water. We went happily to work. Then May 8th, 1945, the war was over – VE Day. The whole world went crazy. A call for Pacific volunteers – of course, I wanted to go so I signed up. Thirty of our boys were called – many of these my good friends – Uppy, Lester Lane, Kelly, etc.

A leave to Utrecht. The boys were always kidding, teasing. The song, Apple Blossom and Chapel Bells – *"You're a good kid Crawf."* We expected to be there for 6 months. New people came – new friendships. There were accidents. Seemed to be working harder than ever. The little Pay Master and my day out, the lovely tea and my gorgeous lilies. The trip to Utrecht to the concert with young "Jimmie." Jeannie had gone on up to Germany. Met Grant and had come back to Canada and was married. I missed her so, but Facey and I still were together.

Met Major Mac. He was so nice and was such a gentleman to me. Corn boils, dinner in Helvirsum, coaxed me to dress up – I did – my blues ready and came off duty to find someone had borrowed by buttons! I had to wear my Khaki. Mac was so disappointed. We had such nice times. Facey and a dental major came along. We went to their mess for refreshments.

I was very busy, but he was such a nice guy. I felt he was safe with me, since there was no drink, no nonsense. Just nicer than being alone. Later I had a leave in Copenhagen. The Col. went too. We had such a great time, matron, Penny, Facey. Several of us, and we had such a lovely time. The beautiful Danish country. A party for us with Danish escorts. Such a nice escort. Facey had a gorgeous naval officer, but a stuffed shirt. We had a great laugh over that. All the sightseeing. Little mermaid. The weather forecast on the Castle, etc. Like a story book. Came back to unit to find plans all changed. Had a 48-hour leave to Vimy which I thoroughly enjoyed to really see history. We were on our way back, the rain, the wind, etc., and to Calais. Back to England. The White Cliffs of Dover. Found I was posted to a Bride ship, the *Scythia*. Dot Godfrey was there too. Crying babies, homesick brides. Halifax. A time to be grateful for so much. So much living and experiencing packed into two years of a lifetime.

I feel that I have been so lucky and now to adjust to the humdrum routine of every day.

They call her Florence Nightingale in jest
But there's an earnestness behind her eyes
That she – High Priestess – does not realize
She only knows she does her simple best
Performing grave mysterious rights.
Aware that often she has
The spark of life to glowing flame
When it is dark and quiet in the woods,
Death walks then
She seems so young to have upon her
Slim proud shoulders
Such a weight of grief and pain
She should be walking thro' a
Or dancing somewhere where the lights are dim
Or should she?
Who to heavy lips must bless
With such profound and utter thankfulness
From my Orderlies at 6 CCS, 1944

Such a fine bunch – eight boys. I had five brothers so got along well with the boys.

Life has not been humdrum. Met and married a veteran so had much to share. Adopted two girls – enjoyed so many things knowing my Army experiences helped me realize how much we had to be grateful for. I lost my husband in 1989, now I have so many more memories!

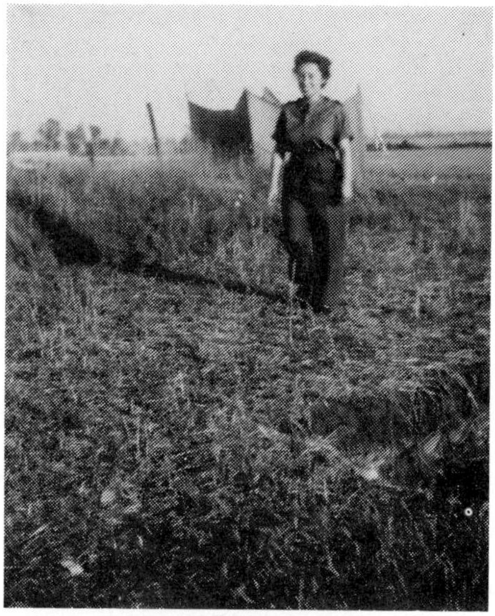

One of the kids
Bayeux, Sept. 1944,
the latest in latrines at that time.

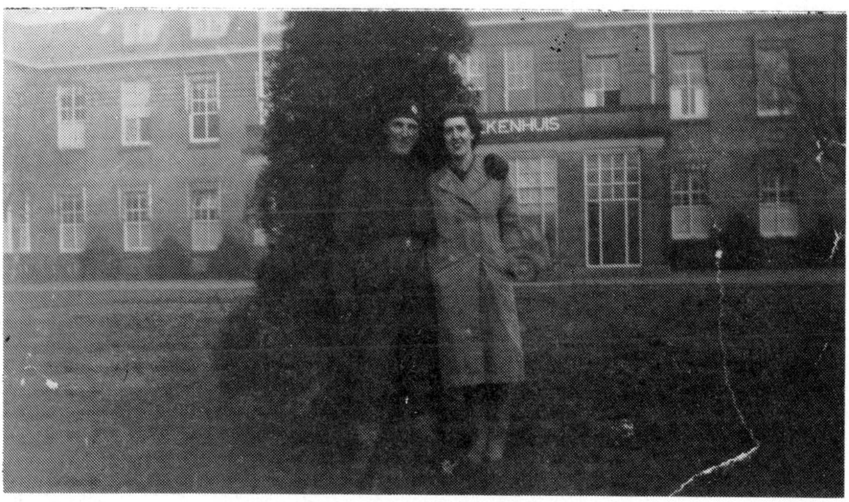

Lt. N/S Crawford
Brother - Pte Ralph Crawford -
mentioned in diary at hospital in Nijmegen. 1945

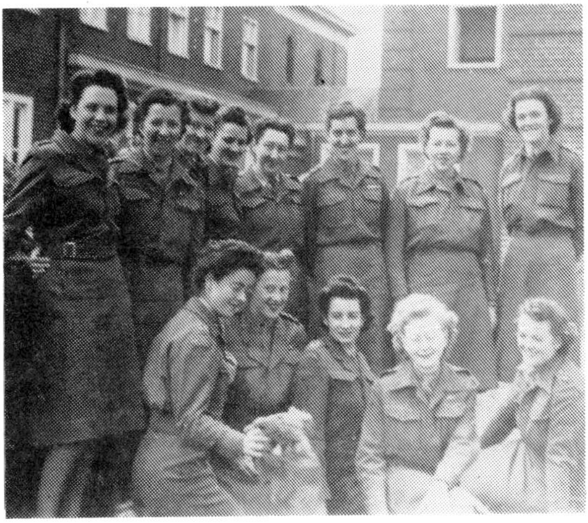

Group of 6 CCS nurses at 'sHertogenbosh Nijmegen, Holland, 1945 – remember some names but have no addresses after almost 50 years.

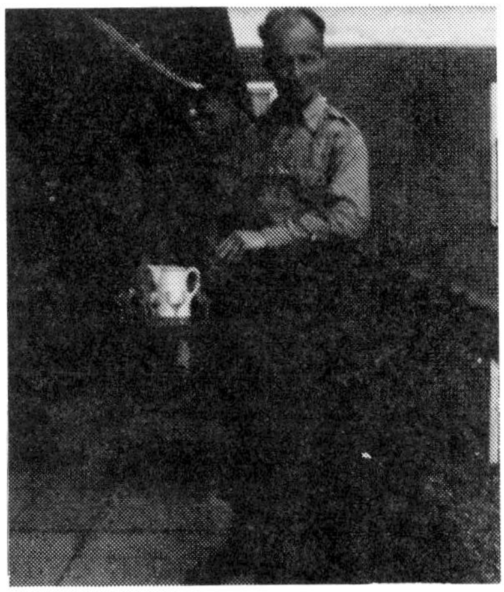

"Bill" - Major Bill Mustard a doctor from Toronto Children's Hospital – famous for his work with hearts. 1944

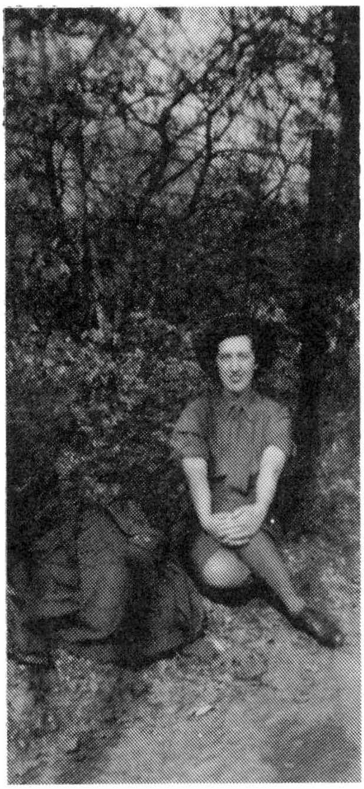

Lt. N/S Crawford Almelo, Holland 1945

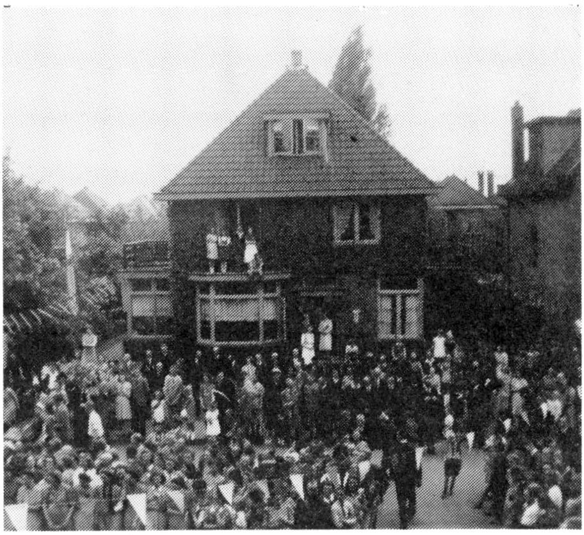

May 1945 – few people out eh? VE Day, Almelo, Holland, I was there.

Arleeta King

Graduated from: Kitchener-Waterloo Hospital School of Nursing. Year: 1937

Military History:

Served: Army

Rank: Captain

Served: 1942 - 1943 South Africa
1943 - 1945 Europe
1948 - 1967 Permanent Force

Margaret A. (Smith) Sparling

Graduated from: Royal Victoria Hospital School of Nursing, Montreal, Quebec. Year: 1932

Military History:

Service: RCAMC

Rank: Captain Matron, 6th Casualty Clearing Station

Served: 22 July 1940 to 1945

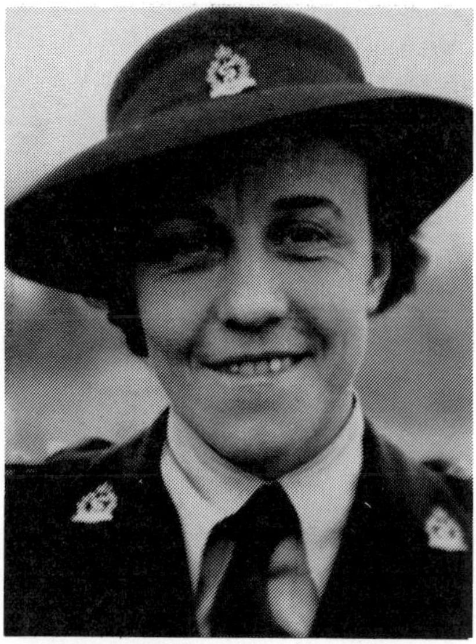

Capt. Matron Margaret (Smith) Sparling
6 CCS RCAMC 1940 -'45

I enlisted in the Canadian Army in July 1941, in Montreal where since graduation in 1932 , I had been a head nurse at the Royal Victorial Hospital. Early in 1942 I went overseas with the rank of Lieutenant, was promoted to Captain on becoming Matron of the hospital of the 6th Casualty Clearing Station. The No. 6 Casualty Clearing Station was formed in Montreal, July 1941. There were matron, (myself) and six nursing sisters, Wilhelmina Bell from Guelph; Kathleen Macleod from Kinross,

P.E.I.; Delia Ouellet, from Montreal; Peggy Hawksworth from Digby, N.S.; Jean Rayworth, Upper Cape, N.B.; and Erma Murray, Stellarton, N.S.

We crossed the English Channel about 10 days after D-Day. We joined our whole unit in France and from then on followed behind the troops looking after casualties from the battle of Caen and Falaise. From there we went to Belgium, Holland and Antwerp.

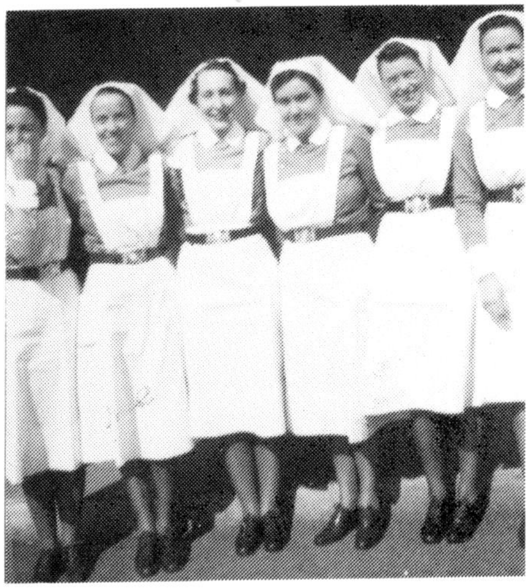

L-R:
Jean Tonary, Shellburne, N.S. No. 7 CGH
Margaret (Smith) Sparling, Matron 6 CCS
Name unknown, No. 7 CGH
Jean Rayworth, No. 6 CCS
Mabel (Glew) Tweddell, No. 8 CGH
P. Sunderland, No. 8 CGH

We had two weddings; nursing sister Hawksworth, married in England. The other wedding was in Nijmegen, Holland. I left November 11, 1944, due to illness. The other sisters were in France until going back to England.

The first penicillin was given in England at our unit. We were lucky we had very good doctors including Dr. Bob Mustard, Dr. Bill Mustard and Dr. W. Bigelow from Toronto, Dr. McLauchlin from London, and Dr. Lirki from Montreal.

I received the Associate Royal Red Cross January, 1944 at Buckingham Palace from King George VI.

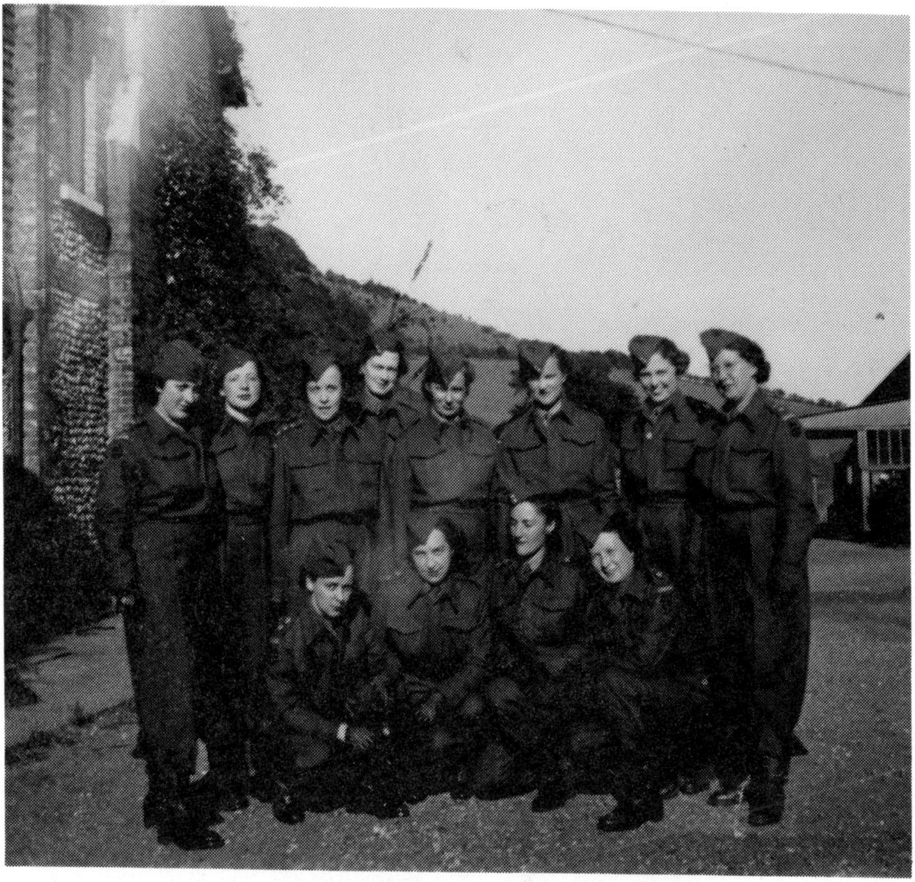

Canadian nursing sisters arrive overseas.
Loaned by Captain Matron Margaret A. (Smith) Sparling

Members of the group photographed in battle dress above are at present attached to the No. 6 Canadian Casualty Clearing Station. They went overseas with Lt.-Col. Clifford Thompson, RCAMC as officer commanding. Included in the group are Nursing Sisters Margaret B. Hawkesworth, Digby, N.S.; Erma Murray, Stellarton, N.S.; Jean Irvine Rayworth, Upper Cape, N.B.; Capt. (Matron) Margaret A. Smith, Moncton, N.B.; Nursing Sisters Kathleen Isabell MacLeod, Kinross, P.E.I.; Wilhelmina Pipe Bell, Guelph, Ontario; Emma Jean Blenkarm, Canning, N.S. and Delia Ann Ouellet, Montreal. Four of the nursing sisters are not identified.

Chapter 4

THE PRISONER NURSES OF HONG KONG

Two members of the RCAMC nursing service sailed from Vancouver, British Columbia, October 27, 1941, as part of the force Canada sent to strengthen the British garrison at Hong Kong. They were imprisoned by the Japanese after the fall of Hong Kong Christmas Day, 1941. The following article is from You Asked Us, *Today Magazine*, 2180 Yonge Street, Suite 1702, Toronto, Ontario, M4S 3A2; it provides a brief description of those two Canadian nursing sisters.

Their Japanese captors let them go after 20 months.

Both nursing sisters, Lieutenant Kay Christie of Toronto and Lieutenant May Waters of Winnipeg, survived their grim ordeal, escaping the atrocities committed when Japanese troops overran the British crown colony. From the fall of Hong Kong on Christmas Day, 1941 until the following August, they were confined to the British Military Hospital, which the Japanese designated prisoner of War Camp "A." Then they were transferred to Stanley Internment Camp on the opposite side of the island. Rumors of their imminent release persisted throughout their internment. But the rumor of July 1943 became fact; they learned they were to be included in a repatriation of all American and Canadian civilians in the Far East, under the auspices of the International Red Cross. On September 23, 1943, they boarded the Japanese exchange ship *Teia Maru.* This former cruise ship, which they called a "floating palace," was designed to accommodate 400 passengers. It presented a vastly different picture when carrying 1530 people. At breakfast, before eating the congee (rice gruel), they sought out the tiny black 'extras' and the white rice worms; they knew only by the shape of the cup whether they were drinking coffee or tea.

After the official exchange at Goa the repatriates boarded the American exchange ship M.S. *Gripsholm*, which had arrived from New York with a corresponding number of Japanese civilian internees. Accommodations and food were markedly improved, and the women experienced considerable weight gains. After six weeks on the *Gripsholm*, they reached New York. On December 2, 1943, the Canadians reached home.

Both nursing sisters continued in the Royal Canadian Army Medical Corps until the end of 1945. May Waters returned to Winnipeg for a time but then worked in hospitals in Oregon and Hawaii. Now retired, she lives in Long Beach, California; she prefers the climate to that of Winnipeg. Not Kay Christie. One of her most vivid memories of the homeward odyssey stems from the morning when she went for her pre-breakfast walk on the deck as the *Gripsholm* steamed far north of Rio de Janeiro. *"I felt that blast of cold, cold December wind and suddenly realized that that was one of the things I'd been missing for those two years,"* she says.

After the war, Kay Christie worked as a medical secretary in Toronto. She and May Waters exchange "annual reports" every year at Christmastime, but they have seen each other only once, in 1966, since they shared this footnote to the drama of Hong Kong.

Both nursing sisters mentioned in the article are now deceased.

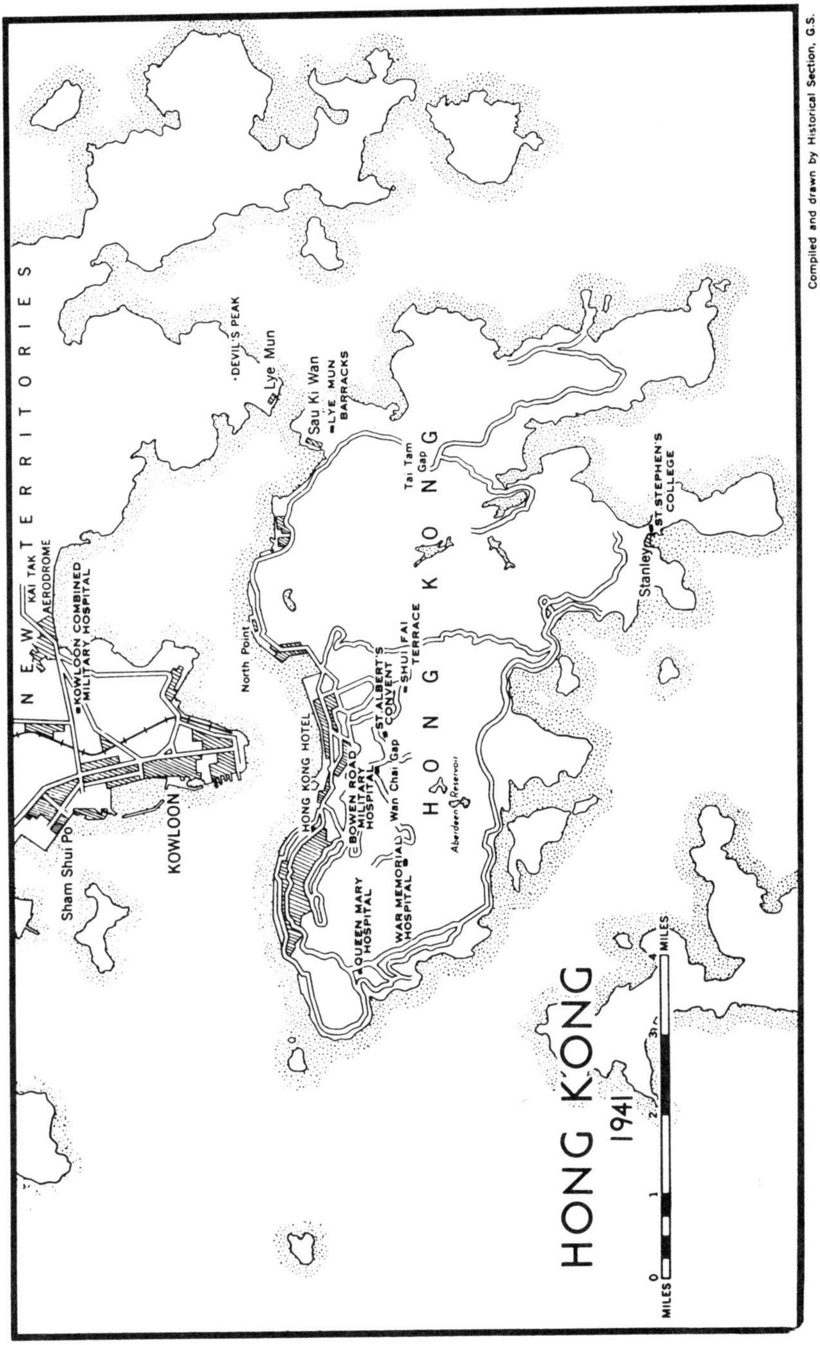

Map of Hong Kong Courtesy: Official History of the Canadian Medical Services 1939 - 1945. Feasby, W. R. p.308.

Chapter 5

CANADIAN GENERAL REINFORCEMENT UNIT, CGRU

Edna (Waugh) Beattie
Kathleen (Rountree) Bowman
Margaret (Middleton) Counter
Margaret Fletcher
Grace Hay
Mary Elizabeth Hindley
Mary McNeil
Elsie (Rauch) McRobert
Eve (Young) Sherwin
Pauline Siddons
Frances (Ferguson) Sutherland

The reinforcement unit was located at Hazelmere; it was the centre for nursing sisters who were assigned as reinforcements.

In addition to CGRU, an advanced Nursing Sisters Reinforcement Pool was formed in north west Europe as field dressing stations and casualty clearing stations with their complement of nursing sisters followed closely behind the advancing troops. Nursing sisters from various hospitals were attached to a small 200-bed hospital in Montreuil, France. From there they were sent wherever their services were most needed.*

* Official History of the Canadian Medical Services, 1939-1945, Edited by W.R. Feasby, published by authority of the Minister of Defence.

Edna O. (Waugh) Beattie

Graduated from: Victoria Hospital School of Nursing, London, Ontario. Year: 1937

Military History:

Service: RCAMC

Rank: Lt. N/S

Served: September 1940 to September 1945

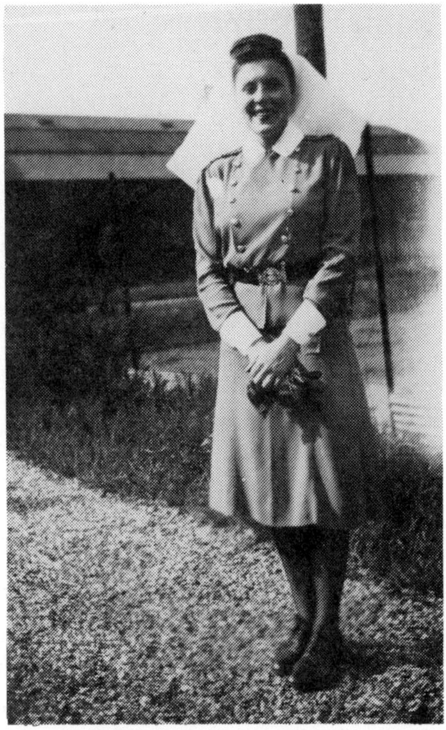

N/S Edna (Waugh) Beattie, 1945

I joined the Army for better salary and a change of lifestyle. I went to England as a replacement in hospitals already established there.

There were about ten of us in the group. We were on a freighter carrying TNT. This boat had been captured earlier from the Germans by the Canadian *Prince Robert*. It was the *Weser*. I can't recall the Canadian name. Anyway, we were chased across the Atlantic by a German submarine and fired on several times. We managed to escape. The nursing sisters on board were obliged to do lookout duty. I was on duty when the submarine was sighted. We finally reached Glasgow, took the train to London but were held up by blown up tracks ahead.

Kathleen (Rowntree) Bowman

Graduated from: St. Joseph's General Hospital School of Nursing, Vegreville, Alberta. Year: 1942

Military History:

Service: RCAMC

Rank: Lt. N/S

Served: November 1943 to February 1946

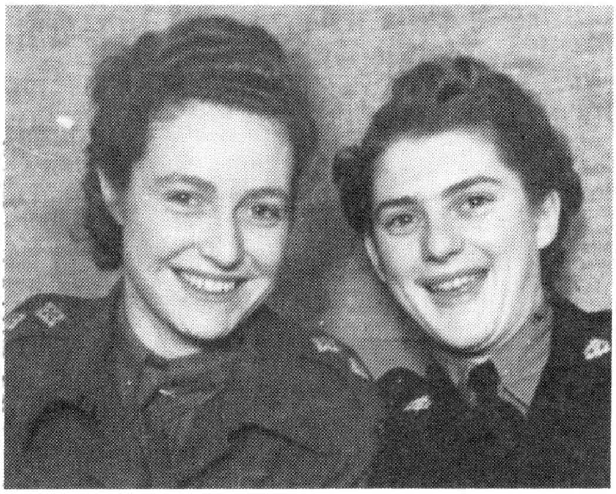

L-R: Kathleen Rountree & Pearl Langille at the Nivanetta Officers Club, Rome. 1944

I chose a military career for adventure, and also because my father had been in the medical corps.

I sailed from Halifax with No. 23 Canadian General Hospital on the *Empress of Scotland* and arrived in England about 2 days after D-Day. We hung around Helmsley, Yorkshire for about two weeks waiting to set up our hospital near London. Whilst in Yorkshire we did a lot of drilling, went for miles on route marches and played softball.

We also spent a few evenings at a neat little pub, "The White Swan," which immediately became known as "The Dirty Duck." There was a dance hall of sorts where we loved to go. One morning I got called into the matron's office and told that "jitterbugging" was not becoming to an officer. That was the first of a few trips to the matron's office, but I survived.

Soon we were off to Watford, just north of London, where our fun days became work days. This was the time of the V-2s and we had some close calls. One landed close enough to knock out some of our windows, but I slept through that.

This was the time of the Big Push in Northwest Europe. We were kept very busy, 12-15 hour shifts were not uncommon. We did manage a few trips to London, a dreary place, everything blacked out. I also purchased a secondhand bike and we had some lovely rides through the beautiful countryside. One ride was nearly my last when I forgot to ride on the "wrong" side of the road. I rounded a bend to come face to face with a huge double-decker bus. The roadside hedge looked a bit more friendly and I ended up in a prickly hedge. The driver stopped the bus, got out and gave me a tongue lashing, using swear words I had never heard before. It was like my trips to the matron's office minus the swear words, of course.

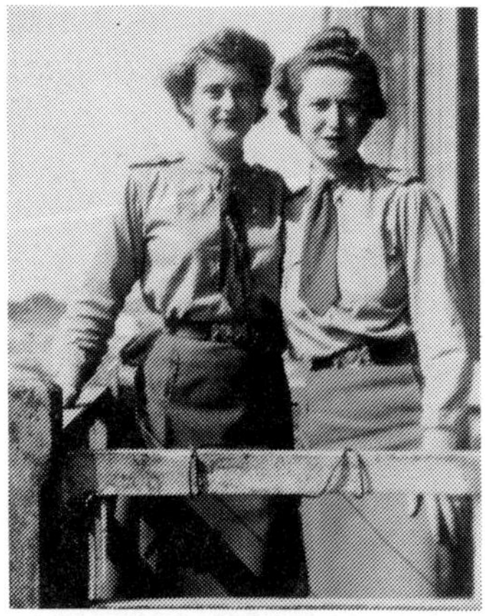
L-R: Pearl (Langille) Conlon. Kathleen (Rowntree) Bowman May 1945, Belgium

After a few months in England, the call went out for reinforcements to No. 5 Canadian General in Rome. Our matron announced that the first group who could gather the khaki overseas issue uniform would go to Italy. My friend Pearl and I moved at lightening speed to assemble the required kit and we were off. We sailed in convoy to Naples. Our bunks were five deep and I, of course, got the top bunk. My face was about 12 inches from the deck above. Grumbling would only fall on deaf ears, so we decided to turn the voyage into fun.

In our khaki kit, we were issued with "bloomers silk," I'm not making this up. They were much like our mothers wore, except for the khaki colour. When pulled up, they came just over our bust line on those of us who were thin. Every night we would don these bloomers and put on a stage show, not exactly Las Vegas style, but we got a lot of laughs and also a few frowns from our "older" sisters.

From Naples we flew on some kind of an old bomber to Rome, the Eternal City, teeming with history. What a marvellous experience, but there was work aplenty. No. 5 Canadian General Hospital was very busy receiving casualties from Rimini, Ravenna, Monte Cassino and other battle areas of Northern Italy. In our precious spare time we did some sightseeing, visited the Vatican chapels, had an audience with the Pope, a very humbling experience.

Our social life went on at a good pace. There were some lovely nightclubs and we tried to visit most of them.

When the war wound down in Italy, we closed No. 5 Canadian General Hospital and left for Naples where we travelled by convoy to Marseilles.

I will always remember our leave taking from Italy, the band at dock side playing "*Retourne Sorrento*" and crowds of Italian people waving us on our way, many with tears streaming down their faces. Seems there were few dry eyes amongst those of us who were leaving.

From Marseilles, we flew to Ghent in Belgium where we were again in a waiting period. This was a pleasant two or three weeks, boating down the canals and just being generally lazy.

Then we were off to join the 16 Canadian General Hospital in Oost Dunkerke, a few miles from Ostend. While there, we experienced VE Day. The long war was over. However, since we were the last overseas we would be the last home. Soon after closing No. 16 Canadian Hospital, Pearl and I were posted to No. 4 CSS in Amsterdam.

Six weeks in Amsterdam, quite busy with mostly medical cases. After 4 CSS closed we were given a 4-day leave to Paris. What fun – saw the "Folies-Bergeres," visited Pigalle, walked on the banks of the Seine. After a few days with our unit, we were posted to No. 1 Canadian General Hospital in Nijmegen. We lived in a huge house called the "White House," simply because it was painted white. It was overrun with mice and we had a great time trying to trap them.

From Nijmegen we took many lovely trips around the countryside and one trip into Germany. On that occasion we met many German children begging chocolate bars and "cigarettes for my brother." One young lad approached my current boyfriend offering to take him to his sister who would give him a "very nice" time. For this he wanted two chocolate bars. Much to my relief, the boyfriend declined the offer, but we gave the kid chocolate bars to reward his ingenuity.

Then it was off to England for repatriation but we stayed at No. 22 Canadian General Hospital in Bramshott for about two months awaiting our turn. Pearl left for Nova Scotia about two weeks before me. I was given the chance to return with a large group of war brides and their children. I and six other nursing sisters were to care for the children who became ill on the voyage. We sailed in February 1946 on the *Mauretania*, a creaky old ship over very rough seas. My "helpmates" all succumbed to seasickness along with many of the passengers, so I was the lone caregiver for up to 10 kids at a time. For this I received the princely sum of $6.00 extra per day. It was called "command pay," I believe.

For all my hopping around, I earned a chest full of medals, enough to put a general to shame!

Margaret H. (Middleton) Counter

Graduated from: Guelph General Hospital School of Nursing, Guelph Ontario. Year: 1943

Military History

Service: RCAMC

Rank: Lt. N/S

Served: February 1944 to March 2, 1946

I joined the Army because all the boys from school and relatives were joining up; it seemed the correct thing to do, go over and nurse them.

In February of 1944 I joined the Army at Trafalgar Military Hospital, London, Ontario. In April of 1944 I was assigned to Ipperwash Military Camp, Ontario, and by the end of May 1944, was off to Debert, Nova Scotia. D-Day was on June 6th. I went over as a reinforcement. We left Halifax June 8th in a 60-ship convoy and arrived Greenock, Scotland, June 25th. By June 26th we arrived at Hazelmere, near Bramshott; No. 22 General Hospital, Canadian General Reinforcement Unit (CGRU).

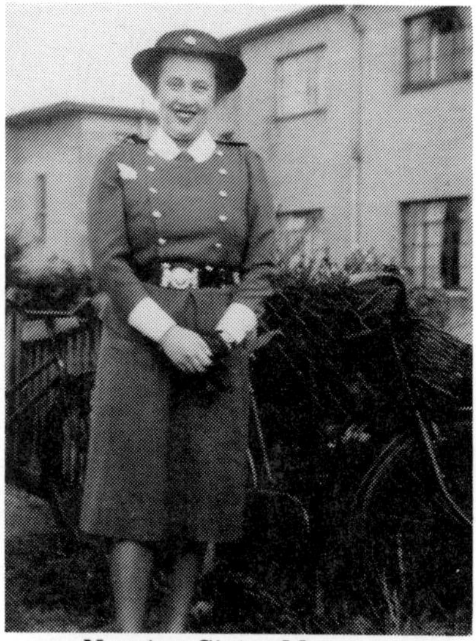

Nursing Sister Margaret Middleton, England

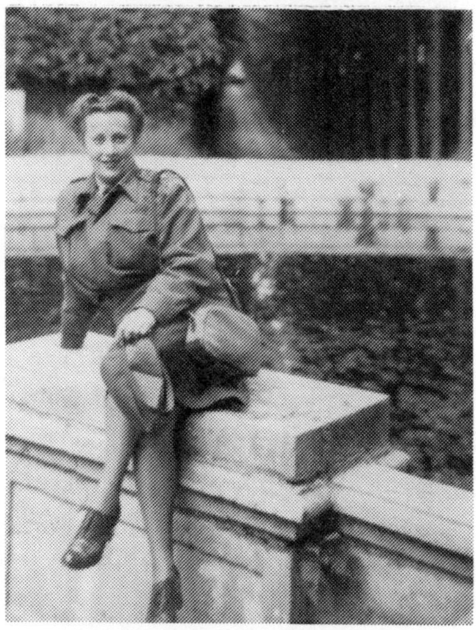

N/S Margaret Middleton at Chateau near Brussels, sitting on a wall of a fish pond in centre of which was a bandstand.

June 28th we went up to Colchester, England, northeast of London just nine miles from Merci and Brightlingsea on the coast. No. 18 Canadian General Hospital had 70 nursing sisters. It was a 600-bed unit although there were often 900 patients. The buildings were made up of six 20-bed wards. There were nine nursing sisters for each "Spider." There was a head nurse and assistant with one nursing sister in charge of each 20-bed ward. One nursing sister plus two orderlies were the night duty staff. Ack-ack, buzz bombs and V-2s seemed to be non-stop.

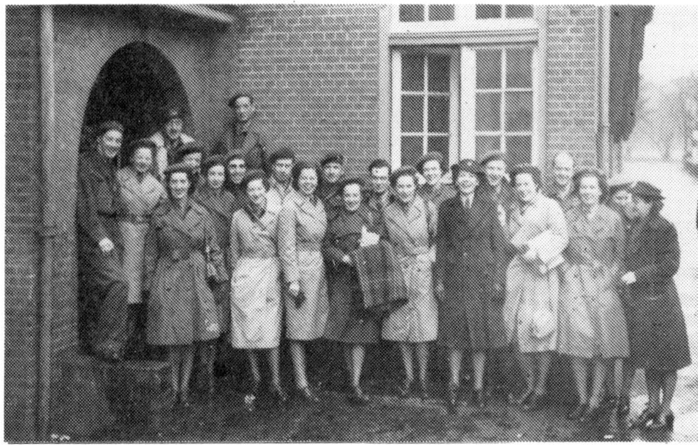

No. 6 CCS staff at Amersfoot, Holland as we are about to leave for England.

Hospital trains would bring 300 new patients and we would get 300 off to a convalescent home a few miles away. I worked 7-7 with three leaves in 10 months in Scotland, Ireland and Torquay in the south of England.

In April 1945 I was back at CGRU at Bramshott. I left Tillbury on a hospital ship that landed at Ostend, from there to Ghent and then to No. 10 Canadian General Hospital, Turnhout, Belgium.

May 8, VE Day, there was much rejoicing. By June 15, 1945 I was posted to No. 1 General Hospital, Nijmegen, Holland, then on to No. 6 Casualty Clearing Station Almelo, Holland 9 miles from the German border. Col. Dr. Bob Mustard was our CO; the staff was 15 nursing sisters and 10 medical officers.

In September I moved to Amersfoort, Holland and left Holland December 28 for Calais. We docked at Dover. I went back to No. 22 CGH and worked with our POWs. I left England at the end of February and arrived in Halifax March 2, 1946, on the *Aquitania* with English war brides. We had to work our way home. Arrived in London, Ontario, had leave and took my discharge.

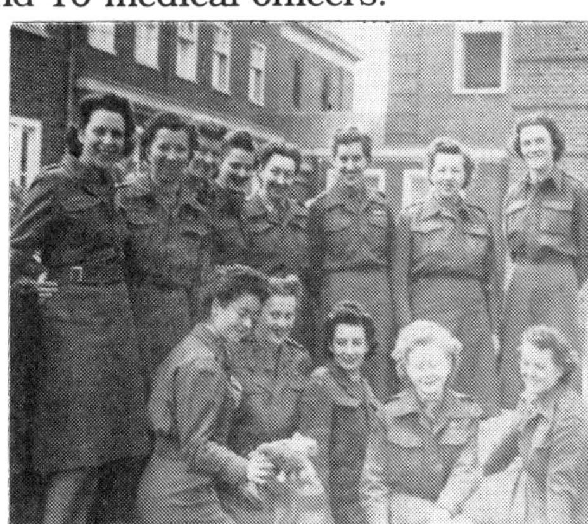

Nursing sister staff of No. 6 CCS, Almelo, Holland

Margaret Fletcher

Graduated from: Royal Jubilee Hospital School of Nursing, Victoria, B.C. Year: 1936

Military History:

Service: RCAMC

Rank: Lt. N/S

Served: 1941 to 1945

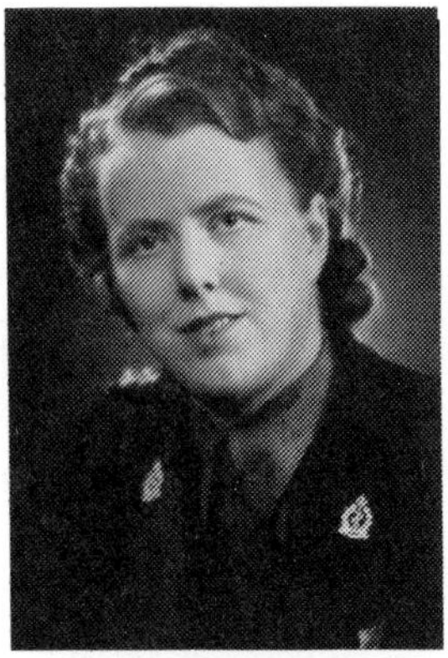

Lt. N/S Margaret Fletcher, No. 2 CCS, Holland 1945

I joined up in Victoria in early January 1941. My brother couldn't go – I felt somebody should so I joined the RCAMC. I was in Esquimalt Military Hospital for six months and then I was sent overseas as a reinforcement. There were six of us; we went together as reinforcements and we were to be sent any place on the Continent or in England where it was busy. We knew we would be transferred from one place to another and we wouldn't have a home hospital as such.

When we landed in Scotland, we came down to England by train and I was stationed in No. 5 General Hospital which had 1200 beds. It was a Red Cross Hospital established on Lady Astors' estate at Cliveden in Taplow, England, I was there until such time as we went across to the Continent. Shortly after the invasion of the Continent I went across on a hospital ship.

The hospitals were general hospitals much like the hospital we had in England that did ordinary everyday hospital work until such time as we went across to the Continent. The General Hospitals were quite large, 1000 to 1200 beds. We had one sister to each ward and then we had an orderly who worked with us. He didn't have any special training but he certainly learned on the job. We also had sergeants who had more training and they were in charge of the ward orderlies. We had our own X-rays, our own operating rooms – just the usual things. At No. 5 General, Lady Astors' estate where I started, the nursing sisters were in the little house across the street. Lady Astor and her husband had the main house – the big house on the estate. The little house across the way was for the next in line for the title until such time as he would move into the big house; so they let us have that house. They added wings to this house for us to use as dormitories. This was fine, except when it was blackout and it was foggy and you tried to find your way across the street to the big hospital – then you really had fun. I got lost more times trying to get from that one place to the other in the fog. Of course, with blackouts, flashlights were not allowed. You just had to get there – that was it. We were on 12-hour shifts – we were supposed to have hours off but whether you got them or not was beside the point. We had one night off in a month – they tried to give us more time than that while we were still in England. If we were working nights we'd get ready the day before – work our night shift – then that next morning we would get off at 7 o'clock, get about five miles down to the station and go to London for the weekend because we'd have 48 hours off.

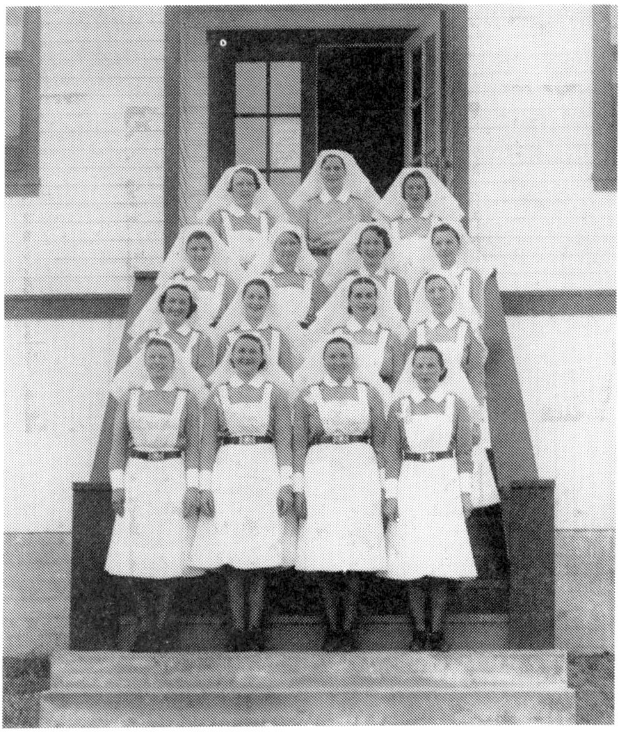

Nanaimo General Hospital – No. 16 Canadian General Hospital. L-R starting at rear: Nursing Sisters Margaret Fletcher; Edna Rossiter; Gamon; Mary Cartright; Nora Allyn; Neary; Kathlen Riley; Kent; Kay Lund; Claser; Falconer; Hutton; Dorothy Buchan; Trimble; McFarlane

When we went to land in Northern Europe they were still bombing just down the coast from where we landed. We went down the side of the ship in scramble nets, of all things, into a landing craft. When we got on shore they put us in vehicles which were flat bed trucks. We were taken to our tent hospital in Normandy – we were 20 to a tent. We'd take our slacks off at night and hang them on the tent pole. By morning, if it had been raining, of course, the rain came right through the top of the tent onto our slacks. They had privies up on the side of the hill – we called them 6-holers, they were just separated by what used to be potato sacks and only waist high. We wondered why all the Canadian airplanes kept coming over. One day we were told.

We were farther north than some of the other hospitals – they were nearer the Coast. They got more of the acute casualties – the flying people and that sort of thing, the bombings. Then when we went across to the Continent, we had smaller hospitals, we also had Casualty Clearing Stations which were smaller still where we took the patients from the Field Dressing Stations, (Field Dressing Stations were the original place where the badly wounded boys went), they then came to us almost immediately, often times without having had anything done to them at all. We had to get them admitted, the dressings done, fed and then decide who needed to go to surgery right away. We kept them there until they were stabilized and then sent them back to the General Hospitals.

Of course, the service was a colossal effort of organization from top to bottom. It was very efficiently done. When I was trying to get evacuated home we'd be evacuated from a hospital ready to go to the next one – we'd just get out in the street and have to come back again. We used to get angry as all get out because we wanted to get home and

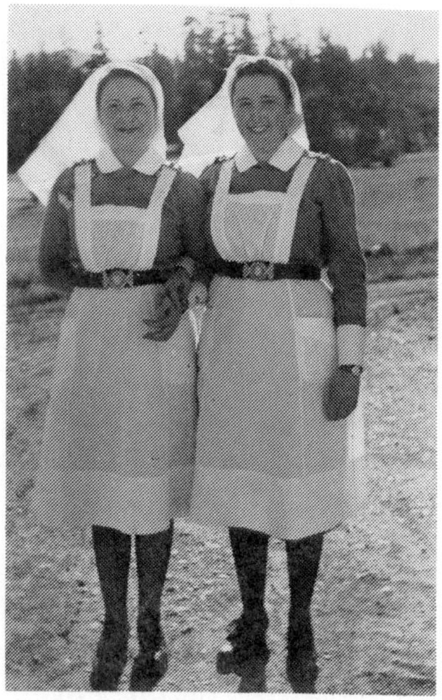

L-R: N/S Dorothy Buchan; N/S Trimble at No. 16 CGH Nanaimo, B.C.

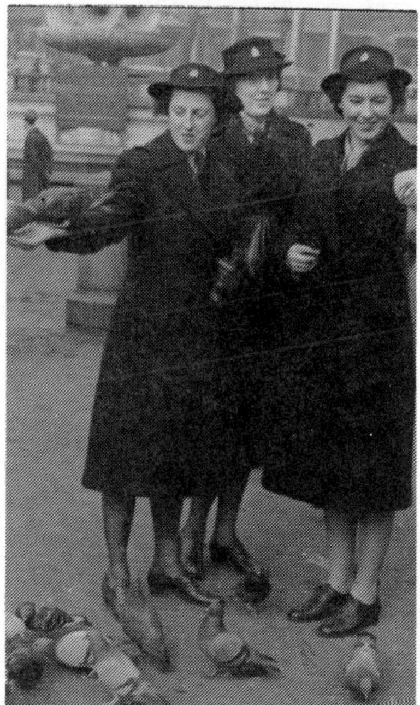

L-R: Nursing Sisters Ellen Wallbridge, Margaret Fletcher, Grace Noble at Trafalgar Square London, 1942

then realized that there had been a bombing raid or something like that – there was always a reason for all these things.

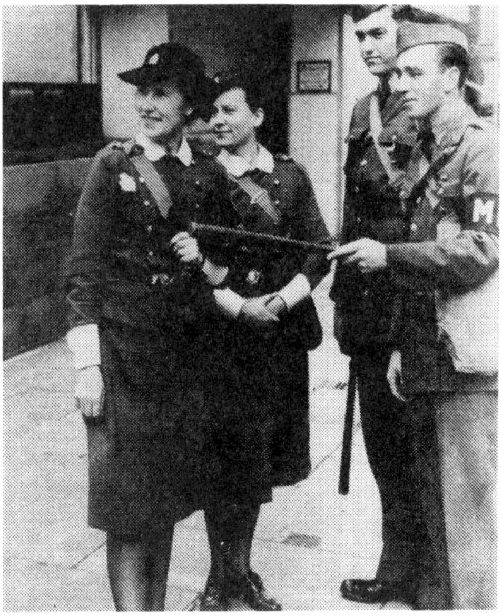

Military Police from most United Nations now patrol London. Here N/S Janet McTavish and N/S Ann Dalrymple ask Pte. Ed Meade, Detroit and T. Fitzpatrick, New York, directions. U.S. Military Police are the only ones to carry nightsticks.
Canadian Forces photo

One of the most interesting things that I experienced when I was there – certain of us were sent down to London to hear a talk from a scientist. We later found out it was Professor Florey who was one of the developers of penicillin – we had never heard of penicillin. We had all these casualties, we were treating them in the usual way and you didn't put casts on infected wounds because you just knew that you'd get gangrene if you did that and that was it – but we went down to see him. We went to the building where he was to give his lecture; however, the night before it had been bombed so they just scraped all the debris off the seats and said, *"Come on in – you're going to have your lecture anyway."* We had our lecture and he showed us pictures; we simply could not imagine that he was telling us the truth. He showed us pictures of what they had been doing in the Mediterranean and it was absolutely astounding.

So time and a half went by and we were allocated a little bit of penicillin for our worst cases. I remember one day we had a consignment of prisoners of war and we had one major who had been quite badly shot up and our major surgeon looked at me and he said, *"Sister, I want you to give so and so so many units of penicillin."* I just looked at him, we had had hate drilled into us for so long – that anything German was evil. I said, *"Do you mean to say you're going to take that penicillin away from our boys who need it and give it to that man?"* He looked at me and said, *"Sister, you damn well do what you are told and don't try to play God."* When I saw how that man got over his wounds in such a short

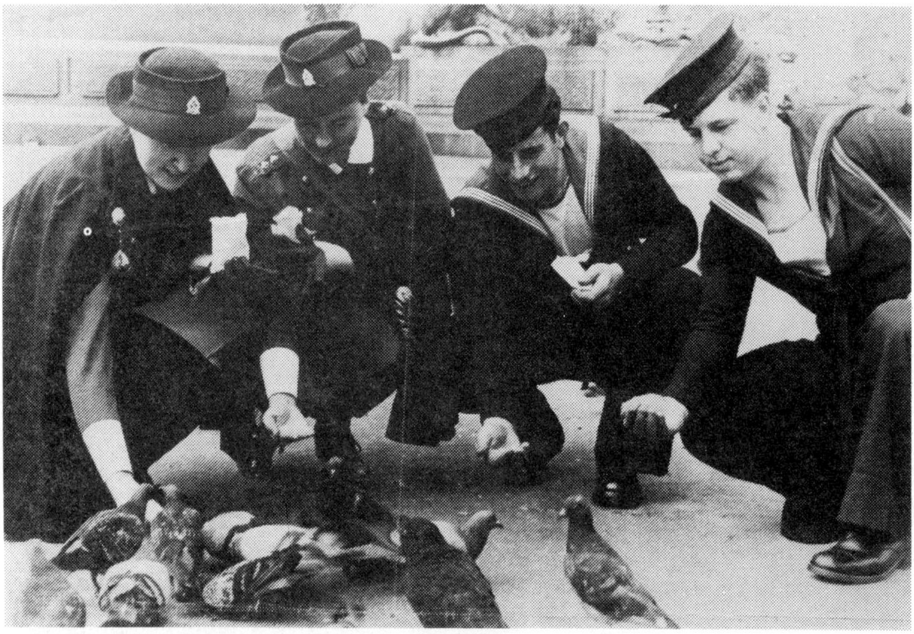

Feeding the pigeons is a must on any sightseeing tour of London. Canadian Army Nursing Sisters Janet McTavish and Ann Dalrymple meet two Canadian Seamen, AB Gordon Gray, Halifax, and AB Gary Arcand, Verdun, and feed pigeons in Trafalgar Square. Canadian Forces photo

time and eventually was able to go back to his family, I said to myself, *"From thereon in you're never going to play God again."*

We went from there to various hospitals. I think I was in almost every hospital and Casualty Clearing Station in Europe. I was there until VE Day at which time I was invalided home.

The six of us who went over as reinforcements were the first B.C. girls that went over – in six months or so we were joined by No. 16 Canadian General Hospital.

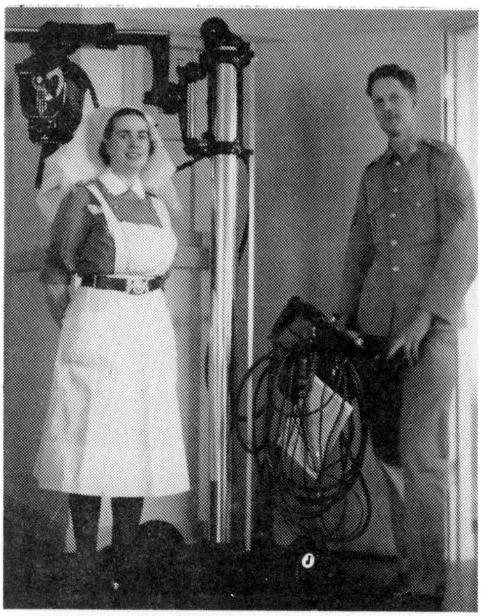

Lt. N/S Olive Clancy, Vancouver and Sgt. Moore, X-ray technician, Nanaimo Military Hospital. 1941

Grace Hay

Written by her friend Jessie Middleton

Graduated from: Royal Columbian Hospital School of Nursing
New Westminster, B.C. Year: 1939

Military History:

Service: RCAMC

Rank: Lt. N/S

Served: July 20, 1942 to April 25, 1946

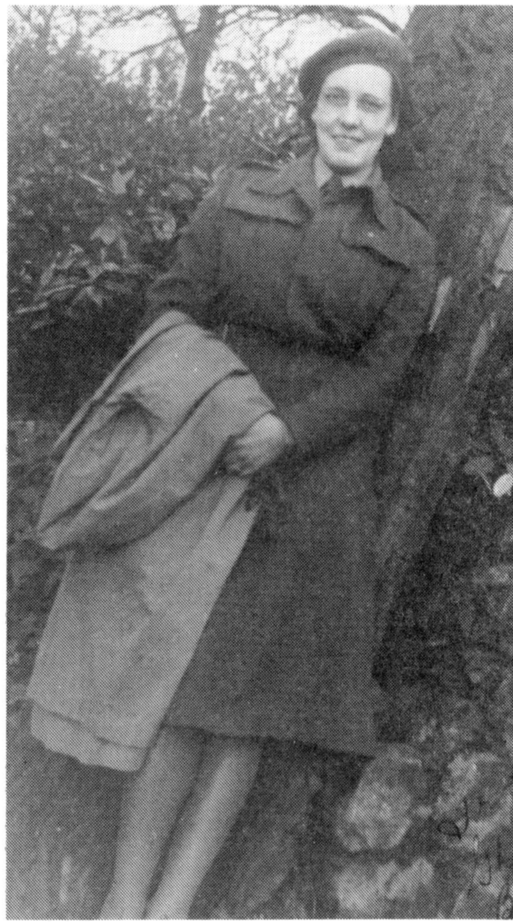

Lt. N/S Grace Hay

Grace's Father had been killed in the First World War. In fact, she was born after he left to go overseas.

The highlight for Grace was surely when she visited her father's grave.

Grace's military experience included; Nanaimo Military Hospital, Prince Rupert Military Hospital, Warnwright Military Hospital.

She went overseas in January 1944 as a reinforcement and served in Northwest Europe.

On her return to Canada, Grace served at the Vernon Military Hospital.

M.E. (Betty) Hindley

Written by her niece, Mrs. Patricia LeMoine

Graduated from: Toronto General Hospital School of Nursing. Year: 1940

Military History:

Service: RCAMC

Rank: Lt. N/S

Service: March 3, 1943 to August 7, 1946

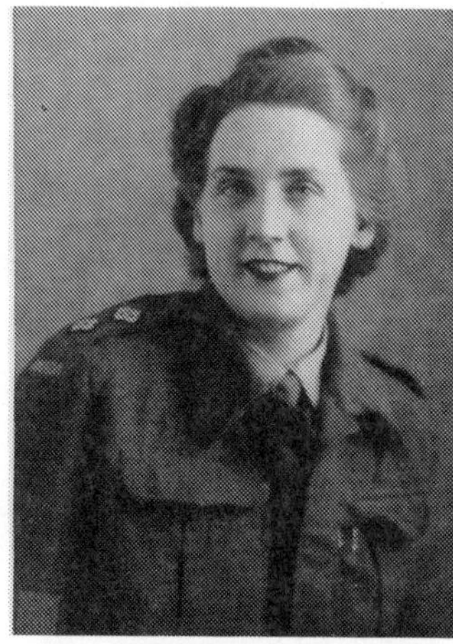

Lt. N/S Mary Elizabeth Hindley

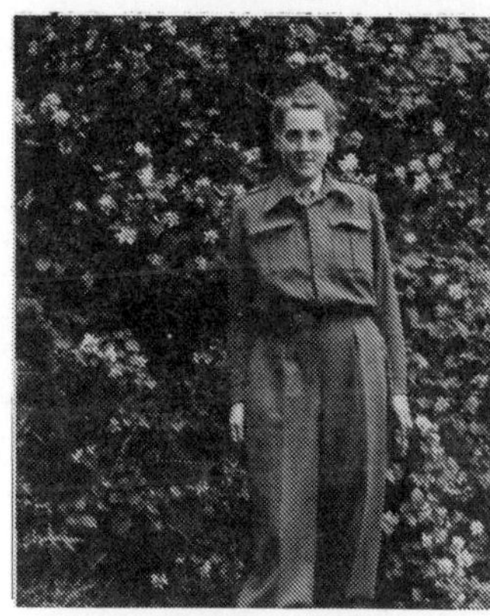

Lt. N/S M.E. Hindley – What a soldier!

From asking other family members, we feel it was the thought of adventure that inspired Betty to choose the Army for a career. Also, her aunt, Alice Hindley, was a nursing sister in World War I and shared her experiences with the family.

Betty did not talk much about her experiences overseas; things like sleeping in orchards, monasteries, washing in their helmets. When she was dying and heavily treated with morphine, she was having nightmares about her war experiences – those thoughts she shared with her cousin who is a minister.

She did speak of the great kindness of the English people and those in Holland. Betty served with Nos. 6, 7, 11, and 22 Canadian General Hospitals in France, Belgium, and Holland. She also served with numerous Field Dressing Stations and with Nos. 2, 3, and 6 Casualty Clearing Stations. Betty was bridesmaid at the wedding of N/S Margaret Lutes Donaldson in Holland.

She returned to Canada in September of 1945 and was assigned to Chorley Park Military Hospital until her discharge from the Army in August of 1946. She then nursed at Sunnybrook

Hospital, Toronto until her retirement in 1974.

Oddly enough, her nursing pals have either died from cancer or have had cancer and are living their lives as best they can. It makes you wonder if there is a link between the cancers!

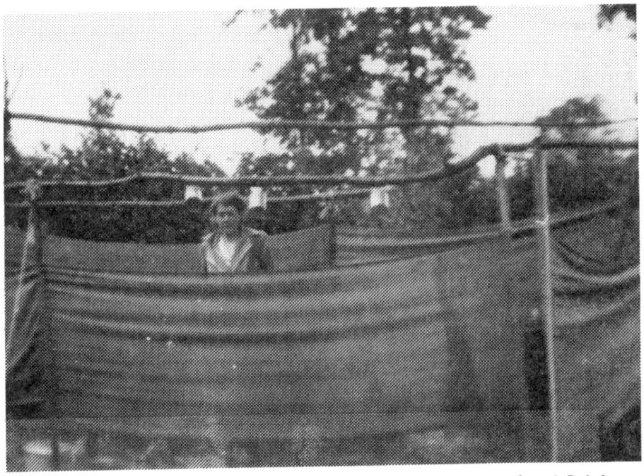

"Normandy Glide," Bayeaux, France. July 1944

Mary F. McNeil

Graduated from: St. Joseph's Hospital School of Nursing, St. John N.B.

Military History:

Service: RCAMC Reinforcement

Rank: Lt. N/S

Served: January 1944 to July 1946

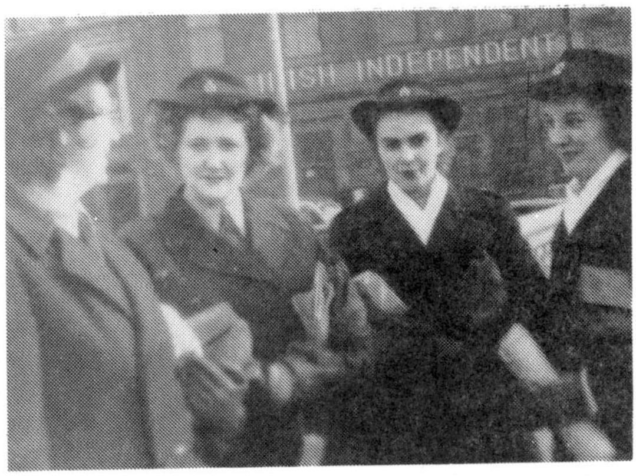

Dublin, Ireland, on leave. L-R: Gertrude Burns Hanley, Saint John, N.B.; Mary McNeil, Saint John, NB; Betty Kneeshaw, Agincourt, ON; Hazel Fitzgerald Arbuthnot, Chateaugay, QC

I chose to join the Army because it was a new field of nursing, plus I wanted adventure.

Since I was sent overseas as a reinforcement I didn't go with a unit. I enlisted in January 1944 and arrived in England in July 1944. I was attached to No. 24 CGH at Horley for only ten days or so when three nurses were required at No. 1 Canadian Special Hospital in Alton, Hants. Annie (Anne) Blacquiere, Helen Fitzgerald, and I reported to the hospital there – convalescents, etc. I remained there until I was sent to Italy where I was stationed at No. 15 CGH in Caserta. My stay there was brief, less than three months.

No. 15 CGH closed in April 1945 and I was on my way back to England, first stop Bramshott. I was posted to Colchester, No. 18 CGH I think. After a leave spent in Ireland, my next posting was No. 23 CGH at Watford. That was May 15th, 1945.

No. 23 CGH closed in July 1945 and I was sent to No. 4 CGH at Farnborough. That was my last move until my return to Canada in March 1946. I was stationed at Fredericton Military Hospital until my discharge in July 1946.

Time spent in the RCAMC was a memorable time for me, interesting work, new friends, new places.

Elsie (Rauch) McRobert

Graduated from: Saskatoon City Hospital School of Nursing.
Year: 1941

Military History:

Service: RCAMC

Rank: Lt. Nursing Sister

Service: February 10, 1944 to June 21, 1946

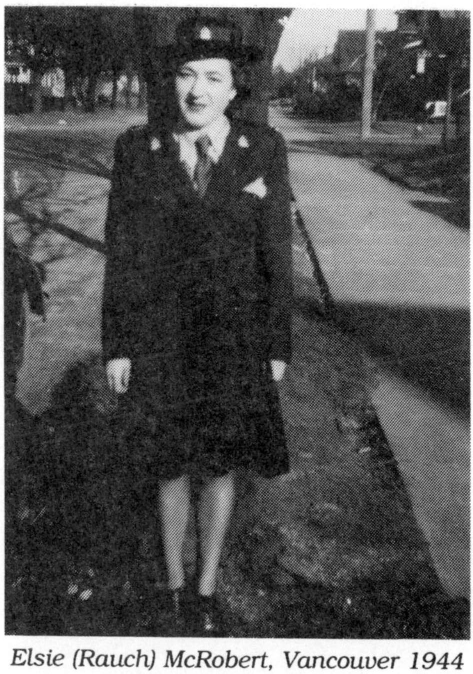

Elsie (Rauch) McRobert, Vancouver 1944

After joining the RCAMC in Vancouver, I was sent to the Victoria Military Hospital for my military qualification. As nursing sister reinforcements were needed overseas. We were soon on our way to Debert, N.S. On June 5th we boarded the MS *Erria* which was in a convoy of 115 ships going overseas. It so happened that my future husband, who was in the Navy, was doing escort duty on one of the ships.

When we arrived in London it was to the sound of air raid sirens and buzz bombs falling, our first taste of the war. I was posted to No. 19 CGH near Marston Green. On my first ward

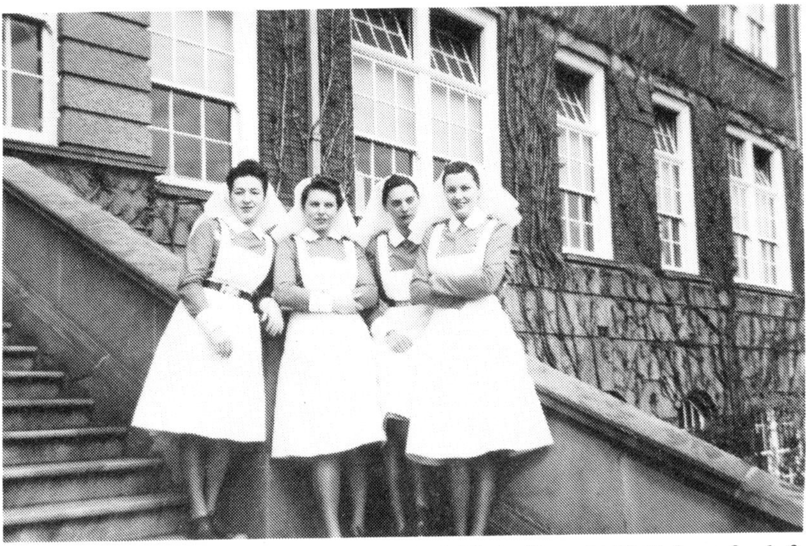
Victoria Military Hospital, Canada, 1944. Elsie (Rauch) McRobert far left.

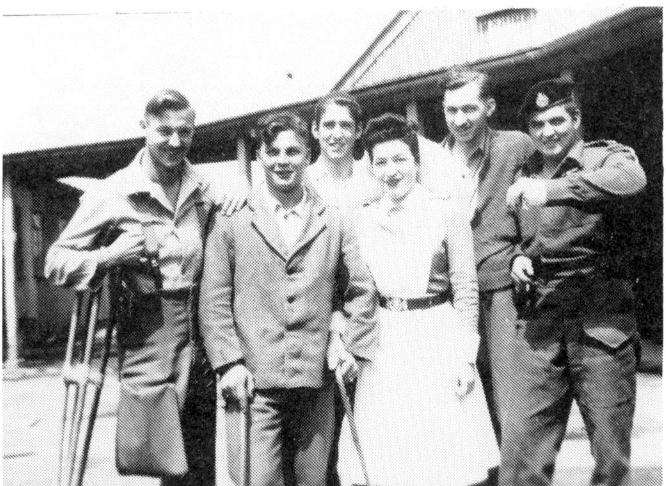
Elsie (Rauch) McRobert, No. 19 CGH and patients 1945

most of the patients were from the Italian Campaign. We also had some Italian prisoners of war as patients. It was at No. 19 that we used to watch the hundreds of planes passing overhead on their bombing missions to various locations. While there, we also took advantage of our leaves to see as much as we could of the British Isles. On VE Day we had 567 patients in our hospital. As most would be repatriated as soon as ships were available, a lot of nursing sisters were assigned to other hospitals or were also repatriated.

I was assigned to No. 16 CGH (near Oldenburg) in Germany

with the Occupation Force where our work was much the same as in England. I was later posted to No. 7 CGH (near Wilhemshaven) where I mostly worked on medical wards. As well as our Canadian patients, we had many other nationalities. When we got our leaves in Germany we used them to go to Brussels, Amsterdam and once to an educational course at the University of Paris.When I was repatriated I went home on the *Ile de France*. Some years after the war both the MS *Erria* that had taken us overseas and the *Ile de France* were destroyed by fire.

Kathryn Eve (Young) Sherwin

Graduated from: Hamilton General Hospital School of Nursing Hamilton, Ontario. Year: 1942

Military History:

Service: RCAMC

Rank: Lieut. N/S

Served: 1943 to 1945

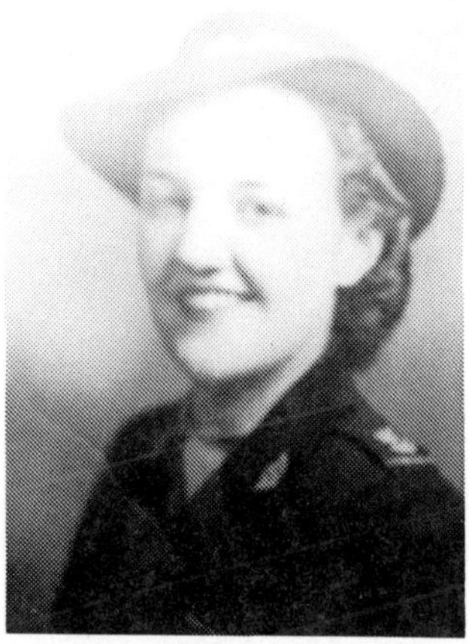

Lt. N/S Kathryn (Young) Sherwin, December, 1943

It was so natural for me to choose a military career as my family had a military background. Father Claire M. Young served in World War I, 1914-18 war and Word War II, 1939-45. He retired as a captain from the First World War and was a major in the Second World War. My brother, Machar, was a Lieutenant in the Militia and my sister, Generva, a staff sergeant. in the CWAC.

After basic training at Sussex Military Hospital, N.B. I was attached to Howe Lake Military Hospital, St. John, N.B., until going overseas in January 1944.

On arrival in England I joined No. 18 CGH in Colchester. When we sailed from Canada to England, we crossed the Atlantic on a British West Indies banana boat called the SS *Cavina*. The crossing was mostly very rough. About three quarters of those aboard were seasick. Fortunately, for me, I was a good sailor. I remember the last appearance of one of the nursing sisters in the dining salon. On being asked what she would like to eat, she replied, *"I don't care as long as it looks pretty coming back."*

When stationed in Colchester, England, there was insufficient room for all of the nursing sisters in the barracks and some of us were billeted in an old home called Blenheim House just down the road from the hospital. Two other nursing sisters and I shared a room with a fireplace. One morning we awoke to find a large bat sprawled on our hearth. Not feeling very friendly about it, we wondered how to get rid of it, when one of us had a bright idea and said, *"Let's call for our Batman."* We did have a batman and he kindly took care of it.

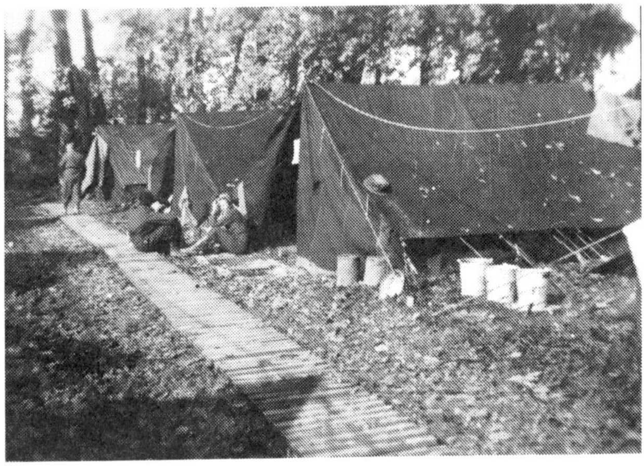

The tents in which we lived at Mesnieres-en-Bray, France

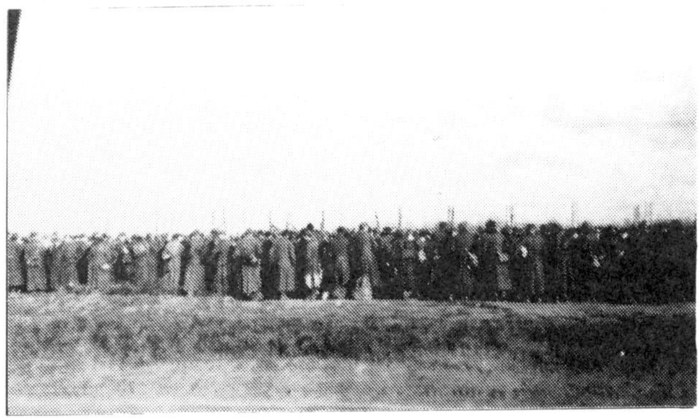

POW enclosure near 21 CGH in 1944 Mesnieres-en-Bray, France

Our first buzz bomb was also encountered there and we awoke to find all three of us with our heads hanging out the window until we came to and then dived under our beds. After that it didn't take long to recognize that sound; apprehension was always there.

In the early fall of 1944 I was sent to the Continent, again, as a reinforcement with No. 21 Canadian General Hospital. We landed at Dieppe and proceeded to Mesnieres-en-Bray where our hospital was set up in an old Chateau with a moat around it. It belonged to a Duke of Orleans. We, the staff, lived in tents. The winter was very cold, wet and sometimes snowy. There were no floors in the tents. We slept with our battle dress carefully pressed under our sleeping bags so they would be warm and dry on rising and our boots nearby ready to plunge our feet into. Our source of heat was a round oil burner.

We had great comradeship. During our off-duty time, as many of us as could would crowd into one tent and sit around the stove trying to keep warm.

Later we were transferred to Turnhout, Belgium, where our hospital and sleeping quarters were in a boys' school which was more comfortable. There, I worked with No. 1 Canadian Mobile Surgical Unit. The Front was on in Nijmegen at that time and we acted as a Casualty Clearing Station. At times we could hear the sounds of battle in the distance.

Our last posting was in Bassum, near Bremerhaven, Germany, where we took over a German military hospital which was very well equipped. The dishes in the officers mess were crested with the Red Cross and Swastika. I still have two of the mugs which I brought home with me. I also have an authentic set of snapshots of the raid on Dieppe when our Forces were defeated, plus a set of the triumphant march through Dieppe when our Forces took possession of it, and an authentic snapshot of Hitler. These were given to me by a POW whom I had as a patient. There was a POW encampment near our hospital at Mesnieres-en-Bray. The trustees did work around the grounds of the camp and we had many of the POWs as patients also.

I returned to Canada in 1945 and took the laboratory technicians course at Hamilton General Hospital and worked at the laboratory there until I married in 1949.

Pauline A. J. Siddons

Graduated from: Saskatoon City Hospital School of Nursing, Year: 1942

Military History

Service: RCAMC

Rank: Lieutenant N/S

Served: 22 February 1944 to 18 June 1946

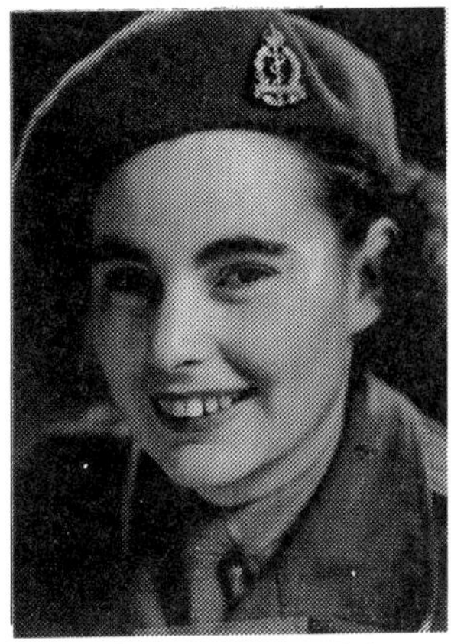

Lt. N/S Pauline Siddons Oldenburg, Germany, 1945. No. 16 CGH

I graduated from high school in 1937 and that summer my mother and I travelled to England to explore the possibility of living and working there. We stayed a year. By the summer of 1938 there was great concern that another war was threatening Europe. One evening I was recruited to assist my uncle, a civil defense officer, in delivering gas masks to homes in his area. We were, in fact, doing this when Prime Minister Neville Chamberlain returned from Munich following the signing of the Munich Pact. We were invited into one of the homes to listen to the broadcast of Chamberlain's message. It was the "Peace in Our Time" address. At the time, there was general relief and optimism. Nevertheless, my mother and I returned home in October.

The "peace" was brief. On September 10, 1939, I entered the Saskatoon City Hospital School of Nursing to begin nurses training. It was the same day that Canada officially entered the war. I decided that day that if the War continued, I would join the Royal Canadian Army Medical Corps as soon as I was qualified!

When the Canadian Women's Army Corps was formed in 1941, I briefly considered leaving nurses' training to enlist in that service. Fortunately, I decided to complete my nurses training. However, by the time I graduated in 1942, there was a temporary freeze on taking nurses from our hospital into the Army. Many had already enlisted and the hospital was experiencing a quite serious staff shortage! I had to wait until February 1944 before my call finally came.

By a strange coincidence, my first posting was to the CWAC Camp at Vermilion, Alberta, where I served in the military hospital from February 26, 1944, to May 15, 1944. I then attended Military Qualifying Course in Calgary and by early June I was on my way to England.

We sailed on the *Lady Nelson* hospital ship, as a group of reinforcements to join Canadian General Hospitals already established in England. We sailed from Halifax and docked in Liverpool. We were unescorted, fully lighted and the vessel was clearly marked with red crosses. We arrived without incident.

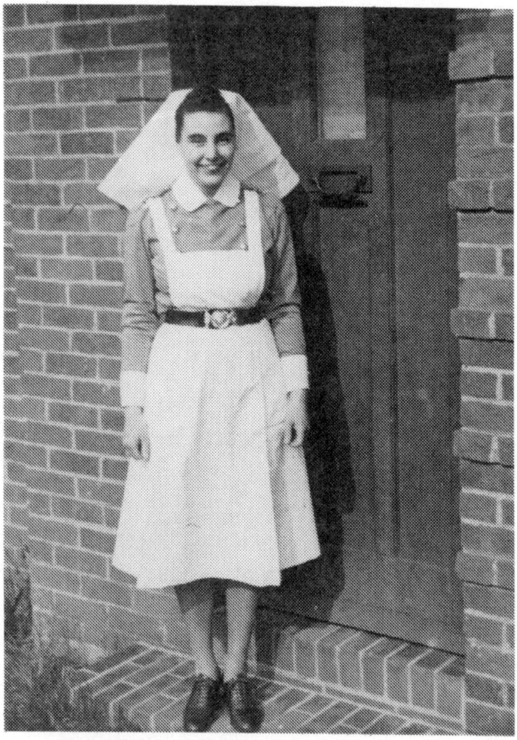

Lt. N/S Pauline Siddons, Farnborough, England 1944. No. 4 CGH

I was among the group posted to No. 4 CGH at Farnborough near Aldershot. At that time No. 4 was a transit hospital. We received large convoys of wounded, many of whom required surgery. Hot meals were served, and patients were bathed and made as comfortable as possible before being moved on to another hospital. It was sometimes a challenge to complete the required services and have patients ready for evacuation before the next convoy arrived. I have memories of halls lined with stretcher patients waiting for a bed, while more loaded ambulances continued to arrive!

This was my initiation into Army nursing and my only experience of the stress one associates with wartime service. Though we worked hard for long hours, we were never in danger. There were occasional buzz bombs and V-2 rockets which came within earshot, but none landed dangerously close to our hospital. One night, shortly after a couple of rockets went over, all was quiet, I was in the nurses' room preparing the next round of medications when suddenly there was a great crash on the ward followed by pandemonium! Dropping a half loaded syringe, I rushed into the ward imagining all manner of disaster. When I put the light on we quickly discovered that one of the wooden blackout shutters had fallen down, fortunately without injuring anyone. Our collective relief did nothing to reduce the noise level. Everyone was telling everyone else what they thought had happened. There was much laughter. Suddenly the duty officer appeared wanting an explanation for all the noise and scolding us severely for having a light on when one of the blackout shutters was down!

By this time the Allied Armies had moved further into Europe and we were no longer a transit hospital. Our patients stayed long enough for us to get to know them! They were not all Canadians; many were British, some American and sometimes we had German prisoners. Following are a few excerpts from my letters home:

August 1944 - *"Most of my patients seem to be in casts, arms, legs, body casts – they need a lot of help with personal care, especially those who can't use their arms. But when they can, they help each other."*

August 1944 – *"We have quite a few POWs on our ward just now and I'm pleased to see that the up patients help to make them comfortable, give them drinks, etc., as they do for each other. Makes me feel that there is still love and compassion in our world."*

October 1944 – *"You will probably be receiving fewer letters from me for a while. I'm on nights. We are doing 13-hour shifts and I haven't been taking any hours off during the night as we have some very sick lads who need constant care. Most of my off-duty time is spent sleeping and eating!"*

January 1945 – *"Work goes on as usual. I have some very nice patients; one boy in particular with both arms in casts can't do much for himself, but has a wonderful sense of humour. He and the boy beside him, who happens to have casts on both legs, carry on the most entertaining conversations. They would make a great comedy act! They keep the ward in stitches. Great for morale – mine too!"*

Finally in a letter written 8 May 1945 at 2 in the morning – *"This is the great day we've all been waiting for. PEACE! Surrender occurred yesterday but the celebration for VE Day is to be today!"*

I spent VE Day in London among the jubilant crowds. I can't remember a great deal about it except that the streets were packed, impassable even on foot; there were flags, streamers, balloons – singing, dancing, laughter and tears too, but mostly excitement, relief and joy. "It's Over," the newspaper headlines screamed!

In August, I was posted to the Canadian Army Occupational Forces in Germany. I was excited to be going to the Continent at last. We crossed the channel at night and travelled by truck and train through Belgium and Holland. We were in Nijmegen on the day the Japanese surrendered and we had another day of celebration. Our journey from Nijmegen to Oldenburg, Germany, was by truck over badly-damaged roads. Again, quoting from a letter home, *"We passed columns and columns of tanks and artillery going out and we crossed many emergency or temporary bridges with the remains of the old ones blown up at the side."*

Number 16 CGH in Oldenburg was situated in a modern hospital just taken over by the Allies. The sisters lived in a wing of the hospital building. Our first job was to clean up and get ready for admissions. My stay with the Occupational Forces was very brief. After just a few weeks I was transferred to Bruges to help close No. 12 CGH. What a beautiful old town Bruges was, and no doubt, still is! We lived in a hotel on the town square facing a two-hundred-year-old clock tower equipped with two sets of beautiful bells. The manual set was played on frequent occasions by a very accomplished bell master. How wonderful that it survived the war.

By the end of November 1945, I was back in England at No. 22 CGH. Everyone was thinking and talking of going home but we had to wait our turn. My turn came in April 1946, and I sailed aboard the troop ship, *Ile de France* to a most joyous "Welcome Home."

Mrs. Jean Frances (Ferguson) Sutherland

Graduated from: The Royal Alexandra Hospital School of Nursing, Edmonton, Alberta. Year: 1938

Military History:

Service: Army

Rank: Lt. N/S

Served: January 1943 to September 1945

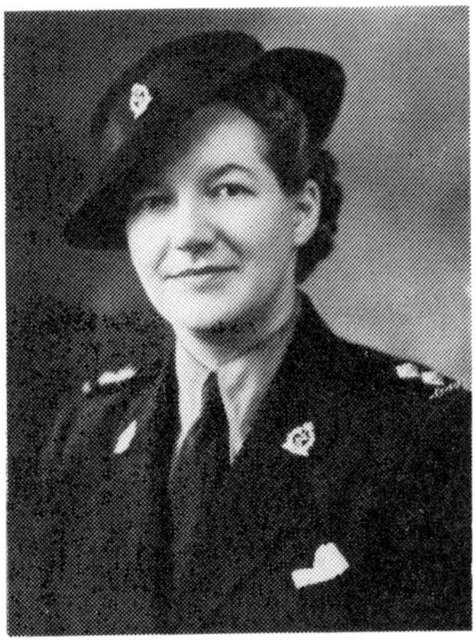

Lt. N/S Jean Frances (Ferguson) Sutherland

I chose a military career because I had a brother in the Air Force, a brother in the Navy, and my father was an engineer in World War I.

Joined RCAMC in Edmonton, served in Edmonton Military Hospital, transferred to Army Basic Training Centre at Camrose, Alberta. Then posted overseas as Reinforcement to No. 12 Canadian General Hospital at Horley, Surrey.

Transferred to No. 7 Canadian General Hospital at Taplow. With No. 7 General to Helmesley, Yorkshire, to await overseas posting. Moved to Southampton with No. 7 CGH to go to France about six weeks after D-Day. No. 7 was a large hospital, about 600 beds.

Moved up to No. 6 Canadian General Hospital, a smaller 200-bed unit. Volunteered to go to No. 6 CCS near Caen and stayed with No. 6 CCS to Nijmegen, Holland.

I was invalided back to No. 10 CGH at Turnhout, Belgium. Back on duty at No. 10 CGH until the end of the war. Then back to Bramshott to go home.

I was discharged in Calgary, September 1945.

Chapter 6

NO.1 NEUROLOGICAL AND PLASTIC SURGERY HOSPITAL AT BASINGSTOKE

June (Plummer) Newton
Margery (Cambon) Quail

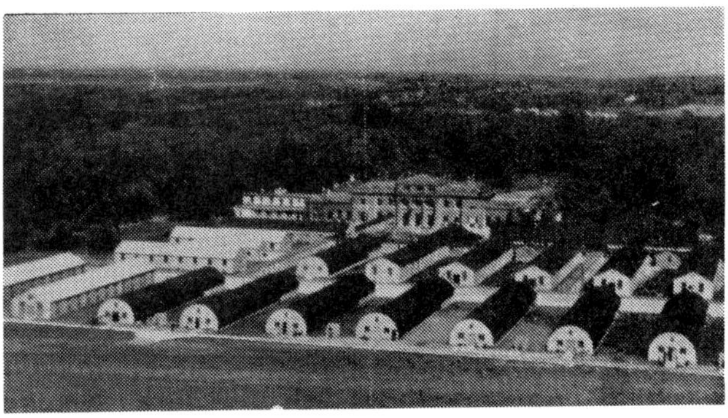

Hackwood House. This was the location of Basingstoke Neurological and Plastic Surgery Hospital, RCAMC, Turnborough. Hackwood House is in the background. The hospital on the lawn accommodated 750 patients. Hackwood itself was the residence of medical and nursing staff. Loaned by June Plummer Newton

Canadian National Defense Headquarters was responsible for the organization of No.1 Neurological Hospital. The mobilization of the new special unit was effective 21 December 1939 at Lansdowne Park Camp, Ottawa. Dr. Wilder Penfield was closely involved in the development of this new unit. Matron M. McDonald was scheduled to go overseas as matron in charge of the nurses who made up the staff of the unit.

The unit moved overseas in June 1940 without the nursing sisters and set up at Hackwood Park near Basingstoke on the estate of Lord Camrose. The nurses arrived in September.

Highly specialized work was carried out in neurosurgery. After the Plastic Surgery Unit moved to No.1 Neurological

Hospital in February of 1943, the unit became known as Basingstoke Neurological and Plastic Surgery Hospital. Specialties now included work with patients who had been badly scarred by burns as well as with those who had undergone surgery of the face and head.

The unit began closing down 31 July 1945.

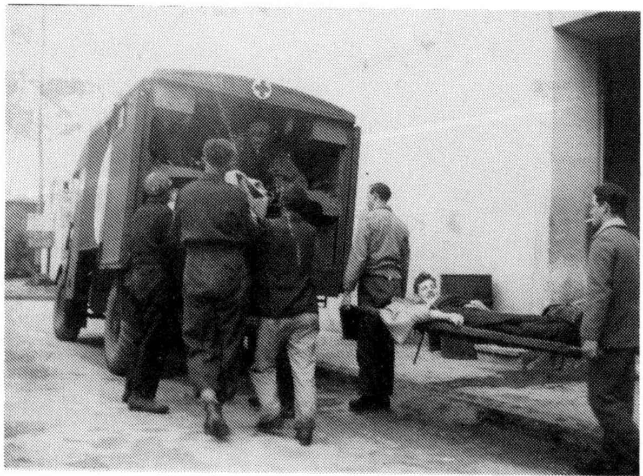

Patients from No. 15 CGH, Caserta were being transferred to a ship to return to England, April 1945.
Loaned by June Plummer Newton

June (Plummer) Newton

Graduated from: Royal Jubilee Hospital School of Nursing, Victoria. Year: 1941

Military History:

Service: Army

Rank: Lieutenant (NS)

Served: January. 1943 to April 1946

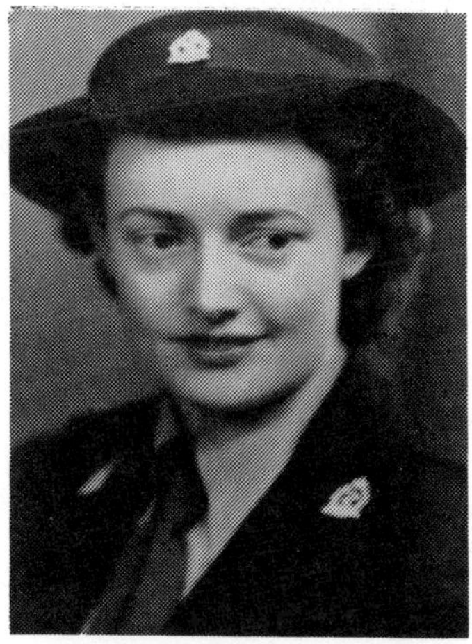

June (Plummer) Newton Lt. N/S Jan. 1943 - April 1946. No. 1 Neurological and Plastic Surgery Hospital in Basingstoke, England.

The Army gave me an opportunity to use my nursing training in a new setting.

I'm sure I was influenced by my father's experiences in World War I. A nurse named "June" saved his foot from amputation by diligent nursing care. I was named "June" partly for this reason.

In January 1944, after four weeks of waiting at Debert, N.S., we boarded the SS *Cavina* bound for

England. Our destination was not known when we boarded, of course. The SS *Cavina* was known to us as a "banana boat." In other words, it was a small ship that travelled between Halifax and the Caribbean before WW II. At the time of our Atlantic crossing it carried no more than 135 passengers. There were two-thirds nursing sisters and the remaining one-third were medical officers. The crew was from England as far as we could discern. The captain may have been Canadian.

Our ship was in the centre of a very large convoy. The month was January, so the sea was very rough and it took us 31 days to reach Liverpool. Our route took us into warmer climes. We gathered from rumours that we were close to the Azores, but a week or two later we were in a very cold climate. It was very stormy. Many years later we heard that two of our destroyers were hit by submarine action and had to be left at Gander Bay, Newfoundland.

Needless to say, we were never told what was happening. One requirement was to sleep fully clothed with water canteen handy ready for evacuation. Somehow I never felt fear, probably attributed to being very young and, I suppose, not really having had any war experience.

There was a fair amount of seasickness which I missed, fortunately. There were very happy times also when we gathered for amateur entertainment evenings. Lifetime friendships were made from that trip.

A group of us arrived at a Canadian Military Hospital where the nursing sisters there gave us a warm welcome. Imagine finding a "ceramic pig" in every bed – hardly what we expected for a war experience.

My next Canadian Military Hospital was No. 1 Neurological and Plastic Surgery Hospital at Basingstoke. There were many patients who had been severely burned during air battles over Britain and Europe.

No. 1 Hospital was situated on an estate in Hampshire – named Hackwood House. This building had many rooms for hospital staff – usually four beds in a room. Our meals were served in the very large dining room of this mansion.

On D-Day we watched hundreds of aircraft towing gliders full of supplies for the invasion.

In a few days we had casualties back in the hospital at Basingstoke. Many Canadians and English soldiers were there. To our surprise, three German Army soldiers arrived with them.

I'm sure there is a story there on the humanitarian act.

In July 1944, I arrived at No. 15 CGH at Caserta, Italy. Our hospital and our billets were both in Mussolini's cavalry barracks. Wards held 30 to 40 patients in each. Most of the patients were so severely injured that they were designated to return to England and then to Canada. Many had arms and legs amputated by land mines and other war machines. The whole hospital was a study in the tragic aftermath of war.

My military experience would be incomplete without paying tribute to the wonderful, brave and grateful patients we were privileged to have in our care.

Margery (Bunny) (Cambon) Quail

Graduated from: Jeffery-Hale Hospital School of Nursing, Quebec City. Year: 1939

Military History:

Service: Army

Rank: Lt. N/S

Served: February 8, 1940 to September 11, 1945

My whole wartime experience was wonderful; so much knowledge was gained, and friendships were made that were very meaningful. Some still exist today after more than 50 years have passed.

I left Quebec in December 1940, and went overseas where I was a reinforcement to the 15th Canadian General Hospital. Doctor Stewart-Gordon, a plastic Surgeon at the 15th General formed a plastic surgery unit. He took two nursing sisters from the 15th General with him; I was one of them.

We went to an EMS Hospital in Basingstoke named Park-Prewett and our unit was stationed at Rooksdown House – the plastic surgery portion of the hospital. Sir Howard Gillies worked from there and that is how our unit started.

Later we moved to No. 1 Canadian Neurological Hospital in Basingstoke and the new title was No. 1 Neurological and Plastic Surgery Hospital, Basingstoke, Hants.

Many amusing things happened and one took each day as it came and was thankful for it. A few of our "Plastic" group still

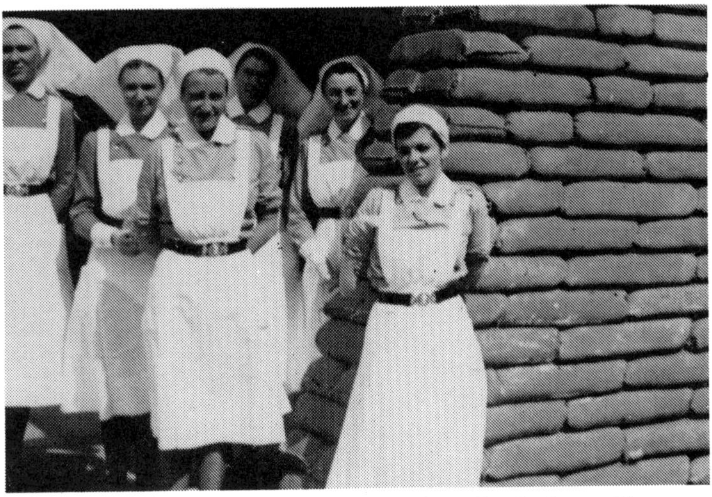

Plastic Surgery Unit first stationed at Rooksdown House EMS hospital in Basingstoke
Our plastic surgeon – Stewart-Gordon
L-R: Nursing Sisters Aileen (Fears) Kent, Dorothy Macham, Freda Dearden, Eva Wannop, Ivy Ackworth, Margery [Bunny] (Cambon) Quail in OR cap – that's me!

meet for lunch occasionally; it is good to keep in touch. I was married in England December 11, 1943, and we celebrated our 50th wedding anniversary in 1993.

Chapter 7

CANADIAN GENERAL HOSPITALS

NO. 1 CANADIAN GENERAL HOSPITAL

Nancy Kennedy-Reid
Velma (Cockerill) McCulloch
Patricia (Moore) Moll
Katherine (Simmons) Ramsey
Elizabeth (Tracy-Gould) Robinson

No. 1 General mobilized at Montreal 1 July 1940 with Col. A.E. Lundon as OC and sailed from Halifax 13 December 1940 for duty at Marston Green near Birmingham, England, 27 December 1940. The hospital opened in January 1941 and took their first military patients 9 January. They took Dieppe casualties in August 1942.

In October 1943, the unit sailed for Italy and were in the convoy bombed in the Mediterranean, 6 November. The nursing sisters sailed later on the British hospital ship *Atlantis* to Algiers and finally to Andria where they arrived ahead of their unit. They opened 1 December at Andria in three buildings that formerly housed a civilian hospital and two schools. In May 1944, they moved to Avellino.

They were at Macerata, south of Florence, for one week before moving to Iesi where they functioned as a large casualty clearing station taking casualties from Corps and evacuating them to other hospitals. In January of 1945, the unit began the move to northwest Europe. By December of 1945 No. 1 General was the only Canadian general hospital under the command of Canadian Forces in the Netherlands, and in January 1946 it was disbanded.

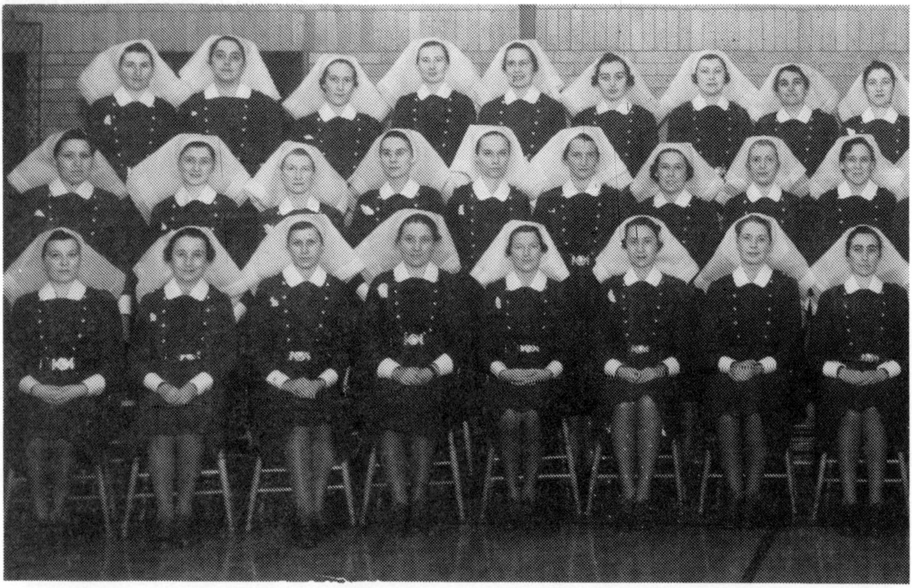

TOP ROW L-R: Levasseur, Rochelle Lachance, Mary Bunbury, Joan Gray, Edith Little, Gertrude Layman, Lil Burri, Mary MacLellan, Cecile Biron.
SECOND ROW L-R: Y. D'Aigre, Lillian Thomson, 2Lt Vera Scott, Home/S, Marian Blackler, Sylvia Fisk, M.W. "Scottie" Douglas, Patricia Moore, Ruth Smith, Laverne Riach.
FRONT ROW L-R: Marie Louise Numainville, Dorothy Murphy, V.I. Fischer Isabel McIver, E.B.Stephen, Muriel Hearn, Anita Springer, Nancy Kennedy-Reid.

Nancy B. Kennedy-Reid

Graduated from: Montreal General Hospital of Nursing, Year: 1929 and diploma as Registered Sick Children's nurse for England and Wales

Military History:

Service: RCAMC

Rank: Lieut. to Major (Matron)

Served: May 1940 to February 1946

No. 1 Canadian General Hospital was mobilized in Montreal in May 1940. On 13 December 1940 I embarked on the *Pasteur* at Halifax for overseas duty. I recall a Christmas tree taken

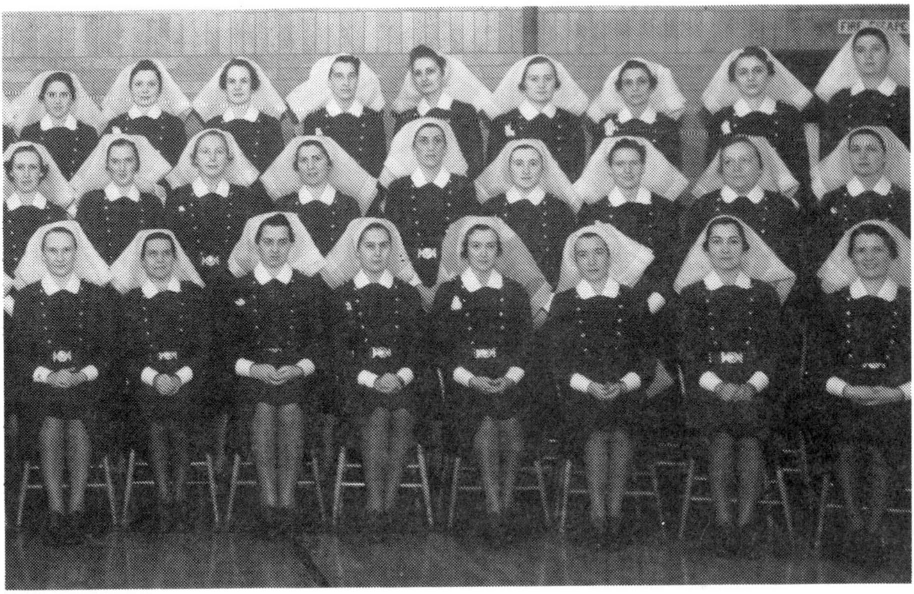

TOP ROW L-R: Trudy Lake,Ruth Sharpe, Elaine Wright, D.V. Carter, Jean Byam, Maddy Farmer, Ede Maquiston, Gwen Hopkins, Elizabeth Tracy-Gould. SECOND ROW L-R:Jean Collins, Terry Hickman, Grace Carter, Christine Cole, Robby Harquail, Doris Watson, Pat De Merral, Marie Jean Latour, Lil Wagar. FRONT ROW L-R: Dorothy MacRae, Ida Henderson, Rita Fulton, Maude Louise Brooks, Mary Maguire, Freda Dearden, Elaine Cornish, Pat Paterson. Nursing Sisters No. 1 Canadian General Hospital, Nov. 18, 1940. Loaned by Patricia Moll, No. 1 Canadian General Hospital

aboard by N/S Doris Watson. At the captain's request, it was hoisted to the top of the mast as we sailed up the River Clyde.

We landed in Gourock 24 December and arrived in Marston Green, near Birmingham, the next day. The bombing raids on the Coventry and Birmingham areas stand out in my mind.

In August of 1942, No. 1 General Hospital received many of the wounded from Dieppe.

The No. 1 nursing sisters remained at Colchester when the unit sailed for Italy in convoy with the *Santa Elena* in October 1943. We sailed later in November on the British hospital ship *Atlantis* and were united with our unit at Andria.

We opened our hospital in December and remained in Italy until the last week of February 1945.

On return from Italy, I was decorated with the Royal Red Cross by King George at Buckingham Palace. I remained in the U.K. as matron of No. 23 General until it closed as a hospital and became Khaki College, then I was at No. 24 General until my return to Canada, December 1945. I arrived in Halifax 1 January 1946 and was discharged from the RCAMC in February.

While I was matron at Ste. Anne de Bellevue, DVA Hospital, Quebec, I received the Queen Elizabeth Coronation Medal.

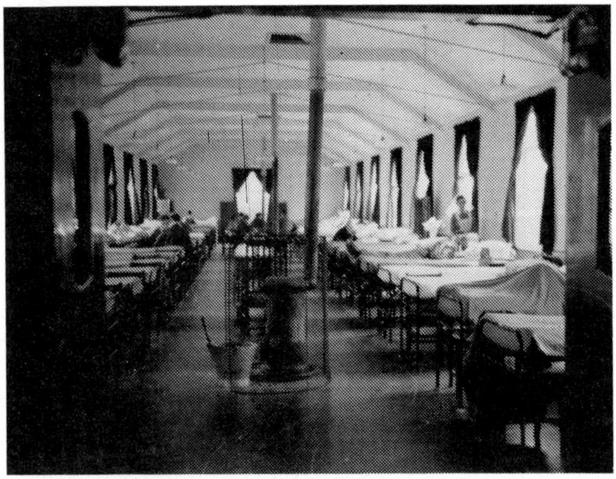

A ward, No. 1 CGH at Marston Green

Velma G. (Cockerill) McCulloch

Graduated from: Misericordia Hospital School of Nursing, Winnipeg, Manitoba.

Military History:

Service: RCAMC

Rank: Lt. N/S

Served: January 1942 to September 1945

My late father was in the Canadian Army in World War I and World War II which inspired me to choose the Army.

My most memorable recollections are the months spent in Italy in 1943 and 1944, especially when I was attached to a Field Dressing Station when we had our Field Surgical Unit at the Hitler Line.

Patricia (Moore) Moll

Graduated from: Homeopathic Hospital (Phillips School of Nursing), Montreal, Quebec. Year: 1939

Military History:

Service: RCAMCRank:

Rank: Lt. N/S

Served: 23 October 1940 to 28 June 1945

September 3, 1939, saw the declaration of war by France and Britain against Germany. Everyone in Canada knew that our lives would take on a new pattern.

September 10, 1940, a proclamation and we were at war with Germany! We in hospitals as nurses waited knowing of mobilization.

I was an RN, a supervisor in a teaching hospital associated with McGill University, I also had a boyfriend hurrying home to Canada from England to join as a medical offfcer.

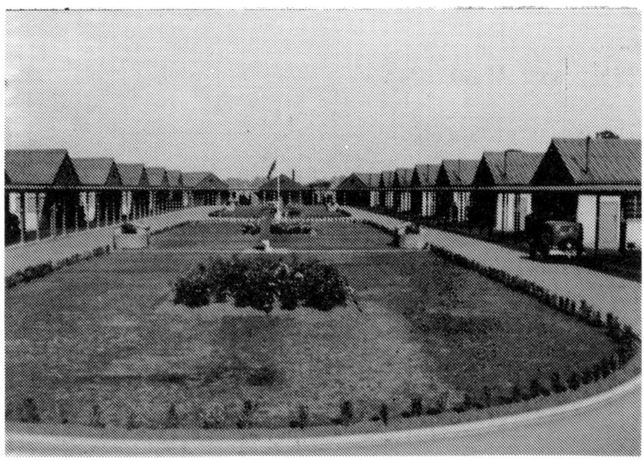

No. 1 Canadian General Hospital, Marston Green 1941

Great excitement on 23 October 1940. I was in the Army – a member of No. 1 Canadian General Hospital – there was a mad rush to have uniforms fitted. A group picture of 58 nurses was taken 18 November 1940.

Enroute to England. There was a division in the groups – the first group under Dorothy McCrae as matron of No. 1 disembarked at Gurock, Scotland, early December 1940. We, the 2nd group, were met at the Halifax docks by the *Pasteur*, a French luxury liner and arrived Christmas Day, 1940, with Matron Kennedy-Reid at the helm.

We were 22 nurses, 250 officers plus 3,000 troops. I even met my younger brother on the deck – great excitement! Amazed at what we found on board; a luxury liner that didn't have time to remove its grandeur, so we walked on wall-to-wall carpeting. French waiters, bartenders, French cuisine – swans on the wall paper in our bathroom – a sleek, beautiful ship – a wonderfully comfortable trip ploughing through the dark Atlantic. The icing on the cake, tea served by a white coated waiter at 7 A.M. each morning.

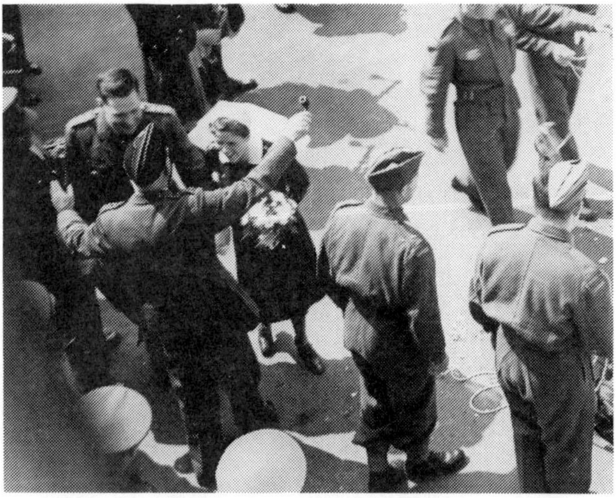

Late John Leishman M.D. and his bride, Trudy Lake. Horsham, England

The train from Guroch to Birmingham took us to Marston Green – a year here. Treating mostly evacuated patients, children, and Air Force men who travelled the skies fighting the German bombers that came over regularly at 6 P.M. One Holy Thursday the Germans dropped 52 bombs around the hospital area – the late Dr. Howard Mitchell, our medical officer, would attest to this – as he repeatedly called through the years to remind me.

Horsham Surrey – our next stop, a lovely little town close to London – the famous "King's Head" pub where we met so frequently, during our stay in Horsham. Muriel Hearn and I were rushed off to Chichester, there to attend a Canadian soldier who was caught between two tanks. He was the nephew of a VIP in the British Air Force; a wonderful 18 year old boy whose injuries were almost indescribeable. I was on night duty; the Germans were bombing Portsmouth, the injured airmen filled the corridors awaiting attention. Our patient developed gangrene; we watched it slowly crawling until the wonder drug penicillin slowly took over to stop it.

Eventually we healed him sufficiently to send him back to No. 1. Back in the OR, when he was wheeled in for dressings before he was anaesthetized, he used to greet us with a huge grin and a "Hello Pat." He left us six months later. While making a ship at occupational therapy he pricked his finger and general septicemia set in.

August 19, 1942 – Dieppe: A planned trip to London to celebrate my birthday on the 21st was abruptly cancelled – no one knew what was up, and why we were all confined to barracks.

P.M. of the 19th saw the casualties arriving in battle dress – just off the boats. Matron Kennedy used to tell the story about how while helping to remove a pair of trousers from a soldier, she said, "I'll just take these off and throw them under the bed." In great anguish he yelled, "No! no! sister, my grenades are in my pockets." And so it went – our first serious working baptism. Ninety-five operations performed in ninteen and one-half hours, stopping only momentarily for food. Dr. Shannon, our orthoepedic man, was seen mopping the floor so he wouldn't slip. We were a terrific team in the operating room; Ida Henderson, Joan Gray, Lil Wagar, Elizabeth Tracy-Gould, Pat Moore (Moll), and Vel Cockerill (McCulloch).

Into the second year our unit became a very special home away from home. We had been tested by "Dieppe" – personnel working as a team – knew things would get worse before it was over.

Colchester: A staging area for No. 1 Canadian General Hospital and No. 14 Canadian General Hospital enroute to Italy.

Rumours had it that nursing sisters from both hospitals would not travel together, (personnel from 1200- and 600-bed hospitals.) They would separate the nursing sisters, and so on 6 November 1943 the Germans bombed the ship carrying No. 14 doctors and nurses. They went to Philippville. We, on a hospital ship to Algiers, all rescued but saw their ship turn over and sink.

It was an exciting time for me as my boyfriend arrived from headquarters with an engagement ring!

Naples: Here I worked relieving in a British hospital, another shocking encounter with battle casualties. Tall, handsome, young guardsmen, the amputee ward – my duty to do the dressings each day. A percentage of them were in the center of the ward were German prisoner amputees. The guardsmen had a little sing song when I first arrived on the ward, "Don't forget the center of the ward."

Andria: Saw No. 1 again with casualties from the Moro River and the fight for Ortona moving on to Avellino; battle casualties arriving daily.

The advance on Rome: Battle of the Liri Valley. Avellino, on 11 May, Major John Leishman, Major B.A. Jackson, N\S Velma Cockerill (McCulloch), and Moore (Moll) set off to the front as a Field Surgical Unit with six orderlies. We were a compact mobile unit able to move fast and go into action with a Field Dressing Station. Only priority cases were done by our unit.

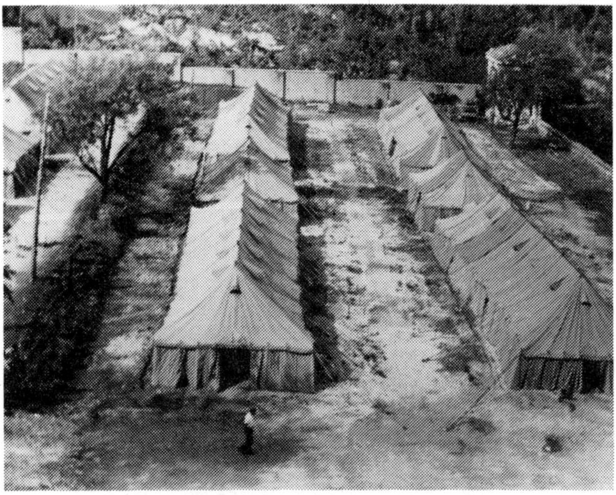

Our tents in Avellino, Italy. 1944

With our 8th Army Patches replacing our pips we moved forward with the First Division. We were called to help at 5 CCS in Pignatora who had heavy casualties from Cassino and the Gustav Line. We were working hard one evening with seven tables going when the Germans made a direct hit on the lighting system. With the auxiliary lights in action, all our seven patients survived. With coming on of the lights I saw a cousin of mine giving anaesthetics. Great meeting!

Passing through Cassino which was in ruins, we travelled through and with the long line of lorries, jeeps and tanks. Everything levelled by shell fire, no people except dead German soldiers hanging in and out of their tanks. There were a few shallow graves with a cross and a helmet on top. We saw dead horses and donkeys – the stench – one could smell it from far off as we approached – a sweet sickly odour that permeated your nostrils and throat. Ahead of the medium light artillery, one felt as

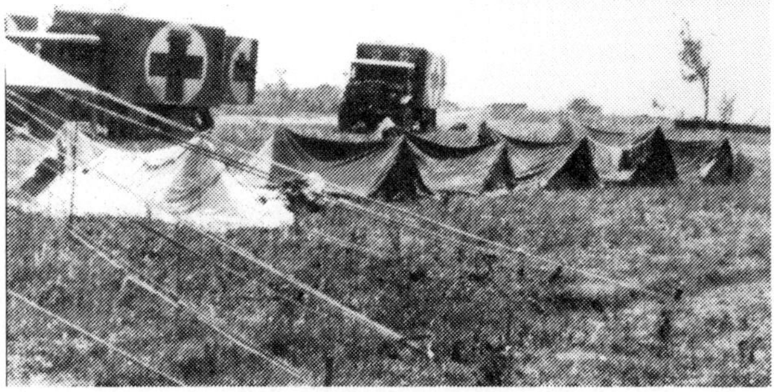

Small pup tents for medical orderlies.

if you could reach up and touch the shells. While there, a "William" target went into action, a concentration of 668 guns firing 3509 rounds or 92 tons of ammunition. The first time in the war that this had been initiated – what a din!

Traveling to Portecorvo throughout the heavily damaged town after its capture, we joined No. 1 Field Dressing Station and were shown the heavily bombed hospital and taken inside. We were told we could choose our room. But having settled on an empty room, we were held back and told to get down on our hands and knees and crawl over to the window. The major said, "Raise your heads slowly and look." There in clear view were German soldiers parading back and forth. Val and I chose the safety of the tarpaulin on the other side. We worked 17 to 18 hours at a time. Early in the morning I watched the gravediggers burying some of our boys who were wrapped in grey blankets; they were lowered ever so gently into the graves to be later moved to a cemetery.

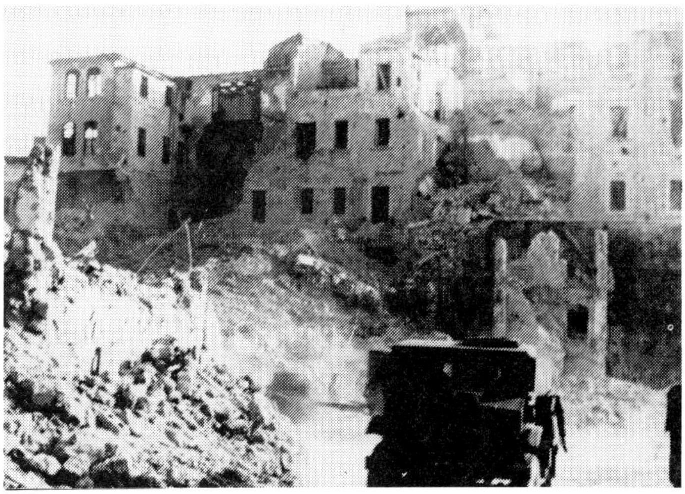

Going through Cassino, Italy, May 1944 enroute to the front.

I was so taken with a memory of the gathering of the bodies of the soldiers. A huge lorry was receiving them and I watched as the soldiers gathering them slowly and carefully placed them one on top of the other, their boots towards the opening of the lorry. The gentleness of the men gathering the soldiers as if it were a sacred duty they were performing, and the poppies in the fields blowing in the wind.

Great disappointment for our team. We thought we would march into Rome but were returned to our unit. Later, when spending a week on leave with Bert, I suddenly became ill. I was moved to No. 15 in Caserta as a patient where I spent seven months before travelling on the Letitia, as a stretcher case, arriving home in time for Christmas. I recovered, waiting for Bert to come back home. We married in 1947. After a wonderful forty-seven years together, sharing many memories of our war years, he died 8 February 1992.

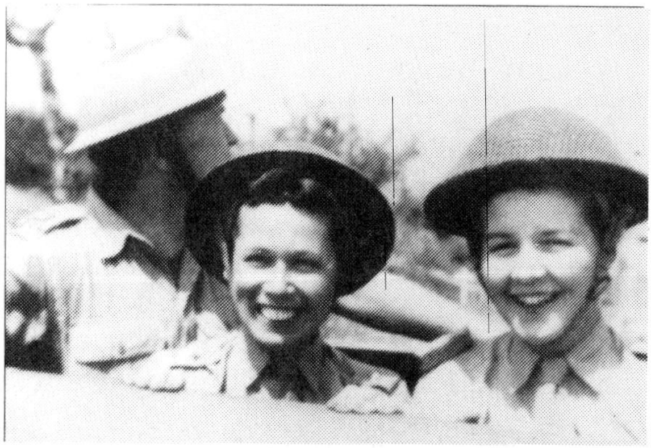

Enroute to the front to set up a Field Surgical Unit passing through Cassino.
Lieut. N/S Patricia (Moore) Moll,
Lieut. N/S Velma (McCulloch) Cockerill

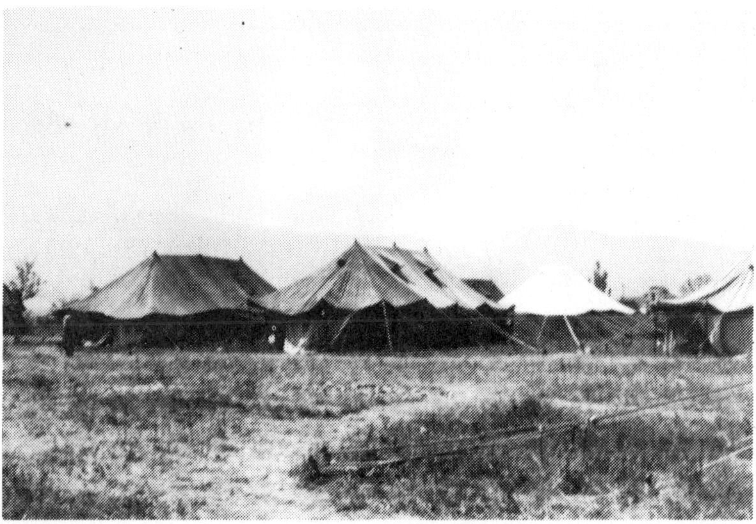

Large group of tents, a hospital CCS, Pontecorva, Italy 23 May 1944

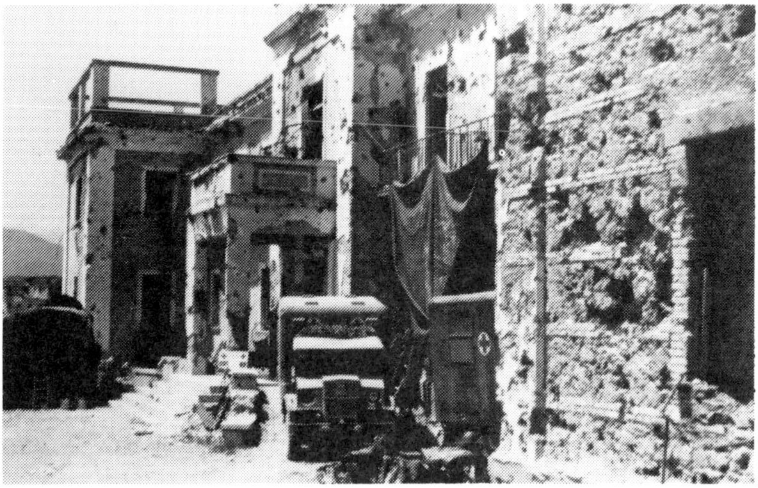

ITALY 1944 In the Hitler Line May 1944
A surgical team of medical officers and nursing sisters; Dr. John Leishman (late), Dr. B.A. Jackson, N/S Patricia Moore, N/S Velma McCulloch from No.1 Canadian General Hospital attached to No. 1 Field Dressing Station in the captured town of Pontecorva, Italy. Here they set up their operating room in a building badly battered by artillery fire.

Kathryn H. (Simmons) Ramsey

Graduated from: Vancouver General Hospital School of Nursing. Year: 1934

Military History:

Service: Royal Canadian Army Medical Corps

Rank: Lt. N/S

Served: 1941 to 1946

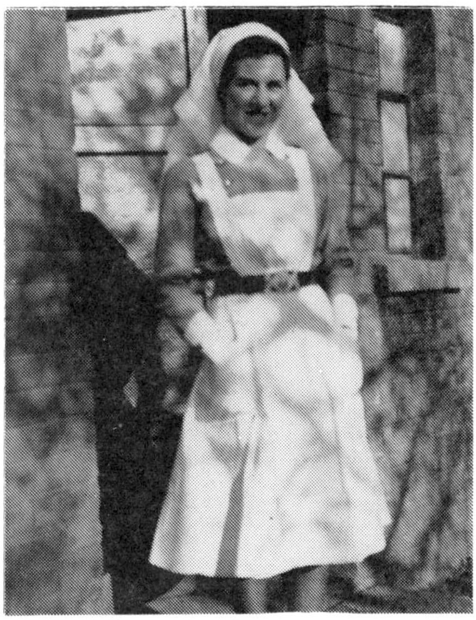

Kathryn H. Ramsay

I joined the Army to serve my country. I believed it would be a great experience. At the time I was nursing in a hospital near a military camp. This influenced me to join; also, the pay was double what I was getting!

One of the greatest challenges for me was when we

were awakened early A.M. (at Horsham, England No. 1 CGH) August 19th, 1942 (probably August 20th) to receive casualties from the Dieppe Raid.

Another experience was when we were in Nijmegen, Holland with No. 1 CGH acting as a CCS in 1945 during the early months when the fighting was all around us. We received such large numbers of casualties each day from many different countries, including 14- and 16-year-old German POWs, just babies, clinging to us and/or dying in our arms. If the casualties lived after returning from the operating room, they were transferred the next day to British hospital ships or carriers or to Canadian General Hospitals in England. It was a very traumatic time for many of us.

Of course, the most momentous time was when we learned that the war was finally at an end, May 8, 1945!

I found the whole five years a very rewarding experience. Travelling to England, Italy, Belgium, Holland and France alone was something we never expected to do in those days. While we worked very hard, we had our 'Leaves' when we could get them. We had good times at parties in officers messes of several different countries: Canadian, British, Australian and New Zealand. All in all, I found it a really good learning experience.

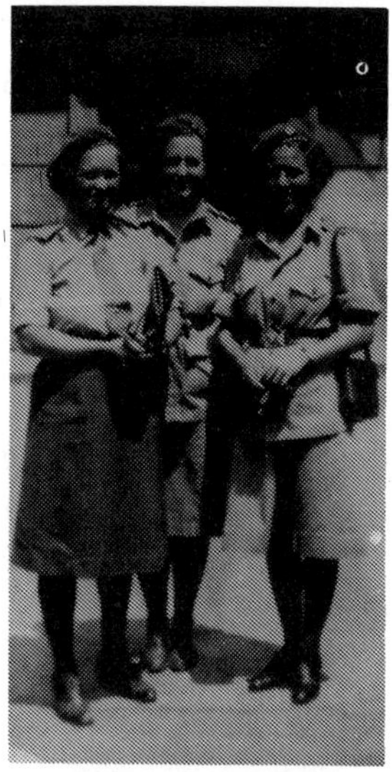

L-R: Madeline E. Farmer, Doris Watson, Kathryn H. Ramsay

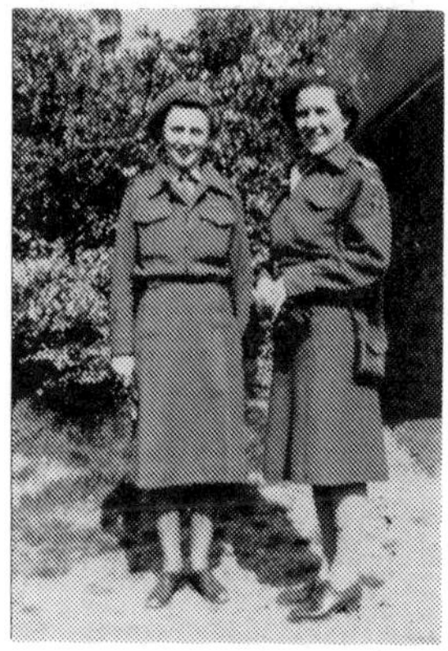

L-R: Gwen Hopkins, Kathryn Ramsay

Elizabeth M. (Tracy-Gould) Robinson

Graduated from: Montreal General Hospital School of Nursing.
Year: 1937

Military History:

Service: Army

Rank: Lieutenant N/S

Served: 1940 to 1945

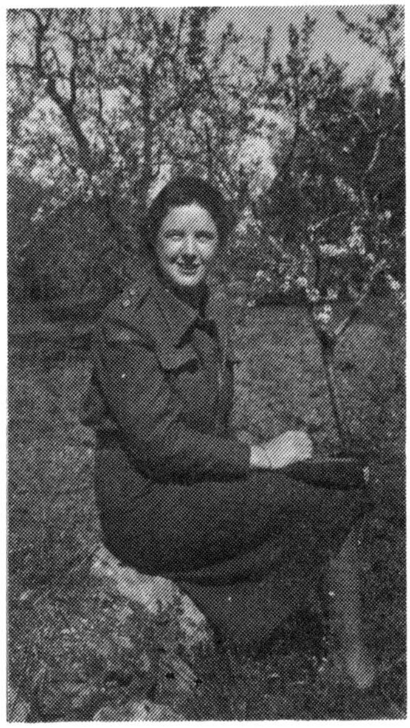

Lt. (N/S) M. Elizabeth (Tracy-Gould) Robinson RCAMC 1940-45 Italy, April 1944 Almond tree in background.

One of our doctors told me a unit was formed with as many as possible from MGH. Naturally, I wanted to stay with my classmates who were going into the Army. I was in OR so was assured of being in the Unit No. 1 CGH.

My military experience began with the trip to Britain in an unescorted 7000-ton Belgian Congo cruise ship in a gale which battered the ship. Seeing the bombing effects on Birmingham; seeing the plays at Stratford; tickets paid by Pady Berd (Custard) or Lady Flowers. Biking everywhere. All this from Marston Green. Then the wonderful move to Horsham, Sussex.

Leaves in such places as Oban, Inverness, Torquay, Cornwall, London, Wales and as many places as one would go for seven days.

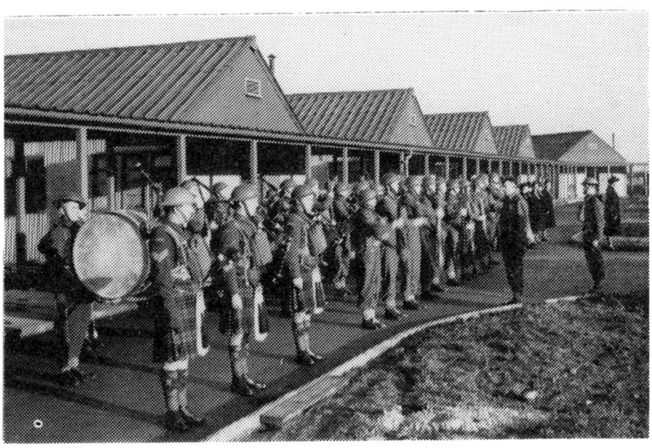

Church Parade Marston Green, England 1941. Col. London, CO and Matron Dorothy MacRae

1943 – our trip, by the Royal Mail Steamer *Atlantis* which was made into a hospital ship; on our way to Italy we were dropped off in Algiers. After three years of blackouts the ship was lighted by the Red Cross with red and green lights all around. Wonderful meals with white bread.

A week in Algiers, then on the Channel Island ferries to Naples (a Sirocco blowing and so many seasick). I managed not to be. Being first into Quisisana in Sorrento; a building full of fleas; then across Italy to Andria. From Andria we went to Avellino, then to Jeri, our last place in Italy. Saw Rome, Florence, Ravenna, Molfetta and Bari. Left Italy spring of 1945, landed in Marseille, ended up in Nijmegen.

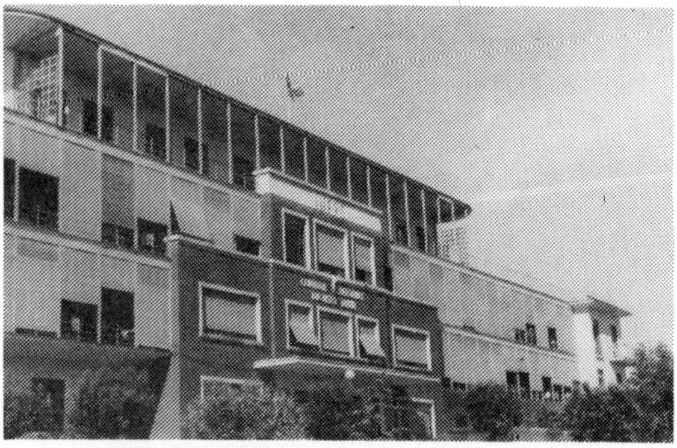

Front of No. 1 CGH, Jesi, Italy

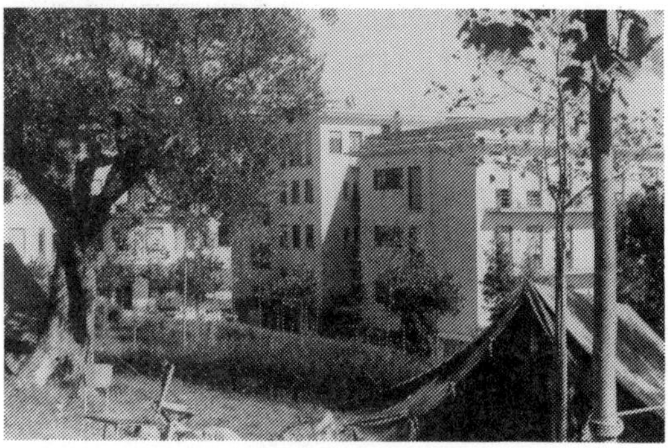

Back of No. 1 Cdn. General Hospital, Jesi, Italy

As an OR nurse, I do not think we had the same contact with patients as the other nurses did. I know I did not.

The last highlight was meeting my husband in Italy and being married in Brussels. He was in the Saskatoon Light Infantry which was Machine Gunners. Came back to Canada by way of Ostend, London, Horsham (No. 9), troop ship *Queen Mary*, New York. Landed – then on to a troop train, with me being the only female from Toronto to Regina but with chaps who had served with my husband.

NO. 2 CANADIAN GENERAL HOSPITAL

Olive Nancy (Squibb) Tysoe

No. 2 Canadian General Hospital arrived in the U.K. in mid-1943 and situated at Bramshott. In June of 1944 they treated casualties from the D-Day invasion then crossed the channel to Normandy in August as a 1200-bed hospital. They became operational at Bayeux. With Matron Agnes MacLeod, the nursing sisters first went on duty at No. 10 General.

No. 2 General moved from France to Ghent, Belgium, where they remained until they disbanded.

Olive Nancy (Squibb) Tysoe

Graduated from: Royal Inland Kamloops Hospital School of Nursing, B.C. Year: 1938

Military History:

Service: RCAMC

Rank: Lieutenant N/S

Served: June 1942 to March 1946

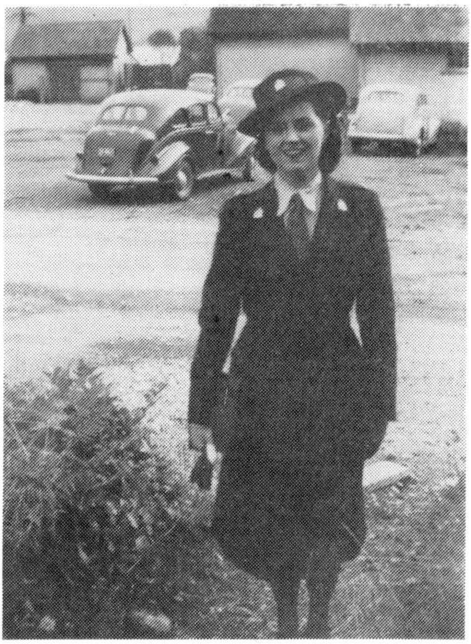

No. 2 CGH
Lt. (N/S) Olive Nancy (Squibb) Tysoe

Patriotism influenced me to choose the Army.

The highlights of my experiences were:

Being on duty No. 2 CGH in Bramshott (England) when the first casualties arrived from Normandy after D-Day.

Going over to Normandy August 1944 on a hospital ship which was filled up with casualties before we were allowed to disembark.

NO. 3 CANADIAN GENERAL HOSPITAL

Ruth Bayne
Jean Dorgan
Helen (Hill) Holmes

No. 3 Canadian General Hospital was organized at Windsor, Ontario and sailed on the *Queen Elizabeth* 13 September 1943 for duty in the U.K. One week later the unit arrived at Dorking; the nursing sisters joined their unit from their temporary quarters at No. 10 CGH.

In January 1944 the unit embarked on the *Lancashire* and after a very rough two weeks at sea, arrived in Italy. After a year of intensive care of casualties and of medical cases, particularly diphtheria, No. 3 was assigned to Northwest Europe. There they remained until mid-July 1945. No. 3 Canadian General Hospital closed at Apeldoorn 17 July 1945.

Anne Ruth Bayne

Graduated from: Brantford General Hospital School of Nursing, Brantford, Ontario. Year; 1940

Military History:

Service: RCAMC

Rank: Lt. N/S

Served: March 1943 to October 1945

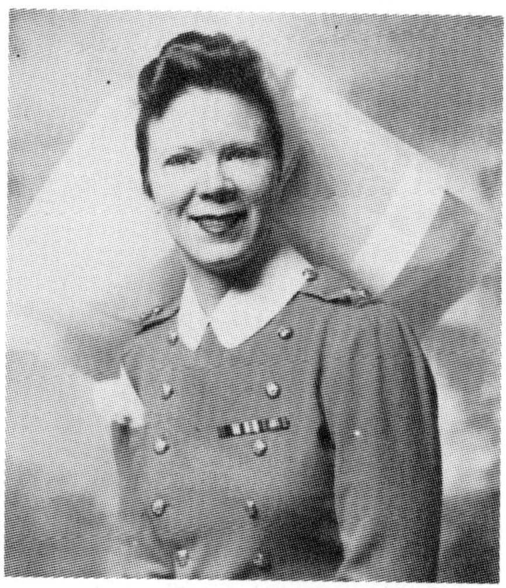

Lt. N/S Anne Ruth Bayne 1943 -1945

I joined the Army to be of service to my country.

My first assignment was Niagara Military Hospital, Niagara-on-the Lake, Ontario. Another BGH graduate, Miss Reta Moffat, was there also. We bought a bicycle between us for transportation from out rooming house to the hospital. We had a great time pedalling our way around. Reta owned the front half and I the back half.

When Reta was assigned to the hospital ship, *Lady Nelson*,

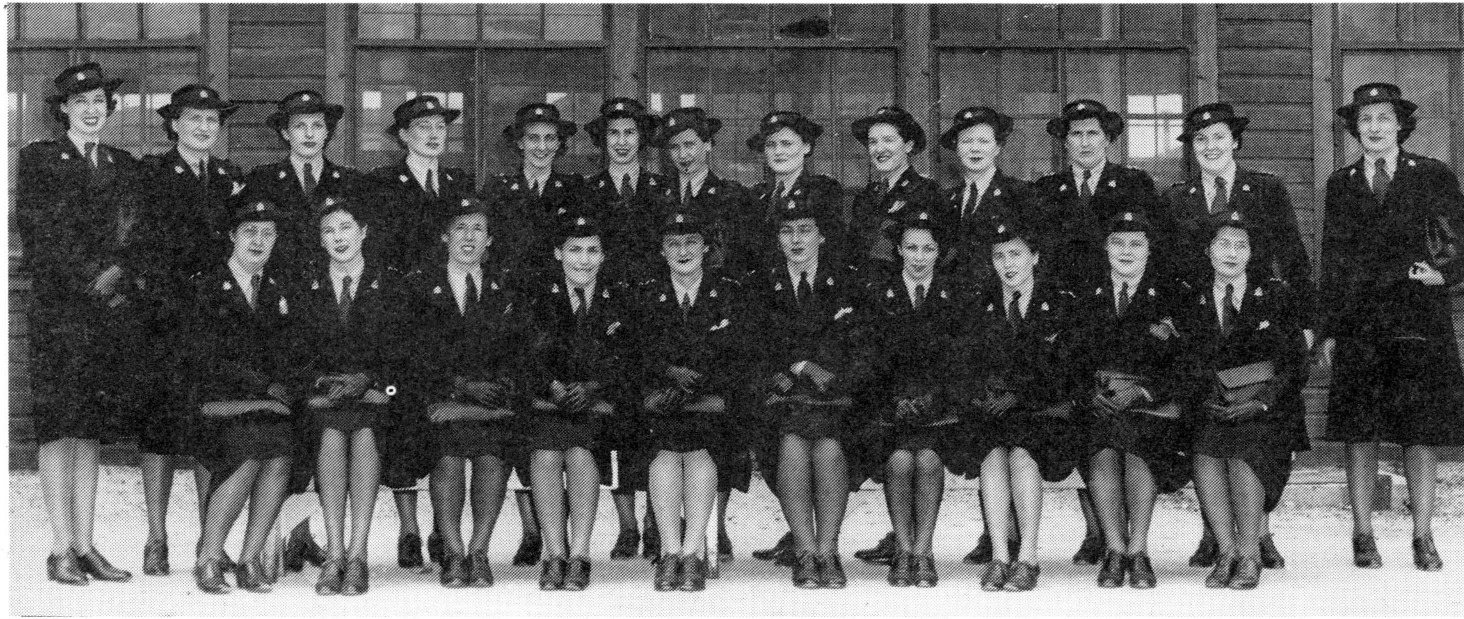

No. 3 Canadian General Hospital (Mobile Surgical) REAR STANDING L-R: 1. Lieut. N/S Eleanor Staple; 2. Lieut. N/S Vandervoort, London, Ont . 3. Lieut. N/S Grace (Tedford) Beresford, Winnipeg; 4. Lieut. N/S Nora Peters, Alberta; 5. Lieut. N/S Margaret Bailey, New Glasgow, Nova Scotia; 6. Lieut. N/S Shirley McLaughlin, London, Ont.; 7. Lieut. N/S Helen (Hill) Holmes, Alberta (now Ottawa); 8. Lieut. N/S Ishbel Gray, B.C.; 9. Lieut. N/S Jean (Buroker) Cusson, B.C.; 10. Lieut. N/S Ruth Bayne, Toronto; 11. Lieut. N/S Marion Palliser, Toronto, Ont.; 12. Lieut. N/S Isabel (Starr) Bizzell, Niagara-On-The-Lake, Ont.,(now living in North Bay Ont.); 13. Lieut. N/S Helen Wells, Toronto. FRONT ROW - seated L-R: 1. Lieut. N/S Marion Ward, Vancouver, B.C. (or Victoria); 2. Lieut. N/S Margaret (McMillan) Finger, Port Arthur, Ont.; 3. Lieut. N/S Jean Dorgan, New Westminster, B.C.; 4. Lieut. N/S Patricia Irwin, Gull Lake, Sask.; 5. Captain Matron Mary Isabel Roach, Montreal, Que.; 6. Helen James, Home Sister, Toronto; 7. Lieut. N/S Evelyn Scott, London, Ont.; 8. Lieut. N/S Elsa Broad, Toronto, Ont.; 9. Lieut. N/S Margaret Medforth, Toronto, Ont.; 10. Lieut. N/S Barbara Ross, Toronto, Ont.; loaned by Jean Dorgan

I think I became full owner of the bike. Shortly after, I was assigned to No. 3 Canadian General Mobile Hospital and was drafted overseas. Our collection point was Windsor, Ontario, where we roughed it for a brief period before going overseas on the *Queen Elizabeth* and then on to Dorking in England.

Jean Dorgan

Graduated from: University of British Columbia, 1934, with a B.App.Sc. Nursing. Year: 1934

Military History:

Service: RCAMC

Rank: Lt. N/S

Served: 1942 to 1945

No. 3 Military Hospital was a 200-bed, mobile surgical unit. It operated in the same fashion as a casualty clearing station. It took medical cases and some general surgery when the Canadian troops were at rest. It was mobilized in Windsor, Ontario, in September 1943.

We left Halifax for England 13 September 1943, one of several Canadian hospitals shipped on the *Queen Elizabeth*. My recollection is that there were thirteen. These had been mobilized in various Ontario towns, and as our train proceeded to Halifax it would stop at these towns and take on more cars containing another hospital.

In Halifax the train proceeded to the docks from which we were immediately marched up the gangplank to our cabins. The nursing sisters were quartered in deluxe cabins which had been stripped of their furnishings and fitted with bunks. There were nine tiers of bunks in our cabin, which meant one had to turn carefully. The suite included a large tiled bathroom in which, I blush to say, we all smoked. We remained in our cabins except for meals for the three days it took to load the troops. I will never forget the sound of marching feet on the gangplank, day and night, until boarding was completed.

We were told that there were 15,000 Army personnel on the ship. Because of the numbers we had just two meal sittings a day. Ours were 7:30 A.M. and 4:30 P.M. We were required to carry our life-preservers at all times. If we forgot, we were ordered back to our cabins to get them.

The enlisted men were in two groups. Half slept on deck, and the other half inside. Every 24 hours the two groups would change places. We would hear, *"Ready for the change-over,"* which was the signal to return to our quarters, if not already there.

The ship changed course every five minutes. It was very fast and could outrun a submarine, but there was always the danger of encountering a lurking "sub" or "wolf pack."

We reached Scotland in four days, docking at Greenoch on the Clyde, thence by train to Dorking. Our hospital took over an estate consisting of three large homes; the hospital in one, the male officers in the second, and the nursing sisters in the third. The enlisted men were in huts on the grounds. The drawing room in the hospital became an operating room, and we began to take surgical patients almost immediately. We had to improvise a great deal, as much of our equipment, linens, etc., had gone astray. Instruments provided for us were unfamiliar and I was asked to catalogue them using names which closely approximated our usage. I recall other oddities such as 24 pairs of bandage scissors and one needle driver for a surgical unit! Instruments were always a problem; they were of poor quality and subject to rusting in the sterilizer.

Our time in Dorking was spent on schemes; patients were nursed on camp cots, we were slated for Italy, although we did not know it at the time, and were being prepared for field conditions.

In December 1943 we were issued battle dress, and by January 1944 we were on our way to Italy, this time in convoy. It was an amazing sight to see all the ships coming over the horizon on cue as they reached the mouth of the Mersey.

Our ship, the *Lancashire*, was the smallest in the convoy, and since we encountered rough seas, we were all very seasick.

We landed in Naples after two weeks at sea. The docks had been destroyed, and we disembarked on planks laid across the hulls of partly submerged ships.

Our first stop was Avellino, a badly-bombed town 60 kilometres from Naples. We took over a convent situated at the foot of Monte Vergine. There was an ancient monastery located at the top of the mountain, which the monks occupied in the winter. In summer they lived in another monastery, located on the flat near our hospital. Here they grew all their produce for the winter.

In Avellino we served the Canadian base reinforcement group, took medical cases, some elective surgery, and some bomb casualties. The building was stone and very cold. The only heat was in the kitchen. The piped water was cold only. Toilets had a drop pipe which went down three storeys to the ground – they did not flush. A bathtub was installed in the cellar for the nurses from which we had to chase the little lizards which were everywhere.

Because the Army was busy unloading guns and ammunition for the final attack on Cassino, we were unable to obtain our hospital supplies and had to improvise gowns, masks, etc. The operating room was heated by a wood stove, so we could not use ether. Spinal anaesthetics were the norm. The nursing sisters provided their own sheets for the one patient we inherited from the previous hospital. I was surprised when coming on duty to see him wearing my "mother hubbard."

On May 11th we were under canvas on Highway No. 6, about 13 kilometres from Cassino. We were one of a number of medical units strung along the highway, prepared for the attack on Cassino and the Gustav Line. The attack began at 11:00 P.M. on schedule. By midnight all staff were on duty. Medical facilities of the Second Polish Corps were too close to the action and had been destroyed, so we took their casualties as well as our own. The fact that we had 200 beds meant nothing. When we ran out of beds we used stretchers.

While we were under canvas in May 1944 the weather was very hot. The nursing sisters were wearing khaki woollen battle dress because their cotton uniforms had not arrived. Seeing khaki shorts at the officer's shop one day we purchased them for wearing in our off duty hours. When the colonel and the matron saw them, they told us to wear them on duty. It seemed sensible at the time. They were knee length and we wore knee length socks with them. The patients didn't even seem to notice.

All went well until the area matron-in-chief decided to visit our hospital. Apparently, there was quite a scene and the shorts disappeared. Fifty years later one wonders at the commotion over such a sensible solution. For some years later, when I was living in Toronto, whenever No. 3 General was mentioned one would hear, *"Oh! Yours was the hospital where the nurses wore shorts."* What a thing to be famous for.

While at Cassino No. 1 Mobile Hygiene Laboratory was attached to our hospital. It did necessary lab tasks and later supervised the distribution of penicillin. I gave one dose of penicillin to a seriously wounded patient but it was all the lab had, but it was too little and too late. This was my first knowledge of penicillin, but very soon after it was available for all our wounded. It was administered by hypodermic into the buttocks and was very painful. The lab stayed with us throughout our time in Italy.

The Allies were now on the offensive and moving quickly. On June 4th, No. 3 was ordered to Farentino. Upon arriving we were instructed to keep going to Anagni. At our destination we were met by two officers who said. *"Nurses! We're just setting up a field dressing station."* Reply: *"Well we are here to set up a hospital."*

We were located in a beautiful building, formerly a school for the sons of Italian officers from the three services. The Germans had departed in haste but not before removing doorknobs and handles from taps. An amputated limb was left on a shelf and I found an anti-personnel mine in a desk drawer. Also, their dead had not been properly buried and the graves opened in the heat.

Shortly after our arrival the Canadians withdrew for rest and regrouping and we were placed under the command of the British. It was an unhappy experience for the most part. British soldiers were used to rigid discipline, and they misunderstood the relationship between the Canadian soldier and his officers. Our soldiers knew what the limits were, and it was possible to maintain a relaxed attitude with them since they never tested the nursing sister's rank and authority. The British soldiers, on the other hand, were insolent and un-cooperative. To add to our unhappiness, a soldier who had been AWL was admitted with a very bad case of smallpox. He had been living with an Italian family

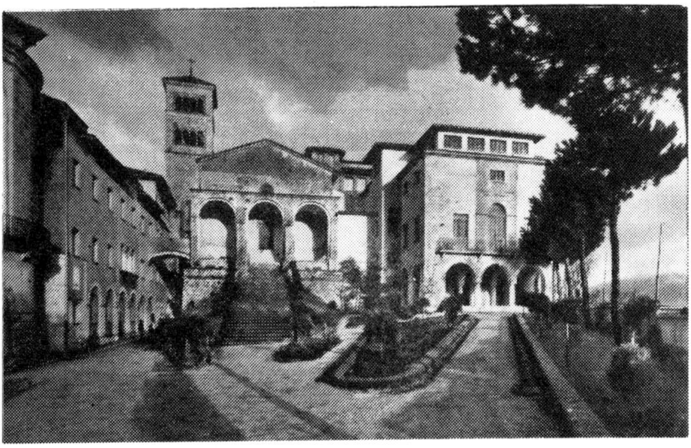

Convitto "Principe Di Piemonte," ANAGNI, No. 3 Mobile Surgical Hospital was stationed here for a time News of D-Day reached us here.

and was apparently a conscientious objector. The hospital was quarantined by the British and it took some time for our colonel to convince the British authorities that there was no such thing as a "conscientious objector" in the Canadian Army. We were all vaccinated. After this the patient was quarantined with two nurses and a medical officer and the hospital was operating again.

During this time, Rome fell to the Allies and we were able to visit. Some of us had audiences with the Pope which was very exciting. We were still in Anagni for D-Day, June 6, 1944.

In July of 1944 the hospital returned to Avellino to occupy the same convent as formerly. We were not happy about the move as we wanted to be in the action.

Morale improved when the hospital was ordered north again on October 1, 1944. This time we were in Riccione on the Adriatic. We established the hospital in buildings owned by the Fiat works and used as a summer resort for their employees.

The weather was cold and rainy and eventually we had wet snow. The grounds were in a sea of mud. Planks were laid from building to building, or we would have walked out of our shoes.

The mobile laboratory, a trailer, sank in the mud up to its hubs and was not hauled out until spring. I remember this as a time of stress for everyone.

The Canadians were inactive when we set up and we were taking medical cases. We admitted many flu cases and diphtheria was occurring at a rate to cause real concern. It was decided that all throat cases would be swabbed on admission and those who tested positive for diphtheria would be moved to an isolation ward.

This meant that staff were involved in moving beds from one ward to another, moving charts, rewriting patient nominal rolls and treatment, sheets every morning as soon as the lab reports were received. I recall it as a nightmare since the turnover was so heavy.

Early in December plans were made to cross the Lamone River. Medical cases were evacuated with 100 beds retained for diphtheria cases. Two additional surgical teams from base, one Canadian and one British were added to our strength.

The British medical officers disapproved of the joint mess at No. 3 General. With the small number of officers on our strength we could not have maintained two messes. They were stiff and unfriendly. Their nursing sisters would not enter the mess in spite of urging, choosing instead to remain in their rather gloomy quarters. They were required to join us for meals otherwise they would not have eaten. We felt sorry for them, they seemed so "brow-beaten."

The wounded were transported down to base hospitals in Perugia, almost on an assembly-line basis. I hated to see them moved on so quickly, but it was necessary. I would raid the Red Cross cupboard of woollens, give them morphine which was recorded on field charts tied to their ankles, and hope they would sleep until they reached their destination.

We spent Christmas in Riccione. While there, Agnes McLeod, Matron-in-Chief, Mediterranean Theatre, visited the hospital and informed us that all nursing sisters who had been in Italy for 18 months would be returned to England. However, shortly after the hospital became part of the 21st Army group destined for the European Theatre. We were moved in convoy to Naples where we boarded a ship for Marseilles, from there by air to Brussels. After leaving London the hospital set up in Tilburg, Holland, again in a convent.

Tilburg was close to the front lines, and we became used to the sound of buzz bombs flying over the hospital each day at dawn. From Tilburg we moved to Utrecht. It was a short stay. After 24 hours, a British hospital took over and we moved into a monastery in Nijmegen. Our patients were in temporary huts throughout the grounds. We were there for VE Day, after which our caseload changed. Released Allied prisoners-of-war walked into the first Canadian establishment they encountered. They were suffering from conditions largely related to malnutrition and poor living conditions and soon picked up. This was not the case with the concentration camp victims, which the Army brought to us. They were in a most appalling state. They were living skeletons, beyond speech, but their eyes were eloquent. They understood that they were safe at last, but it was too late. None who reached our hospital survived.

The civilians were starving, and the hospital fed many, but it was heartbreaking to be unable to assist with some serious medical conditions, such as diabetes, as we had no insulin.

From Nijmegen we moved to Apeldoorn, where Capt. N/S Kay Lunn came to us as matron. Here our hospital was inactive, and in June 1945 it was disbanded. I was among the nursing sisters scheduled for Canada. After a short stay in Ghent we returned to England, and on July 8, 1945 we were shipped to

Canada on the *Nieuw Amsterdam*, then by troop train to British Columbia.

I had volunteered for the Pacific Theatre, but while I was on leave VJ Day signaled the end of the war. I then asked for my discharge and left for Toronto to study social work at the University of Toronto.

I believe it was reassuring to our soldiers to have women in the services. We could bring some warmth and kindness to what was essentially a grim situation. One could not, however, maintain the professional detachment of civilian life. Every man and woman in the Army was your brother or sister; if they died, you grieved. Few who managed to reach a hospital died, but when they did, it was difficult to accept, and the sadness pervaded the whole hospital.

Helen (Hill) Holmes

Graduated from: Galt Hospital School of Nursing, Lethbridge, Alberta.

Military History:

Service: RCAMC

Rank: Lt. N/S

Served: Two years

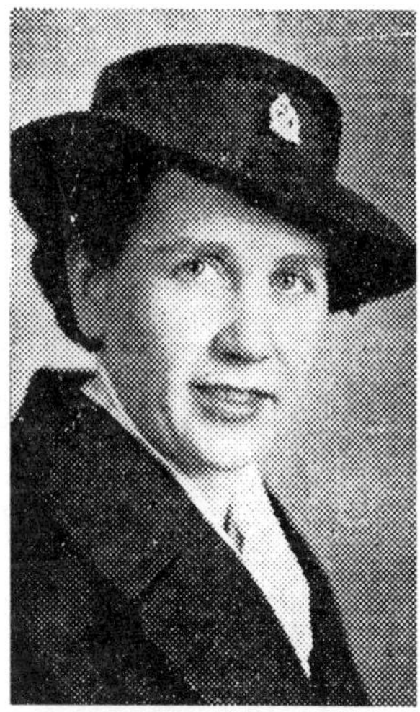

Lt. N/S Helen (Hill) Holmes

Love of my country influenced me to choose a military career.

I was with the British 8th Army at Cassino. Anything and everything was used for a hospital. Sometimes it would be an old convent, but in spite of all this, the courage and cheerfulness of the boys was really wonderful.

There was little or no recreation for the patients. All the magazines were back-dated number the boys read over and over again. There was one radio and it was in very poor condition.

When a ward of soldiers was all set to go home, they all stood at their beds, shook hands and said, *"Good-bye sister – you've been a sister and a nursing sister to us."*

I was lucky to meet movie star Marlene Dietrich when she

was guest of honour at a cocktail party.

While in Rome I met two Lethbridge men, Lt. Col. A. H. Warr and Major Earl Clemis. I was present at an audience of Pope Pius. I also was present when Mount Vesuvius erupted. It was a most spectacular sight with surprisingly few casualties.

However, the thing that impressed me the most was how wonderful our Canadian soldiers were. They were "tops"!

After I got home from the war I took my uniform to the war museum in Ottawa. Later I went back to see if they had displayed it. I asked a young chap who worked there to find it and he said, "Which war ma'am?"

I was glad to go overseas. I spent a year in England and a year in Italy. I was glad to stay put for a while at Suffield, Alberta, when I got home.

I married a year later to a perfect man. He died in 1989. We had four children. Our first died at birth; our second, a daughter, died at the age of seven from leukemia; our third child, a son is healthy; and our fourth, a daughter, suffered brain damage at birth.

NO. 4 CANADIAN GENERAL HOSPITAL

Theresa (Vidal) Gallacher
Margaret (Ross) Ward

Authority was granted on 13 December 1943 for the formation of No. 4 Canadian General Hospital as a 600-bed hospital for service overseas. The unit was mobilized in Sherbrooke, Quebec, and personnel were drawn from military districts across Canada.

Matron Helen L. Shanks and nursing sisters began arriving in February 1944.

The unit along with Nos. 19 and 20 General Hospitals embarked on the *Empress of Scotland* 3 May 1944 and arrived in Liverpool a week later to be assigned to Aldershot.

No. 4 General was designated as a railway transit hospital. It had the role of transit hospital for the flow of casualties evacuated from the other side of the channel after D-Day.

The unit remained in England until October 1945.

Theresa M. (Vidal) Gallagher

Graduated from: Holy Cross Hospital School of Nursing, Calgary, Alberta. Year: 1939

Military History:

Service: RCAMC

Rank: Lt. N/S

Served: June 1943 to August 1946

I chose a military career because I hoped as a nurse I would be of help caring for the sick and wounded from the Armed Services.

After I joined the RCAMC in June 1943, I was stationed at Currie Barracks, Calgary, Alberta. From there I was attached to No. 4 Canadian General Hospital. We spent six weeks in Sherbrooke, Quebec, waiting for transport overseas.

We (my sister Barbara Vidal and I) were billeted at a private home, which proved to be very enjoyable. No. 4 CGH finally arrived in Farnborough, Sussex, where we took over from No. 8 General.

The highlight of my stay there was when we were a CCS following D-Day. I was an OR nurse; we had 60 patients a day (following D-Day) to be attended to before they were shipped on to a base hospital. We worked 12-hour shifts with teams of an MO and nurse. It was exciting, exacting and tiring, but we were so thankful to have experienced all of this.

My sister and I were next in line, once we were a base hospital, to go to the Continent. However, by this time the powers-to-be had received a request from the American Medical Corps for 50 nursing sisters who had overseas experience to join the AMC and hospital units to go to the Pacific Region.

We were sent to Bramshott to wait to mobilize for this next venture, as they were drawing nursing sisters from the different zones – Italy, the Continent and England. After a month in Bramshott we sailed for Canada, but enroute "the bomb" was dropped, so that was the end of our careers as nursing sisters in or near action.

After a leave, I worked in Calgary and Edmonton until I obtained my discharge in August 1946. My sister went on to

Public Health at which she was active until her death from cancer in 1969.

We both felt we were most fortunate to have served as nursing sisters. Besides the interesting and rewarding duties we were able to perform, we made many friends and saw as much of England and Ireland as we could with the travel bans in force. It was all unforgettable and we were very grateful for this opportunity in our lives.

Margaret Elizabeth (Ross) Ward

Graduated from: Regina General Hospital School of Nursing.
Year: 1941

Military History:

Service: RCAMC

Rank: Lt. N/S

Served: 14 January 1944 to April 1946

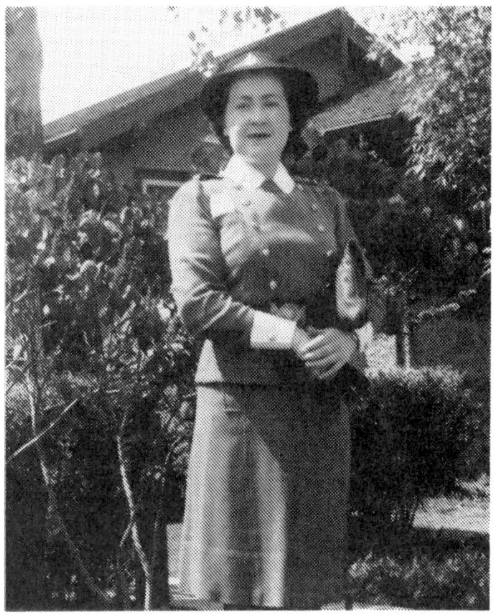

Lt. N/S Margaret (Ross) Ward

No. 4 Canadian General at Farnborough, Hants, England, was the Duke of Connaught Hospital used by Florence Nightingale in the Crimean War. It was old and creaky and cold with only fireplaces for heat.

After D-Day convoys came in with wounded on stretchers. We did not have enough beds so stretchers were lined on the floor. We worked 12 hours with no days off for several months after D-Day. We gave massive doses of penicillin every 4 hours, most times the only ID we had to work with was their field card.

On a lighter note:

I met my husband, he was then a patient who had been injured in Italy. Incidentally, he was English but in the Canadian Army. He asked me to go home with him one weekend, so I told the girls who lived in the cottage. They were horrified and said, "An Englishman never asks a girl home unless he intends to marry her." There was no such intention at that time.

However, he was transferred and I was repatriated. We wrote each other but never got any letters.

After the war, I came out to Vancouver for my discharge – faked a holiday intending to go to McGill in the fall. It so happened the fellow in charge of discharging knew my husband and knew me; so consequently, he gave Les my phone number. Forty-six years after we are still Mr. & Mrs. Ward.

Itinerary:

Left Regina, arrived in Truro, Nova Scotia (a mud hole), left Halifax; boarded Hospital Ship *Lady Nelson*. Miss Rossiter was matron.

I was seasick the whole trip, so sat out on deck most of the time. A private from the laundry staff used to bring me crackers and jelly. One nurse had to have IVs for her seasickness.

Arrived in Liverpool, Euston Station, then Bramshott and then Aldershot.

Came home on the *Nieuw Amsterdam*, a beautiful crossing, not a ripple.

Looking back over the years, I think it was an invaluable experience and I have many happy memories.

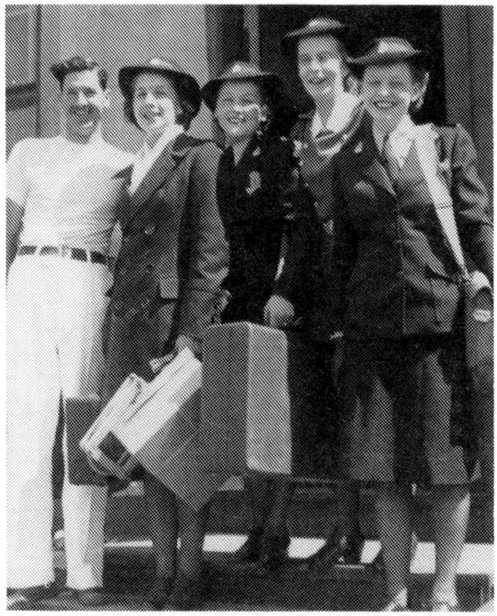

L-R: Marc, Lts. N/S Grace Porter, Laura Anderson, Ann Townsend, and Mary Taber enroute from Camp Dundurn, Saskatchewan

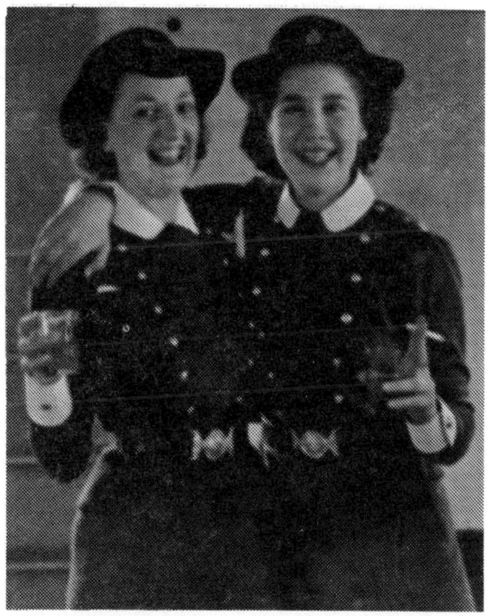

Clarice Steeves and Grace Porter at a party in the mess at No. 4 CGH

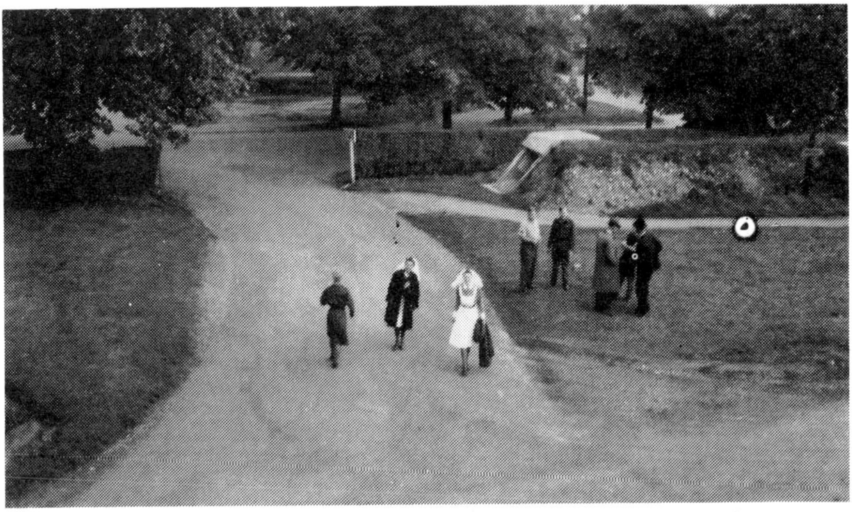

Going on duty, No. 4 CGH, Duke of Connaught Hospital, Farnborough, Hants, England. Used by Florence Nightingale in the Crimean War. It was old and creaky and cold, just fireplaces for heat.

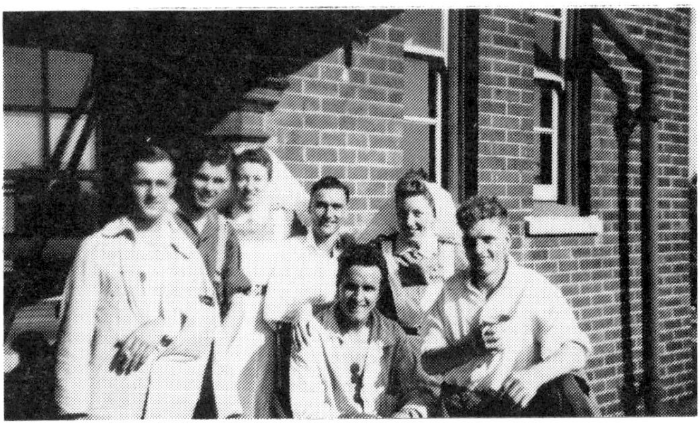

D-Day casualties, No. 4 CGH

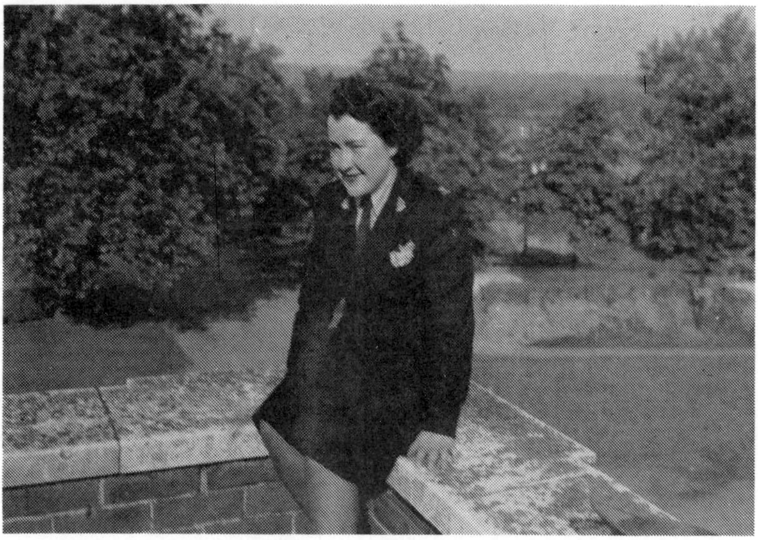

Margaret (Ross) Ward on roof of hospital at No. 4 CGH

NO. 5 CANADIAN GENERAL HOSPITAL

Muriel (Cascaden) Guyot
Elizabeth (Burnham) Lawson Lowe
Helen (Ross) O'Brien
Anna (Allen) Swail
(Dolly) Mabel (Vincent) Watkins

No. 5 Canadian General Hospital mobilized as a 600-bed unit in Winnipeg, September of 1939, and arrived in Halifax January 1940, to embark on the *Monarch of Bermuda.* They left Halifax for the U.K. and officially opened their hospital at the Cliveden estate of Lord and Lady Astor. It had been equipped by the Canadian Red Cross Society and handed over to the Army in 1940.

In July of 1943 the unit embarked on the SS *Franconia* and sailed in convoy for Italy. By the end of July they were operating a 400-bed hospital in Syracus, Sicily. Six months later they were enroute to Italy and set up their hospital in Andria, moving as often as the situation demanded.

As the campaign in Italy wound down, No. 5 General prepared to move to north west Europe. By March of 1945 they were located in Belgium acting as a base hospital. In September of 1945 the hospital was disbanded at Turnhout.

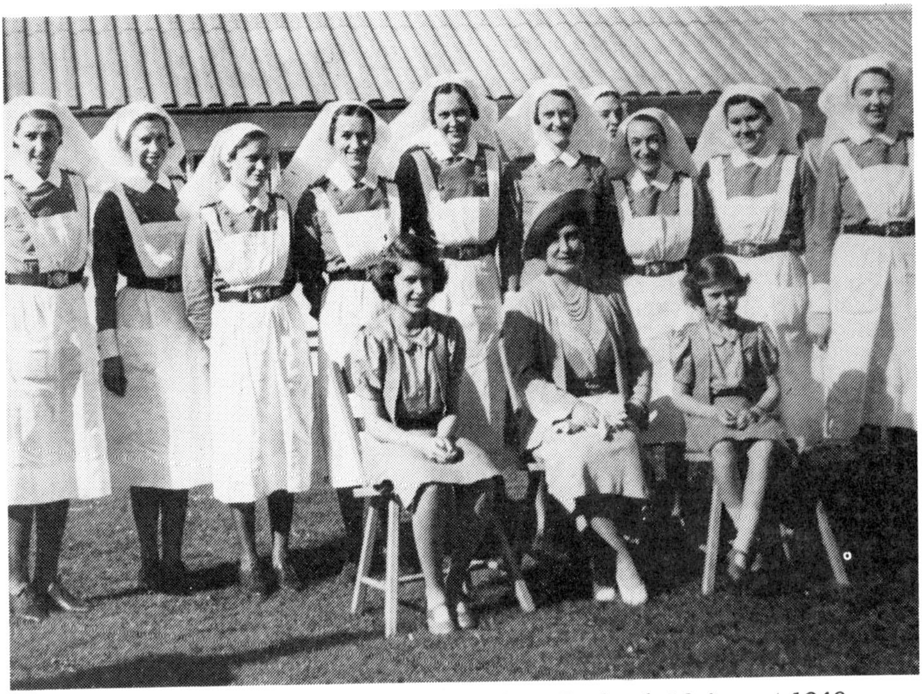

No. 5 Canadian General Hospital, Taplow, England, 10 August 1940.
BACK ROW, L-R: Nursing Sisters Pearl Lungren; Frances Wait; M. Stanley; Dorothy Lowe; Ann Miller; Kay Lunn; F. McLeod; A. Clake; Muriel Cascaden; Anna (Allen) Swail (partly hidden).
Princess Elizabeth, Queen Elizabeth, and Princess Margaret.
Loaned by Muriel Cascaden Guyot, No. 5 CGH

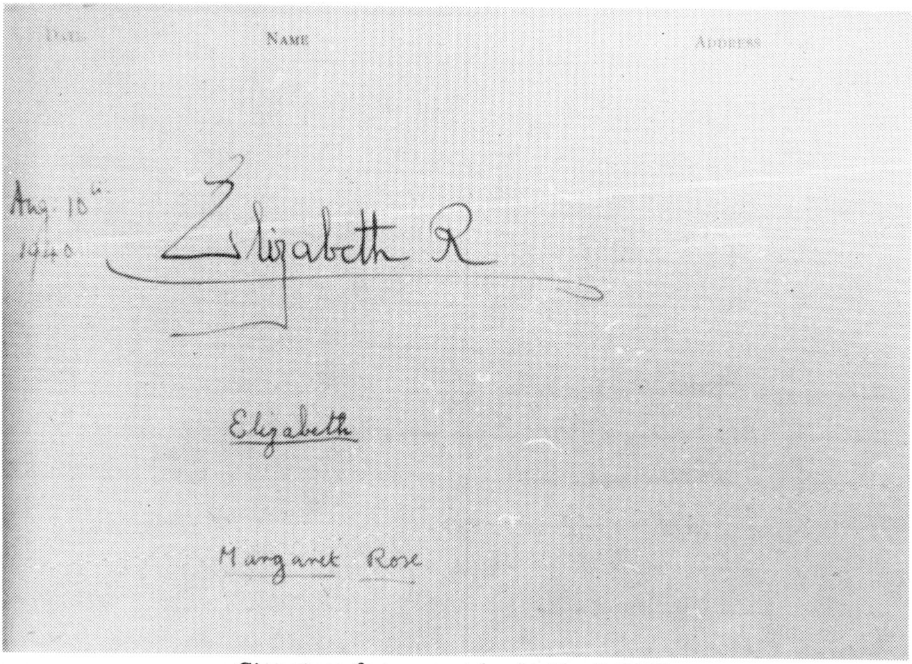

Signature from guest book, No. 5 CGH

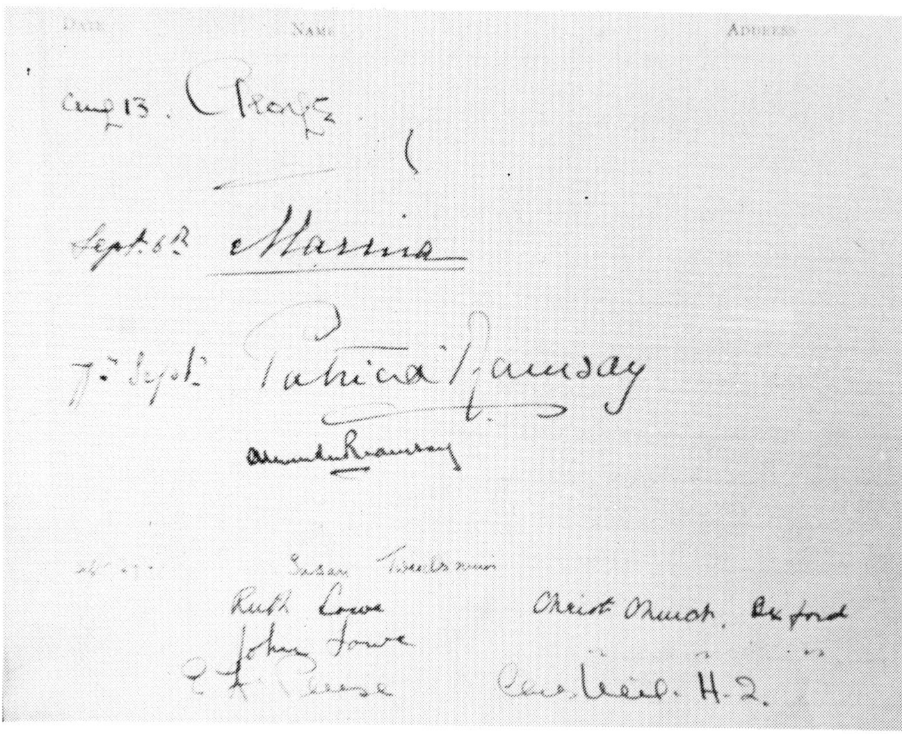

Signature from guest book No. 5 CGH

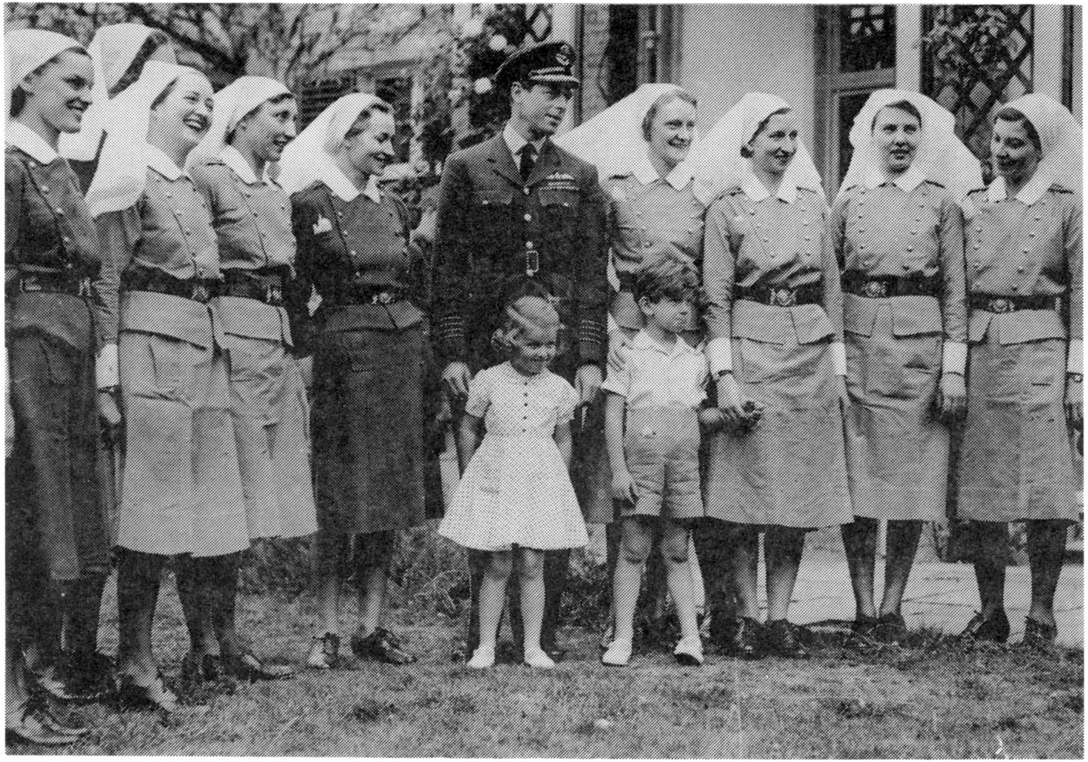

No. 5 Canadian General Hospital, Taplow, England.
Nursing Sisters with the Duke of Kent, 1940. Nursing Sisters L-R: Grandy; Irene Lang; Alice Nicholson; Dorothy Lowe; George Duke of Kent; Matron Lunn; Olive Meadows; Muriel Cascaden; Clare Brazier.
FRONT ROW: Princess Alexandra, Prince Edward, present Duke of Kent.
Loaned by Muriel Cascaden Guyot, No. 5 CGH

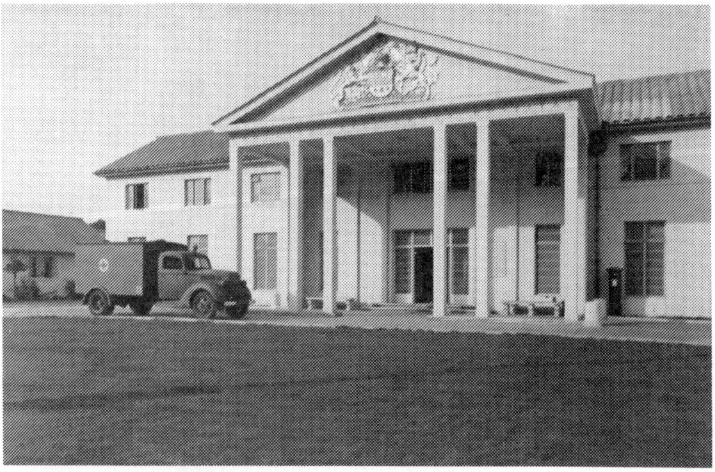

Ambulance arrives

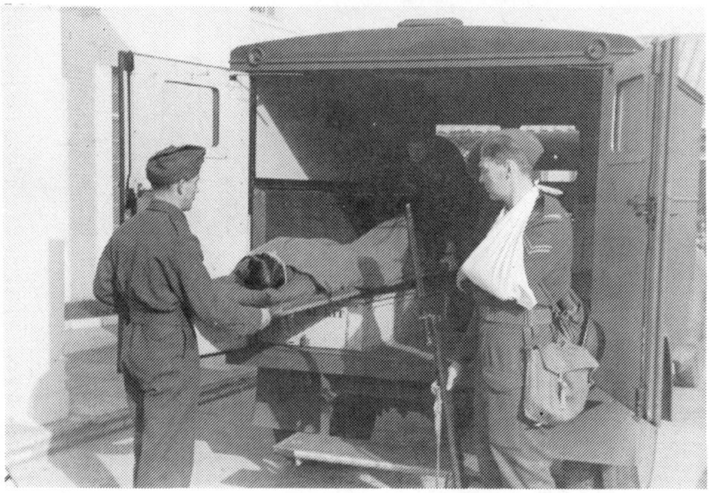

One stretcher case and one walking case

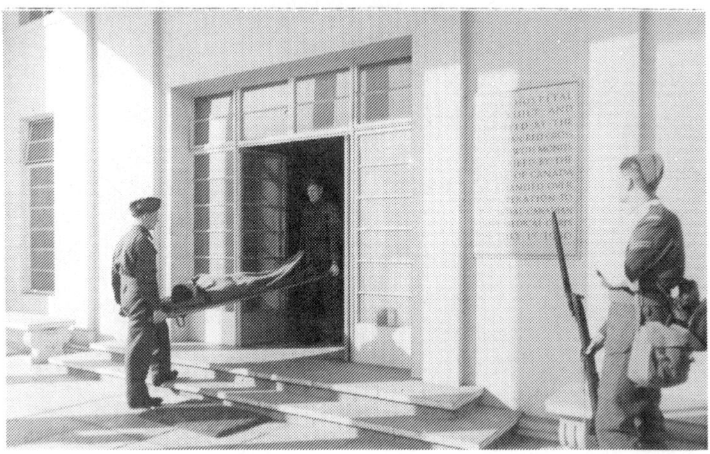

One goes in and one pauses

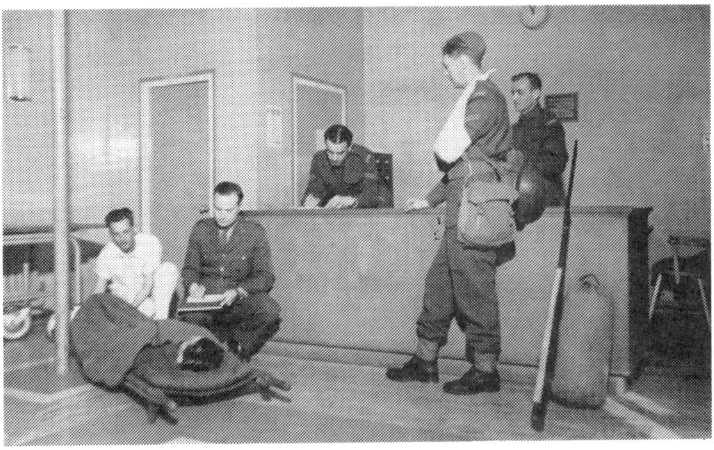

The admitting room

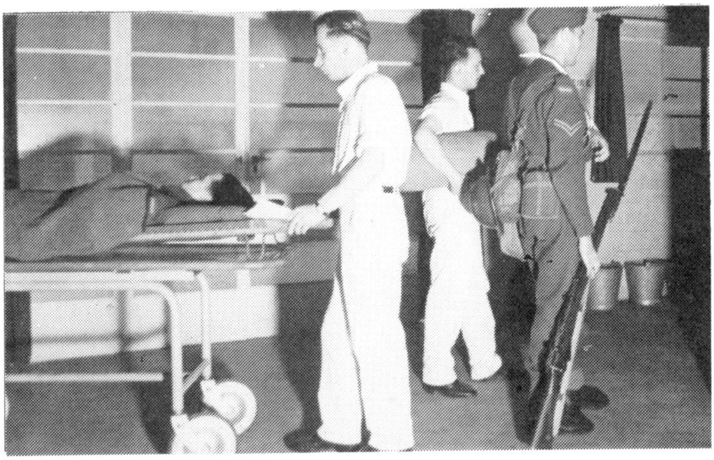

Stretcher case to ward and walking case to pack strores

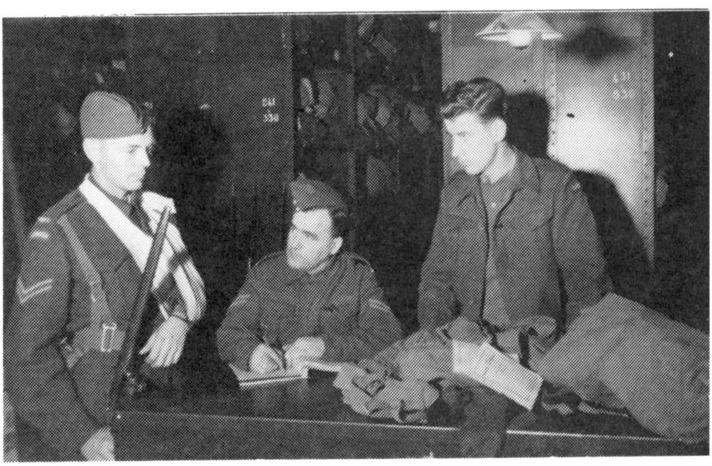

Turns in his pack

Draws his hospital blues

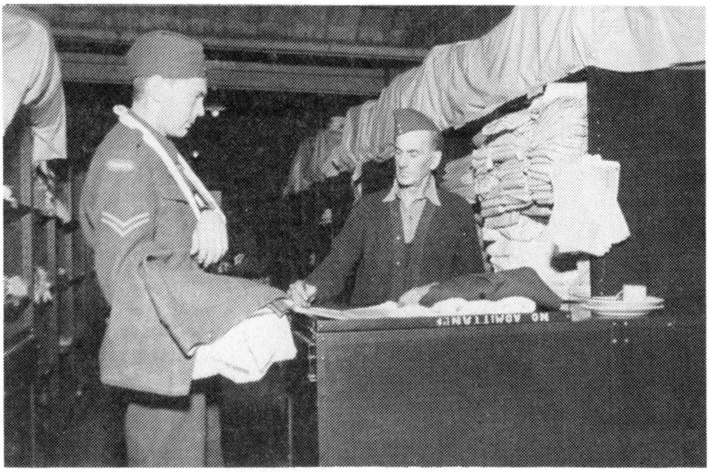

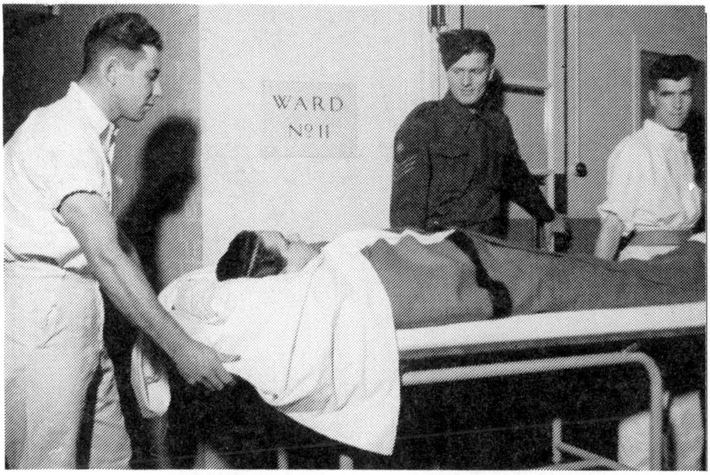

Stretcher case reaches ...

The ward

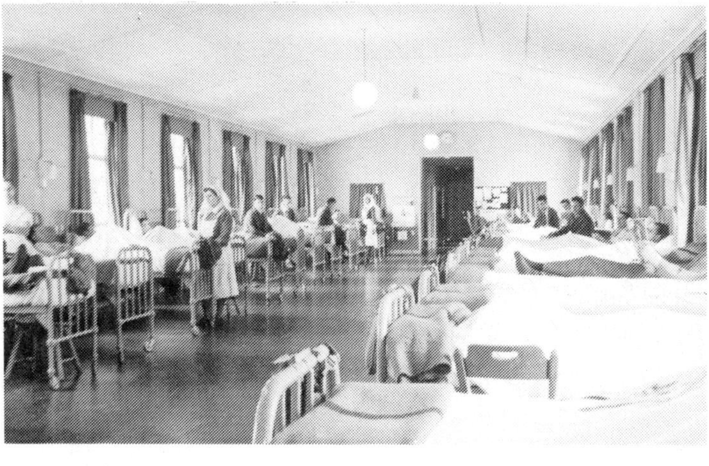

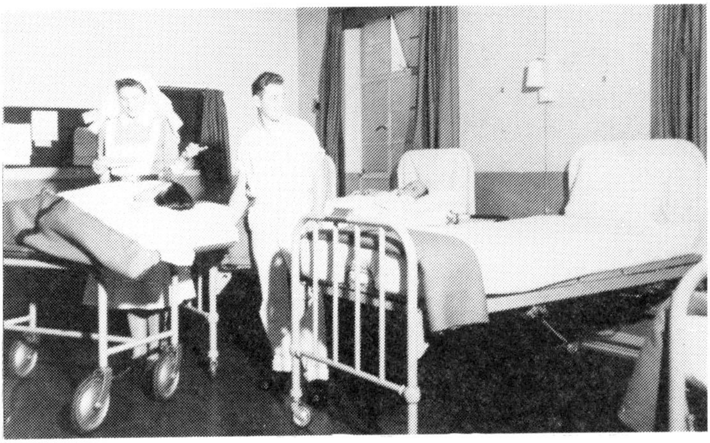

The empty bed

The examination

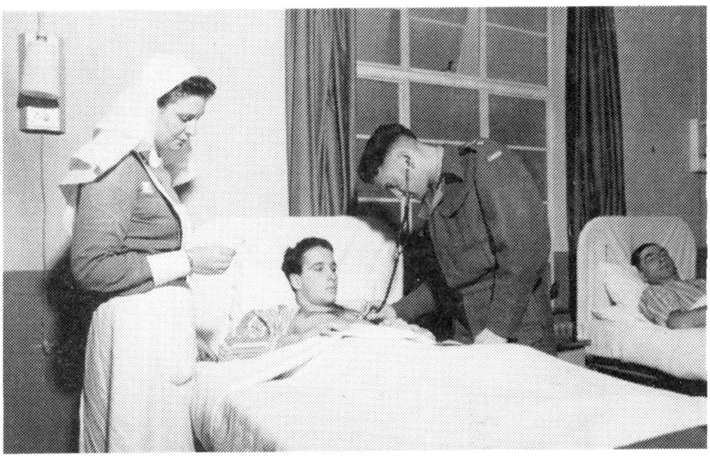

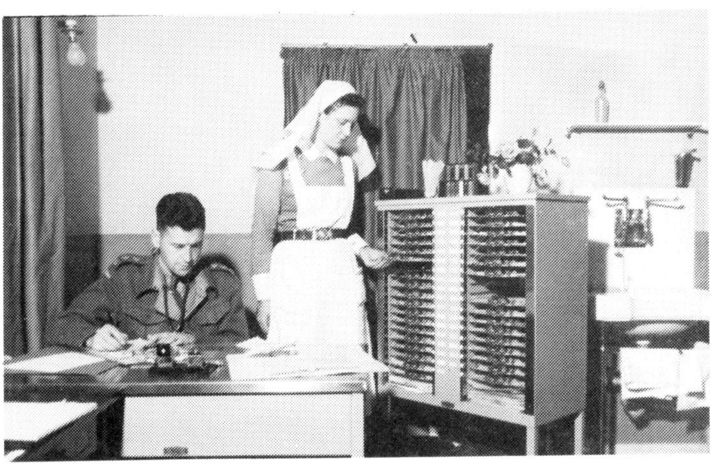

The history and orders

Technician takes blood

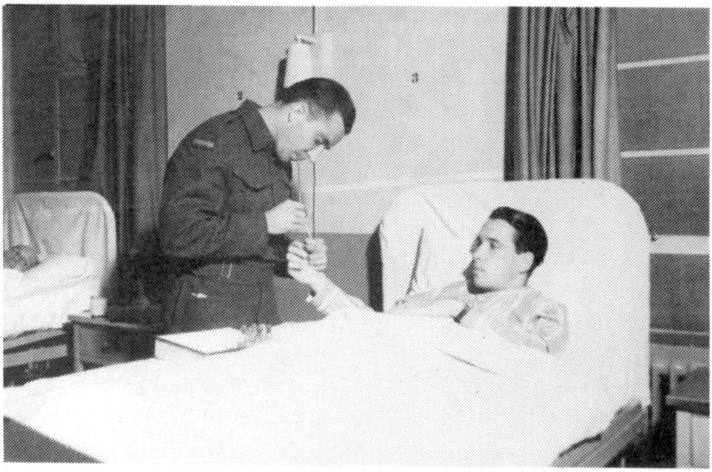

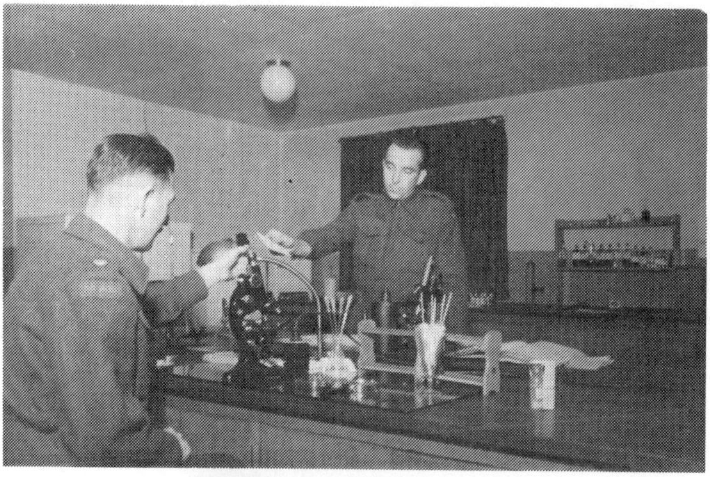

The pathology laboratory reports findings

The Canadian Red Cross visitor gives him a can of soup

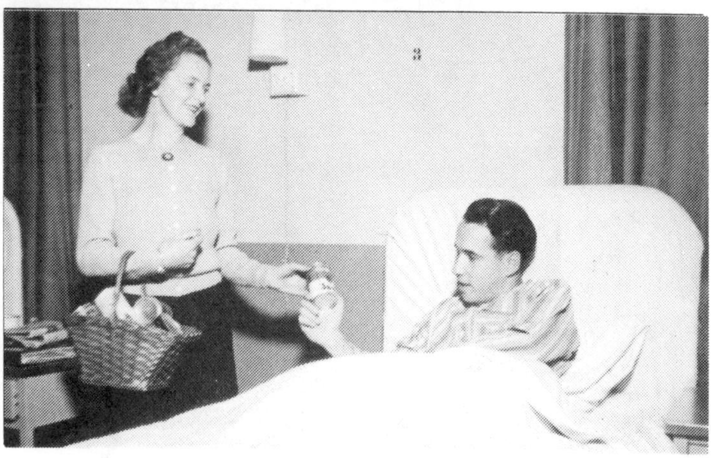

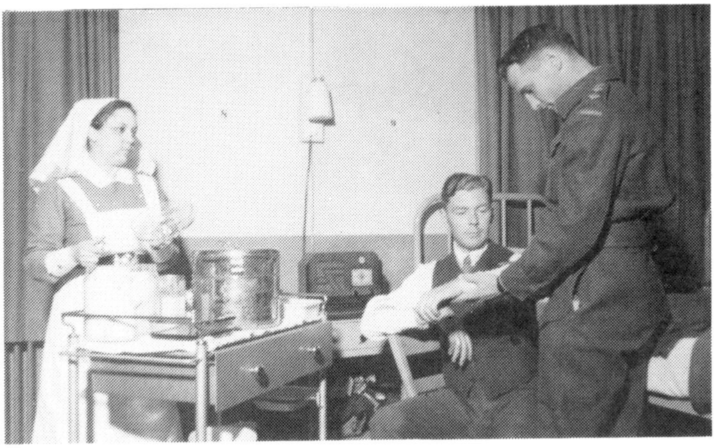

Walking case on the ward. The MO removes the dressing

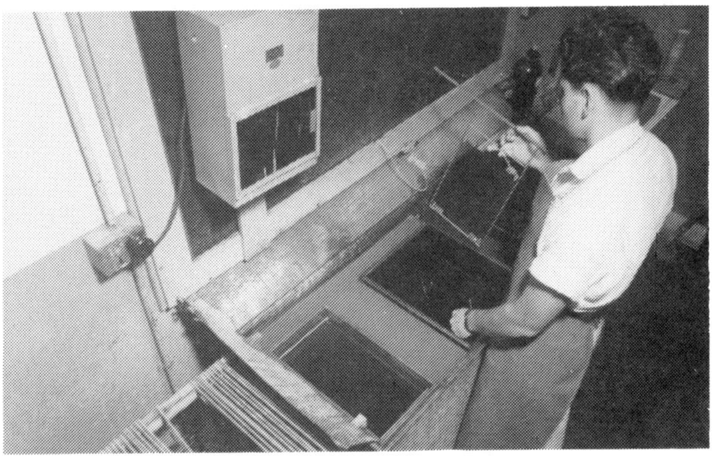

X-ray is made, developed and checked

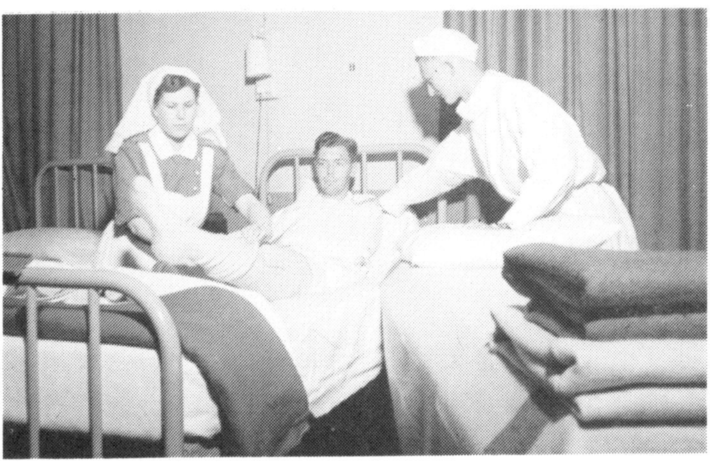

"It's the operating room for you!"

Operating room supplies are made

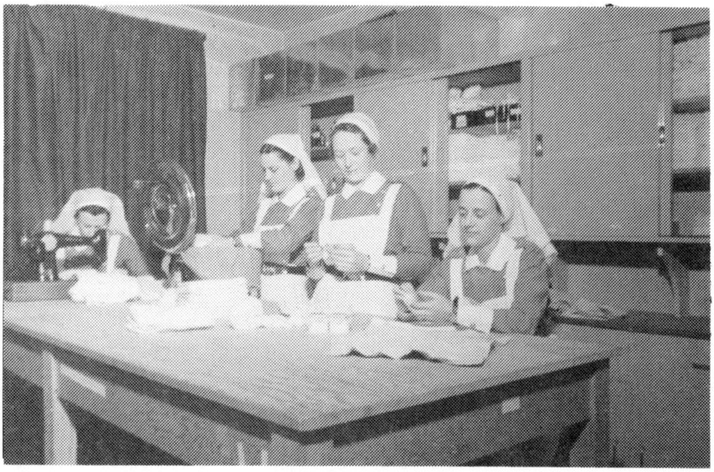

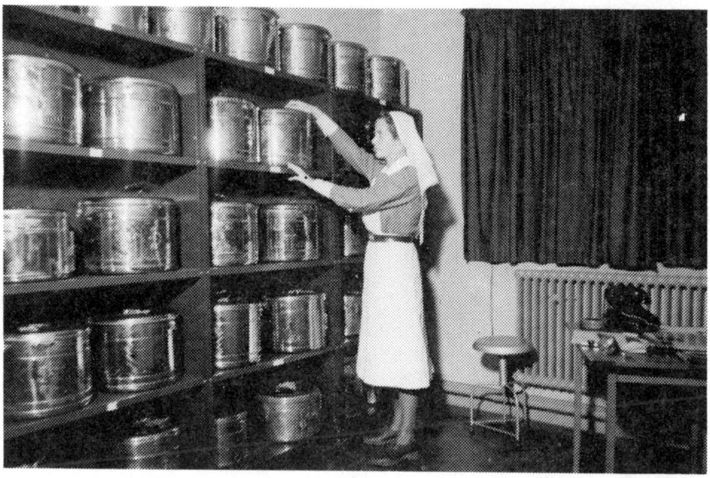

Sterile supplies for the operating room

After boiling, the instruments are given to the "surgical sister"

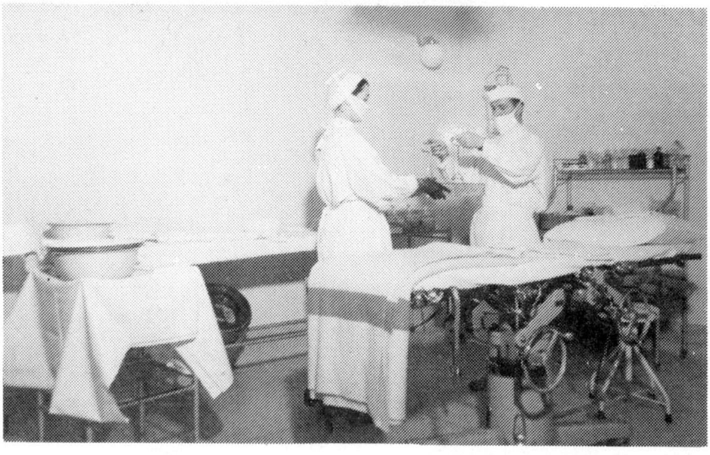

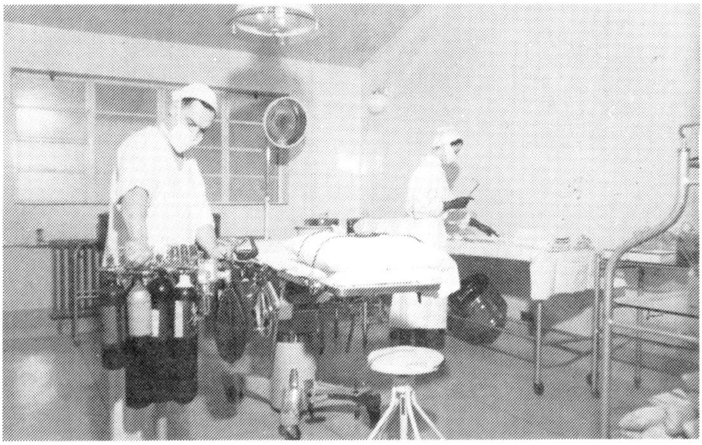

Gettting ready for the operation

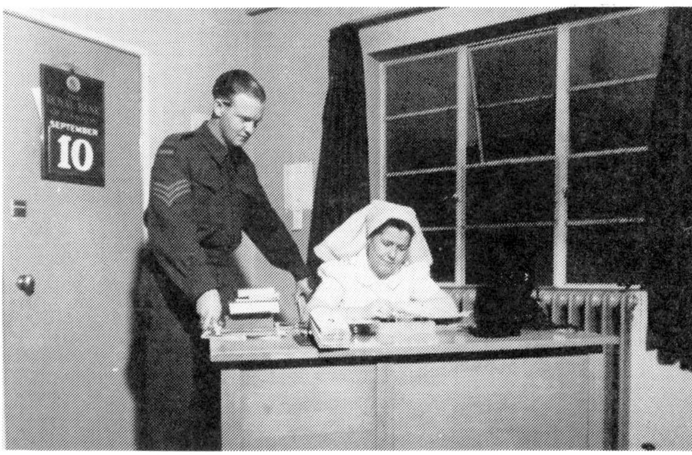

Dietitian and steward make up the diets

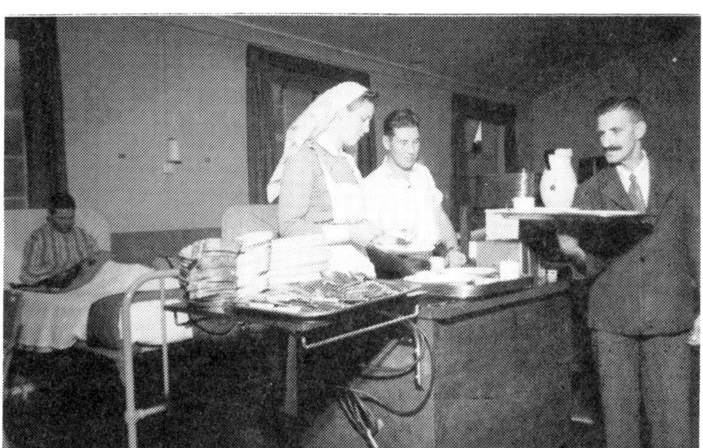

Dinner is served on the wards

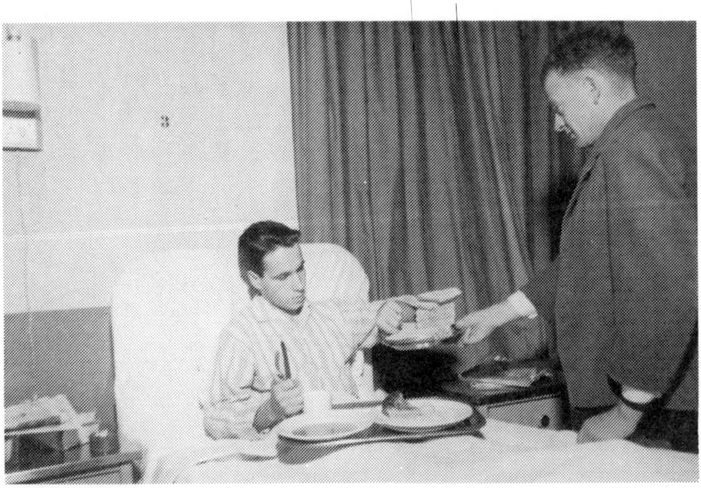

Patients appetite has returned

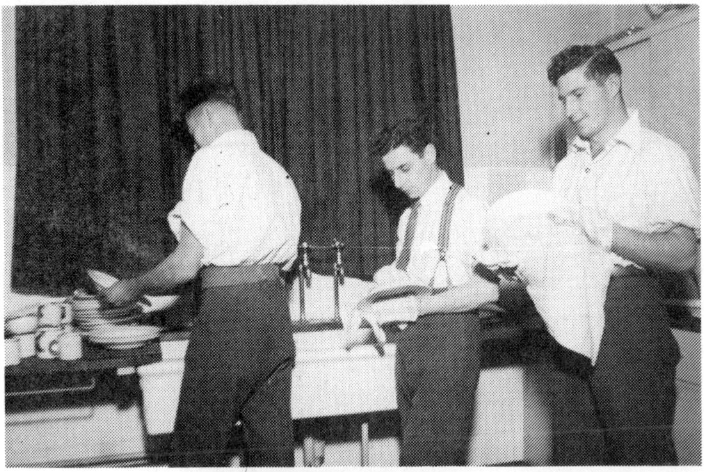

Our patient will help, too, in a few days

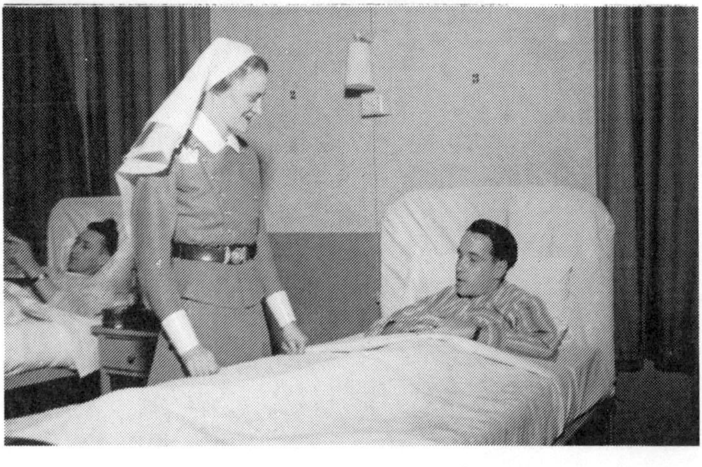

Matron Kay Lunn makes her rounds

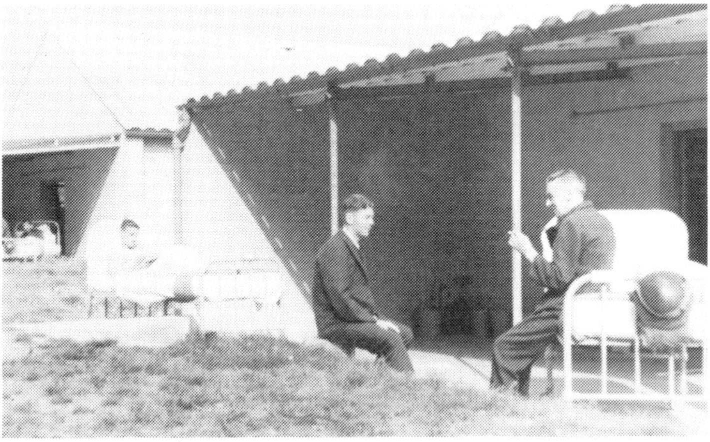

Gossip on the ward's back porch

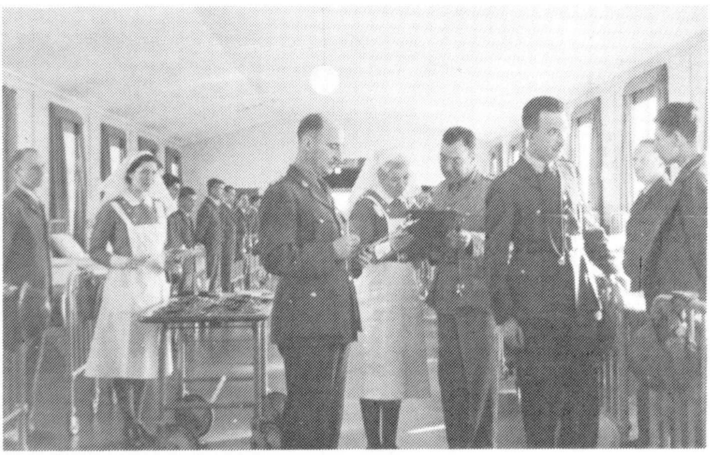

Medical officers ward rounds

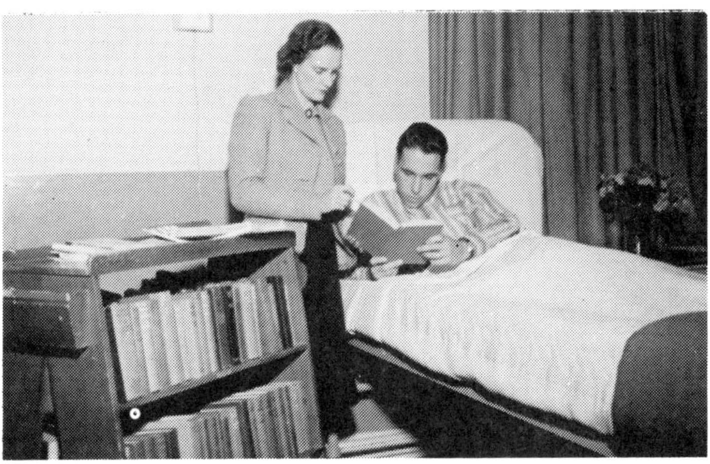

Red Cross librarian offers a book

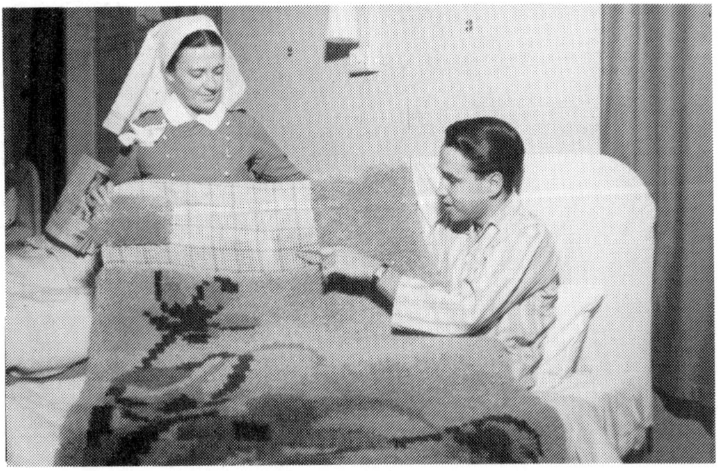

Assistant Matron Anna (Allen) Swail finds patients almost finished handicraft provided by Canadian Red Cross

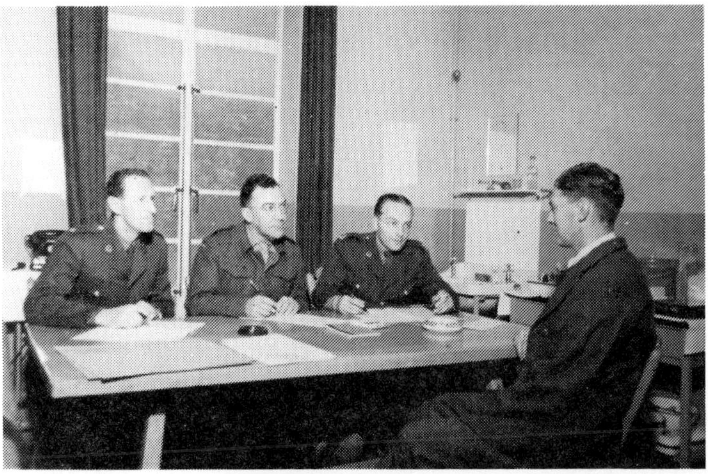

The medical board review his category

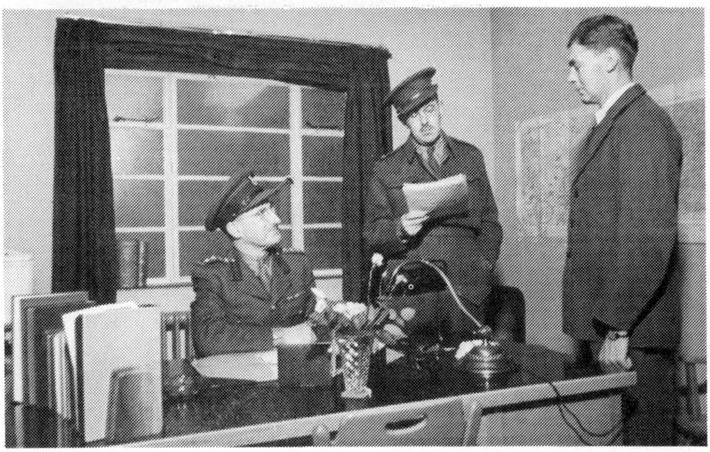

Commanding officer's interview before patient leaves the hospital

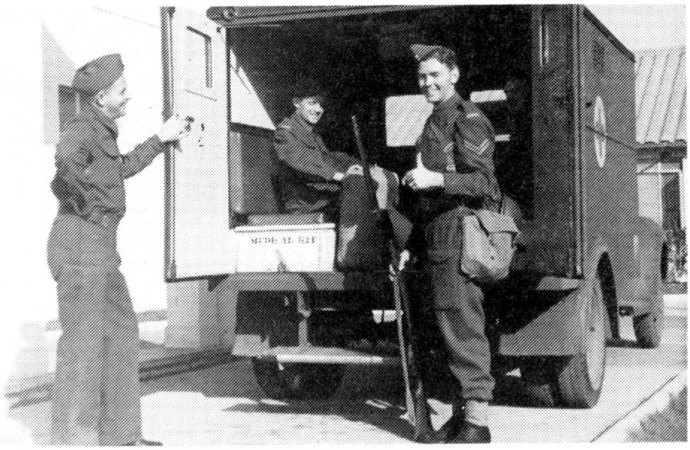

Goodbye and good luck

Muriel (Cascaden) Guyot

Graduated from: The Brandon Hospital School of Nursing, Manitoba. Year: 1938

Military History:

Service: RCAMC

Rank Lt. N/S

Served: December 1939 to July 1946

I joined No. 5 Canadian General Hospital in Winnipeg, Manitoba. I worked periodically at Deer Lodge Hospital until June 1940 when we left for England. No. 5 General was located at Taplow, Bucks, on the Astor estate called Cliveden.

In 1943 No. 5 was sent to Sicily. I was stationed at Catania, Sicily from August 1943 to January 1944 when we were air lifted to Bari, Italy. We proceeded north to Andria. Here we worked in tents. From Andria I was sent up to 5th Casualty Clearing Station. From there to Field Surgical Unit with Helen Dycke and Alice Ecland, where we worked in the Field Dressing Station following the lines of battle as they progressed.

I returned to Canada in 1945 and was discharged in 1946.

Elizabeth L. (Burnham) Lowe

Graduated from: Saint John General Hospital School of Nursing, Saint John, N.B. Year: 1939

Military History:

Service: RCAMC

Rank: Lt. N/S

Service: August 1940 to June 1945

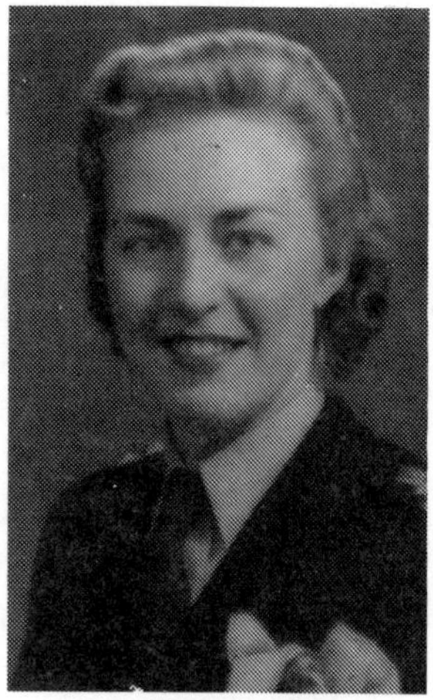

Lt N/S Elizabeth (Burnham) Lawson

When I graduated in January 1939 it never occurred to me not to sign up for "war and disaster." If Canada was going to be at war, I felt that is where I would want to be. I joined up, the first of three nursing sisters to be enlisted in New Brunswick. I was lucky to be able to go on to No. 5 CGH in England four months later.

We had had three glorious years in England enjoying the facilities of the Astor Estate in Cliveden, punting on the Thames and spending our days off in London. I had arrived Christmas Eve 1940 with the first reinforcements to join 5th CGH, a Winnipeg Unit which, with the No. 15 CGH from Toronto, were the first military hospitals to arrive in England six months earlier. No. 5 CGH was stationed in Taplow in a well-equipped hospital outfitted by the Canadian Red Cross. We were busy enough on duty as the troops were going through extensive training and along with the usual illnesses, travelling the narrow English roads in the blackout during schemes resulted in a heavy toll of fractures. However, it seemed that we Canadians were never to take part in the War and we settled down to a pretty normal life. In January 1943, nursing sisters were finally allowed to remain in the service if they married. I, and several others, took advantage of this and although we didn't become "Mrs." we went on orders as having a name change and I became Lieut. N/S Lawson instead of Burnham.

In May 1943, our easy life came to a sudden halt. Almost overnight our patients were transferred to other hospitals in southern England and our staff went under canvas. We nurses were given lectures on tropical diseases and taught the intricacies of drill and route marching, along with saluting. Rumors were rampant as we all knew our inactive role was to end, but where and when the invasion would be was the big question.

On Dominion Day we found ourselves sailing the Mediterranean on one of the finest of troop ships, the *Franconia*, where we enjoyed sunning on the decks and sumptuous meals after our plain fare in England. At Algiers we joined up with many other Allied ships and waved to other women on decks nearby who turned out to be nursing sisters of No. 15 General Hospital enroute to North Africa.

On July 10 we finally heard news of the invasion of Sicily by Canadian and other Allied troops. With our men in action the war became more real to us and we felt excited at being able to take part. We then continued on our journey and, on July 19, nine days after the invasion, we were loaded onto landing crafts at Augusta, four miles from the front.

On the beach we were greeted with considerable consternation by those in charge as they hadn't expected nursing sisters with the first advance medical unit. We were rushed back by lorries to Syracuse and the cheers and greetings by the soldiers we passed enroute dispelled any reservations we may have felt about our situation. At this time we were still in our blue uniform, and with tin hats, packs and duffel bags, we must have been a startling sight to the soldiers passing us in the heat and dust.

We were taken to a hospital building at a mental institution and our first night was one I will never forget. We were put up in one large ward, fifty-five of us, the beds having just been vacated by the Germans who, unfortunately for us, had left the beds infested with creepy crawlies. We were given one bucket of water for our ablutions, but this time all we wanted was to settle down for the night. Heavy shelling kept on all night which didn't make us feel very relaxed. Many of us developed gyppy tummy from the oppressive heat and odd diet, and we must have been a strange sight for the guard at the front door as we filed out towards the biffy, set in the center of a clear field some distance from the hospital, dressed in housecoat and tin hat which we had kept on even in bed. One girl lit a cigarette to try and relax and we all sat up and screamed at her to douse the light. I think we were a bit overwhelmed by the constant shelling although we had gotten used to the bombing in England.

When we landed in Augusta harbour we were greeted by a large explosion which sent our dinner plates flying and we discovered that the ship nearby which was carrying our supplies had been bombed.

A British medical unit had been operating the hospital as best they could as their nursing sisters were still in North Africa. As our drugs and supplies had been lost, we had to make do with what could be confiscated from the enemy or Italians who at that time were not our allies, but co-belligerents. We had many wounded Sicilians, mainly children, who came in contact with booby traps. Their families moved right in with them to make sure we gave them good care and all enjoyed our sparse fare.

The hospital was greatly overcrowded and many patients were left on stretchers under tarpaulins outside; our 600-bed hospital soon cared for over 1000. Longer-term patients were evacuated to No. 15 General in North Africa by plane or hospital ship and there were a steady stream of admissions and discharges. In the two weeks preceding the fall of Catania, the middle of August, we admitted 3600 patients under very poor working conditions. The nurses, as well as the staff, adapted very well considering the very humid temperatures of over 90 degrees, severely rationed water, and shortage of staff. We depended on our large number of prisoners-of-war to carry out many duties. The Italian Red Cross workers remained with the hospital throughout our stay in Sicily.

After we landed, some of us were loaned out to British field ambulance units. I and five others were sent to a British air evacuation center where patients waited for transfer to the base hospital in North Africa. The patients remained on stretchers in small tents which made nursing them quite difficult. Among them were many POWs and I often wondered how they would be controlled, if necessary, by our unarmed medical staff. Our own tents were put up at a respectable distance from the men's tents, but I've questioned this decision as we were adjacent to an old road which was used by snipers.

A building adjacent to the hospital was soon made available for the nursing sisters and we were more comfortable. Those of us loaned out returned to settle into our busy routine. Some of the mental patients were in the adjacent building and they peered at us through the fence. One, a former opera singer, kept us awake in the wee hours warbling operatic lyrics. We were now wearing men's khaki bush shirts and trousers which were usually too big on top and too tight on the seat. Eventually our battle dress arrived and we felt more civilized. We also wore our blues, and when the weather became cooler in the fall, brought out our suits and berets.

After the fall of Catania, the middle of August, we moved to a fairly new hospital which had been well equipped except that the Germans had managed to rip out plumbing and destroy as much as they could before evacuating. However, we soon settled down to our role as a general hospital. Since the fighting was more severe as the Canadians moved up into Italy, we soon became overcrowded again with patients in corridors and also on the roof under canvas. Alone on the roof on night duty with many shell-shocked and mental patients, I often wondered about our safety in this wartime nursing.

An unplanned holiday in Palermo:

I never expected to go AWOL in the Army but one experience could have put me in this category.

While in Catania, Sicily, the American Air Force approached our matron offering to give a couple of nursing sisters a day off in Palermo, as they went daily across the Island. We would return by British Air Force. Dorothy Quehl and I were coming off night duty and applied for the trip. It was to be a day's excursion so the pay officer didn't think it necessitated any advance pay, although we hoped to shop.

We left about 8 A.M. and had a great trip. Neither of us had flown before and the scenery over the mountains and along the coast was beautiful. On arranging our trip back we found out that all seats were filled with VIPs and we would have to stay overnight. As we had only a little money and not even a toothbrush, this was quite a shock. We thumbed a ride into Palermo and located the American Red Cross. They were very helpful and took us to rooms in the rear of a Sicilian flat which they had reserved for the U.S. Army nurses on leave.

That problem settled, we decided to see the city and luckily ran into a British Navy officer whom Dorothy had met before. He and the American Air Force officer with him took care of our meal problems. Our stay turned out to be five days instead of five hours as the weather changed and the next day we had quite a storm.

After wiring our unit, I can't say we were overly worried. Each day we bounced out to the airport in a truck and after hearing, "No planes today!" drove back for more sightseeing. We had most of our meals in the American officers' mess and enjoyed the entertainment along with the U.S. Army nurses we met there. We visited the catacombs and went through some of the worst slums I had ever encountered. Long, narrow and crowded streets, many buildings bombed, laundry hanging from one side of the street to the opposite and pigs and chickens coming out of the doorways.

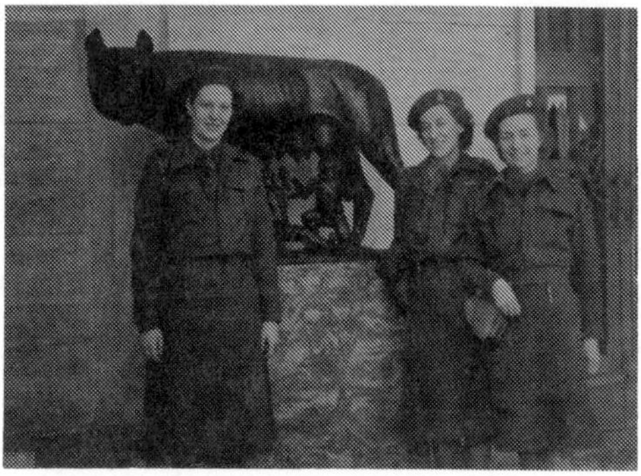

Rome 1945
Connie Clark, Betty Brown, Lib Lawson
Romulus & Remus

Our own rooms were clean enough but had been quite shaken up during the bombing; we had some reservations going through the family's rooms since we couldn't communicate with them. Finally we were able to hitch a ride back to Catania and, needless to say, this adventure put an end to any other nurses seeing Palermo.

Our unit was the first to follow the invasion of Sicily. In December of 1944 the authorities decided to return to England all nursing sisters who were married or who were over forty. You can imagine our reaction to that, especially to me. My husband was with the 4th Recce; Princess Louise Dragoon Guards, and we could have been together during the lull in action all the way through Italy. I returned to No. 13 CGH and he was killed in action on the Gothic Line, September 1, 1944. I returned to my old unit in Rome. In March 1945, returned to England and home in June 1945. My husband was Major J. Bruce Lawson.

Helen M. (Ross) O'Brien

Graduated from: Winnipeg General Hospital School of Nursing. Year: 1934

Military History:

Service: RCAMC

Rank: Lt. N/S

Served: December 1939 to May 1945

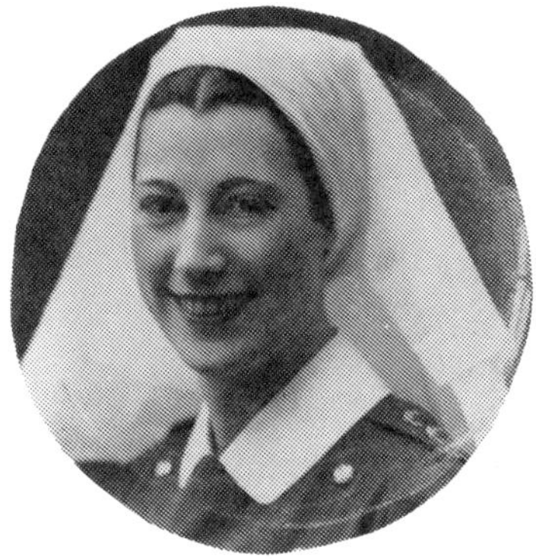

Helen Ross O'Brien, at No. 5 CGH, Taplow, England. 1941

I was influenced to choose a military career because I wished to emulate nursing sisters of the First World War who were close friends. It was also an opportunity to travel and return to nursing after doing clerical work as a medical records librarian at WGH.

I joined the Army in 1939 and soon found myself at Taplow with No. 5 CGH. While in Taplow air raids were common; we had shelters adjoining the wards and patients and beds were quickly moved to them. We went to London on days off duty and were subject to many bomb scares. We enjoyed the theatres while we were there.

After 3 years in England, we were part of the huge original convoy which went to the Mediterranean. Our ship, the Franconia, was dive bombed just out of Malta enroute to Sicily and almost immediately after disembarking at Augusta, Sicily, the Agusta harbour was bombed.

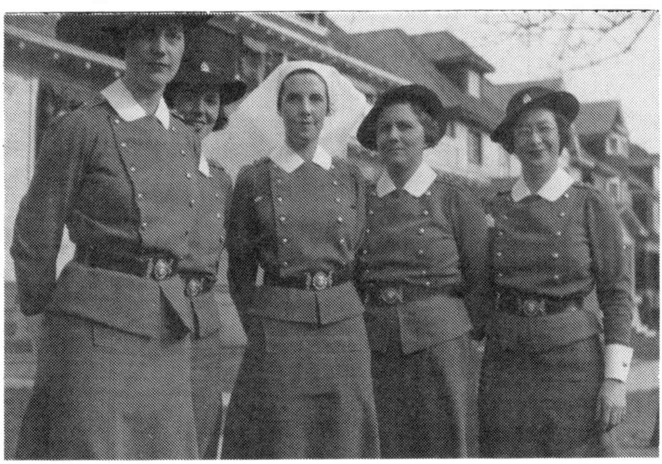

Winnipeg, June 1940
Helen Ross, Phyllis Bennest, Elva Honey, Alice Clake, Edna Leishman

Most of our medical supplies were lost, also KD (Khaki Duty) uniforms for nursing sisters.

Camp was set up in Syracuse. I was in a motor accident (a head-on-collision after dark). My steel helmet fell forward and cut my right eyelid requiring 8 sutures. A mix-up in a British First Aid Station resulted in me being given tetanus anti-toxin which reacted conversely with tetanus toxoid which had been given in Canada. Consequently, I was hospitalized with one allergy after another. Most of the time we were stationed in Syracuse prior to going to Catania.

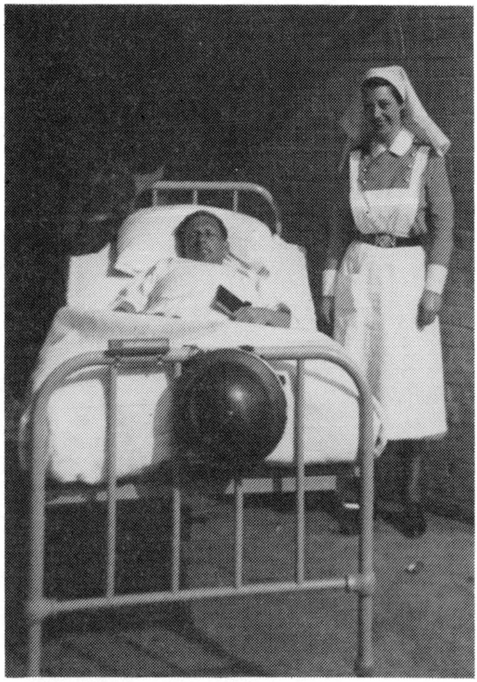

Helen Ross at No. 5 CGH Taplow, Bucks, England 1941, Gnr. H.J. Graham, 53RD Field Battery, RCA, Toronto

Our last 9 months in Italy were spent in Rome at a former military academy quite close to St. Peters and the Vatican. The nursing sisters' residence was formerly a private girls' school, directly across the Tiber from the Castello San Angelo.

Opportunities for sightseeing were many, as the fighting was reaching an end in Italy. My entire five years with the No. 5 Canadian General Hospital were a marvellous experience, memories of which I still treasure.

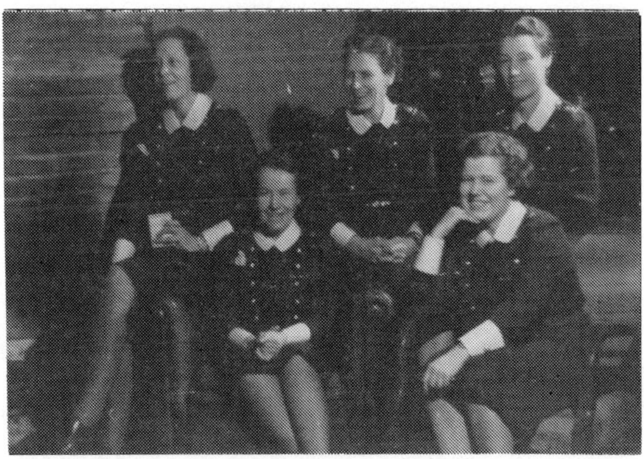

No. 5 CGH at Cliveden
Fron:; Matron Agnes MacLeod, Dietitian Catherine McDole. Back; Anna Millar, Matron Marjorie Rutherford, Helen Ross

Anna M. (Allen) Swail

Graduated from: Winnipeg General Hospital School of Nursing, Manitoba. Year: 1928

Military History:

Service: RCAMC

Rank: Major (P/M)

Served: December 1939 to August 1946 (London 1940-1944)

I joined the military because of money. During the Depression, $5.00 a day and board looked awfully good.

The highlights of my military career are as follows:

Received the Royal Red Cross Medal in 1945 from King George.

In Germany in a bombed-out nunnery with our capes used for curtains.

Being guarded by Polish soldiers and not really knowing which side they were on.

Taking over a German hospital and having to deal with German officers as patients! (Approx. 1944).

Ostend, Belgium (1944) seeing the German underground hospital! The operating room was lit in such a way that there were no shadows. (Built in 1938 for Hitler's Navy).

Being somewhere in Europe and having General Montgomery in for treatment after a little accident.

Sitting in the hospital yard, 1940, and watching the fires in London from all the bombing.

Watching "dog fights" between two planes.

Seeing houses ripped apart.

Being in the underground stations in London where people hid out.

Having tea in soup cans or whatever they had. They offered it to "share."

"Business as Usual" signs in front of bombed out stores.

Overcrowded hospitals in Britain for they never turned patients away – no matter what!

Taking over a German hospital from pathetic little nuns who obviously hadn't eaten in a long time. They had no supplies and were using paper as bandages by then.

Hearing the Italian prisoners of war singing their hearts out down the road.

Seeing Russian prisoners of war who had obviously been very poorly treated. We took over the camp – there were something like 200 deaths the first day. They had no food, no clothing, etc. We had a little Russian priest as interpreter.

We came home on the *Ile de France* – 14,000 or 15,000 troops and a bunch of British war brides with their babies. The trip took only four days. Twelve to fifteen of us per state room – each in our own cot. The weather was god-awful. We were packed in like sardines and many people seemed scared. There was a sick bay on the ship. They fed us two meals a day – there were too many people to be able to manage three meals each day.

"Whatever you think of war, it's just gruesome, gruesome. I don't think we won anything!"

(Dolly) Mabel M.J. (Vincent) Watkins

Graduated from: Winnipeg General Hospital School of Nursing. Year: 1934

Military History:

Served: RCAMC

Rank: Lt. N/S

Served: May 1940 to November 1945

Chiefly patriotic upbringing and the idea of overseas service influenced me to join the RCAMC. I joined as Lieut. nursing sister in May 1940 and went overseas directly with No. 5 Canadian General Hospital, from Winnipeg, Manitoba. We arrived in England June 1940.

I spent four years nursing in England, the greater part of time at Cliveden, Lord and Lady Astor's estate near Taplow. The 500-bed hospital was built by the Canadian Red Cross and given for Army use.

The highlight of my experience in the medical corps was most definitely the last year overseas. I went to France shortly after the invasion with No. 7 CGH from PEI and Nova Scotia. We were the first Canadian hospital to land after the invasion in June 1944. We went to Bayeux, France, and shortly after I was sent to No. 3 CCS Carpiquet Airport near Caen.

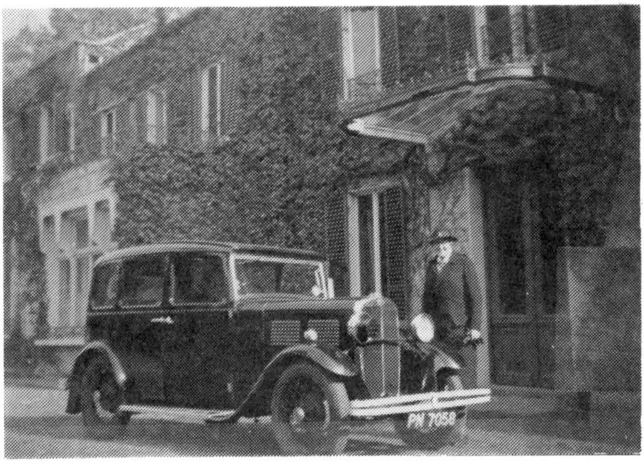

Matron-in-Chief Emma Pense at No. 5 CGH, Taplow, Summer 1940

We were extremely busy with dreadful cases to care for, nursing in tents. Our IVs, plasma, suctions, etc., pinned to the seams of the tent. Only severe cases were held; others were sent further back from the front, then back to England.

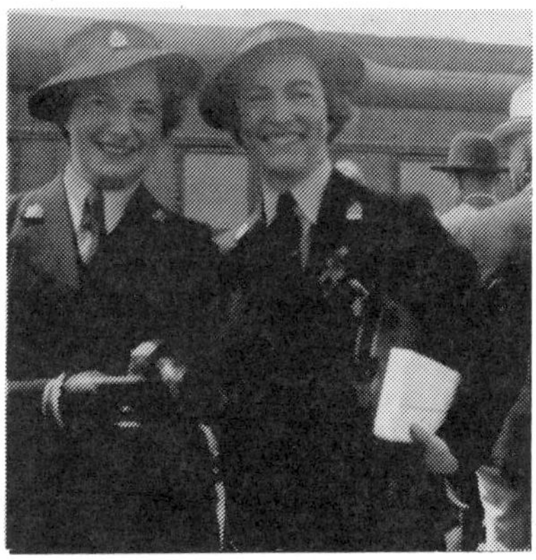

Marjory McCulloch and Dolly Vincent ready to go overseas to Caen, France 1944

One instance I remember, we had been working several weeks without a break. An invitation came from No. 2 Division at Caen for two sisters for dinner. I was one chosen to go. After dinner I was asked to accompany an officer to a church service to be held outdoors and to be conducted by the late Lieut. Col. C. Stone. As we approached, we passed a Canadian mobile bath being used by a British unit. Someone suddenly realized there was a woman in the jeep! What a scramble of naked men for cover! It made a good cartoon for the Canadian paper!

As we went further north, I was privileged to visit Vimy Ridge Memorial with its beautiful monument.

We joined No. 6 Field Dressing Station with surgical teams attached, and served air evacuation during the winter in Holland near Eindhoven for some weeks. While there, I witnessed the Germans' last real raid New Year's morning 1945, little destruction – lost part of the chimney and a few windows.

We pushed further north through Belgium, Holland and into

Germany. On our last move from Almelo, Holland, we two sisters and the advance unit were given one hour to prepare to move.

We set up our hospital in a bombed church in Germany then received orders to return to Canada!

I arrived home in Vancouver June 1945, after 5 years overseas.

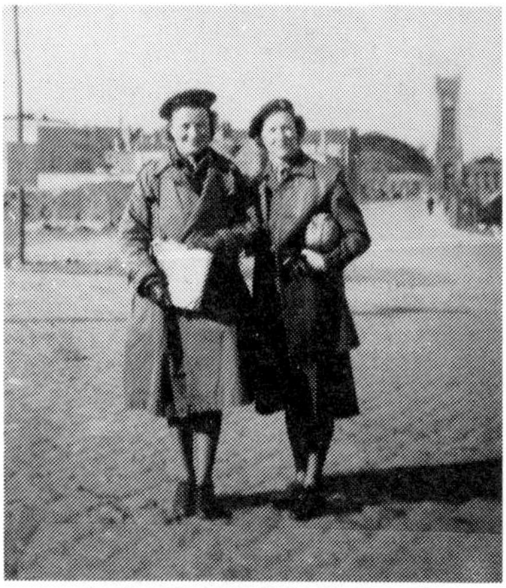

Ostende, Belgium, 1945
Ready to go home
L-R: Marjory McCulloch, Dolly Vincent

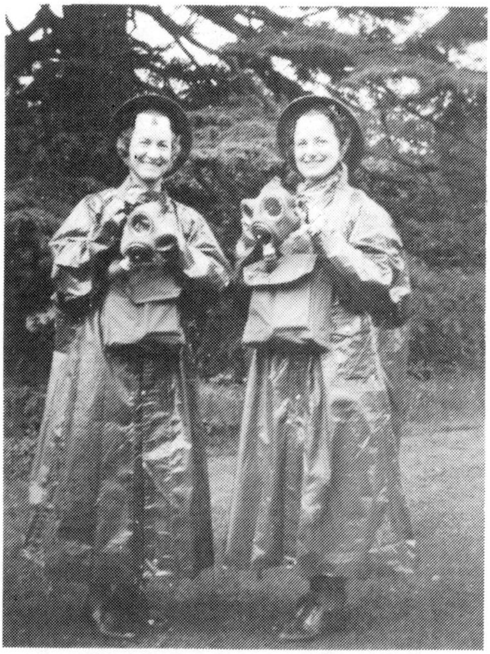

Marjory McCulloch and Dolly Vincent, mustard capes, eye shields, respirators and tin hats all ready for "Jerry," England

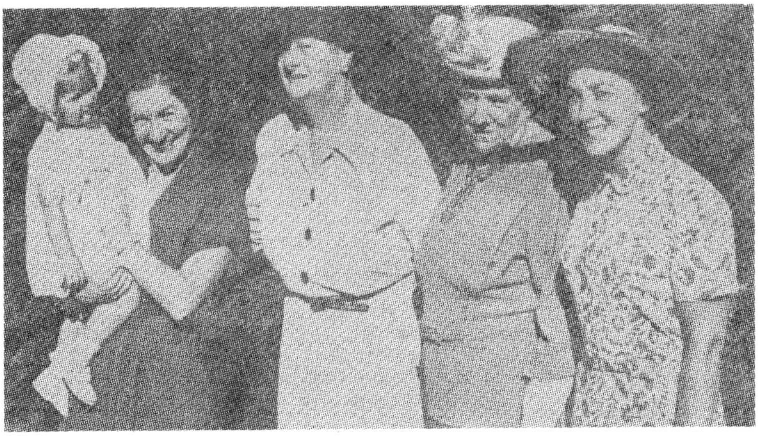

OVERSEAS SERVICE IN THREE WARS REPRESENTED
1950
N/S Dolly (Vincent) Watkins with daughter Pamela, WW II
N/S Marnie Hearn, WW I and WW II
N/S R.A. McLennan, Boer War
N/S Marjory Lownds, WW II and UNRRA

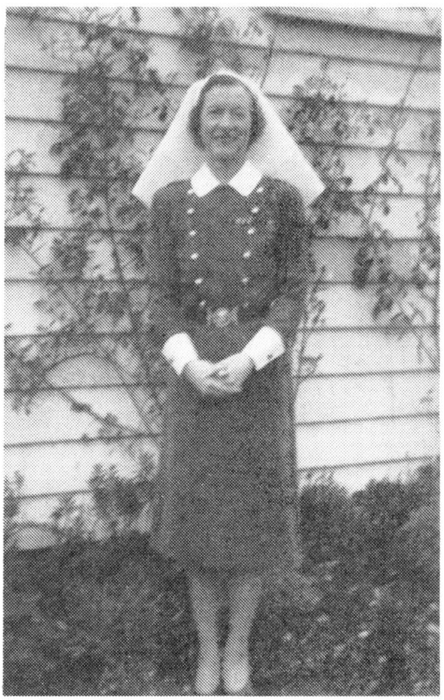

Dolly Vincent Watkkins, 5 CGH
June 1945, just returned home after
five years overseas

NO. 7 CANADIAN GENERAL HOSPITAL

Diana (Harrison) McKay
Elizabeth (Gillespie) Jeffrey Williamson

No. 7 Canadian General Hospital mobilized in Halifax, Nova Scotia in May 1940 and reached England early in December of 1941 where they succeeded No. 1 General at Marston Green with Moya MacDonald as matron. On July of 1943 they were situated at Taplow on the Cliveden Estate.

On 13 July 1944 the nursing sisters of No. 7 CGH arrived in Southampton. They boarded the troopship *Princess Astrid* and the next morning transferred to an Landing Ship Tank to be taken close inshore where they transferred to special shore landing barges that took them ashore at Gold Beach in France.

By midnight they were assigned to the field near Bayeux. The next day the nursing sisters arrived from the British Hospitals where they had been working since their arrival 14 July. They took care of casualties and moved from France to Belgium to Holland and then Germany as the Allies progressed through northwest Europe. They were in Bassum near Bremen in Germany for VE Day and were notified that No. 7 would be one of the occupation hospitals.

Major (P/M) Wilson from No. 11 GCH, who had replaced Matron Moya MacDonald in mid-February 1945, now went to No. 10 General at Turnhout. Matron M. Boutilier came to No. 7 GCG in June.

Canadian occupation forces were to leave Germany 1 April 1946 and plans were made to close the hospital. No. 7 Canadian General Hospital was officially disbanded 8 June 1946.

Diana H. (Harrison) McKay

Graduated from: Winnipeg General Hospital School of Nursing.

Military History:

Service: RCAMC

Rank: Lieutenant N/S

Served: 1942 to 1945

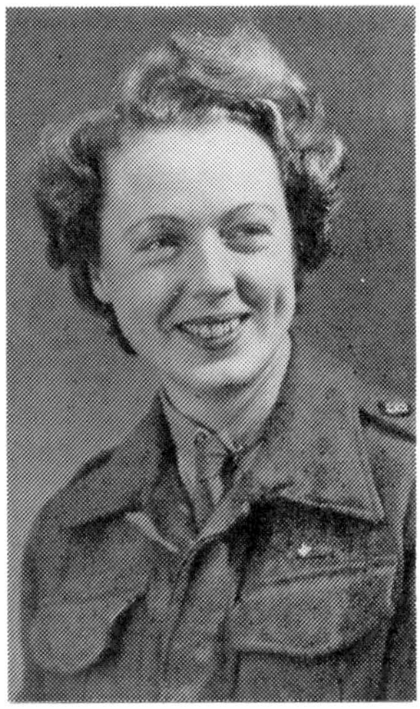

Lt. N/S Diana Harrison

I enlisted in the RCAMC in 1942, at Fort Osborne, Winnipeg. Later I was assigned to Camp Shilo, Manitoba – we learned to survive with sand in our food. I was posted overseas; we went over on a banana boat, part of a large convoy that took such a long time – there were a few scares of U-boats. We landed in Oban, Scotland in February. Cold! I always remember the waitresses at the hotel, elderly and wearing real button boots. The Wrens took us to visit the McDougals of Donally, a darling elderly couple living in one room of an enormous mansion full of ancient treasures, suits of armour, shields, a framed letter by a Lady to her husband in the Crusades, etc.!

Then on to London, to Horsley, then to No. 7 CGH. Our field training took place in Helmsley,

Eventually the fighting moved on; we moved to Dieppe, we had some German POWs, all sent to England. It was November and cold and rainy; we were in tents on the lawn of a lovely old manor house. We slept in our clothes and made trenches through our tents. Some of us were sent ahead as reinforcements to other hospitals.

In Antwerp, the V-2 rockets were so bad the back of our apartment was blown off. A constant stream of black hearses filled the streets.

I went to Nijmegen with No. 1 and worked in neurosurgery. We met up with hospitals and troops from Italy. We all returned to No. 7 in Turnhout, Belgium; spent Christmas there. The patients made decorations from silver paper from cigarette packs and our white cotton swabs. We all joined in singing carols.

We ended up in Hahn, Germany, in a hospital that had not been abandoned very long by the Germans. We had "our" POWs; men of all nationalities. They had had no contact with the outside world for four years or more; some were so thin they were literally human skeletons. The mobile ones rushed out to forage in the garbage cans – absolutely heart breaking.

Finally – back to England and then Home! I gained 10 pounds from Halifax to Winnipeg, we were fed so well.

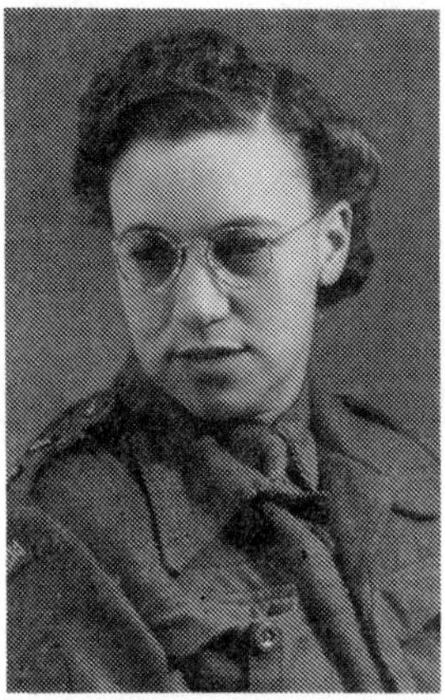

Lt. N/S
Phyllis Hadland

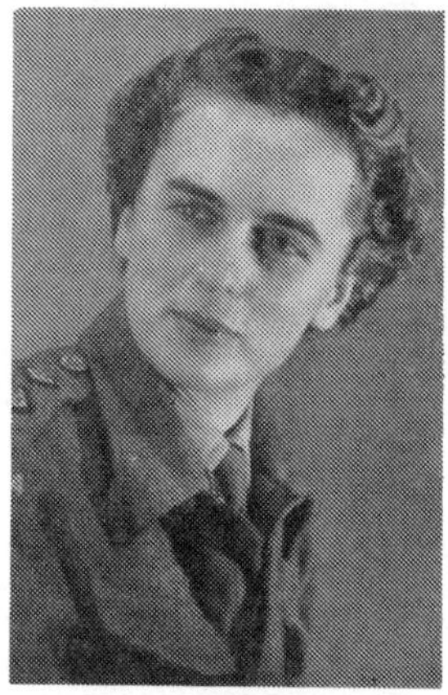

Lt. N/S
Erica Gifford

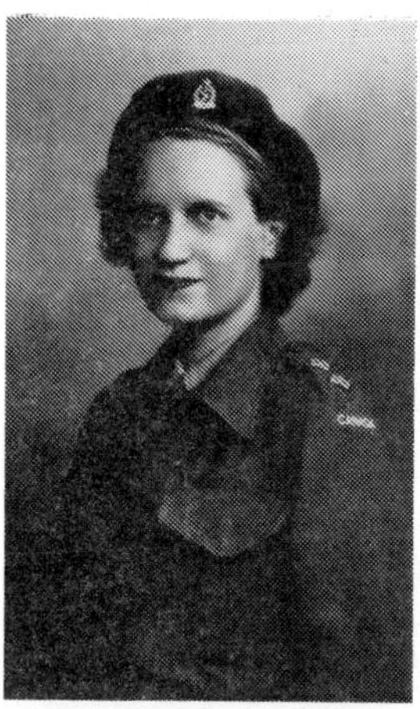

Lt. N/S Pearl Graham

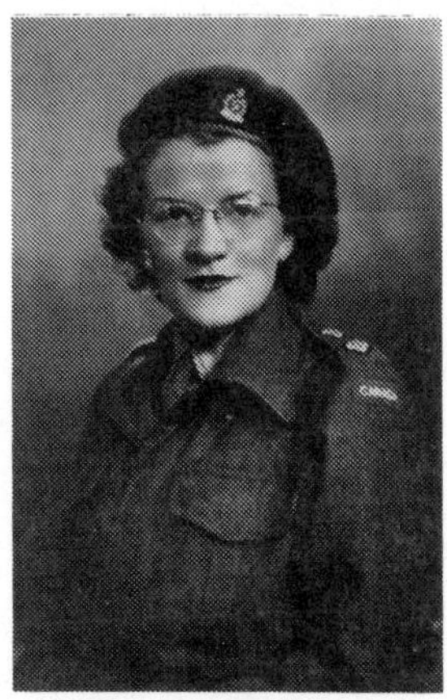

Lt. N/S
Mary Jane Elliot

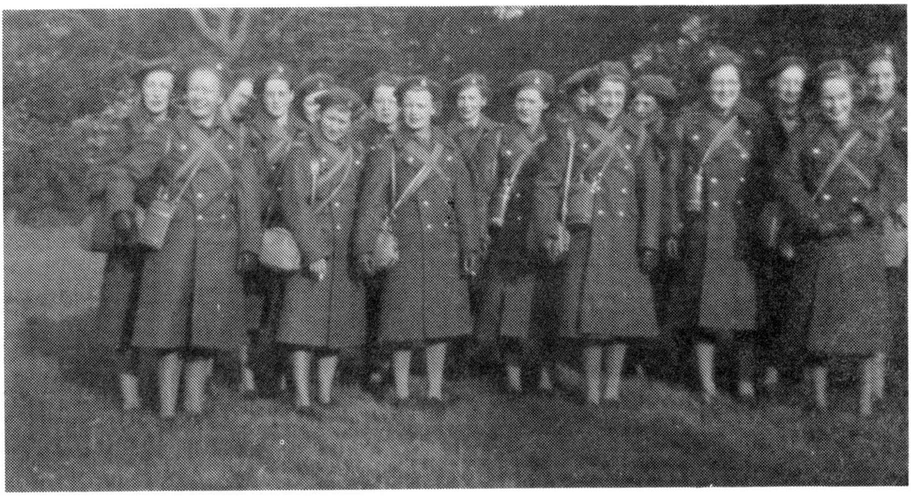

Field Training, No. 7 CGH, Helmsley, Yorkshire, England

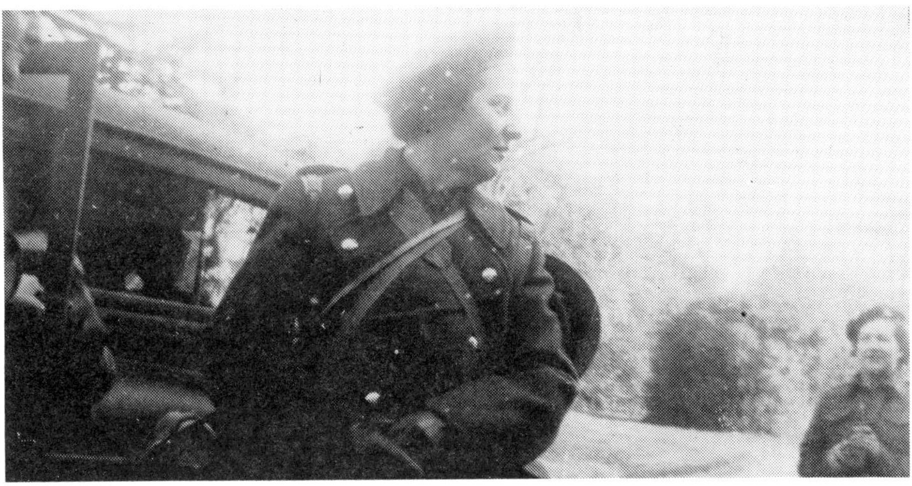

Assistant Matron Boutillier

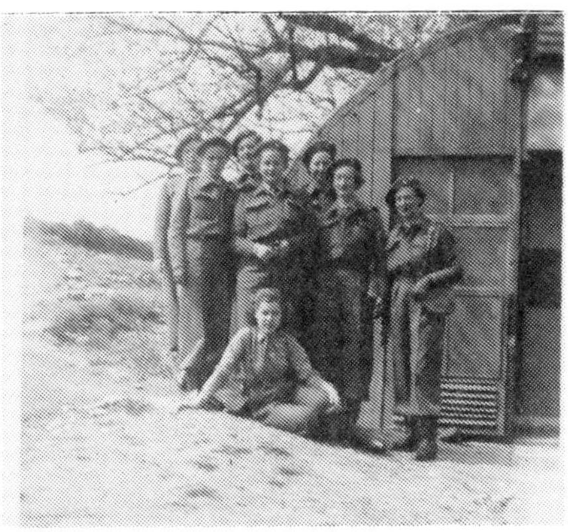

*Lillian Docherill, Muriel Graham,
May Heartz, Jerry England,
Margo Dussault, Matron MacDonald*

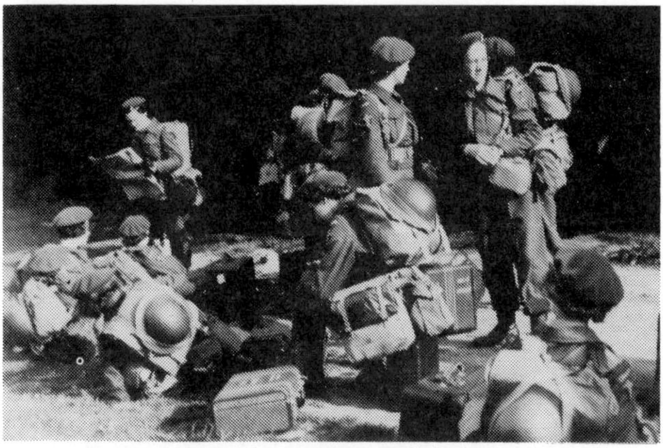

Field training Helmesley, 17 June 1944

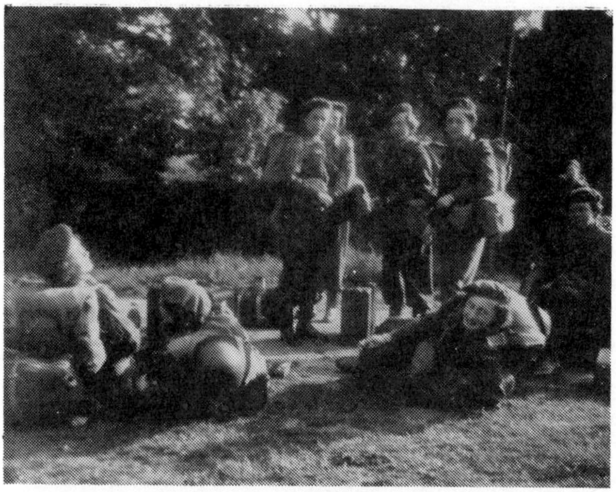

Field training Helmesley, 17 June 1944

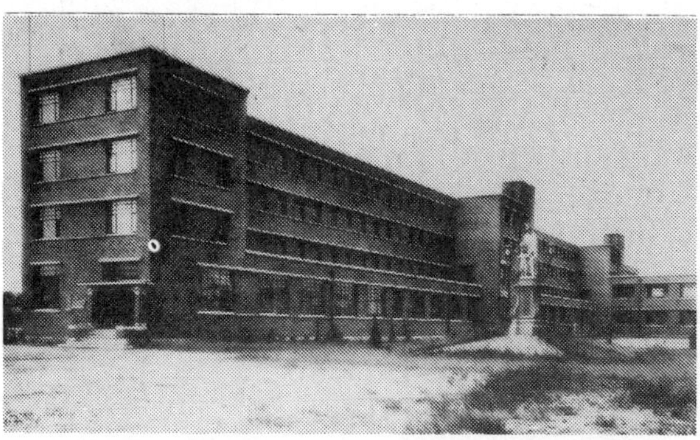

Turnhout, Belgium. This building was a boys' school before No. 7 CGH was located there.

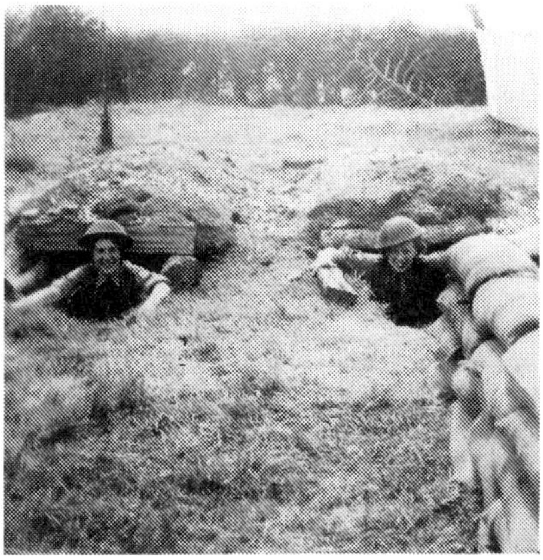

Bunker at Bayeux

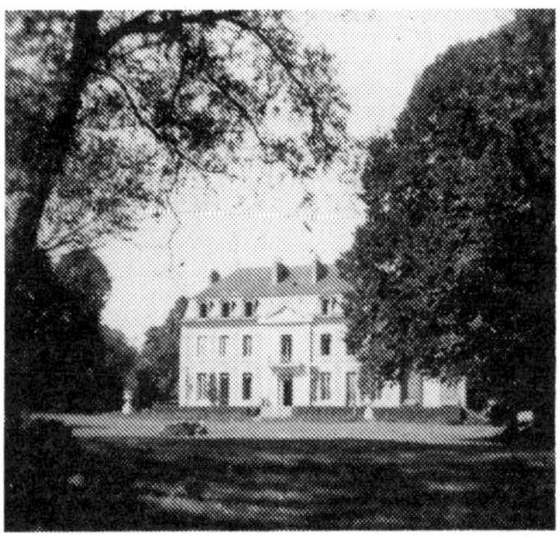

Chateau of Madame Ste. Claire of Martigny (a village) near Arquis la Battille (a small town) eight Km. from Dieppe. Some of the nursing sisters lived in the Chateau, the rest lived in tents on the lawn of the Chateau.

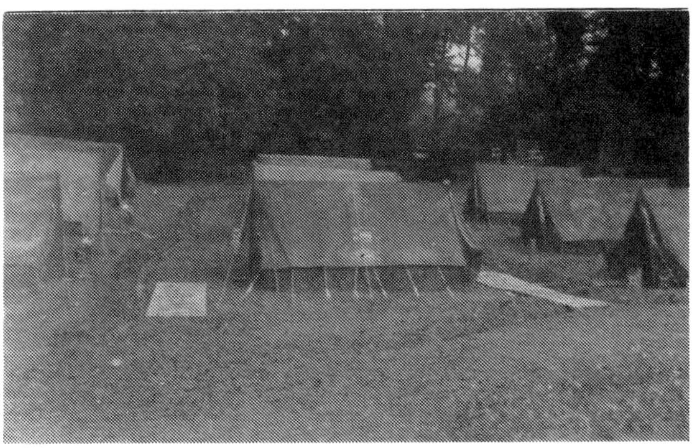

Tents on lawn of chateau

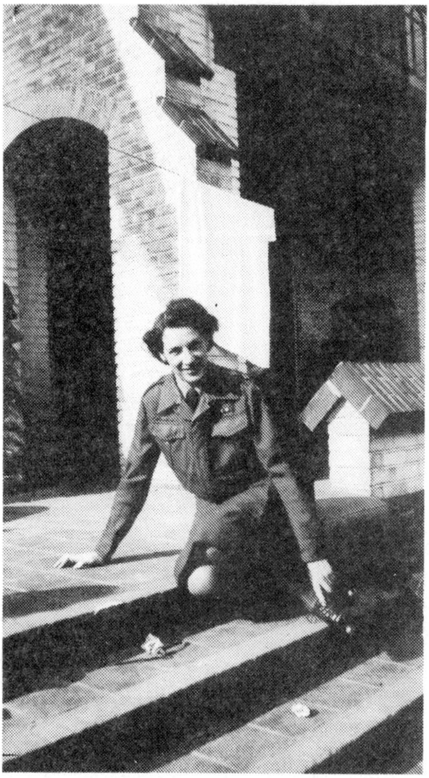

Lt. N/S Terry McDonald

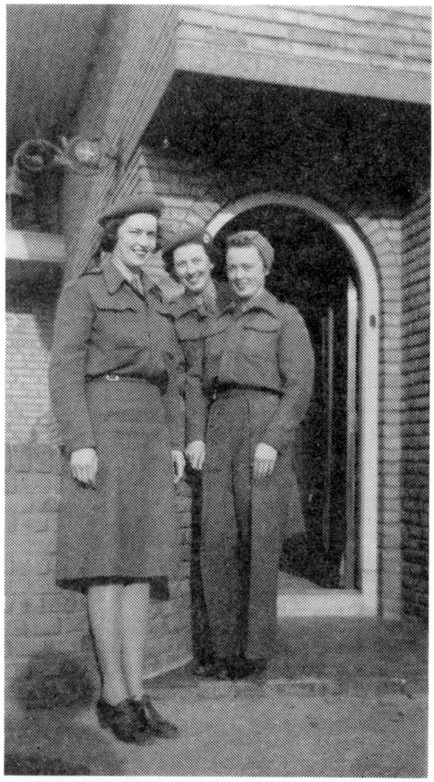

Connie Harrison, Marj Harvie Cdn. Red Cross, N/S Diana Harrison, Nijmegen, Holland

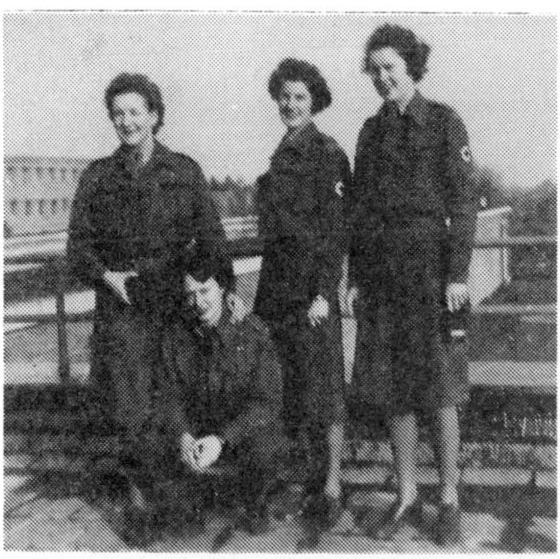

N/S Jean Frances Ferguson, N/S Betty Hanlon, Jean Ellis, Connie Harrison, CRC

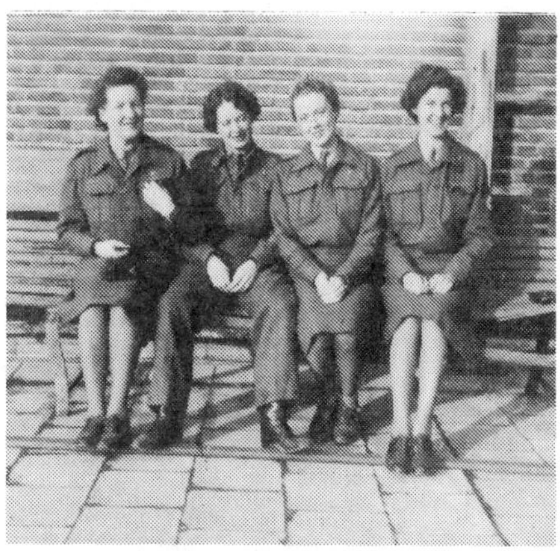

December 1945
L-R: Frances Ferguson, Betty Hanlon, Diana Harrison, Jean Ellis

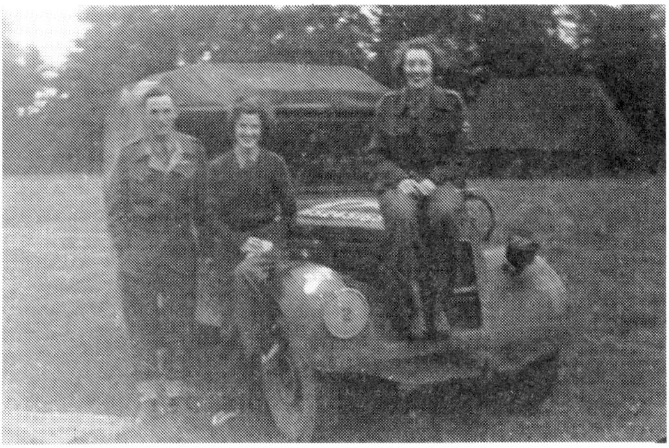

L-R: Major Tabbie Bethune, Adjutant, Jean Ellis & Connie Harrison, CRC

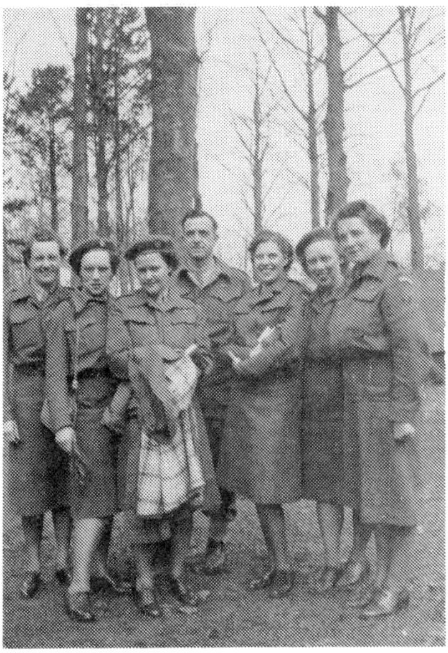

At s'Hetrtogenbosch, Holland Nursing sisters name unknown, Phyllis Hadland, Kay McLean, Major C. Trask, Matron Hunter, Robbie Robinson, Dorothy Kaulback

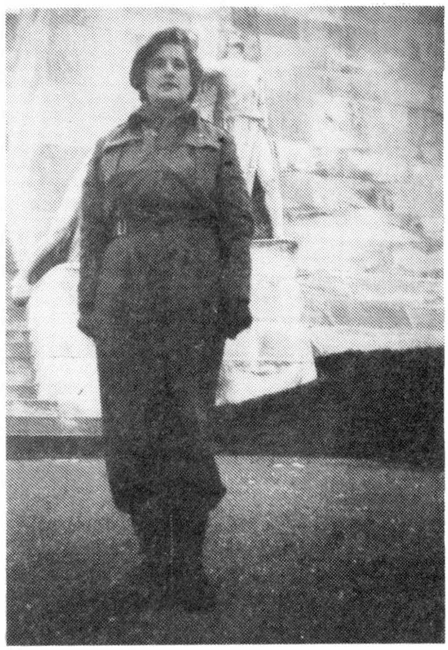

Lt. (N/S) Dorothy Kaulback standing at attention, Vimy Ridge

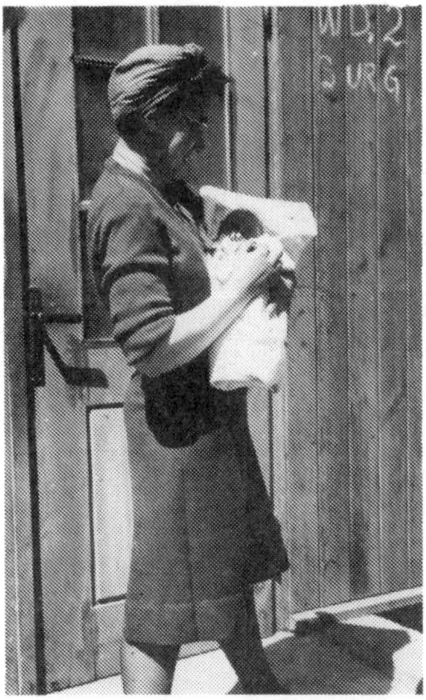

VE Day, Hahn, Germany. Phyllis Hadland with baby born to a civilian woman on VE Day at No. 7 CGH & named Victoria Elizabeth

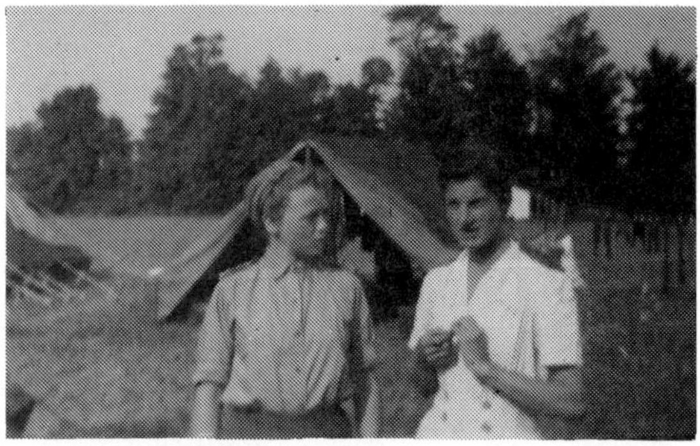

N/S Diana Harrison, Jean Ellis, CRC

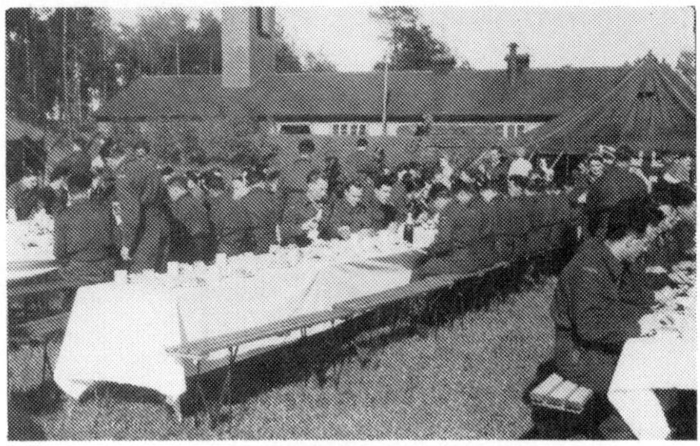

VE Day, Hahn, Germany

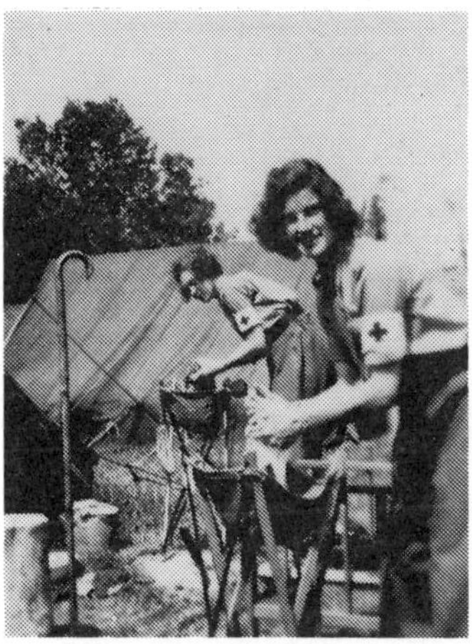

Connie Harrison, Jean Ellis, CRC

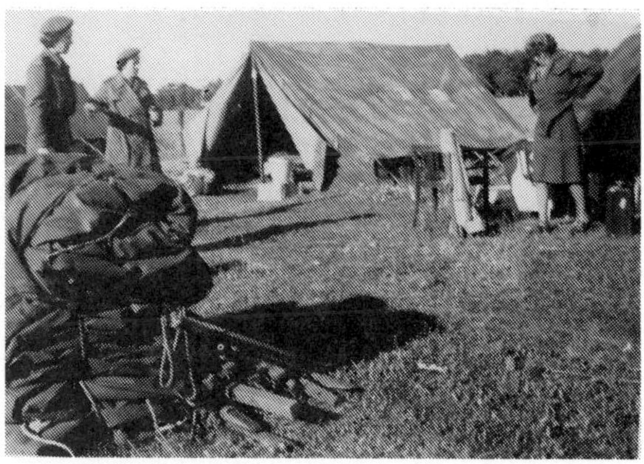

The day we left Bassum for Canada, July 1945

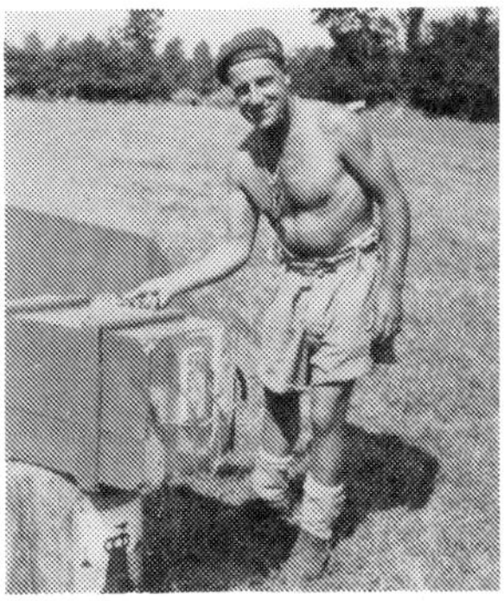

Our dear sergeant

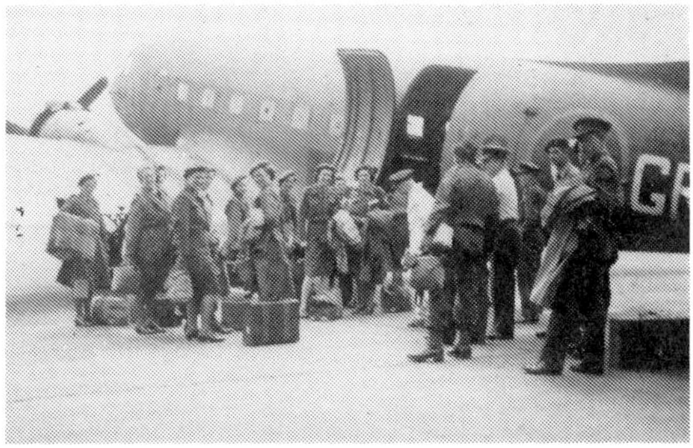

Ready to go home

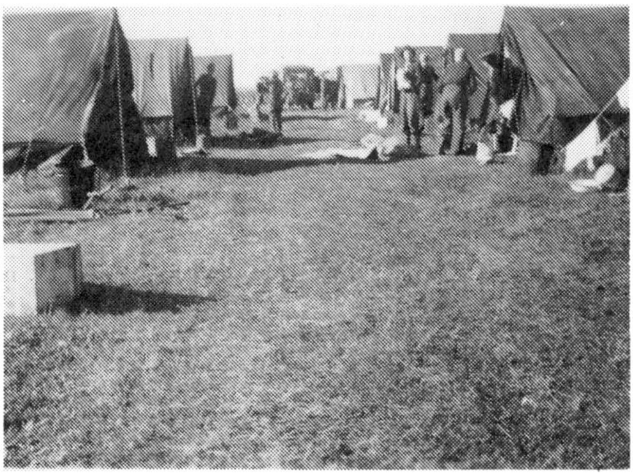

Bassum, June 1945

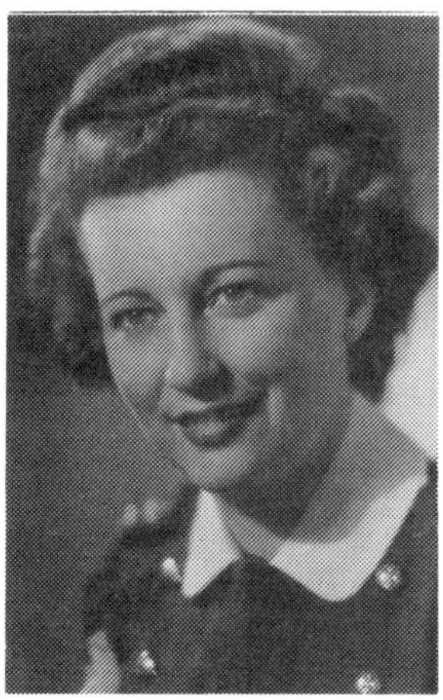

No. 7 CGH
Florence (Glidden) Pentland

Elizabeth Jeffrey (Gillespie) Williamson

Graduated from: Royal Columbian Hospital School of Nursing, New Westminster, B.C. Year: 1939

Military History:

Service: RCAMC

Rank: 2 Lt. to 1st Lieutenant

Served: 2 January 1942 to January 1946

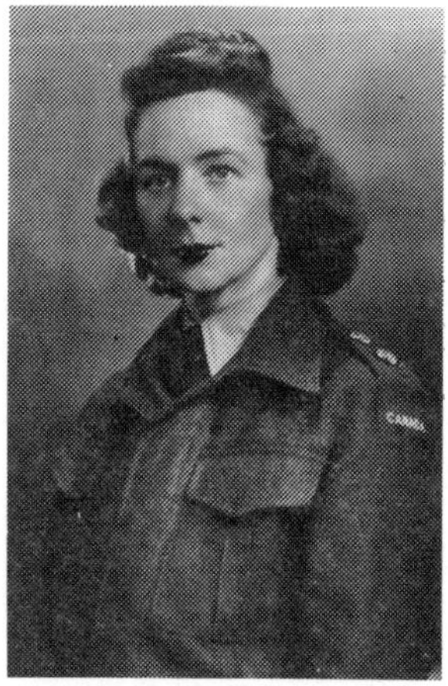

Lt. N/S Elizabeth Jeffrey

My husband, Lt. Jeffrey, died overseas so I felt I had to go.

The highlights of my military experience were:

Basic training, Victoria Military Hospital.

England No. 7 CGH, Reinforcement.

France, Battle of Normandy.

Belgium, Battle of the Scheldt.

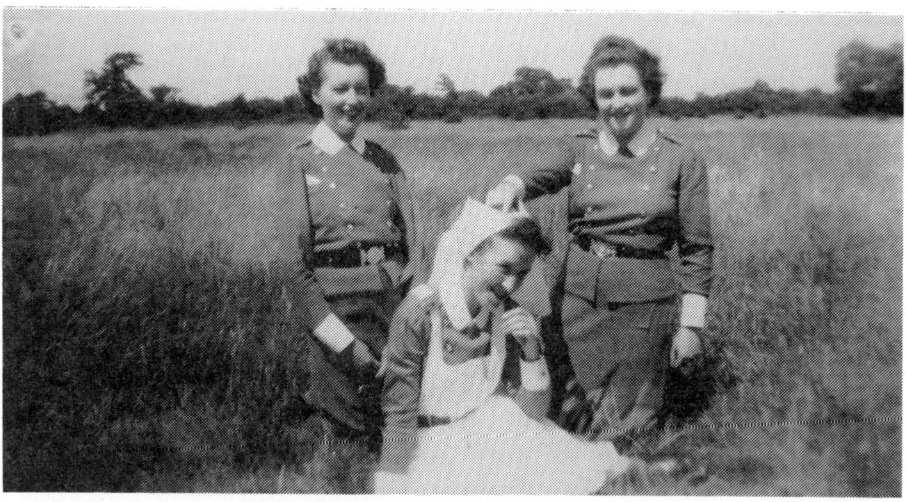

No. 7 CGH Hanley, England, August 1944.
L-R:Florence (Glidden) Pentland, Evangeline Currie, May (Parks) Kaye

NO. 8 CANADIAN GENERAL HOSPITAL

Helen (Bright) Armstrong
Frances Copeman
Corinne Lettner
Beth (Andreas) McIntosh
Harriet J. T. Sloan
Mabel (Glew) Tweddell
Marion (Thompson) Wolstein

No. 8 Canadian General Hospital was mobilized at Regina in July of 1940 and disbanded effective 16 July 1945 having been in operation in Canada, England, France, Belgium, and Holland five years and three days.

On 25 January 1942 No. 8 attempted to leave Canada on the *George Washington* but the ship did not leave Halifax harbour and No. 8 returned to Debert, N.S. On 13 March they boarded the *Empress of Canada* and this time sailed to the U.K. situating near Crowthorne, Berkshire with Dorothy M. Ritches as matron and D. F. Ballantine as assistant matron.

The nursing sisters were in battle dress and performing route marches in the field in May 1944, and on 18 July the unit sailed into Arromanches and disembarked on special improvised docks near Bayeux. They cared for casualties and for numerous illnesses as they moved from France through Belgium to Holland until the unit disbanded.

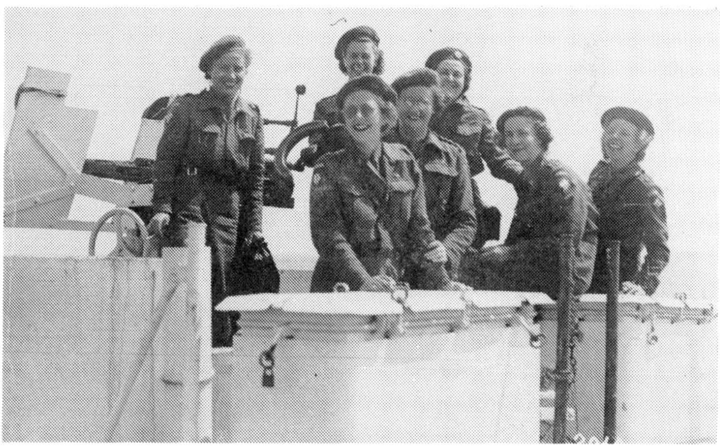

From left to right back row – N/S N.E. Harburn, Lt (P/A) Clarke & 2/Lt W.O. Mundy, Cdn. Red Cross. Front row – N/S Molly Spohn, Mary Arnot, M.J. Steele, & Claire Pethick on forward part of LCI just before leaving Portsmouth on 18 July 1944.
Canadian Forces photo

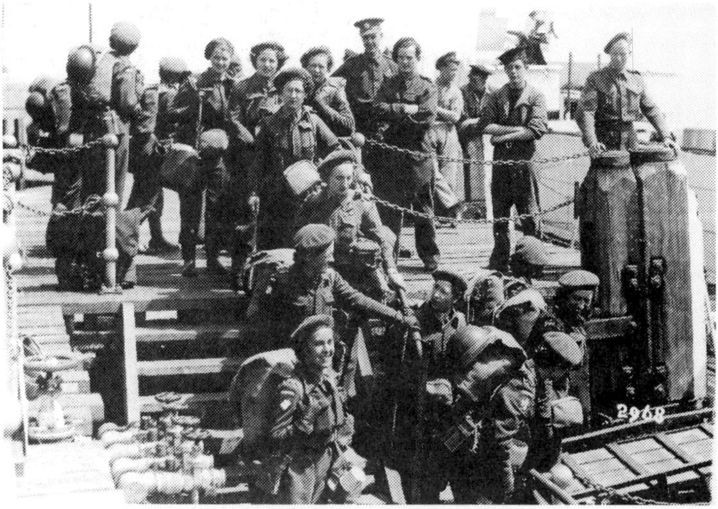

Nursing sisters going on board LCI at Portsmouth 18 July 1944 enroute to Normandy. The sisters facing craft starting from rear of group are: Frances Copeman, A.J.N. Whytock, R.M. Muldoon, M.E. Fitzpatrick, M.K. Beaton, M.E. Herringer, J.B. Dube. On right of railing: M.J. Smyth, K.M. Morton, (Diet) N.M. Attree
Canadian Forces photo

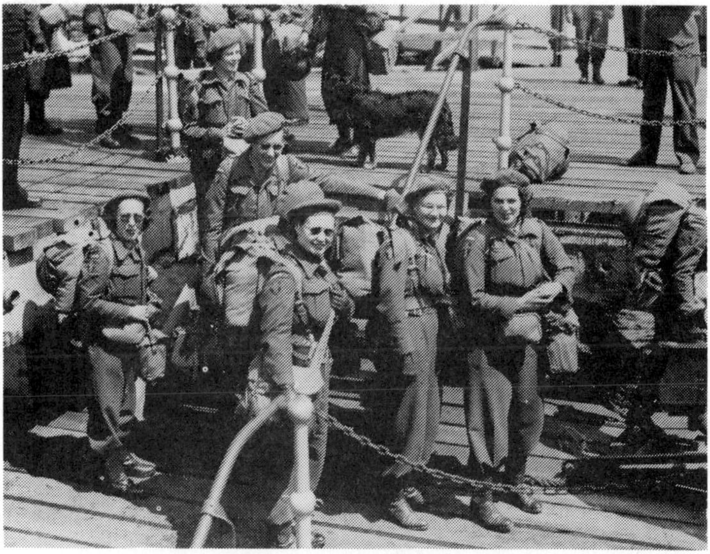

Rear Lt (P/A) Clarke
in front of person in rear: N/S Helen Bright
front row: N/S N. Patricia O'Connor, Anne Chudy, Lillian Dahl, K.E. McKinnon
Canadian Forces photo

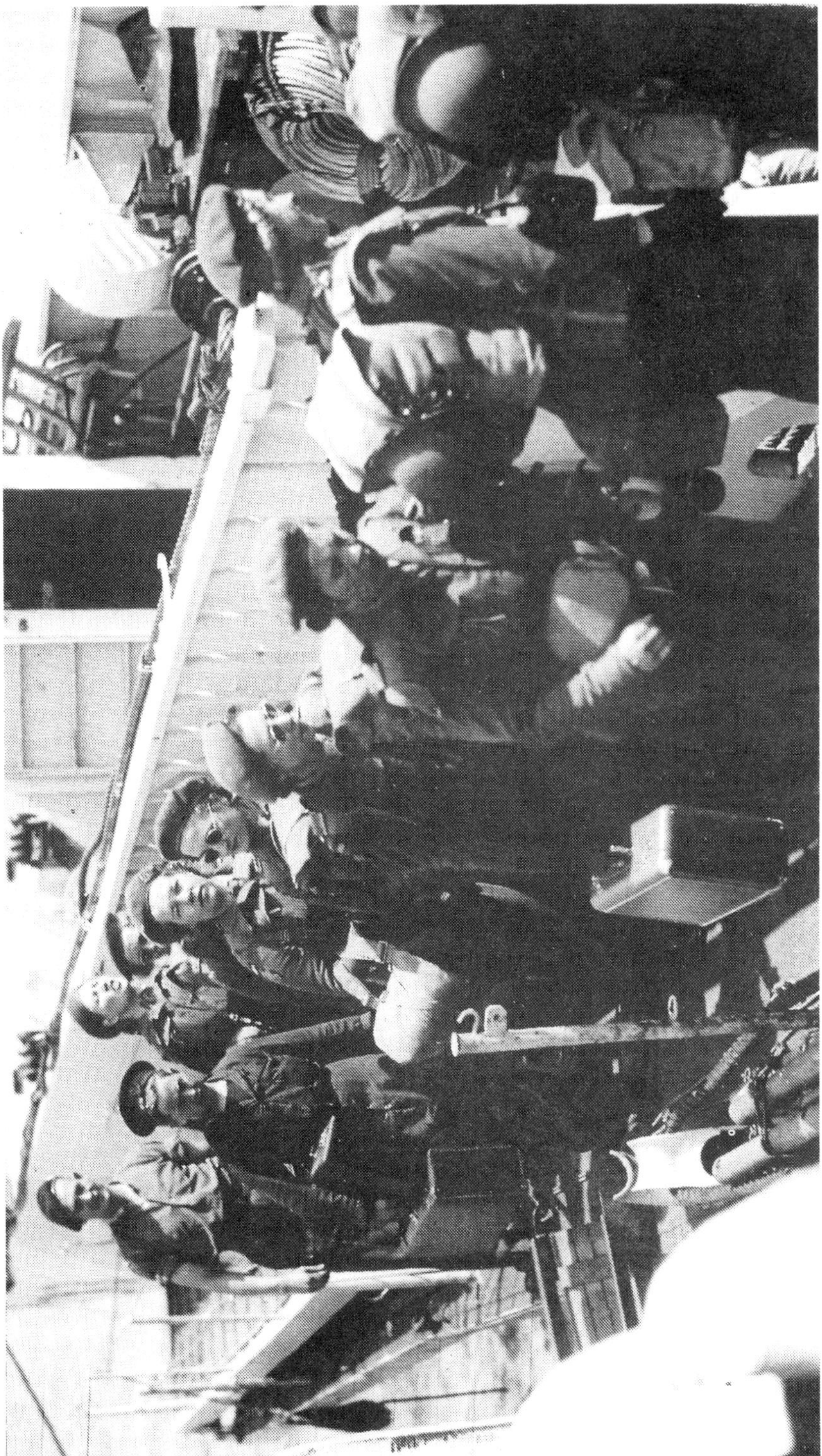

Enroute Portsmouth to Normandy. From rear: Nursing Sisters Claire Pethick, Margaret Lutes, Beth Andreas, E.A. Andrews, Ethel M. Jamieson, Mary Elizabeth Hindley (reinforcement)
Canadian Forces photo

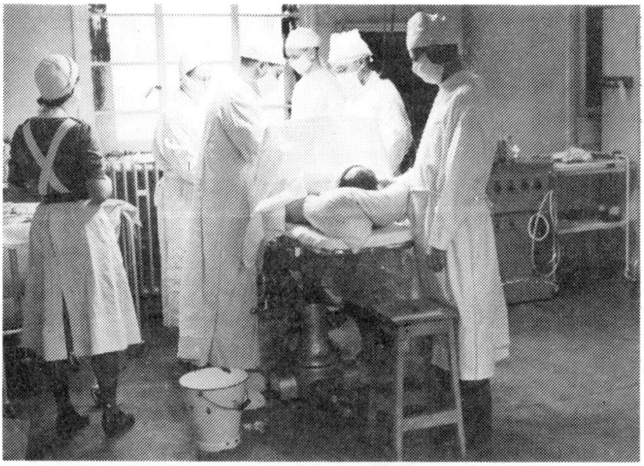

Operating room at Pinewood, England
L-R: N/S Trudy (Keohane) Mills, Mary Arnot, Major Campbell, Major Schroeder, Major McCutcheon

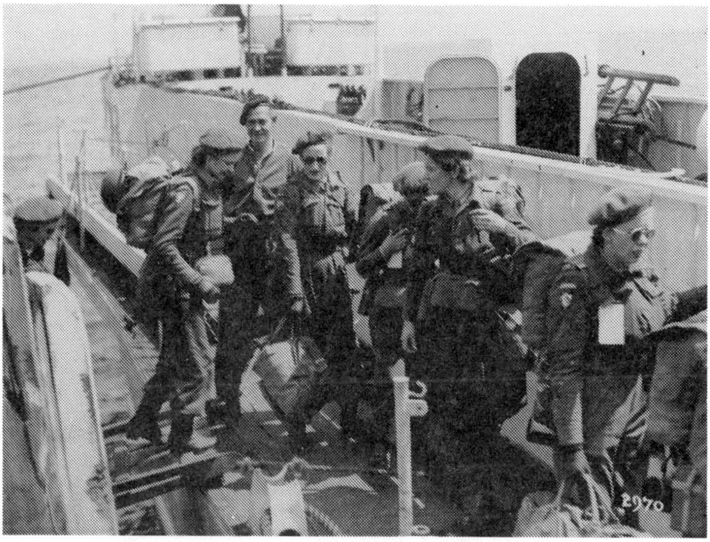

L-R: Lt's (N/S) M. Lennox, F.E.Welsh, J.B. Dube, Molly Boyd (Home Sister) M.J. McLellan stepping on LCI [TLC] enroute from Portsmouth to Normandy 18 July 1944
Canadian Forces photo

Helen (Bright) Armstrong

Graduated from: Regina General Hospital School of Nursing, Regina Saskatchewan. Year: 1935

Military History:

Service: RCAMC

Rank: Lt. Nursing Sister

Served: 1941 to 1945

This story was written soon after I returned to Canada from overseas.

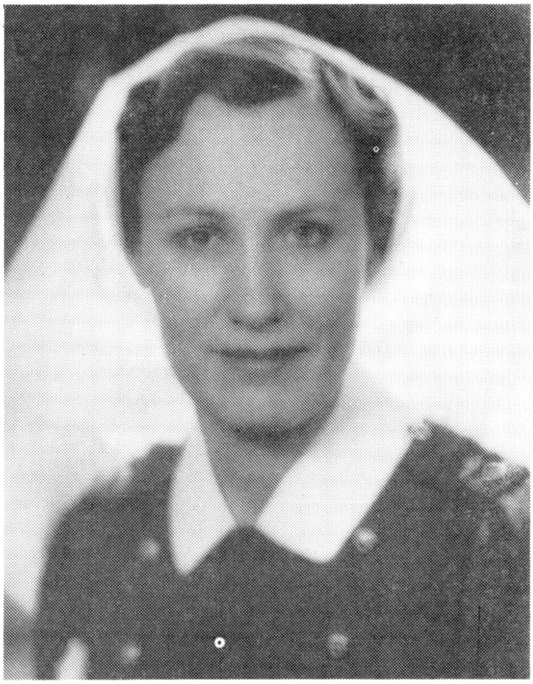

Lt. N/S Helen (Bright) Armstrong
No. 8 CGH, London 1943

On 8 September 1944 six nursing sisters left our hospital unit, which was, at that time, under canvas at Rouen, France, for a pool at a small mobile hospital of two hundred beds at Montreiul, France. There we met other nursing sisters from various hospital units who had been sent, like ourselves, to the pool.

A day later, eight of us from the pool proceeded by transport to a Casualty Clearing Station which was about two miles from the Belgian border. It was under canvas near a small town called Steenvoorde. Here four of the nursing sisters were put on duty while the remaining four waited to be called to Field Dressing Stations. Three days later the call came. Again we separated, two of the nursing sisters going to a Field Dressing Station near Calais, while the two of us who were left were sent to one in Dixmude, Belgium.

It was nearly five o'clock in the afternoon when we arrived at our destination somewhat weary, as we had been travelling for twelve hours. After dinner we met the officer commanding, a major who had seen service in both Italy and Dieppe. We were told the unit was moving the following day to Eecloo, a small village on the Leopold Canal. We were to remain with the rear party for a day or two.

Dixmude was the first place since our arrival on the Continent where we lived and worked in a building. It was a large stone structure which in peacetime had been operated by nuns as a home for the aged. However, during the German occupation it was used by the Germans as a headquarters. In the front entrance hall were murals of German despatch riders and a huge swastika painted over the door. In the courtyard were huge cement air-raid shelters which had been built by the Germans. Our rooms were on the second floor just over the part which served as a hospital, while the ORs and the medical officers were housed in another wing. Although we were in a building again, we had no running water or electric lights. However, the wards were illuminated with electricity supplied by a small portable generator.

The civilians were exceptionally kind both to the patients and to the members of the unit.

We joined the unit at Eecloo. It was occupying a small portion of what had been an exclusive girls' school operated by the Bequine Order of Sisters of Charity. The convent consisted of modern buildings surrounded by beautiful gardens.

The advance surgical unit, consisting of the Field Dressing Station, two mobile dental units, one mobile Blood Transfusion Team, together with the two sisters, occupied two of the buildings. One building we used for patients. One room on the ground floor we used for admission and discharge purposes as well as for medical inspections. Another room we used for a ward for patients with compound fractures. On the second floor were the two operating rooms of the surgical teams and the resuscitation room where the Blood Transfusion Unit worked. The remaining six rooms were used for post-operative wards, a utility room and a small serving room, while some of the ORs lived on the third floor.

The other buildings we used for living quarters and mess rooms. On the ground floor the officer commanding had his office and sleeping quarters. Here also were the officers,' sergeants,' and men's messes. The second floor was used for the officers' quarters. All the rooms were single and complete with built-in furniture – cupboards, shelves, folding beds, desks and chairs, as well as a basin with cold running water. Our rooms were at one end of this hall. You can imagine how delighted we were when we saw this "Savoy" setup, even though it was complete with "air-conditioning" through glassless windows. Here we had our first real bath in a tub in several months. The water was heated in the kitchen and carried upstairs for us. The non-commissioned officers and the remaining ORs of the unit occupied the rooms on the third floor.

There was no place suitable for a kitchen in either building, so two tents were pitched between the buildings; one serving as a kitchen and the other as a storeroom.

At first, we had only a few patients, as the regiments in the sector were holding the line until the division which was fighting in the Calais area moved forward. During this slack time, we had the opportunity of becoming acquainted with the orderlies with whom we were to work and to feel our way into the unit which had never had nursing sisters before.

The standard equipment in a small unit like a Field Dressing Station was very limited. It consisted of beds, grey blankets, and a limited supply of pyjamas and towels. We had no sheets whatever. The nuns loaned us tables to use as bedside tables, one table serving two beds. They also loaned us boards and blankets to substitute for glass in the windows. Several of the sisters of the school spoke English very well. They were kind to us and to the patients.

We were delighted with the opportunity when one of the sisters offered to teach us French. She was a tiny little nun of seventy-six years, and when she spoke French it sounded just like music. Our French lessons were brief, however, for on October 6th, the Battle of Leopold Canal began. Then the patients began coming in quickly. We worked in twelve-hour shifts. We became extremely busy so we kept only the patients who were seriously wounded and required priority surgery: those with abdominal and chest wounds, amputations and compound fractures.

Our procedure in nursing care was as close to civilian methods as possible, in spite of the fact that we had so little with which to work. Our first and foremost thought and duty was to keep the various "tubes" and bottles working, intravenous solutions of glucose and saline, sulpha drugs, plasma, and blood, drip penicillin, gastric suctions and Miller-Abbott suctions. To keep these going kept us constantly alert, e.g., in just one small room of six patients there were twenty-one bottles and tubes. We would bathe and fix the patients between treatments and keep the bottles going.

The patients were gradually becoming fewer and fewer and our work, of course, becoming less each day until November 6th when we four nursing sisters received orders to join a Casualty Clearing Station which was east of Antwerp, and to move with them the following day to Nijmegen. It took the convoy sixteen hours to arrive at our destination. It didn't take us long to roll our camp beds and crawl in that night.

We remained at the Casualty Clearing Station nearly three weeks. Then we were recalled to our original Field Dressing Station which was to act as an Air Evacuation Centre. The entire unit was billeted temporarily in a somewhat war torn school in Zeelst, a small town close to a large airport near Eindhoven, Holland. The next day the medical officers moved into billets in nearby houses. The officer commanding had arranged for billets for the nurses, as well as for the location of the officers' mess in the home of a wealthy manufacturer.

A one-storey building which had been a private school was to serve as our wards. When we first saw it we wondered how we could transform it into a place suitable for patients. There were numerous windows missing, especially in the corridors, which had to be repaired in some way. There was also a lot of rubble and dust from an explosion which had taken place next door prior to our arrival. Another important thing was to find some method of heating the rooms. The OC secured small stoves from the burgomaster, one was set up in the admitting room, one in each of the five rooms we used as wards, one in the treatment room, one in the office room, and one in the operating room. When everything was clean and the stoves installed, the beds were made up with grey blankets only, and we were ready to go to work. A British CCS at the other end of town was doing air evacuation until we were ready to take over. We could accommodate about seventy-five patients. We had beds in four of the wards while the fifth ward had racks on which to place stretchers.

The Field Dressing Station was acting as an air evacuating centre. The patients were brought from the advanced surgical units and Casualty Clearing Stations to be evacuated back to base hospitals in Antwerp, Brussels, or England, depending on the extent of their wounds. Our ambulances would drive up beside the planes for loading. Sparrow planes were used to transport the patients to hospitals in Europe, while Dakotas were used to transport them to England.

Airport evacuation operations were most interesting. It looked like a lake and the road signs like buoys on its surface. Earlier in the war, the Allies had done a good job of bombing this airport as not one building stood in its entirety. In fact, the Air Force officers were under canvas, and some of the tents had a second floor which they were forced to use on account of the water.

The nursing care of these patients was much simpler than it was when we operated as an ASU. The patients, being nearly all post-operatives of several days, required mainly penicillin and sulpha drugs and routine nursing care. Some of them, of course, required special treatments, but nothing difficult.

We worked eight-hour shifts except during bad flying weather. When we became bogged down with patients it was necessary, of course, to arrange our time differently. On duty we wore our slacks because the corridors were cold and draughty, even though the wards were warm. We had to use the corridors to go from ward to ward.

Our OC came to dinner one evening and told us about a Dutch family that had been evacuated from the north. The parents, with eight children, the youngest being twins, had lost everything and were now living in two tiny rooms. The twins were six months old but were only the size of newborn babies. Their complete wardrobe consisted of one sweater which had been cut in two to make a garment for each twin. We decided to make a set of clothes for each twin and to send a box of food over to the family including tinned milk for the babies. Everyone in the mess made contributions for this purpose. The food was delivered immediately, but it was nearly Christmas before we could complete the two tiny wardrobes, as, of course, we could only work in our spare time. Really, it was a pleasure to see how grateful these people were when they saw the clothes.

By the time it was nearing the Christmas season the unit was making plans for a party for the village children in the afternoon of December 24th, and the party for the Dutch people with whom we were billeted, for Christmas Eve. The boys of the unit were planning to have their Christmas party the Friday before Christmas, and they asked us to help with their decorations. Therefore, our off duty hours until Christmas were well filled. Christmas was celebrated in true Canadian fashion.

About 9:30 o'clock New Year's morning, "Jerry" paid a visit

to our airport. Out of every window we looked we could see planes with big swastikas on them. Some were so close we could see the pilots. We could see the shellfire over the port, and as the planes circled around they strafed the civilian houses. One plane came three times to strafe a house back of us. Fortunately, nobody was hurt, but the bullets made a mess of the house. Some of the bullets hit an ammunition dump at the airport. Loud explosions kept occurring. The blast blew off tiles from the roof and several windows in the house where we lived, besides cutting off our electricity. The building occupied by the ORs also lost a few windows. Fortunately, just a small amount of plaster came down in the primary school where the patients were.

Although we wished to return to our hospital unit sometime, when the time came, we felt sorry to leave the Field Dressing Station for, after nearly four months, we had become part of it.

Frances Copeman

Graduated from: Regina General Hospital School of Nursing.
Year: 1935

Military History:

Service: RCAMC

Rank: Lt. N/S

Served: 24 May 1940 to May 1945

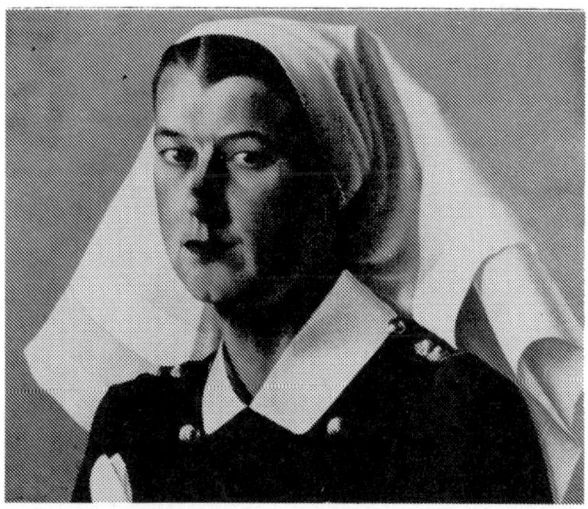

Lt. N/S Frances M. Copeman, No. 8 CGH

I joined the Army in May 1945 and went to Dundurn Military Hospital which I helped open. While there I helped open what was the beginning of No. 8 Canadian General Hospital. Next, I went to Debert, Nova Scotia. From there we went overseas in November 1941; I was stationed at Farnborough. My service on the Continent took me to Bayeux, Caen, Antwerp, and Holland. On my return home in May 1945 I took a position instructing at Regina General Hospital.

Corinne Lettner

Graduated from: General Hospital School of Nursing, Sault Ste. Marie, Ont. Year: 1935

Military History:

Service: Royal Canadian Army Medical Care

Rank: Lieutenant N/S

Served: 15 October 1941 to 22 July 1946

No. 8 Can. Gen. Hosp. 15 Oct. 41 Regina, Sask.

No. 8 Can. Gen. Hosp. 5 Nov. 41 to 14 March - Debert, Nova Scotia

No. 8 Can. Gen. Hosp. 25 March 42 to Pinewood, England

No. 8 Can. Gen. Hosp. 1942 to 1 Nov. 43 - Farnborough, England

No. 5 Can. Gen. Hosp. 13 Nov. 43 to 26 Jan. 44 - Catania, Sicily

No. 5 Can. Gen. Hosp. 26 Jan. 44 to 22 March 44 - Andria, Italy

No. 14 Can. Gen. Hosp. 23 March 44 to 8 April 44 - Caserta, Italy (a patient there)

To England on Hospital ship *Atlantis* 8 April to 16 April
No. 17 Can. Gen. Hosp. 4 July 44 to 24 May 45 - Pinewood
Left England 29 May 45 on the *Volendam*
Arrived Halifax 7 June 45
Arrived Regina 11 June 45
Regina Military Hosp. 13 July 45 to 23 July 46
Discharge 23 July 46

Directions given to me by an Englishman to get from Knightsbridge to Trafalgar Square; The following directions will enable you to reach your destination: Take the first turning on the right towards the left of the right hand side of the turning. Turning left of the right side of the left side of the right hand side of the right street.

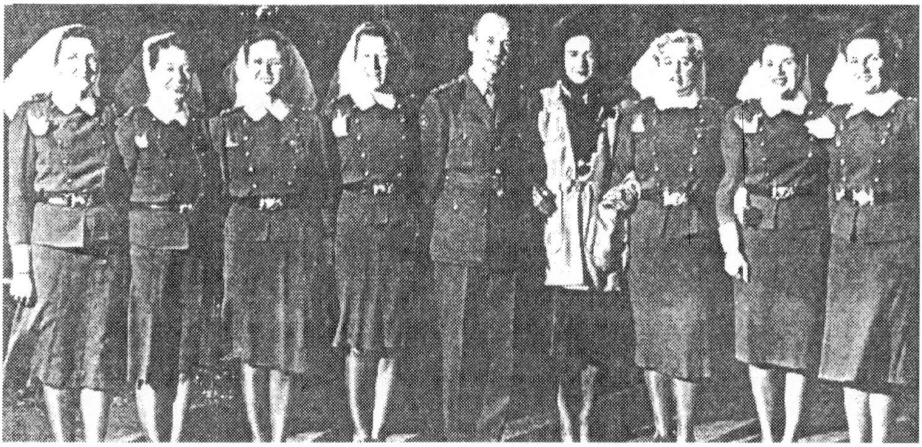

French Countess Visits Canadians in England 14 February 1945:
La Comtesse de Hauteclouque, wife of the French Ambassador-Designate to Ottawa, was cordially received at a French-Canadian military general hospital in England, which she recently visited in order to meet representative Canadians. She had tea in the nursing sister's mess and this photo shows her with a number of these sisters. L-R: Lieut. N/S Kathleen Wadden, Westville, NS; Lieut. N/S Ruby Soper, Edmonton, Alta.; Lieut. N/S Corinne Lettner, Nokomis, Sask.; Lieut. N/S Elinor Peatt, Victoria, BC; Col. C.P. Gaboury, DSO, ED, Montreal, the Countess, who is a veteran of the French liberation movement; Matron Giroux, RRC, Trois-Rivieres, Que.; Lieut. N/S Olive Flint-Jackson, Toronto, Ont. and Lieut. N/S Grace Breau, Moncton, NB.
Canadian Forces photo

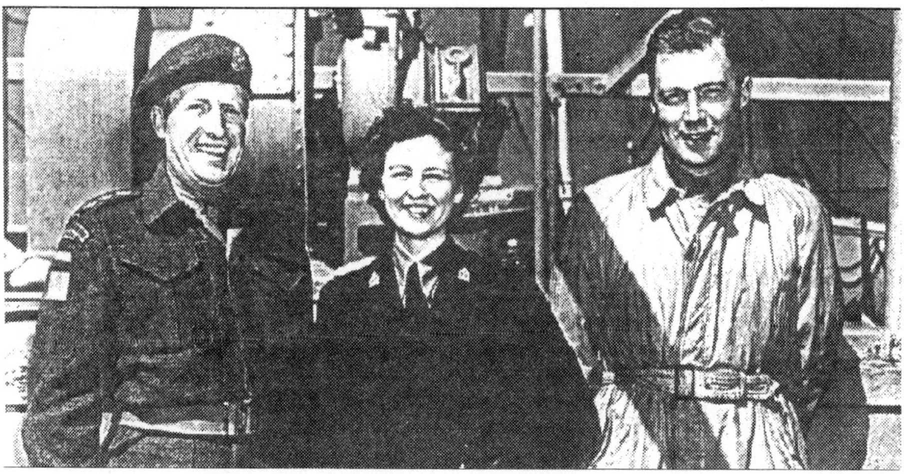

Three Saskatchewan officers on the boat deck of their troop ship Volendam *near the end of a long journey home from overseas. Left to right: Capt. H.S. Robinson, Regina, who commanded headquarters company of the Loyal Edmonton Regiment from Sicily to Holland; Lt. N/S Corinne Lettner, Nokomis, with No. 5 CGH in Sicily and Italy; and Lt. G.C. Scowcraft, Saskatoon, with the 4th Armoured Division from France to the Leopold Canal.*
Canadian Forces photo

Elizabeth (Andreas) McIntosh

Graduated from: Regina General Hospital School of Nursing.
Year: 1938

Military History:

Service: Army

Rank: Lt. to Major

Served: August 1940 to January 1964

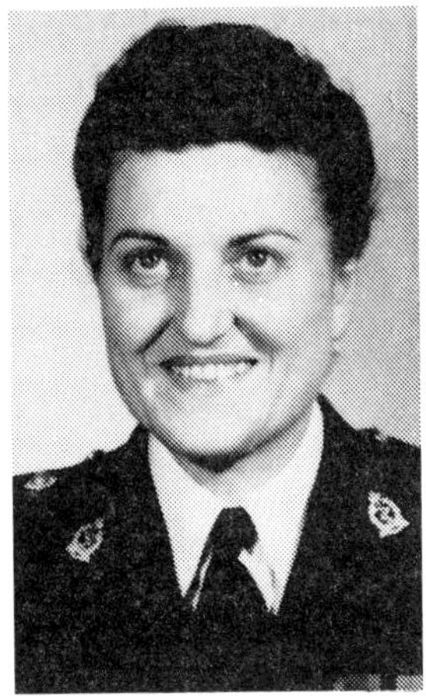

N/S Elizabeth (Andreas) McIntosh, No. 8 CGH who was chosen to represent Canadian nursing sisters at the coronation of Queen Elizabeth 6 February 1952

During the European campaign I was one of the 60 nursing sisters with No. 8 General Hospital, a Saskatchewan Unit.

Prior to the invasion of Normandy, our unit was sent to Yorkshire, England, for field training. We were issued with a field kit which consisted of a water bottle, gas mask, canvas pail, canvas tub and basin, khaki tam, shirt, jacket, heavy boots, sleeping bag, folding camp cot and a tin helmet. We learned how to pack our gear and how to carry it. We learned to pitch tents and how to live under camping conditions using the gear we had.

Following field training we were transported by train, overnight, to London, and then to the south coast of England to a staging area in a forest near Southampton. During this period the buzz bombs (V-1) were frequent disturbances as they were directed at London during the night hours. As it was double daylight saving in Britain, it was not really dark till near midnight. We were loaded onto an ICL (Infantry Landing Craft) in daylight but did not leave Southampton until midnight 18 July 1944.

The 60 nursing sisters were assigned to one of the holds with stacks of bunks, four deep. There were not enough bunks to accommodate all 60, so in more than one instance two people shared a narrow bunk. We had a choice of using a blanket from our bed roll but rather than face the misery of re-rolling the bed roll, most of us slept on the bare planks. The one toilet and the diesel engine were in close proximity to the bunks. The smell and the lack of ventilation was overwhelming. About 3 A.M. our ICL either ran into or was run into by an object (we were told it was an oil tanker). The engines stopped immediately. Prior to lying down, someone left a canvas pail of water beside the lowest bunk. With the jolt of the sudden stop, the pail of water upset. The nursing sister on the outside of the lowest bunk (6 inches from the floor) put her hand in the water. She jumped to her feet and yelled, *"Girls we will have to swim for it."* Everyone was out of their bunks. There was no further thought of sleep but the vomit bags were well used.

By mid-morning on 19 July 1944 we docked at Arromanches on the coast of France. A temporary harbour and dock had been made at the location by towing sunken ships into position. The British were in charge of the dock and the good old "Tommies" had tea brewing on the open dock. They offered us some, and since we carried our own mugs, the tea was greatly appreciated.

As we were loaded onto lorries, we noticed the ground was chewed up from heavy traffic. It was very dusty. The few trees and shrubs were laden with dust. We were transported to our hospital site which was in a field about three or four miles east of Bayeux. There were Canadian soldiers (possibly Engineer Corp) working on the roads; cheering us as we went by.

No. 7 General Hospital preceded us to France and they already had their tent erected in the field very close to our site. We were given accommodation in one of the big tents for two or three nights before our equipment was located and established. By 26 July 1944 our tents were set up in record time and we were operational.

Casualties were heavy. The patients were brought in by ambulance. They were placed in a triage area where they were assessed, documented and directed appropriately. Since the majority had wounds, they were directed through to the operating room and attended to according to priority. The wounds were cleansed, debrided, sprinkled with sulpha powder and, where appropriate, loosely sutured. Limbs were put in bi-valved casts for transportation back to Canadian hospitals in England. The rest period for these patients in the ward tents was very short as the beds had to be cleared and made ready for the next casualties.

The surgical teams were able to operate at night by light provided by a generator. Hurricane lanterns were used in patient tents.

After the first day and night of operating, my staff and I realized that we could not function efficiently with tarpaulin floors. It was difficult to walk; it was hard to transfer instrument trays and very difficult to mop up water spills. It was chaotic! Our priority request was for cement floors under the operating room tents. The engineers provided this, as if by magic, and our work became much more efficient.

The nursing sisters' tents were pitched in an apple orchard. The latrines were dug beside a hedge. There were canvas walls to give privacy but no roof. The path to the latrine was slippery with mud from recent rains so flashlights were a necessity. One flashlight was dropped into the hole accidentally and it stayed lit till the battery ran down.

The nights were disturbed by the ack ack guns and shrapnel fell around the area. When we heard the ack ack we slept on our bed rolls under our cots with our tin helmets over our face.

At the beginning of September our hospital was moved closer to the front lines. Again, we were under canvas near a village just north of Rouen. By now it was getting colder and damp for tent living. It was in mid-October 1944 when we finally settled in Antwerp in buildings.

Harriet J. T. Sloan

Graduated from: Vancouver General Hospital. Year: 1940

Military History:

Service: RCAMC 1943 to 1959 and CFMS 1959 to 1968

Rank: Lt. Colonel, Matron-in-Chief 1964 to 1968

Served: 1943 to 1968

A Tribute

A company of British Pioneers was attached to our general hospital near Bayeux in Normandy. These men were not physically fit for duty with the fighting arms but no group of men anywhere worked harder.

They off-loaded the ambulances. They carried the wounded

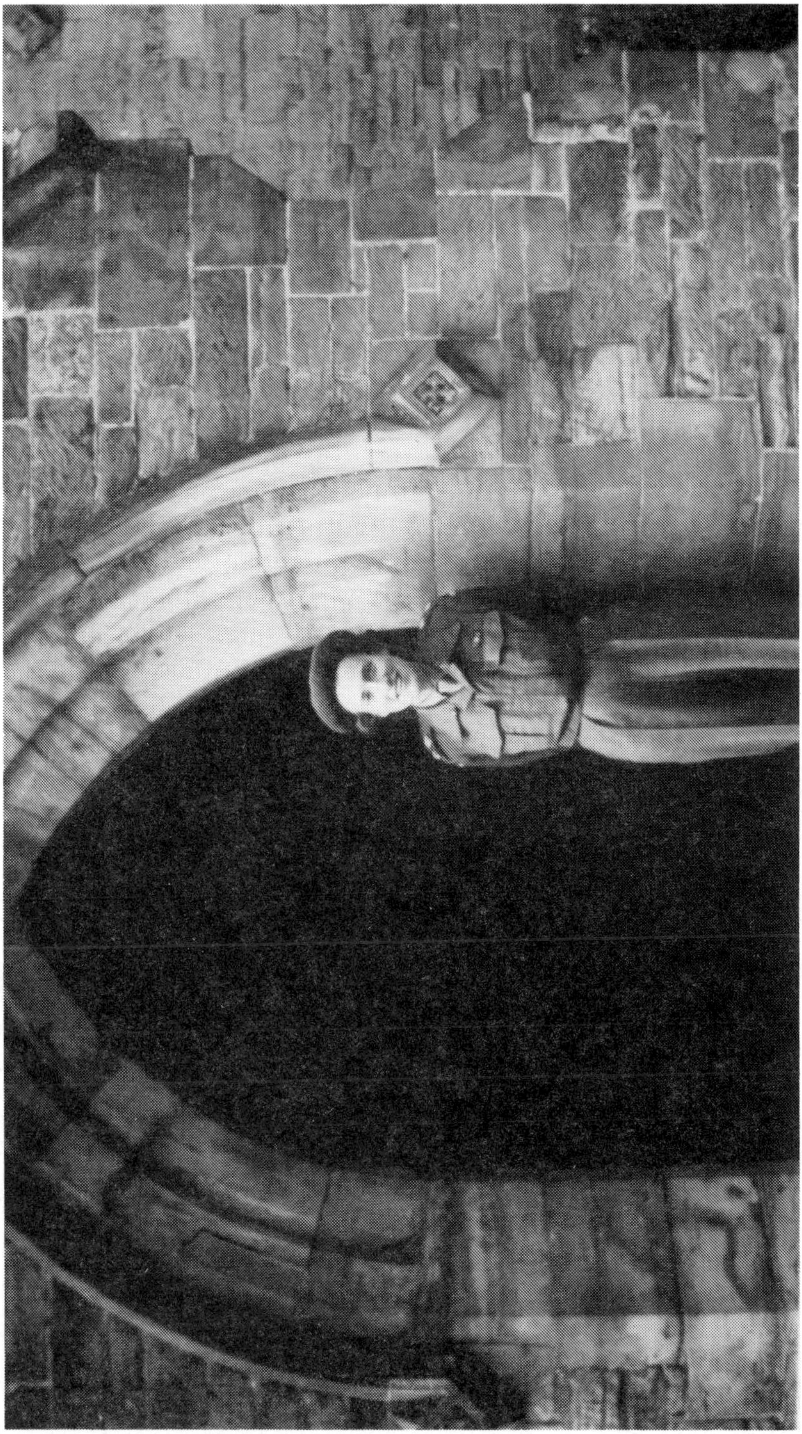

Lieut. N/S Hallie Sloan in battle dress, 1944
Richmond Castle, Richmond, Yorkshire, England

to triage, X-ray, operating room as required, and finally, to the wards. They worked indefatigably around the clock over rough terrain. Tent guy lines must have been a menace, especially at night. There were no lights.

When the mud made it impossible for the ambulances to reach the unit, the Pioneers provided the solution. They unrolled heavy bales of large mesh metal tracks. Through the mesh they wove tree branches, and thus provided a solid base for the ambulance.

They were so cheerful. If you asked them how they managed the long hours of back-breaking work they just grinned and said, *"All right Sister."* And so we gave them yet another mug of "compo" tea. I admired and respected them. They were special.

Mabel (Glew) Tweddell

Graduated from: Regina General Hospital School of Nursing, Regina, Saskatchewan. Year: 1939

Military History:

Service: RCAMC.

Rank: Lt. N/S

Served: From 1941 to 1945

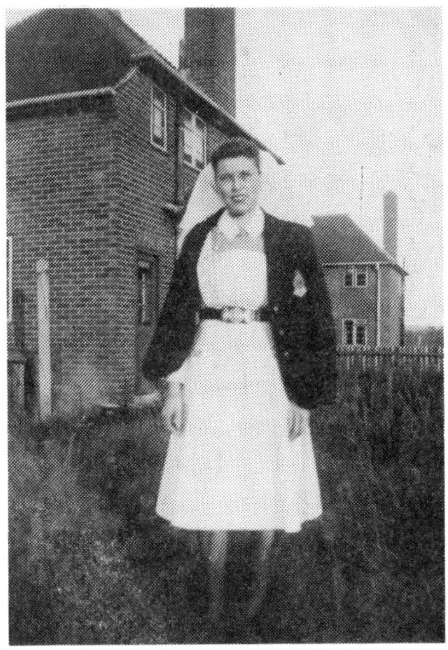

Mabel (Glew) Tweddell living quarters at Farnborough No. 8 CGH, later No. 4 CGH

After graduation from Regina General hospital in 1939 I joined the reserves. It was just a lark, you know. We went out to Dundurn and just had a ball for two weeks. Then in September war broke out. I was in the reserves and was called up.

Through a series of circumstances, I didn't go overseas immediately. In fact, it wasn't until New Year's Eve 1941 that I found myself on a train which eventually wound up in Halifax. At 23 years old, I wasn't really worried until we got on the boat, and then all of us were sure we would never get over there, that we'd be torpedoed. But you know how it is when you're young, we really couldn't care less.

We started out on a ship called the *George Washington*. It had been a ship captured during the First World War by the Americans and then mothballed. The Canadian government bought it, and that's how we went on our way. We just got out of Halifax harbour and the boilers all went kerflooey. So we stayed out there for three days before we managed to get back, and it was five months before we could get another ship to take us over. We finally left for England on the *Empress of Canada*. I was sent to Marston Green near Manchester. Our hospital was right near Aldershot.

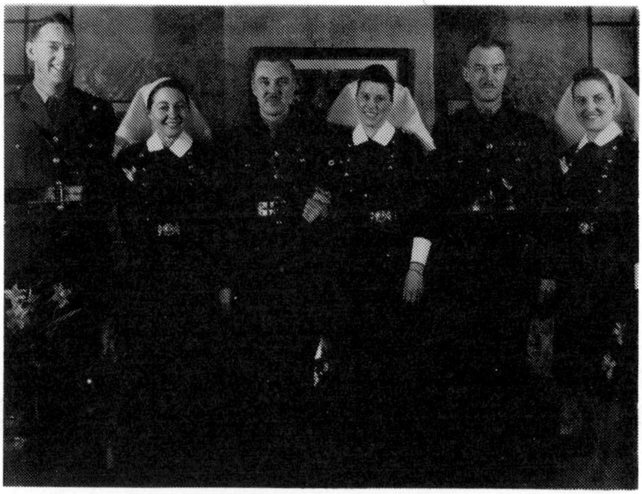

Aldershot 1944, No. 8 CGH.
L-R: Major Fairbairn; Lt. N/S Kay Morton; Major Tweddell; Lt. N/S Mabel (Glew) Tweddell; Major Findley; Lt. N/S Beth (Andreas) McIntosh

In October of 1942 I was in the operating room of a hospital near Aldershot. We used to get these doctors coming in off the field, and we'd say, *"Oh, here's another Joe, another new guy, wonder what he wants?"* So when Tom Tweddell came in we had something, a hernia or something, and someone said, *"Mable, you'd better scrub for him."* I did and that was the start. We were married in February 1944. Tom was insistent that I not go overseas, so I stayed in England for the rest of the war.

In March of 1945 Tom was able to get leave and we went to London and stayed at the Savoy. It was so deluxe and they pampered us. We rode the double-decker buses all over London. We went to all the shows and movies. And then Tom had to go back to cover the crossing of the Rhine at the end of March.

Tom came back to Canada three days before me in July 1945. What sticks out in my mind is what it was like to come home. We'd been living Army life – I'd been four years over there – and it was a different life entirely. You came back here and you'd be amazed how hard it was to get back. They (the people at home) didn't know anything about war. All they knew was that the war was over. They didn't realize what we had been through. I was a nervous wreck when I got back. But it is an experience I wouldn't have missed. We made so many good friends.

Marion I. (Thompson) Wolstein

Graduated from: Regina General Hospital School of Nursing, Regina Saskatchewan. Year: 1935

Military History:

Service: Army

Rank: Lt. N/S

Served: October 1941 to September 1945

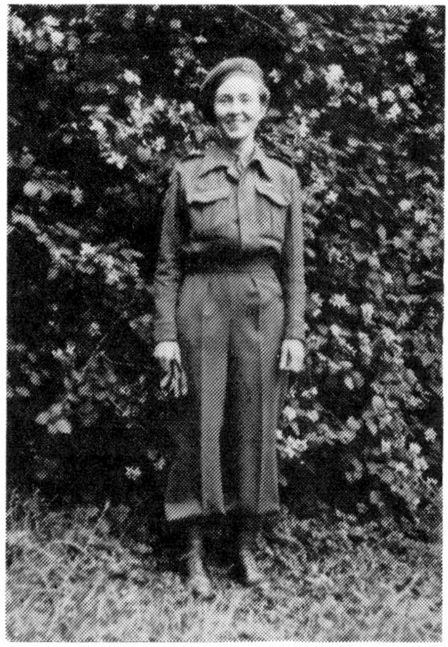

Marion (Thompson) Wolstein, No. 8 CGH 1941- 1945 Yorkshire, England before going to France.

I joined No 8 CGH in Regina in October 1941. I spent October in Dundurn, Saskatchewan and November and December in Debert, Nova Scotia. We began our trip overseas early in January 1942 aboard the *George Washington*, the ship that had carried President Wilson to the Peace Conference in 1918 and had been in dry-dock in Philadelphia ever since. She had been refurbished and painted etc., but sat at such a list in harbour that some passengers got seasick just walking the deck. We were aboard some three exciting weeks during which time we (5000 troops) experienced: 1). a very severe blizzard which froze all the plumbing on board. 2) A banana boat exploded and burned beside us in the harbour. 3) The Glasgow crew decided they weren't about to sail the Atlantic in that ship and staged a full fledged shooting riot on board.

We did eventually set sail, however, and luckily the boilers blew before we got out of Bedford Basin into the U-boats and were ignominiously returned to Debert by train.

Early in March we sailed on the *Empress of Canada*, two

troopships without convoy. The following two and a half years we were stationed in Pinewood and Farnborough in England, then one year plus in France, Belgium and Holland. I was chosen one of the first two nursing sisters sent to serve with a Field Dressing Station (No. 6 FDS) from September 1944 to mid-January, 1945 in Dixmude and Eecloo in Belgium and Zealst in Holland. We worked hard, long hours, one of us on days and one on nights. Many patients were too severely wounded to be evacuated. I still marvel at how efficient the other ranks were, trained by the officers of the FDS – dedicated heroes all.

There was a lull in operations at the end of December 1945 and the officer commanding decided we could all use a break so he organized a "skate." There was lots of ice in the vicinity and he borrowed wooden skates that strapped over our Army boots from friendly visitors. We all looked forward to the treat! However, early in the morning of the first of January, we had a visit from the Luftwaffe. They destroyed our air ambulances on the ground and strafed the residence where we were billeted, flying so low we could see the faces of the pilots. Needless to say, we didn't skate. The windows, chimney and floor slates were smashed. No light, no heat and New Year's dinner was cold bully beef. But no one was injured and we were glad to be alive!

NO. 9 CANADIAN GENERAL HOSPITAL

Bertha (Herr) Hull
Pauline (Glew) Kaleal

No. 9 Canadian General Hospital was mobilized at St. Johns, Quebec and began its function as a unit 1 July 1942. A month later they departed for Debert, Nova Scotia.

The nursing sisters reported to the unit 1 September 1943 from many areas across Canada. The principal matron was M.B. Nelson. On 13 September the unit embarked on the *Queen Elizabeth* at Halifax and sailed the next day. They were situated at Horsham in the U.K. as a 600-bed hospital. They were classified as a coastal hospital and received casualties from the D-Day invasion.

No. 9 Canadian General hospital disbanded 22 September 1945.

Bertha A. (Herr) Hull

Graduated from: Winnipeg General Hospital School of Nursing. Year: 1940

Military History:

Service: RCAMC

Rank: Lieutenant N/S

Served: 3 September 1942 to 30 May 1946

I joined the Army because it just seemed the thing to do. My brother was in the Air Force and my best friend had joined.

I went to Camp Shilo with Matron Roberts to staff the hospital. Matron Roberts was a nursing sister in World War I.

Our accommodations were wooden huts covered with tar paper. We had a stove in each bedroom with the chimney going out the window. Orderlies came in the middle of the night and stoked our fires. Matron Roberts got permission from headquar-

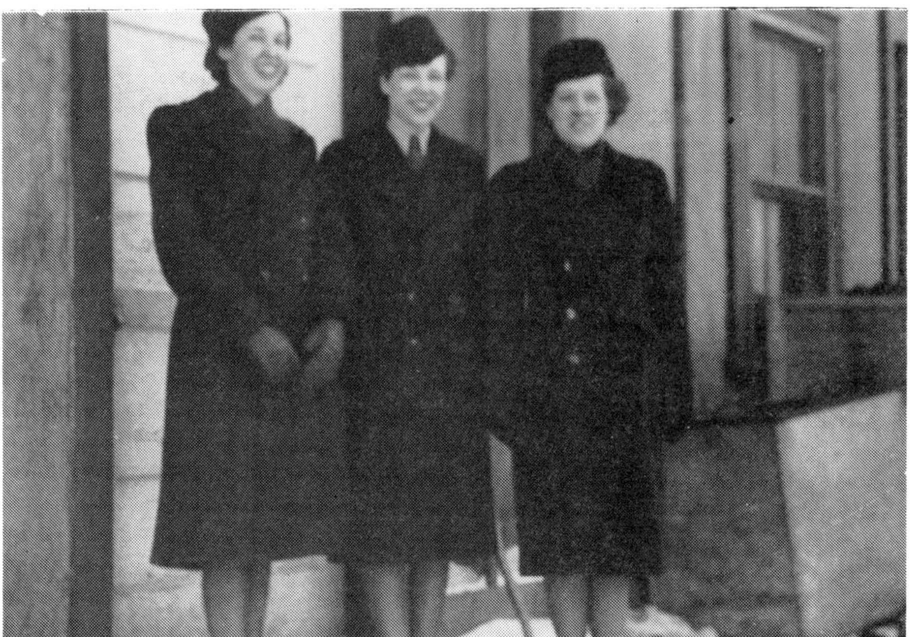

Camp Shilo Manitoba, Winter 1942
Nursing Sisters Stapes; K. Simpson; D. Simpson

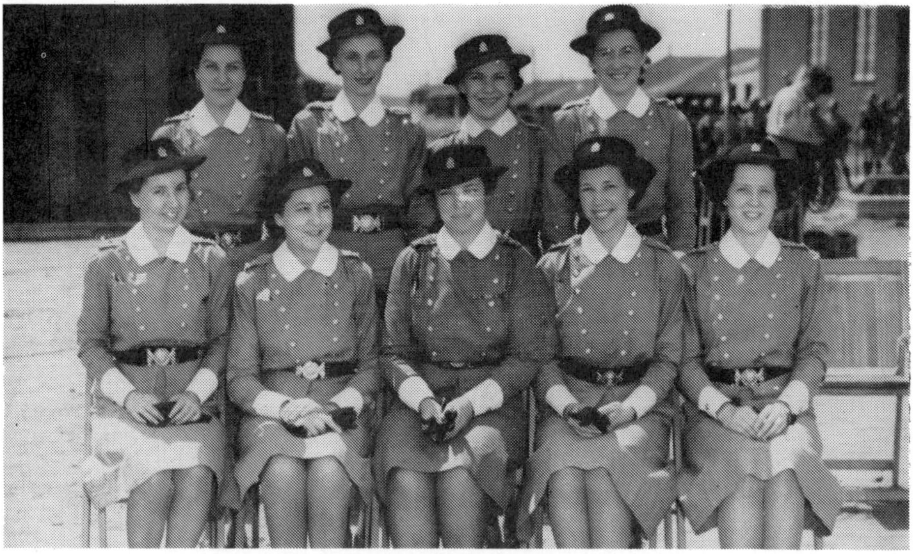

Camp Shilo Manitoba 1943
BACK ROW: Nursing Sisters Berna Tuckwell, Erna Bauman, Arthran, Hains
FRONT ROW: D. Simpson, Matron Roberts, Bertha Herr, Margaret Perley

ters so we could wear Persian lamb hats because of the cold weather in Manitoba – and it was cold!

My mother kept some of my letters – the ones I wrote on leave. Of course, we could not write home too much of what and where we were – also, I didn't want her to worry about me but she was concerned when she heard about the "buzz bombs."

I was at Horsham with No. 9 CGH at that time and we did not know what they were when they first went over. It was strange and frightening, but when the papers came out with the explanation as to what they were, we were not as concerned. Christ Church nearly had a hit and I recall working all night in surgery on the civilians. At that time I was surgical nurse.

The week before the invasion was terrible – waiting and preparing – then it was horrible receiving the wounded – sometimes men that had been injured in France in the morning were back to us being operated on at 4 P.M. Some of them we had socialized with.

Before Christmas 1944 I was sent to No. 20 CGH at Scotch Corner, England, north near the border of Scotland. Isabelle Nicholson and I were sent on as added strength. The unit had been there some time waiting to go over to Belgium. Right after our arrival it was decided we should go for a march with our packs. We had never been training so the Sgt. Maj. had us all

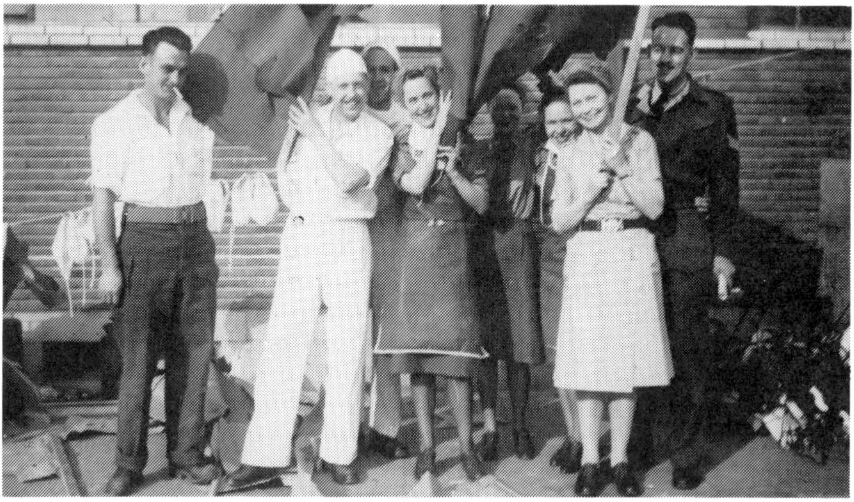

Operating room staff "throw out" blackouts.
Sgt. George May, Winnipeg, N/Ss Jannette Foster, Erna Bowman, Doris Linscott, Kathy Napier, George Taylor, N/Ss Murphy and Donaldson

line up in our battle dress with packs on. One particularly well endowed nurse did not have her straps right so the Sgt. changed them only to have her shift them back saying, "When I'm built like you, I'll wear them that way." He just blushed and went on his way.

No. 20 CGH was stationed at Turnhout, Belgium. I recall that we had a shower once a week, so I used to wash my hair, myself, and my laundry at the same time. While there I was sent to Gaile, Holland with Isabelle Nicholson to relieve a couple of British nurses for leave. I was billeted with a Dutch family that did not speak English so we used our language dictionaries. The hospital was a couple of blocks away in a school. I was there for two weeks. I attended a concert the people put on for the liberating forces.

VE Day was a great day. We tore up the blackout curtains. The Germans that were patients at the time were quite apprehensive when they heard the bagpipes being played through the halls.

Christmas 1944 at No. 20 CGH

We had not been there very long. I recall that we had high windows along the corridors (it was a school) and we made some cut-outs of houses from black paper that came with the X-ray films, then put cotton on them for snow. We covered lids, etc., with foil from cigarettes. Each ward tried to do something.

At one point, while on night duty in my ward, I had

Canadian patients, a Russian and two or three Germans. I used to start at one end of the ward and fix them up for the night, then spent some time with a paralyzed lad getting him to sleep. This particular night the German Sgt. (typical Nazi) started fussing. He had abdominal wounds and had been taken off hypos and put on oral pain killers. He started fussing and making noises, and not wanting him to wake my paralyzed patient, I told him, *"You call yourself the master race, act like it."* He kept quiet. I realized later that I had emphasized the point by shaking my flashlight to him and as he did not understand English, he thought I was going to hit him.

Pauline (Glew) Kaleal

Graduated from: Regina General Hospital School of Nursing. Year: 1942

Military History:

Service: RCAMC

Rank: Lt. N/S

Served: August 1943 to April 1946

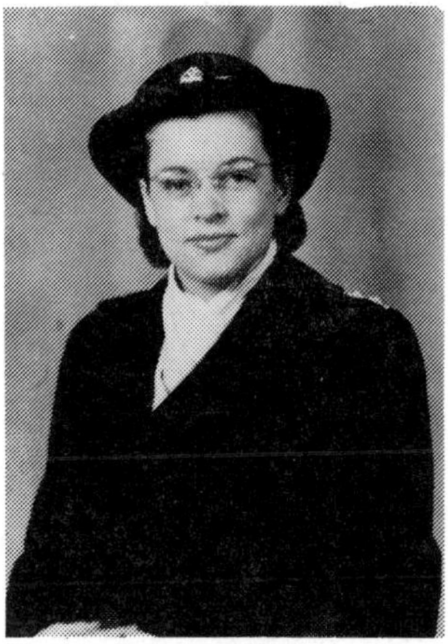

Lt. N/S Pauline Glew
No. 9 CGH

I wanted to join up because my father who, as chairman for the National War Finance Committee, worked hard to achieve the quota needed for the Victory Loans. Three brothers were in the Army and my sister was with the RCAMC.

My military experience was brief but rewarding. I met many interesting people and visited many different places.

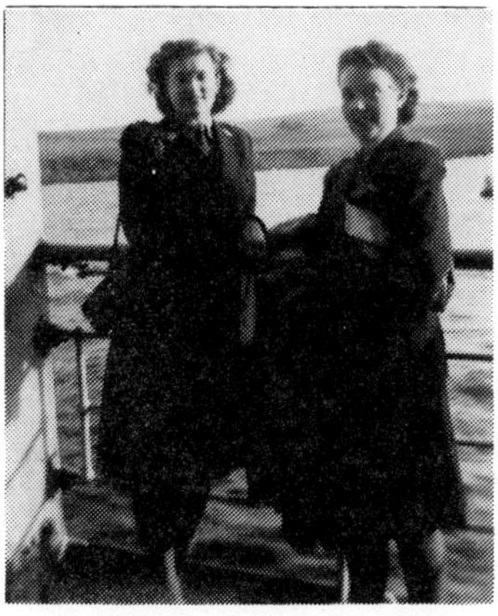

Pauline Glew and Vivien Bergen on leave to Ireland.

NO. 10 CANADIAN GENERAL HOSPITAL

Alexandra Bury
Marie Cantin
Margaret (Lutes) Donaldson
Jean (McIntosh) Elleker
Erna (Penner) Janzen
Margaret (Anderson) Keel
Louise (Sovereign) Marquette
Irene (Stephenson) Mercier
Jessie Morrison
Eleanor (Robinson) Schneider
Eleanor (Winnett) Turvey
Teresa (Woolsey) Weir
Madge Wheaton
Jean (Scrimgeour) Wilson

No. 10 Canadian General Hospital received authority to mobilize at Wolsey Barracks with Col. H.P. Hamilton as commanding officer 1 August 1943.

Matron E. Dick, Ottawa and N/S D.F. Harris, London Military Hospital conducted interviews at London Military Hospital and by 17 August nursing sisters were secured and documented. Ten days later nursing sisters from other military districts began arriving.

Nursing sisters were billeted in private homes when the unit moved to MacLagen Barracks at Stratford, Ontario in mid-October.

They proceeded overseas almost immediately. The unit boarded the *Queen Elizabeth* 11 December 1943 and arrived in Greenock, Scotland, a week later. Their destination was Leavesden, England, just outside Watford.

In March 1944 the nursing sisters were issued battle dress and took part in exercises in the field.

By 22 July the unit sailed in convoy and landed in Arromanches the next day. The nursing sisters sailed 0430 hours and arrived off the coast of France by noon. They were taken off in a small landing craft and began the ride to Bayeux. No. 10 General was located in a hospital area known as "Harley Street."

By the end of August most of the canvas was up and patients began arriving.

No. 10 General began the move to Turnhout, Belgium, at the

end of November. The nursing sisters arrived 30 November 1944 and were pleased to be out of the mud. Matron M. Maclaren replaced Matron Dick and remained at No.10 until mid-February 1945 when Matron Moya MacDonald replaced her.

Casualties were received in great numbers until May 1945 when Churchill announced the war was officially over.

German prisoners of war now replaced Allied soldiers as patients.

Major (P/Matron) Helen Wilson replaced Moya MacDonald as matron.

On 27 July 1945 a British Field Ambulance Unit moved in and removed all the white sand and red bricks from the famous Red Cross on the parade square. All the patients had gone, and by the end of August 1945, No. 10 Canadian General Hospital was awaiting instructions for disbandment.

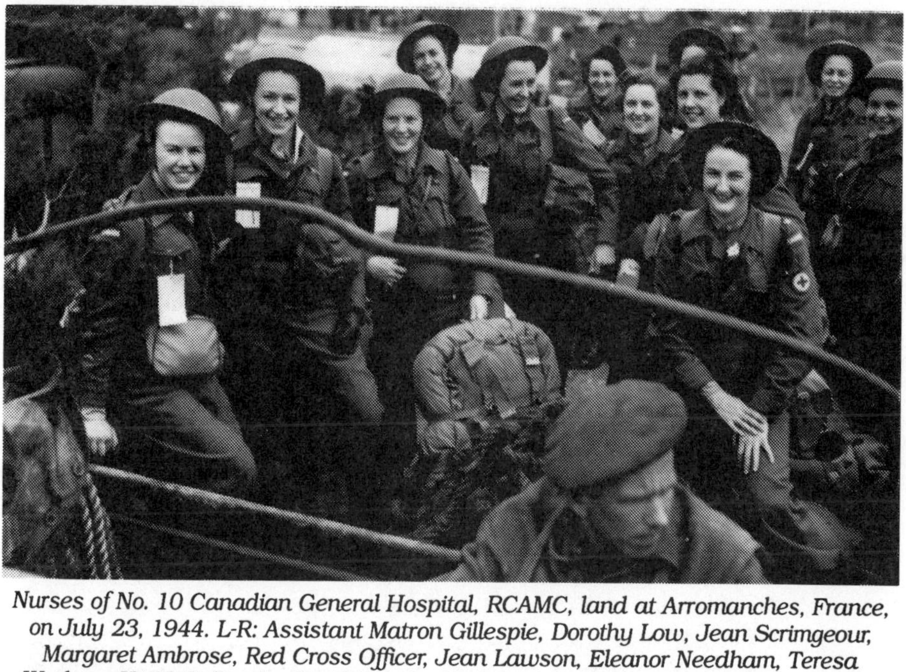

Nurses of No. 10 Canadian General Hospital, RCAMC, land at Arromanches, France, on July 23, 1944. L-R: Assistant Matron Gillespie, Dorothy Low, Jean Scrimgeour, Margaret Ambrose, Red Cross Officer, Jean Lawson, Eleanor Needham, Teresa Woolsey; Kit McCullough, Sue Edwards, Red Cross Officer; Madge Wheaton, Grace Mason. Photographer: Harold G. Aikman, National Archives of Canada, PA108174. The following description of DUKW courtesy of Canadian Military History, Wilfred Laurier University, Waterloo. The photo shows nurses riding in a DUKW. The United States developed a two and a half ton swimming truck capable of carrying fifty men or equivalent load of supplies from ship to shore. It was equipped with six driving wheels and conventional steering gear for use on land and marine propeller and rudder for use in water. The name was given by engineers of General Motors Corporation: D for 1942, U for utility, K for front-wheel drive, and W for two rear driving axles. It was frequently called Duck.

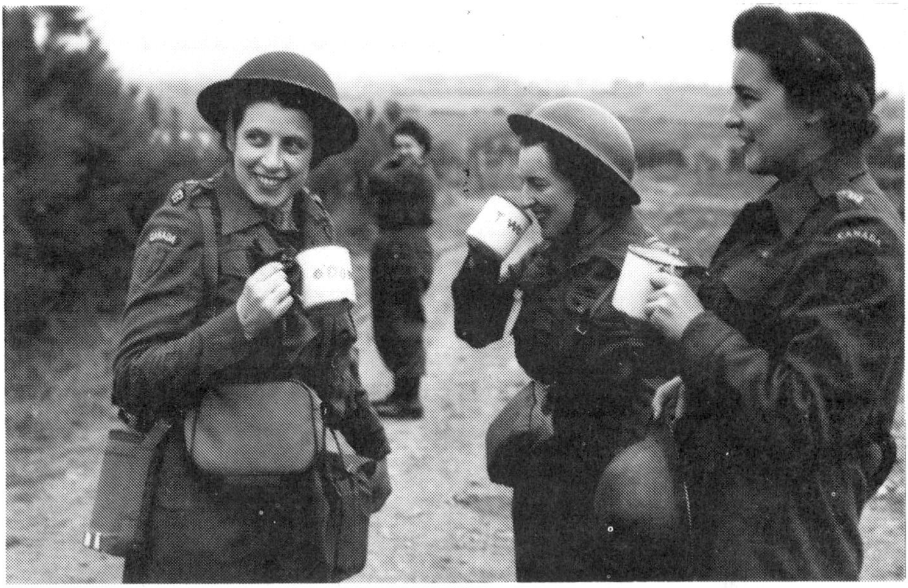

Nursing sisters with No. 10 Canadian General Hospital having a cup of tea upon landing in France at Arromanches Beach, France 23 July 1944: Hazel O'Donnell; Teresa Woolsey and J. MacKenzie. Photographer: Harold G. Aikman, National Archives of Canada, PA132851

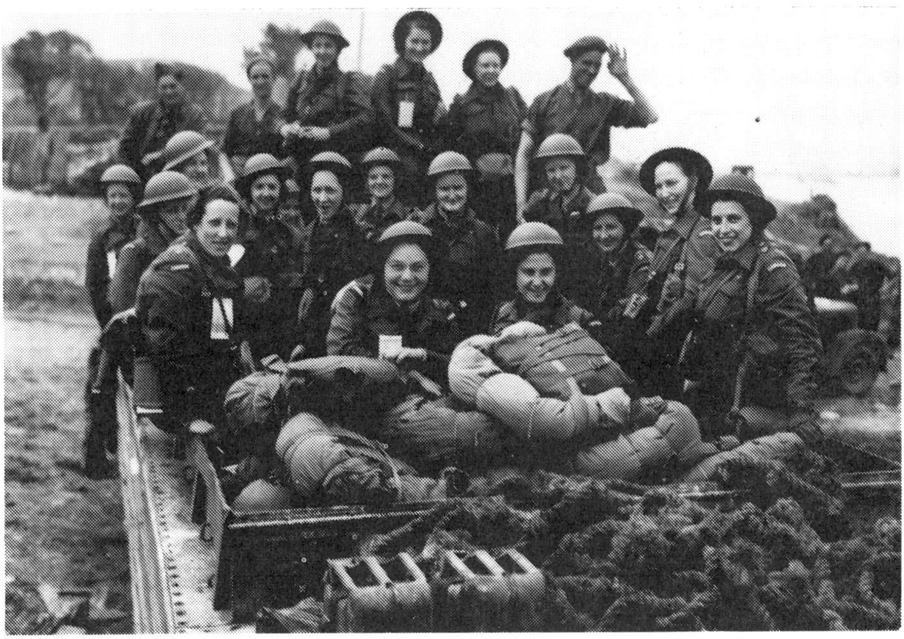

Nursing sisters of No. 10 CGH, RCAMC landing at Arromanches, France 23 July 1944 L: Seated on edge of landing craft: Neta Moore, R: seated on edge of landing craft: Hazel O'Donnell, Jean McIntosh, Alexandra Bury, Margaret Stewart. Photo: Harold G. Aikman, National Archives of Canada, PA108172

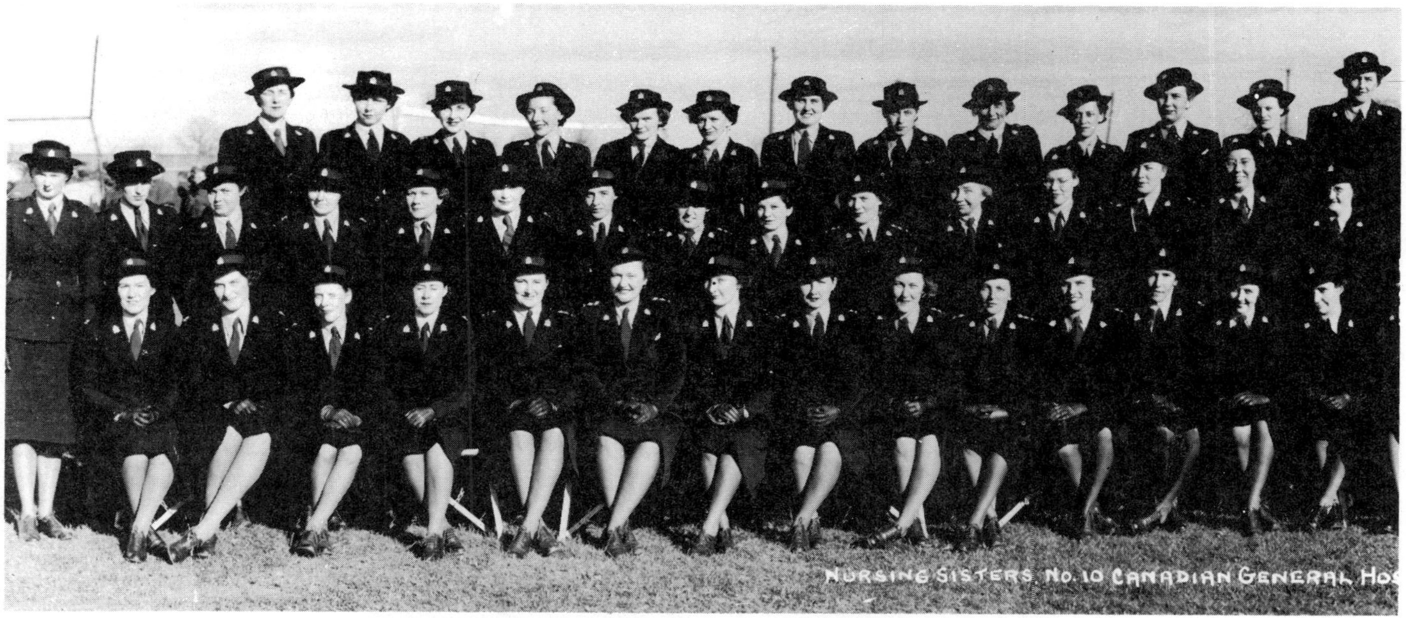

No. 10 Canadian Nursing Sisters November 1942
LEFT REAR; 1. J.A. Atcheson, 2. I.M. Atkin, 3. J.M. Bateman; 4. P.R. Bell; 5. M.M. Bell; 6. K.J. Black; 7. M.H. Black; 8. B. Bowles; 9. B.W. Bradley; 10. M.T.G. Brown; 11. J.M. Burt; 12. A. Butler; 13. A.D. Campbell; 14. M.H. Campbell; RIGHT REAR; 15. M.R. Cantin; 16. L.M. Cardwell; 17. J.M. Chapman; 18. E.D. Chesman; 19. L.M. Climie; 20. A.M. Conroy 21. V.G. Coons; 22. E.J. Cram; 23. C.E. Cummins; 24. M.A. Dean; 25. E.M. Ellacott; 26. F.E. Field; 27. T.M. Finlayson; LEFT MIDDLE; 28. M.E. Forbes; 29. H.M. Grieve; 30. V. Harper; 31. P.F Harris; 32. M.G. Harwood; 33. P.E. Hebb;34. A.J. Henderson; 35. G. Hilock; 36. E. Holfield; 37. C.C. Hull; 38. M. Inches; 39. L.A. Cadwell; 40. P.M. Kersey;41. D.M. King; 42. M. Klassen; 43. K.M. Laird. RIGHT MIDDLE; 44. L.T. Larson; 45. S.D. Legate; 46. N.E. Little; 47. H. Little; 48. E.B. Love; 49. K. Lyne; 50. A.V Macklin; 51. M.S. MacWhirter; 52. A. L. Malone; 53. K.E. Martin; 54. A.J. Martin; 55. I.G. Mason; 56. J.I. MacKenzie;

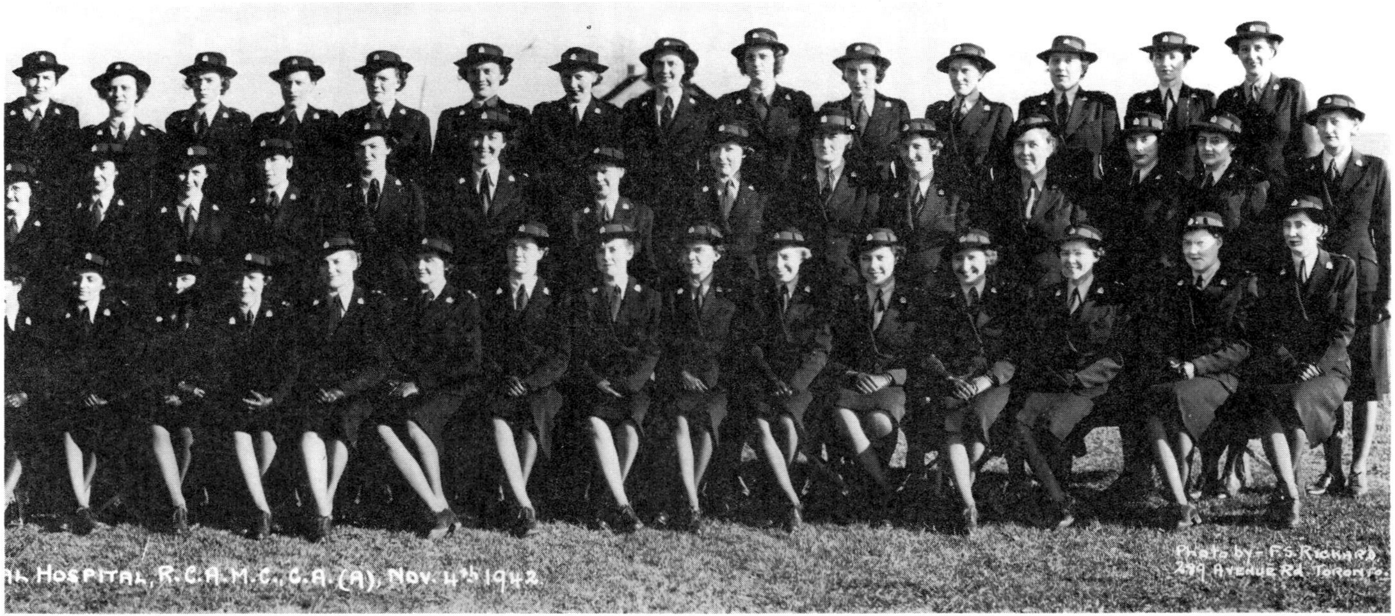

LEFT FRONT; 57. K.B. McCullough; 58. M.M. McManus; 59. M.V. Moore; 60. A.I. Morrison; 61. J.G. Morrison; 62. E.M. Needham; 63. H.M. O'Donnell; 64. M.J. Perkins; 65. M.M. Proctor; 66. E.M. Robinson; 67. E.M. Schmidt; 68. L.M. Schummer; 69. J.D. Scrimgeour; 70. E. Smith; 71. E.J. C. Smith; RIGHT FRONT; 72. L.G. Sovereign; 73. M.I. Stephenson; 74. M.L. Sturdevant; 75. B.A. Syerson; 76. E.R. Truman; 77. D.G. White; 78. L.M. Wilks; 79. A.E. Zumach;

THE NEXT FIVE NAMES ARE PHYSIOTHERAPISTS, DIETITIAN, HOME SISTER; 80. M.I. Miller; 81. E.M. Oliver; 82. P. Wakefield; 83. A.P. McGuigan; 84. I. L. Wellwood; 85. Matron E.R. Dick.

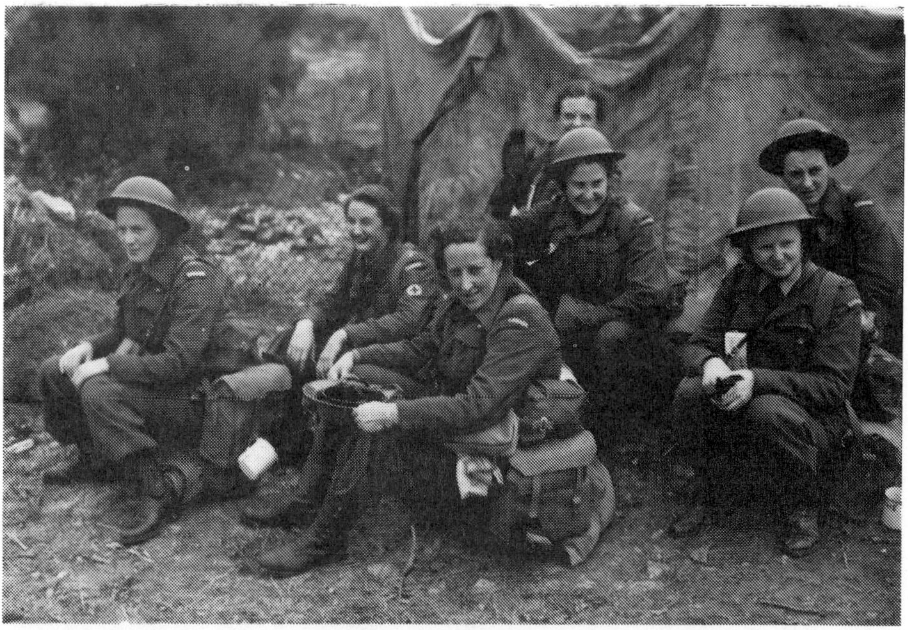

Nursing sisters of No. 10 CGH, RCAMC at Arromanches, France 23 July 1944
L-R: Jean Scrimgeour, Susan Edwards, Neta Moore,
Leona Whitmore, Margaret Stewart.
Photographer: Harold G. Aikman, National Archives of Canada, PA108173

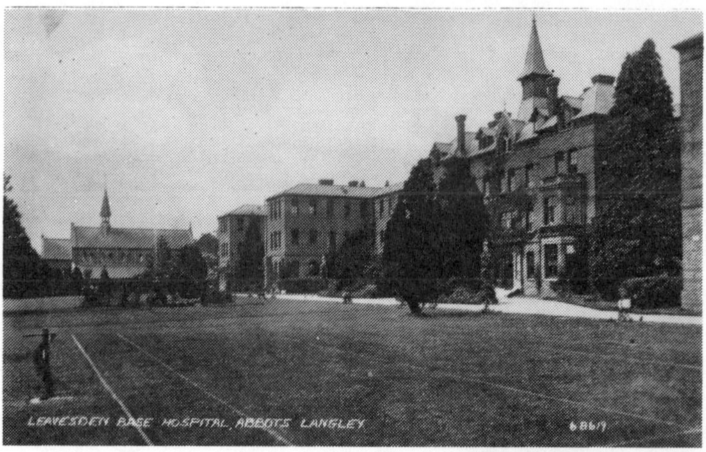

No. 10 CGH at Leavesden near Watford, December 1942

No. 10 CGH at Leavesden near Watford, December 1942

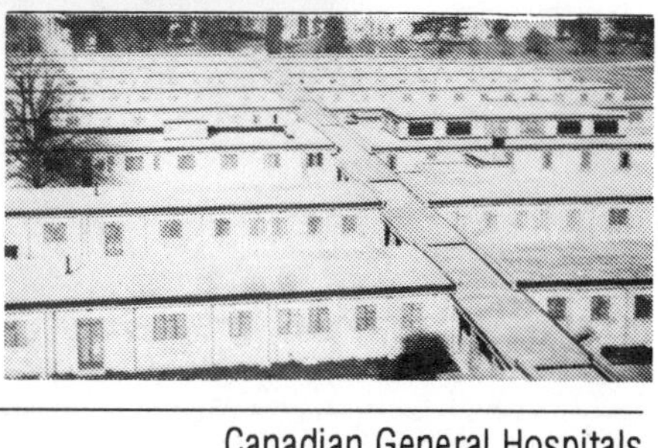

Alexandra Bury

Graduated from: Misericordia Hospital School of Nursing, Edmonton, Alberta. Year: 1931

Other: Registered Medical Records Librarian

Military History:

Service: SAMNS and RCAMC

Rank: Lieut. Nursing Sister

Served: November 1941 to March 1946

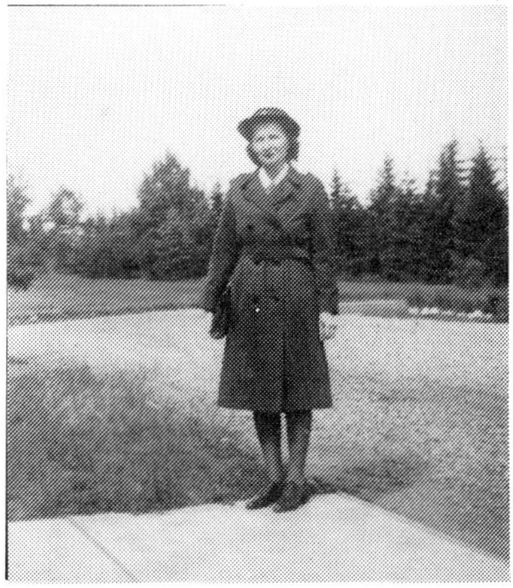

Lt. N/S Alexandra Bury
No. 10 CGH

A sense of duty and wanting to help, as well as travel, all influenced me to choose a military career.

Nursing casualties during WW II was a very meaningful experience for me; for short periods in South Africa and England, but mostly in France. In July 1944, I was with the No. 10 Canadian General Hospital when it was moved to Normandy, south of Bayeux. There, on six fields of cow pasture, large tents were set up for a 1200-bed acute care hospital and small ones for some 300 staff members, of whom about ninety-five were nurses. We were two to a tent. Everyone worked – nurses scrubbing and making up beds, dressing and chart holders.

In early August, convoys of patients began to arrive. When ward beds were filled, other stretcher cases were placed on the floor. The men had injuries to various parts of their bodies – head, chest, abdomen, missing limbs, and so on. Nurses and orderlies worked at a steady pace. On nights during a 12-hour shift I recall giving more than one hundred injections of penicillin and morphine, boiling needles between hypos. For some weeks it was intensive nursing with a fast turnover – patients who came one day were usually flown to a base hospital in England the next day (their medical records, I was told, went with them). During this time we heard the crackle of anti-aircraft, and shrapnel fell through the roof onto beds, making us nervous; some patients shuddered involuntarily. Nights were bright with fireworks and searchlights swaying. Daytime skies were impressive when bombers and fighter planes roared overhead.

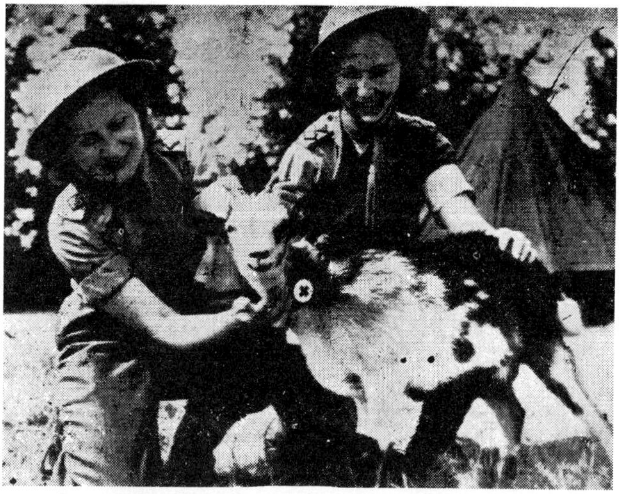

August 1944. "Chewey" the goat, wandered into the area where a Canadian general hospital was being set up in France, and stayed. Now the best of friends are Lt. N/S Alexe Bury, Edmonton; Lt. N/S Jean MacIntosh, Calgary and the goat.
Canadian Forces photo

The wounded were a mixture of nationalities and ranks, most in their teens to mid-thirties. All were the best of patients, polite and easy to look after. Enduring their injuries bravely, I remember many of them fondly and sadly – the blue-eyed teenager from Saskatchewan, terribly nervous but cheerful; the bonny young Scot writing poetry to nurses; the officer who showed us snaps of his wife and baby and gave me a recipe for Yorkshire pudding; a silent young soldier who had lost his right foot; the lad from England who spoke a dialect I didn't understand – an orderly had to help me out; another English chap who didn't finish his dinner and when I asked him why, he said it was for pigs (the one time we had corn as a treat); the young German, recently married, anxious to know if he would walk again – one of our chaplains was with him before he died that night because of the hideous wounds to his lower back (later, the minister himself became a patient when he developed stomach ulcers); also, two German youngsters, nicknamed Hans and Fritz, who cheerfully helped with carrying water, sweeping floors and other chores.

On Saturdays our three chaplains made ward rounds to tell us about Sunday services which at times were held outdoors. Some mobile patients attended. I went to Mass, usually with my friend Terry Woolsey.

As the front advanced, our work eased up. Once when Madge Wheaton and I were walking on the country road, a jeep rattled by – there was General Montgomery standing up, waving to us. We waved back.

In the fall we were transported to Belgium by lorry, and along the way we saw a lot of buildings in ruins. In Turnhout we were set up in brick buildings, and some thirty of us were crowded in a large room. Again, we nursed young men, most of whom were exhausted and anxious to get back home. They missed families and "home life" as well as fresh eggs – we were all tired of powdered eggs.

On time-off we went out, often shopping, trading cigarettes from home for paintings of windmills, wooden shoes and such. My friend, Jean McIntosh, and I met a hospitable Belgian family who spoke English, fed us goodies and we took them refreshments from the mess. One day we went to a cemetery of white crosses (Canadians and unknowns) where Jean placed flowers on the grave of a family friend. Once two Canadian officers took us for a drive in a jeep and stopped by a river. We got out to look across at Germany, which appeared as benign as the ground we stood on. At that time we knew nothing about the gruesome goings-on in places like Buchenwald.

After coming home to Vancouver, B.C., in the fall of 1945, I went to the military hospital in Victoria, B.C., where we nursed ex-POWs returning from Japan – men who had survived prolonged trauma.

Though I mourned the death of friends (those lost at sea and those killed in Europe), I was very thankful my two brothers returned home after years overseas. And I am glad I had the privilege of nursing our valiant veterans who did so much for us and paid so dearly for our freedom.

Marie R. J. Cantin

Graduated from: Misericordia Hospital School of Nursing, Winnipeg. Year: 1936

Military History:

Service: RCAMC

Rank: Captain

Served: March 1942 to December 1962

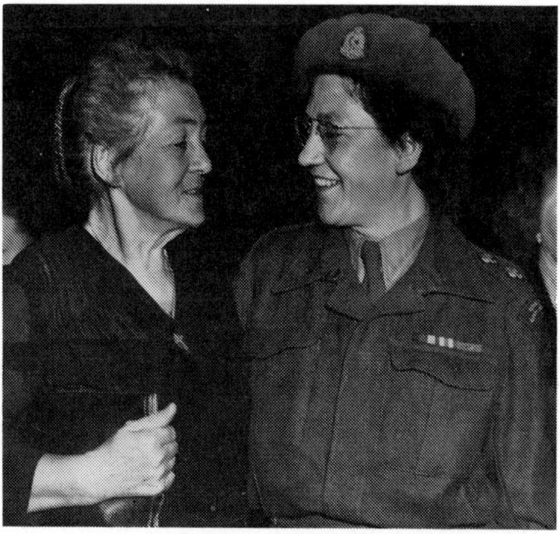

Captain Marie R. J. Cantin, RCAMC March 1942-December 1962 with her mother Julienne M. Cantin in Winnipeg on her return from overseas in July 1945. Loaned by her brother, Albert J. Cantin

During World War II, the total family of 10 children (1 girl, 9 boys) served in the Armed Services.

The following information has been supplied by her brother, Albert Cantin.Marie is in the Personal Care Home at McCreary, Manitoba.

Marie spent her entire career in the RCAMC as an operating room nurse. She was stationed at Fort Osborne Military Hospital until October 1942 when she was transferred to No. 10 Canadian General in Toronto. The unit moved to the U.K. in December 1942. After D-Day in 1944, No. 10 CGH moved to the Continent and was located in western Belgium from April 1945 to July of that year. She was attached to the RCAMC operating out of front line field dressing stations from Holland to Germany.

Following her return to Canada, Marie joined the permanent force. From 1946 to 1950 she was stationed in Toronto. She served at the Quebec Military Hospital until June 1955, when she was transferred to Shilo, Manitoba. Her final posting was to the Winnipeg Military Hospital in 1957 until her retirement in 1962.

After retirement Marie worked briefly in British Columbia but returned to McCreary, Manitoba, to look after her parents. She currently resides at McCreary.

The highlight of her career would be the period of service overseas and especially her involvement at Field Dressing Stations on the Continent. She remains very proud of her family's involvement during WW II and looked forward to frequent visits with her brothers while overseas.

Margaret M. (Lutes) Donaldson

Graduated from: Kitchener-Waterloo Hospital School of Nursing, Kitchener, Ontario

Military History:

Service: RCAMC

Rank: Lt. N/S

Served: August 16, 1942 to December 1945

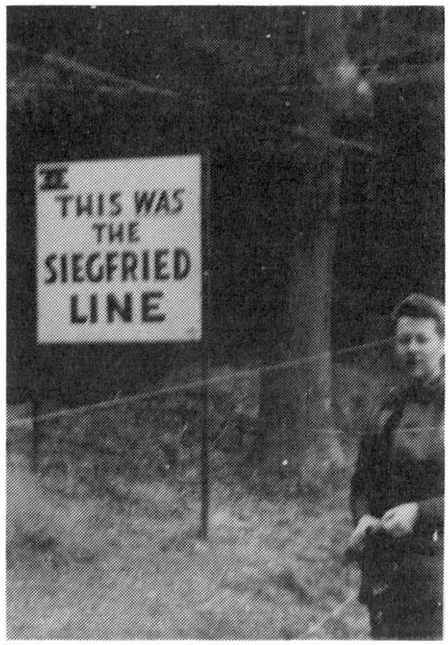

Margaret (Lutes) Donaldson near Cleves, Germany April 1945

Dr. Hamilton of K-W Hospital was recruiting nurses to form No. 10 Canadian General Hospital. He was to be the OC. I joined the RCAMC along with many of my K-W nursing friends.

The highlights of my military experience were:

No. 13 CGH Canada - England
No. 8 CGH France, Belgium, Holland
No. 5 CCS No. 5 FDS
No. 6 CCS No. 6 FDS
No. 2 CCS

I was married at s'Hertogenbosch, Holland, 24 May 1945 to Capt. Robert H. Donaldson of South Alberta Regt.

Jean (McIntosh) Elleker

Graduated from: Holy Cross Hospital School Of Nursing, Calgary. Year: 1937

Military History:

Service: SAMNS and RCAMC

Rank: Lieutenant N/S

Served: 1941 to 1945

I chose a military career for travel and excitement.

My military experience was something I would not have missed. From sunny Africa to Red Deer, Canada, then to England, France, then Belgium.

Highlights were: Working at 2 CCS in France when they were bombing Carpiquet Airport. The flowers in Africa. Africa in general. It was beautiful.

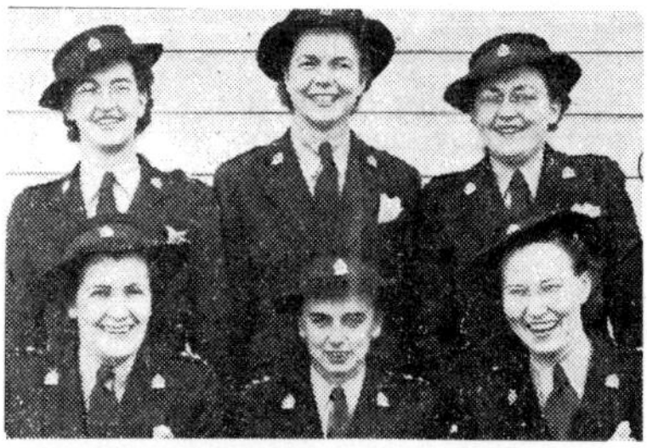

Six nursing sisters from Calgary were included in a group of nursing sisters whose safe arrival overseas has been announced. L-R: Front Row: Ruth Hooper, Lethbridge; Erica Gifford, Calgary; Jean McIntosh, Calgary; 2nd Row: Letitia Simmons, Calgary; Elsie May Smith, Calgary; Eileen Corbett, Calgary. Canadian Forces photo

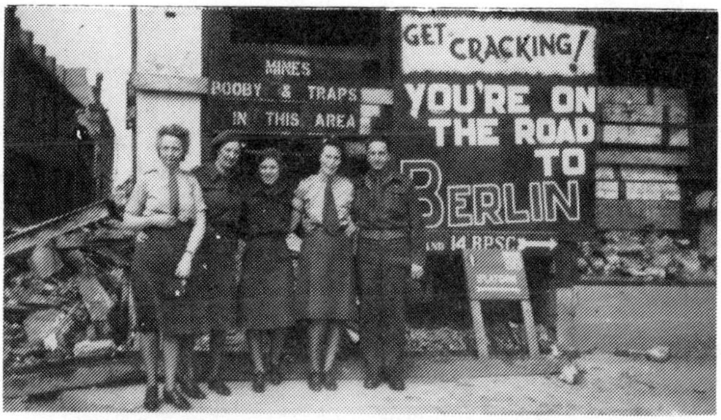

August 1944 No. 10 CGH on the way from Normandy to Belgium; Marjory Hooper 3rd from left, Jean McIntosh 4th from left and our lorry driver

Erna E. (Penner) Janzen

Graduated from: Women's College Hospital School of Nursing, Toronto, Ontario. Year: 1938

Military History:

Service: RCAMC

Rank: Lt. N/S

Served: December 1942 to July 1946

It was wartime and nurses were joining up and I wanted to be a party to it. I was a trained nurse and I think I felt a sense of duty for the war effort. The possibility of travel, seeing the country and, of course, the uniform had some appeal too.

Camp Borden Military Hospital, Ontario. One year – 1943.

The highlights of my military experience were:

No. 10 CGH, Watford, England, January to June 1944.

No. 10 CGH, Turnhout, Belgium, July 1944 to June 1945.

Chorley Park Hospital, Toronto, July 1945 to July 1946.

After my military service I took a course in public health nursing and did community nursing until my marriage in 1949.

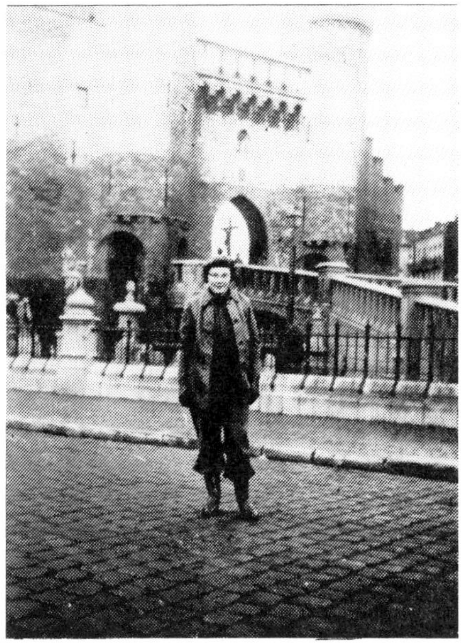

Lt. N/S Erna Penner. Christmas Day 1944, Turnhout, Belgium

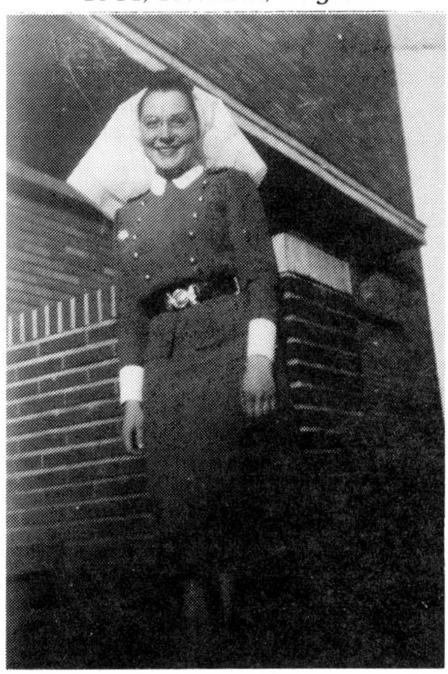

Lt. N/S Erna (Penner) Janzen; Antwerp, Belgium 1944

Margaret B. (Anderson) Keel

Graduated from: Orillia Memorial Hospital (Soldiers) School of Nursing, Orillia, Ontario. Year: 1940

Military History:

Served: RCAMC

Rank: Lieut. Nursing Sister

Served: 1 August 1943 to February, 1946

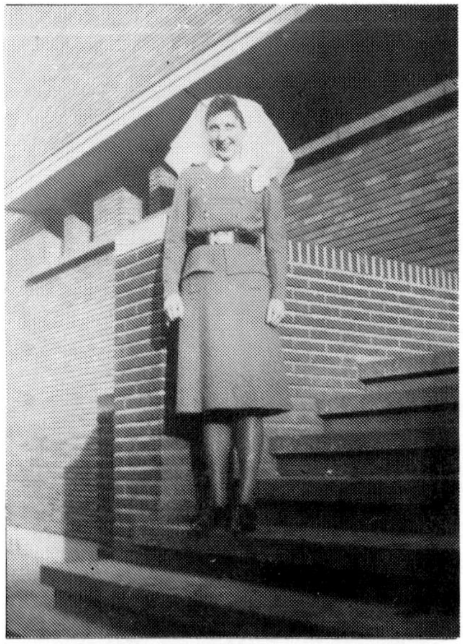

N/S Margaret (Anderson) Keel Turnhout, Belgium, Christmas 1944. No. 10 CGH, front entrance to our mess.

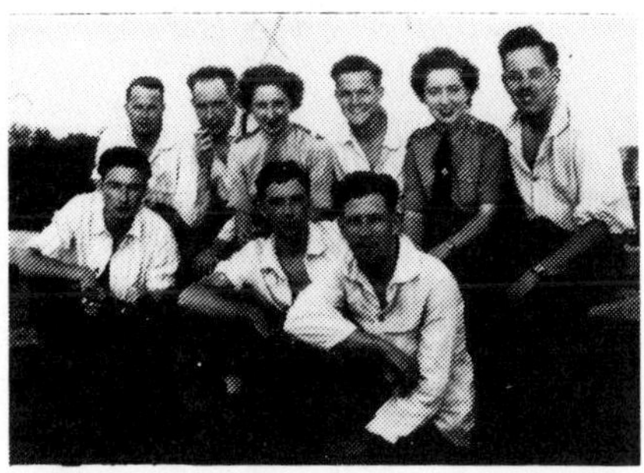

N/S Margaret (Anderson) Keel and Pearl Bloomfield This is Pearl & me up on the roof of our hospital with some of our Canadian patients in Turnhout, Belgium, close to the Holland border. We were 15 miles from Antwerp, Belgium. We wore khaki uniforms on the continent, our blues in England.

I had several friends in the RCAMC. I had a boyfriend that had gone overseas in 1942. My cousin, whom I grew up with was in the Army, went overseas in November 1940 and was killed at Ravenna, Italy, Christmas Eve 1944. All of this influenced me to choose a military career.

I went to Bayeux, France with two of the patients who had passes. We ate at one of the eating places and started to hitchhike back to No. 10 Canadian General Hospital - about three miles. It happened that Field Marshall Montgomery was in our area and came upon the three of us walking. He had his driver stop. I was asked to sit with him in the back seat and the boys in the front. I recognized all the braid and the flag on the car and nearly had a heart attack! I fully expected he would tell Col. Hamilton and Matron Captain Edith Dick. I thought I'd be sent home dishonourably discharged. We drove into the hospital grounds, they let us out, that was it.

There were lots of interesting times. It was a wonderful experience.

Louise G. (Sovereign) Marquette

Graduated from: Victoria Hospital School of Nursing, London, Ontario. Year: 1940

Military History:

Service: RCAMC

Rank: Lt. N/S

Served: August 1942 to September 1945

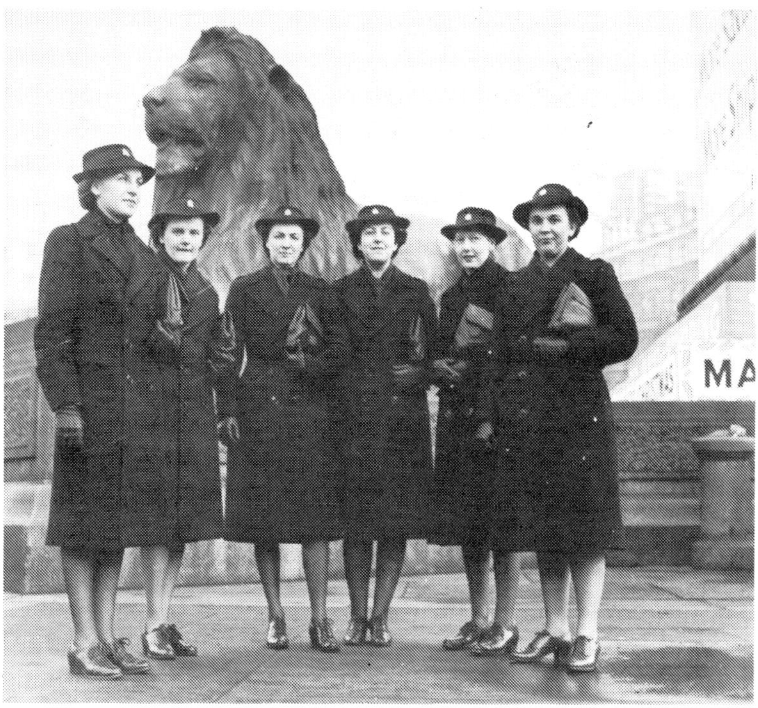

L-R: Nursing Sisters Mary Proctor, Margaret (Forbes) McCallum, Louise (Sturdevant) Graham, Eleanor (Robinson) Schneider, Louise (Sovereign) Marquette, Flora Fields
Canadian Forces photo

Irene (Stephenson) Mercier

Graduated from: Kitchener-Waterloo Hospital School of Nursing. Year: 1941

Military History:

Served: RCAMC

Rank: Lieutenant (N/S)

Served: August 1942 to July 1946

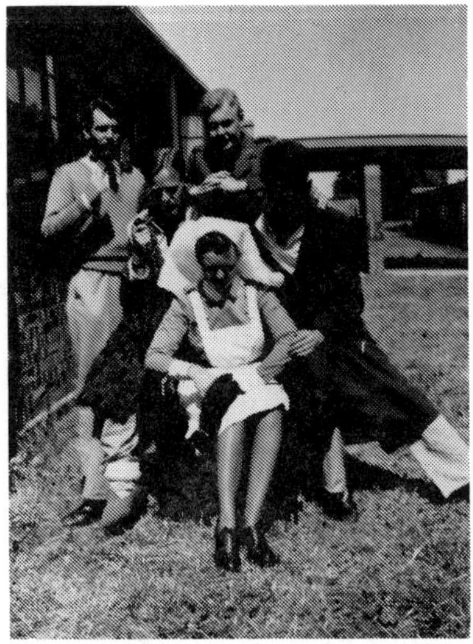

Irene Stephenson with patients and kitten at Leavesden, 1943. No. 10 CGH

When No. 10 CGH was recruited in our area, it was natural for me to sign up. Also, I wanted to be with the boys.

It was the summer of 1942. Two friends, also nurses, and I had rented a cottage at Grand Bend on Lake Huron for the month of July. It was my first real holiday in four years. Our country was at war and things weren't going well. There had been the blitz in London, and the fall of Dunkirk. There was the fall of Hong Kong and all Canadians taken prisoner by the Japanese, including two Canadian nursing sisters, May Waters of Winnipeg, and Kay Christie of Toronto; they would remain prisoners for almost two years.

Other disasters would be the Dieppe raid (August 19th, 1942). Also a Canadian Nursing Sister, Agnes Wilkie, drowned when the *Caribou* was torpedoed on the way to Newfoundland. The Germans had taken most of Europe.

Here on the beach we seemed removed from war news. The Americans had come into the war in December 1941 when Pearl Harbor was bombed and U.S. servicemen were appearing at the beach. We swam during the day and at night went dancing to the big bands at the casino. In the midst of this I received a call from Kitchener telling me of a hospital unit being formed to go overseas almost immediately. This was No. 10 CGH, a 1200-bed unit being recruited with many from the London and K-W area.

My story is also the story of No. 10 as I remained with this unit until the war ended and returned home with them. The minimum age limit for Canadian nurses to go overseas had just been reduced from 25 to 23 years of age, and I had turned 23 in March and had my RN diploma. I couldn't wait to sign up. I took the bus to London and became a member of No. 10.

Nurses' training in those days was very thorough. We had to scrub up and assist at a number of major and minor operations in the OR and similarly in the caseroom. Sterile technique was very important; no penicillin in those days. A crack on the knuckles from a sterile forcep wielded by a circulating nurse was a sharp reminder. Just the threat of it was enough to keep us on our toes. Nevertheless, they thought we needed more training in a military hospital. I was one of those sent to Kingston Military Hospital. Our living conditions were very poor, or perhaps I just hit a particularly poor boarding house. Coupled with this, I was assigned to a ward full of pneumonia patients. Eventually I came down with pneumonia myself, violent chills, temperature of 105, and severe chest pains. I was sent to hospital by ambulance. All I remember is the terrible chest pains and wanting an oxygen tent which never materialized, probably because the hospital didn't have one. I was very ill but recovered and was able to move on the with rest to Stratford when the order came.

While in Kingston we went up to Montreal to buy uniforms from Simpson's; there were two greatcoats, navy blue with cherry lining for winter, one for summer as well as navy blue trenchcoat. A beautiful cape with cherry lining, a navy blue suit with medium blue shirt pleated in front, with navy tie and hat, a navy purse and brown leather shoes. There was a lovely medium blue crepe dress for summer and a similar one in wool for winter, complete with brass buttons, stiff white collar and cuffs. All our uniforms had epaulets to which we attached our rank of Second Lieutenant. In six months we would receive a second "pip" when we would be promoted to First Lieutenant. Our working uniform was similar to the blue dress, only in cotton, complete with white aprons and bibs and a white organdy veil.

We had to buy a steamer trunk and a steamer rug also. On the list was another curious item – a pair of fine white kid gloves. We were told that this was in case we met the Queen. As officers we had to buy our own uniforms, but were given a $250 clothing allowance. The bill was more like $500, and we had to make up the difference. Our salary was $150 a month, so I was in debt to Simpson's for a while.

Also in Kingston we met a couple of fellows who were dressed like French gendarmes and said they were from Paris, France. They never let their guard down, and it was years later I became aware they were French-Canadians being trained for the French Resistance, probably at Camp X as we were near there. I met one of them after the war, Pierre Meunier, and he talked a little bit about his experiences in the underground. To me, that was one of the most difficult assignments in WW II.

From Kingston we moved to Stratford, Ontario, and for the first time our whole hospital unit was together. Our commanding officer was Col. H.P. Hamilton, M.C. ED; a Kitchener doctor and a veteran of the First World War. In a newspaper interview he said he would have a total of 225 personnel including 85 nurses and 33 doctors and be equipped to handle 1200 beds. He expected to go overseas soon.

Our matron was Edith Dick, former inspector of training schools in Ontario. She was a wonderful lady, very kind and considerate and much liked by all the nurses. Years later, after her death, nurses who had been with No. 10 journeyed to her home town of Milton to present and dedicate a plaque in her honour to be hung on her church wall.

In Stratford we did a lot of route marching around town. We stayed in private homes. I had a nice warm boarding house and great meals. I couldn't get enough of my landlady's cabbage salad. I really appreciated her good care, especially after our experiences in Kingston.

In December we boarded the train for the East Coast. The troop train was blacked out, but I remember going through Riviere du Loup. On arrival in Halifax we discovered we would sail on the *Queen Elizabeth*, that wonderful ship that was so fast she needed no escort.

It was said at the time that there were 17,000 troops on board, the same number as the city of Stratford at that time. There were even tiers of bunks in the swimming pool. We set sail around mid-December. History records it as one of the roughest crossings the *Queen E* ever made as a troopship. Waves were very high. Rumours abounded such as the ship was listing dangerously and that someone was washed overboard in the night. About half way across the Atlantic we had an alarm that an unidentified aircraft was overhead. We were ordered to our posts, but soon the all-clear sounded and we were told the plane turned out to be one of ours. We zigged and zagged to fool the U-boats, and finally landed in Scotland.

We took a train to London, then to Watford and out to Abbots Langley, to Leavesden Hospital, which had been nicely prepared for us. There was one large building, and the rest consisted of numerous huts for staff and patients. It was nearly Christmas. Everything was green. I remember especially the green holly. No, it was not a white Christmas, but we were happy and excited to be in England.

Our hospital was located close to London. We could take a cab into Watford and from there the underground into London. Charlie Young's Chinese restaurant on Wardour Street became a favourite. We saw the terrible ruins in the East End, a result of the relentless German air raids.

Something which greatly surprised us was to find actual television sets in some of the stores. This was unheard of at home. However, we never saw a working set. A few invitations came in for a reception to be held at the Mansion House in London given by the Lord Mayor of London, Sir Samuel Joseph. I was able to attend. I thought, if only the folks at home could see me now, entertained at the Mansion House by the Lord Mayor of London. I was also able to attend a Bob Hope concert at a nearby American base. Bob had his English grandfather up on stage with him. His grandfather looked confused, but Bob sure knew how to crack jokes that really hit home.

In London we became adept at getting around in the blackout. We saw stage plays, such as "The Doctor's Dilemma" and stars performing on stage, such as Vivien Leigh. Different groups came out to Leavesden to entertain the patients and staff. I remember The Tin Hats. I remember the songs – like *"This is the Army, Mr. Jones - no private rooms or telephones; you had your breakfast in bed before, but you won't get it there anymore."* There were poignant songs like *"I threw a kiss to the ocean – it floated out to the sea – and from the ocean a voice came back – 'twas my bluejacket answering me."* And an Air Force song, *"Coming in on a wing and a prayer."* And the rollicking song "*Wish me luck as you wave me goodbye – with a cheer not a tear, make it gay – give me a smile I can keep all the while – in my heart while I'm away. Till we meet once again, you and I, wish me luck as you wave me goodbye.*"

I was moved to write a poem myself, and a patient encouraged me to send it in to *Blighty* magazine, and I received a small prize – one or two pounds, I believe. Here is the poem.

An Ode to the Air Force by Irene Stephenson, 1943

While all the world is deep in slumber
And the stars come out in number,
And the search lights stretch their arms across the sky,
While I give myself to dreaming,
You are up there planning, scheming,
And the fates are tossing if you'll live or die.

With the dusk may come the warning,
You may fight on through till morning,
It's your duty and you do not question why.
Although the coming of the morrow
May bring happiness or sorrow,
Tonight you are the master of the sky.

From foreign lands you are returning
From the havoc fires burning,
Yet you're singing to the tune of throbbing plane.
Though your heart is quickly beating
All our songs you keep repeating
Until you've reached Old Blighty once again.

Another day is dawning
As I wake up with the morning
I wish to offer up my thanks to you.
Your silver wings I am saluting
And your awesome sense of duty
Which guards me while I'm sleeping all night through.

I recall the bombing of the cathedral town of Coventry, England, with its massive loss of innocent life, which some historians rarely question today in their eagerness to talk about the bombing of Dresden, which occurred much later. There were so many innocent victims on both sides.

In England, we were given leave every three months with a free ticket to anywhere in the British Isles. I went from Cornwall in Devon, on the south coast, to Loch Lomond and Edinburgh in Scotland, and even up to South Uist in the Hebrides, and many points in between. We bought English bikes and toured the countryside. It might appear we never did any work, but such was far from the case. My first assignment at Leavesden was to the officers' ward. It was Nissen hut No. 32, but the patients called it Club 32. There was a lot of camaraderie, and after work it was a common sight to see in the local pubs, patients in airplane splints, leg casts, crutches or canes, drinking Pyms with nursing sisters. One night we received 500 patients from Sicily. Most were well on their way to recovery but some were still quite ill. Some needed a lot of surgery such as bone grafts. No. 10 was fortunate in having some great doctors on staff who excelled again in peacetime. There was one surgical head, Dr. Angus McLaughlin, of London, Dr. Frank Brien, Dr. Charlie Thompson, Dr. Cam Grey, and Dr. George Pennell, to name a few. I worked on the officers' ward for six months and it was a happy assignment. We had 48-hour leaves when we could visit London. Garfield Weston had loaned his London home to the Canadian nursing sisters as a home away from home. It was a large dwelling, complete with open lift (elevator), so we always had a cheap, reliable place to stay in London. We also had the use of an estate in southern England. It was harder to get to. I only remember going there once, and I slept in a canopy bed.

After six months on the officers' ward, the assistant matron informed me I was being assigned to the operating room. At first I objected, saying I didn't have a postgraduate course in OR but she said, *"You'll get along just fine."* Since there didn't seem to be any way of getting out of it, I determined to make the best of it and observe some operations to refresh my memory. I was dismayed, on my first morning in the OR, to find only the doctor and myself scrubbed up. At this point I was grateful for my training in sterile technique at K-W hospital, and to the nurse with the unpredictable sterile forceps. Before two months were up, I was scrubbing in bone graft surgery for Dr. McLaughlin. We used Lane's technique, everything doubly sterile, two gowns, two pairs of gloves, etc., until we got into the bone, then shedding the outer garments and becoming sterile again. Any doctors who had free time would come to the OR to observe Dr. McLaughlin's work, such was his reputation as a surgeon. I began to really enjoy the OR when a notice was posted offering an exchange for two months at a Canadian hospital in southern England. Two of us volunteered and spent two months there.

On our return to No. 10 there were lots of rumours of No. 10 moving, and speculation about a second front. We always knew our stay in England was only temporary and sooner or later we would be moving to the Continent, or Italy, or elsewhere. There was much interest in what was coming into QM stores. Was it mosquito netting, or something more suited to the climate of France? The popular song was:

> *"We don't know where we're going until we're there*
> *We only know the move is in the air.*
> *We heard the sergeant say, you're on the move today,*
> *Oh, we don't know where we're going until we're there."*

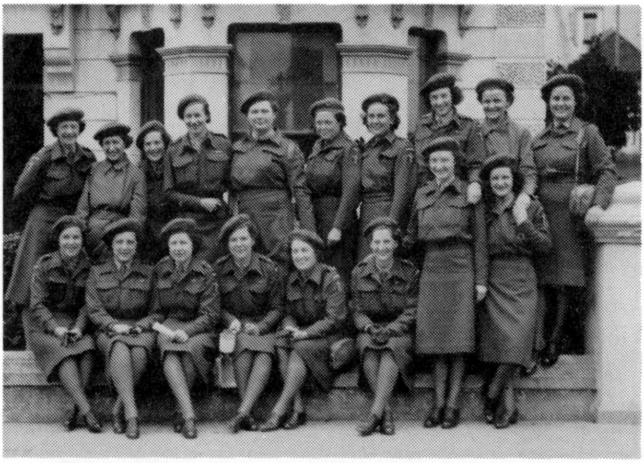

Ready for Normandy 1944; Some No. 10 CGH nursing sisters. L-R , Bottom row; Marjorie Hooper, Kit McCullough, Agnes Conroy, Nora Bell, Terry Woolsey, Ev Zumach, Hilaire Little, Maggie Campbell. Top Row: Rae Adams, Betty Smith, Jean Scrimgeour, Dorothy Low, Ida Rothwell, Kay Martin, Flora Field, Mary McWhirter, Margie Forbes, Elizabeth Cram.

Since gas was used by the enemy in WW I, we were always being prepared for gas attacks. We had to spend time working on the wards with gas masks on. Finally, new battle dress uniforms arrived for us in QM stores. There were khaki English ATS uniforms and all had been treated for gas attacks, making them very rough. There were shirts, skirts, jackets and trousers, greatcoats and berets, also high leather field boots with gaiters around the top, ground sheets and bedrolls and canvas buckets, steel helmets, etc.

It was all deadly serious from now on. The ship carrying a large Canadian General Hospital unit had been torpedoed near Gibraltar. Fortunately, all the nurses were rescued by another ship. A few nurses from No. 10 who were going as reinforcements were also on board. A sobering thought, "What could one expect from an enemy who torpedoed hospital ships or were they aware of who was on board?"

We spent time trying on our new khaki uniforms. Soon it was time to pack away our lovely blue uniforms. We were now in khaki battle dress and ready for anything. We were sent to Yorkshire for field training and billeted in the Scotch Corner Hotel near Darlington. We went on long route marches, sometimes five miles with our packs on our backs. Odds and ends were stuffed in the blouses of our tunics. We looked quite busty at times. We were near an Air Force base from which airmen took off nightly on raids, and some buzzed low over the hotel on their return. This wasn't appreciated by some of the medical officers, who said, *"Tell your boyfriends to cut it out."* A couple of us met two Canadian pilots who were stationed nearby with either the Ghost or the Moose Squadron. They used to bike over to see us with a little black Scottie dog in each bicycle basket. Those puppies were so cute. These boys promised to take us with them on a raid some night, but we left before it happened.

Years later I met a padre who had been taken twice on raids by these squadrons, so I guess they really meant it. My friend, Wally Dumas, survived the war. Another pilot friend from Winnipeg wasn't so lucky. He was killed on a raid. Later on I would receive a prisoner of war card from a friend who was an American pilot. He stated he was a prisoner of war across the channel, shot down just after I went north. His card was dated, simply, February. It took many months to reach me and I never heard from him again. His name was Joseph Kenneth Robbins. I hope he made it out. He was a very nice person. I still have the POW card.

We left Darlington for the south coast. It was now past D-Day. We stayed in Brighton first and then went into seclusion somewhere on the coast where we were in tents. Here I had my first experience with a V-1 buzz bomb. Hitler had developed a V-1 buzz bomb and a V-II rocket. The buzz bombs were being launched from ramps on the coast of France and directed to London. They were pilotless and shaped somewhat like a plane. They had enough fuel to reach London and its environs. The motor was very loud, with a different sound than an airplane. As long as the motor could be heard, it wouldn't explode, but when the motor stopped it would fall to the ground and explode. They caused massive destruction in London. We were aware of all this, so when I heard the loud peculiar noise, and it stopped, I knew what it was and hit the ground. I wasn't sorry we were leaving England and the buzz bombs.

We weren't long here, and soon boarded a ship to cross the channel. It was about six weeks after D-Day. We were one of the first Canadian hospitals into France. We had to wait until the fall of Caen before they would send us over. Montgomery's plan had been to take Caen the first day. A month later Caen was still not taken. There was much fierce fighting by British and Canadian troops, but the city was defended just as fiercely by the Germans. Finally, Monty called in the bombers. We would later see the results of all the bombing. Even then there were still pockets of resistance. Finally Caen was taken and we were on our way. Except for one emergency call to our stations, the trip was uneventful. We landed on the famous Mulberry harbour at Arromanches. This was the huge harbour that had been floated over from England. We came ashore in landing craft (ducks), and there are several pictures in war history books showing No. 10 hospital nurses landing on the coast of France in these unique landing craft. So we were now on the beachhead in France and a soldier was waiting with a large boiler full of tea. That mug of tea was very welcome.

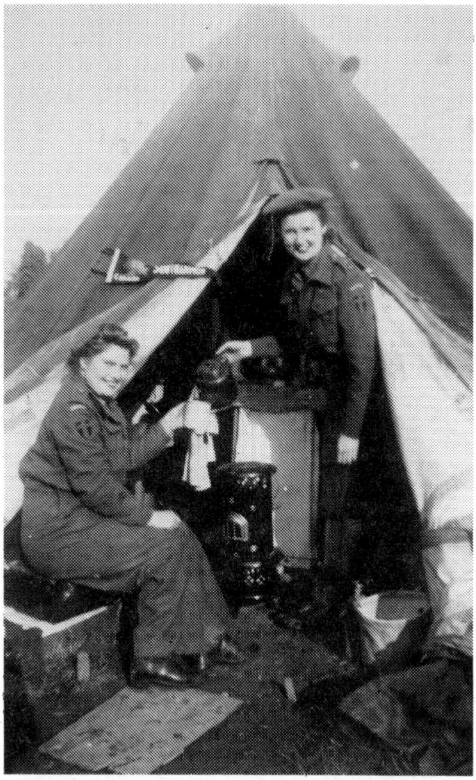

R - standing pouring tea, Lt. N/S Irene Stephenson. L - seated is Edna Ellacott, No. 10 CGH. Littry Road, Normandy July 1944. Note kerosene stove, canvas bucket, 21st army patch on sleeves, pennant on tent reads Southampton.

Then it was into the trucks and across the dusty roads to Bayeux. I felt like I was about to save the world until we passed a group in a field and an elderly woman pointed to her bandaged knee and shook her fist at us. I guess she connected us to her injury somehow, and dressed in khaki battle dress and steel helmets we all looked like soldiers anyway.

When we got to Bayeux we were taken out to the Littry Road which would be dubbed Harley Street because of all the ten hospitals which would eventually set up in the fields and orchards.

Years later, on an anniversary trip, I went out to Bayeux and, sure enough, there was a sign, "The Littry Road." I didn't have time to explore to see what had replaced the hospital tents along the Littry Road in Normandy.

We were not allowed into Bayeux at first without an armed guard. We also had to wear a Red Cross armband. I imagined a sniper behind every tree. We soon had our hospital ready. Everything was under canvas. We lived in bell tents, two to a tent. There were only dirt floors which became muddy whenever it rained. The tents were old and sprang leaks, and they put another tent with holes in different places over the first one. Sometimes there were puddles of water in the beds. I thought of what I had read of the WW I nurses at Gallipoli with their large tents, wooden floors, and batmen bringing them hot tea.

One night we were awakened by screaming. Ida Rothwell was awakened by a large form rubbing against her bed through the tent. It turned out to be an old cow that had wandered into the compound and was having a good scratch on the side of the tent. The only heat in the tents came from a portable kerosene stove with a handle on top. I saw a similar one in an antique store a while ago and it brought back memories. One day mine caught fire and I carried it outside and poured water on it (not recommended) but the fire went out. All of my worldly possessions were in the tent – namely, a trunkful of uniforms.

The mess tent served up dehydrated food. The pot of jam on the table usually had honeybees in it. You had to dig around the bees to get the jam out. We never saw a fresh egg, tomato, or an orange. Canned Spam was a great standby. We took vitamins. Everyone had dysentery. We called it the Normandy Glide. I remember taking large doses of Sulphaquanidine for it. The latrines were open to the elements. We washed from water in a canvas bucket. One of our nurses used to sing a naughty song called, *"Home presents a dismal picture."* It did describe the situation quite well.

When our hospital was operational I was assigned to the resuscitation war and would remain on this ward until the end of the war. We would have the worst cases, mostly on the SI and DI lists (Seriously Ill and Dangerously Ill). In those days it was 12-hour shifts every day. All the patients got penicillin every three hours, and sulfa drugs every four hours. We were the first to use penicillin. People in Canada still couldn't get it. It was all by injection and, of course, there were no disposable syringes and needles then, so everything had to be boiled up on the coal oil stove. We were also short of equipment, with few syringes and needles. Sometimes we were so short-staffed, even the dentists would come in to help. We had a very good orderly on our resuscitation ward, Carl, from Kitchener.

We were operating as a 1200-bed field hospital with 85 nursing sisters. We had a dietitian, home sister, three physiotherapists, an occupational therapist, and 33 doctors; the rest were registered nurses. The remaining were other ranks who took care of the myriad other details of running the hospital, such as transporting the equipment and patients, running the pharmacy, X-ray, QM stores, kitchens, orderlies on wards, stretcher bearers, etc. This team ran smoothly – it had to. We admitted 500 patients at a time. There would be a steady stream of ambulances until 500 were admitted. Then another hospital in the area would admit. We kept our capacity of 1200 patients, all the while sending stabilized patients back to England by ship and admitting new ones, a constant process. We always hoped the ships would reach England safely. More urgent cases were evacuated by air from an airstrip nearby.

The patients were always very grateful for their care, never complaining. We also had some patients from the Free Polish Army, and even some German POWs who received the same care as our boys. They even got penicillin. We followed the Geneva Convention. We thought it would be followed, also, by the other side, but when we heard about the Canadian POWs who were executed in cold blood by Kurt Meyer and his SS, we lost hope.

I remember the death of one POW on our ward in France. He died of tetanus. We had given him antitoxin but it was too late for him. He had probably not been immunized previously with tetanus toxoid which takes time to build up an immunity. That was one of the first things a raw recruit in the Canadian forces encountered. It was called TABT (typhoid, paratyphoid A and B, and tetanus toxoid). It packed a wallop. Later, in Belgium, during the flooding at the Scheldt, we had many diphtheria cases, and later diphtheria was added. It was now TABTD, and it packed a double wallop.

Our Canadian patients were a joy, even on this resuscitation ward, presenting the most grievous casualties. Some stand out in my memory, even today. There was the patient entirely swathed in bandages who had a marvelous personality. Although we never saw his face, his spirit came shining through.

Another one was entirely encased in plaster except for his hands and parts of his face. He could neither see nor hear. He could only feel cold plaster wherever he touched. He kept shouting in the night, *"I'm turned to stone, I'm turned to stone."* He had probably been in some kind of explosion. Another memorable patient had gas gangrene, and it was horrifying to watch it creeping up. One of the first things we checked on a new patient was his gas gangrene serum record, to make sure he had it, which I recall was 5 cc of very sticky fluid given intramuscularly, and also to make sure he got his tetanus antitoxin and toxoid booster. We were constantly washing and boiling syringes and needles on the coal oil stove. It was in the ward so we could keep an eye on patients and stove at the same time.

We worked long hours with few staff, but when at night the Canadians would come in big trucks to take nurses to a party we were all ready to go, and the closer to the front we went, the better, or so we thought, until the night of the First Hussar's party. It was right up at the front line. We sat around in a circle in this house, plates of food on knees, looking white and scared while the shells pounded around outside. We heard the house was shelled next day, and demolished, but I still had the silver fork I took as a souvenir and a reminder that the evening had really happened.

One night we were coming home from one of these outings and we came to a crossroad where we were stopped for hours due to Canadian soldiers moving up to the front. They must have just landed, and it seemed like a whole division was moving up. It went on for hours and we had a front row seat. It lives in my memory – the darkness, the noise of movement, the general apprehension and thoughts of what these boys would soon face. Across the road was a tiny light in the very top of a tall house, and furtive shadows moving behind it. Was it friend or foe?

Another night when arriving home at our tent compound, we were met by a rain of ack ack. We crawled under our camp cots and hoped for the best. I felt sure the ground would be covered with shrapnel next day, but when I looked I didn't see any. Our hospital wasn't marked by any big red cross, as it would be later in Belgium. Of course, the British and Canadians knew we were there. I hoped the Americans did, too, because of the day the Flying Fortresses came right over us. On that day I trudged to work in battle dress with bandage scissors dangling from binder twine at my side. I heard the heavy drone of airplanes overhead. I looked up to see hundreds of Flying Fortresses (American bomber planes) coming in from the direction of the channel and heading towards the front lines, passing directly overhead. This was the new era of the 1000-bomber raids. No planes had flown over us, either before or after, in France and in such numbers. I wondered what was up.

The Battle of Normandy raged on. August 7th the Caen to Falaise assault began by Canadian, British and Polish forces. There were successful RAF bomber raids, then the Americans were asked to bomb. Many of their planes bombed short, decimating the Canadian lines. The troops were also engaging SS troops. These were Hitler's so-called "elite" troops. They were deadly adversaries, especially Kurt Meyer and his SS troops. After the war he would be tried and sentenced to death for being involved in the execution of Canadian POWs. Eventually he went free. On August 14th the RAF were asked to bomb on a daylight raid. However, the airmen weren't aware the yellow markers were Allied positions, and thinking it their target, they dropped their bombs on them. Again, Canadians had many casualties from our own Allied planes. The battlefields were filled with dead soldiers and horses. Amazingly, the Germans, although with the best military equipment, still used horses and wagons to pull equipment. On August 17th the Canadians took Falaise. The town was now in ruins – another Caen. The German army was soon trapped in the Falaise pocket from which half of them would escape to fight again another day.

This, then, was the background to what we were doing in our tent hospital on the Littry Road outside Bayeux. We were all working unbelievably hard. I remember working 17 hours one day on the resuscitation ward. I didn't even have time to comb my hair. The heat in the tents was severe. The patients had the most horrendous wounds. There were no textbooks preparing our doctors for this kind of surgery. We ran out of tent ropes to hang the plasma on. We had a portable oxygen tank we wheeled around the tent for the patients needing it. I remember a British boy with most of his face missing, begging for a cup of tea. I can still see him today. Was this what Churchill meant when he promised only Blood, Sweat and Tears?

The front moved on rapidly. We had been working steadily and for long hours since our arrival in France, and now we were able to have leave. I was with a group of our nurses who were given three days' leave at the Normandy Hotel in Deauville – a very posh hotel where the Duke of Duchess of Windsor were reported to have spent their honeymoon. The hotel was beautiful; the bedrooms were papered with heavy paper showing teams of oxen, done in a lovely burgundy colour. The headboards were upholstered in material to match. No one could figure out what the second toilet (bidet) was for. The dining room was lined with mirrors. The French chefs did marvelous things with our army rations. The beaches were mined and signs warned us not to walk on the beach, but we couldn't resist walking down to the water.

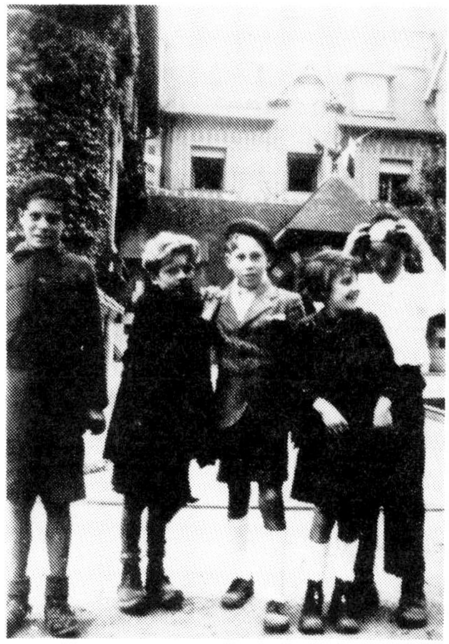

French children in front of Normandy Hotel, Deauville August 1944

Canadian officers were also back here from the front lines, and Doug Kennedy, an officer in the HLI from Galt, Ontario, joined our K-W group. I had met his brother Pete when he came to our hospital at Leavesden to see Col. Hamilton, but I hadn't met Doug before. Col. Hamilton was very fond of them, and very proud of them. This was to be Doug's last few days on earth. When he returned to his regiment, he learned his brother Pete had been killed in his absence. A few days later Doug was killed, also by a sniper. How can a family cope with such news?

We were saddened that Col. Hamilton was leaving us to go home. He would be replaced by Dr. Jones of Kingston. We gave him an afternoon tea party as a send-off. I still have the clipping from the local newspaper when he was interviewed on his arrival home. He said in part, *"Tank and infantry men lived under appalling conditions, and these conditions are even worse now than at the invasion time."* The HLI were fighting almost continuously from D-Day until D+60 when they had their first rest. Heavy fighting around the Falaise area cleared the way for a major advance. He said No. 10 welcomed visitors from the K-W area. Placed near Caen in Normandy, the hospital rendered aid to many wounded personnel. However, before Col. Hamilton left France, he said the battleline had stretched far ahead of the hospital, and plans were being completed to move the unit forward. He also paid tribute to his staff and mentioned his K-W nurses.

I sometimes wondered how the people of Normandy could endure so much; first the long occupation, and now their country was being torn apart. We had seen the total destruction in the city of Caen. We had walked in the rubble and found a set of steps which was all that was left of a building. The whole city was in ruins. Seeing the beautiful cattle of France today at fairs and ploughing matches, I often wondered what happened to those beautiful animals during the Battle of Normandy. I remember the fields with their hedgerows and pleasant orchards, and the destruction in Caen. I wrote the following poem about it.

Normandy 1944, by Irene (Stephenson) Mercier

Hedgerows blasted in the noonday sun
Burned-out tanks with broken twisted guns,
Bloated cattle lying upturned in the sun.
I want to flee but there's no place to run
O Normandy, O Normandy, pray look thee what's been done.

These broken fields which once my plough ran through,
And turned the earthy furrows straight and true.
Gone is my dream of skies of azure blue
And fragrant meadows wet with morning dew.
O Normandy, O Normandy, pray tell me what to do.

Bombers race across the windless sky
While dropping deadly peril from on high
Buildings fall like matchsticks tinder-dry.
I want to cry but all my tears are dry.
O Normandy, O Normandy, pray tell me, tell me why.

So many battles waged on thy dear face
Have faded into nothing without trace
And so I pray this scene will be erased
And peace again will beautify this place.
O Normandy, O Normandy, beloved by all thy race.

As Dr. Hamilton had said, the front had moved far forward, and we were still in Normandy. On September 17th the operation Market-Garden was launched. This was a combined airdrop and a push by ground forces with a plan to link up. On this day thousands of paratroopers took to the skies in planes and gliders. Their drop zone was in and around Arnhem in Holland. It was thought this area was not heavily defended. Such was not the case. Troops and supplies were pouring in, including the dreaded SS troops. Many paratroopers were killed or wounded on landing. American and British forces were pushing up from Belgium, eventually taking the Nijmegen bridge, but they were never able to get to Arnhem. For nine days the paratroopers held on until what was left of them were finally evacuated. The Dutch people had such high hopes of liberation when the assault began, but such was not to be until over six months had passed, and then their country would be liberated by the Canadians. This explains the high regard the Dutch have for the Canadians; how they never forgot who liberated them, and they teach their children on down through the generations about the Canadians who came from a far country they had scarcely heard of, and set their people free.

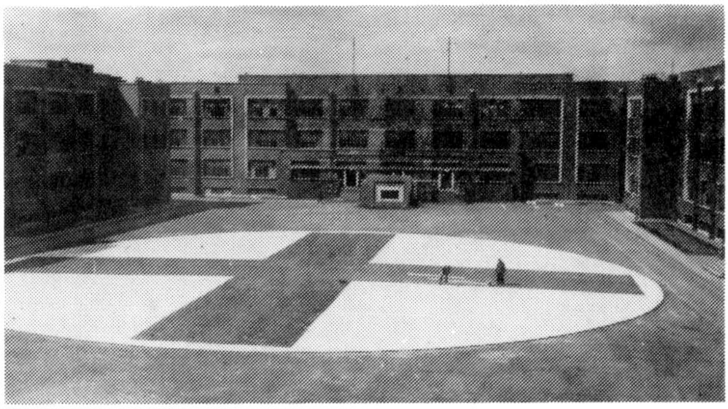

No. 10 CGH and the famous Red Cross Turnhout, Belgium, 1944

In Normandy the weather turned cold and rainy. Mud was everywhere. We prepared to move on. Our destination was Turnhout in northern Belgium, near Antwerp and the Dutch border. We travelled in convoy, bag and baggage, the whole hospital. The first night we stayed overnight in a barracks near Rouen. They showed the movie *Joan of Arc*. It was quite fitting to see the movie, *Joan of Arc*, in France. The next night we reached Brussels. We stayed in a nice hotel and felt very out of place in battle dress and caked in mud. The next day we reached Turnhout and our hospital site. There were five buildings of three storeys each. Four of them were set to form an enormous square. Our new OC, Col. Jones, had a gigantic cross made of red bricks, set in white sand, erected in this square. We were not supposed to walk on it or stir up the white sand. Belgian workmen worked diligently sweeping it off. Sometimes at night nurses would have company and go out and dance on the red cross, but not without repercussions. We thought it funny and named it "*Jones' Folly*" until one day a visiting airman told us how much they appreciated it. He said it was a wonderful landmark, and when they saw the red cross they knew they were on the right way home.

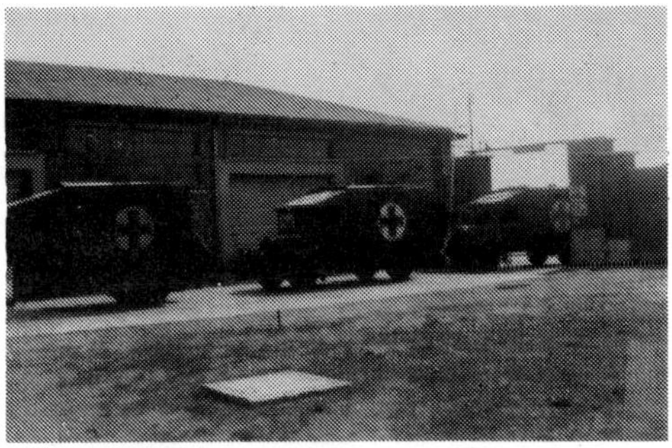

A convoy of patients coming in.
No. 10 CGH, Turnhout, Belgium 1944

We decided to have a party – a sort of open house. Surrounding regiments were informed. I was on the committee, so got transport to Antwerp to look for a band. I succeeded in engaging a popular band. It was said at the time that Antwerp was the recipient of 70 buzz bombs a day, but I sincerely believed the band would appear as promised. The great evening arrived, but not the band. I'll never know what happened to them, but by then Antwerp was being besieged by V-2 rockets as well as the buzz bombs. The regiments didn't fail us. Large numbers of guests arrived. There was food and drink, and everyone had a great time. I was amazed when a tall officer walked up to me and introduced himself. He had been a student at Port Elgin school at the same time I was. Imagine meeting someone from your home school in Turnhout, Belgium, in the middle of a war. It was a happy reunion.

In the meantime, Hitler was not idle and was planning an enormous breakthrough. Having survived an assassination attempt by his own officers and having had a number of suicides among his generals, he was not deterred. He took no chances and everything was done in extreme secrecy. Troops were carefully screened. The build-up in the Ardennes went on for months. This was the American sector, and American Intelligence did not seem to be aware of what was happening so close to them. The resulting surprise attack known as "The Battle of the Bulge" very nearly succeeded in Hitler's favour. He had several armies, and one very large SS army was pointing straight our way. We were aware of the crisis and knew we were in danger of being cut off. We had been ordered to evacuate our patients and be ready to move at a moment's notice. All the equipment went back to QM stores. This would be our strangest Christmas in a strange land. Even Santa Claus was different. He wore a tall hat and had a helper called Black Peter who carried a switch for bad boys and girls. I remember wondering if I should open Christmas presents from home, or would the Germans get them anyway. On Christmas day we each received a bottle of champagne from the mess. The Americans were fighting a great battle. Monty's 21st Army Group joined in. This was the group we belonged to and we wore the 21st Army patch with pride. Our hospital unit was ordered to stand by for 24 hours. Then an order came to stand by for a second 24 hours. At the end of this period, an order came through to be ready to admit patients in the morning. We worked all night setting up the wards, getting our special equipment for the resuscitation ward, and were ready when morning came. The hospital filled with patients and overflowed. They were straight from battle. They had cards around their neck telling what first aid they had received. The halls were filled with stretchers. We went up to 1800 patients with the same number of staff as before. We now wore red rubber aprons on our ward. Some patients' veins were so flat it was difficult to find veins for the intravenous. I still remember the first time I saw a patient transfused via the jugular vein. The patient took it all in stride as though this were an everyday occurrence and he got along just fine.

The Americans had tremendous casualties. The Battle of the Bulge is a large part of the history of WW II, yet today, when you mention the Battle of the Bulge, some people think you are on a diet. Even in our own parliament a few years ago, when Kay Christie asked if there were plans for nursing home beds for nursing sisters, one MP asked, *"Who were the nursing sisters? Was it some kind of religious order?"* Our full title was Lieutenant N/S copied after the British system. Patients called us "sister" with the utmost respect.

After the Battle of the Bulge, things settled down somewhat. Towards the end of March, Elizabeth Cram and I were given leave. We chose to go to Ireland. We flew to England and crossed by boat to Belfast. We went to Londonderry and there we met some British naval officers. It was my birthday; the third away from Canada and the most memorable. The British naval officers gave me a lovely birthday party on board their ship, anchored offshore. They also typed out and stamped a rather illegible permission to cross over to Dublin, which was neutral. It was enough to get us across the two borders after we had taken off our pips and Canadian insignia and donned sweaters so as to appear as civilians. Enroute to Dublin we met a lovely lady who invited us to her home for lunch. She had a beautiful home, and there were two maids in formal black and white serving the meal. She had relatives in the British Army. We feasted on ice cream in the ice creams parlours which seemed to be outdoing each other in their lovely green decors. We rode in a cart pulled by a lovely Irish horse. My roots are Irish, but I didn't get to kiss the Blarney stone – it was too far away. Goodbye Ireland – we had a lovely visit, but now it is back to Belgium.

Organizations from Canada sent us parcels including cigarettes. For those of us who didn't smoke they were used as barter. It was easier to buy something with cigarettes than with money. When we had time off we would set off, often hitchhiking, with our cigarettes up to Rotterdam and Amsterdam. Rotterdam was in ruins, but we found a jewelry shop and bought rings and later oil paintings. The proprietor came out to the front of the store and said, *"There's nothing for sale today. Go."* Through an opening in a curtain we saw a German officer in full uniform seated at a table. Obviously they were having some kind of dealings. When the owner yelled at us a second time to get out we didn't lose any time doing so. Just as in peacetime, there wan't a policeman when you needed one. In each country there were collaborators (locals who sided with the Germans and sold out their countrymen).

Some would transmit messages to the enemy but would have to keep moving in order not to be caught. Often they used baby carriages to push their equipment around while sending messages. One day in Turnhout, I was coming down main street and ahead of us was a peculiar group. There was a little old lady in a long invalid cart and three or four attendants in uniform – both men and women. I felt sure they were sending messages. I followed them to the edge of town hoping a military policeman would appear. I gave up on the edge of town as the road ahead looked very spooky.

My friend, Margaret Lutes, was planning her wedding to Bob Donaldson of the South Alberta Regiment. She was stationed in s'Hertogenbosch, Holland. She asked me to be a bridesmaid. I was delighted to do so. It was a military wedding. We were all in uniform. Tables for the reception were decorated in white sheets with gauze garlands tinted pink with small amounts of red ink and fastened with fresh flowers. It was a happy occasion.

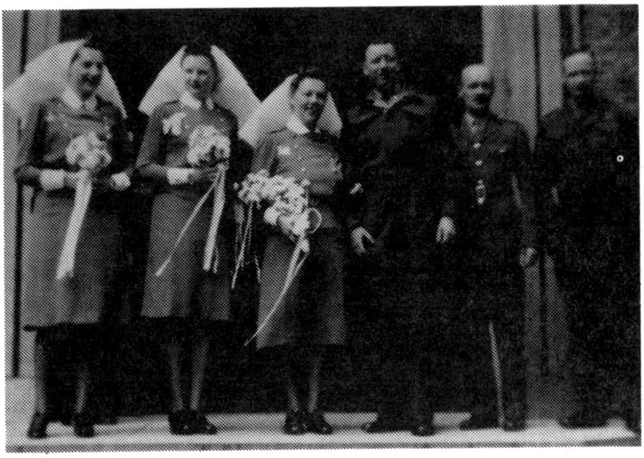

Wedding of Margaret Lutes and Bob Donaldson, s'Hertogenbosch, Spring of 1945. L-R: Betty Hindley, bridesmaid. Bride, Margaret Lutes, groom Bob Donaldson

As more and more places were being liberated we heard about the concentration camps. Our *Maple Leaf* paper had stories of terrible findings. One day we were able to go to the Vught concentration camp in northern Holland, near the German border. We didn't see bodies but we saw the stretchers lying on the ground near the ovens. It was shocking. I have never had any difficulty in knowing the Holocaust happened. In 1980, on an anniversary visit to Holland, I was asked what I would like to do. I had only two requests. To go back to Vught, and to see the old hospital in Turnhout. First we went to the Vught camp. It was still there surrounded by barbed wire. Refugees were living in the huts. There was a sign stating that the ovens were only opened once a year. I can see it as plain as if it were yesterday. In a nearby clearing in a forest there was a wall of names. In the centre of the wall, on the top, was a cross made of tree limbs so it was very uneven. It was truly the *old rugged cross*. It was a truly memorable sight. Wreaths of flowers adorned the wall. These people were not forgotten.

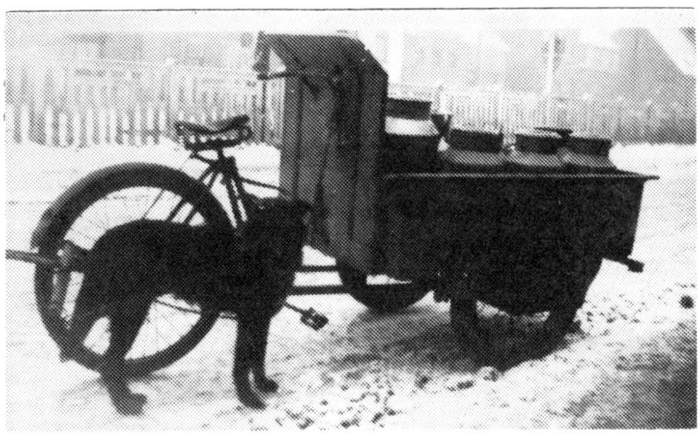

Guarding the milk. Turnhout, Belgium 1945

We drove to Turnhout, Belgium. We sampled the best chocolates I have ever eaten anywhere. Then we set out to find the old hospital. No one could remember it until we met some nurses who directed us to the barracks. I recognized it instantly; the only difference was the red cross was gone but the large square remained. Soldiers were training. It had reverted to a barracks once more. On this trip we went to Amsterdam, went over the battlefields of Arnhem and stood in the centre of the famous highway bridge at Nijmegen. Our wonderful hosts added to the warm feeling of belonging.

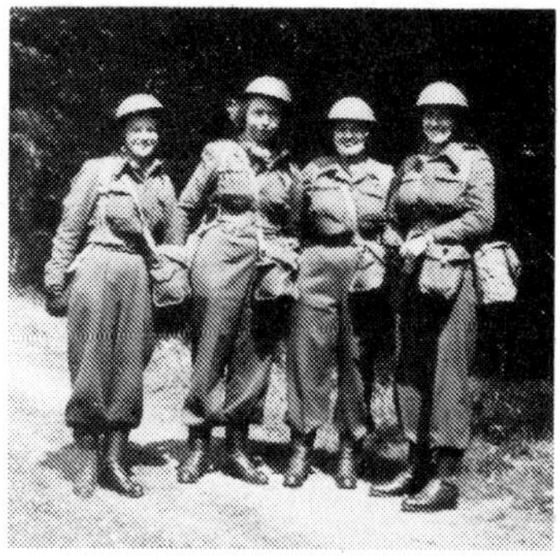

L-R: Daisy King, Mae Caldwell, Edna Ellacott, Jean McKenzie

Even though we knew it was nearing the end of the war, VE Day on May 8, 1945 was a shock. I had to work so couldn't celebrate. Those who could went to Brussels to celebrate.

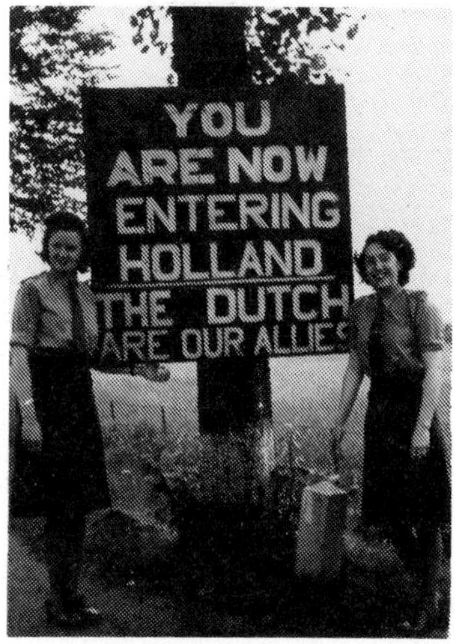
YOU
ARE NOW
ENTERING
HOLLAND
THE DUTCH
ARE OUR ALLIES

Dutch German border. L-R: Irene Stephenson Melba Lister (Dietitian)

Soon I received leave to go to Paris. I went with Jean McKenzie from Tiverton. We stayed in a nice hotel. The air smelled like perfume – as though someone had dumped perfume in the streets. We went to a racetrack to see a horse-race. We went to see the Folies-Bergeres. I remember the floor opening up and a girl on a white horse rose up with the floor. We went to the most beautiful ballet at the opera house. All the girls were in snow-white dresses. We were with a couple of Canadian officers. As we left the opera house in the wee hours, a French driver in a carriage was waiting outside. One of the officers and I hopped up on the horse's back and rode around the Place de l'Opera. I was finally celebrating VE Day. Afterwards, whenever I heard the song, *"The last time I saw Paris her heart was young and gay,"* I remembered how her streets smelled of perfume and I didn't know if her heart was young and gay but mine surely was on that day.

At the end of the war our Canadian patients had all returned to England and the hospitals were filled with German prisoners of war. In fairness, I would say they were very well behaved and although we had guards on each landing, they had no desire to escape. They knew they were well off in the hospital. They seemed to be all Werhmacht troops (German Army troops) and were different from SS troops. One in particular I remember, a smiling cheerful fellow who was very helpful to the other patients. He had had some medical training. They seemed to have accepted the fact that the war was over and they had lost.

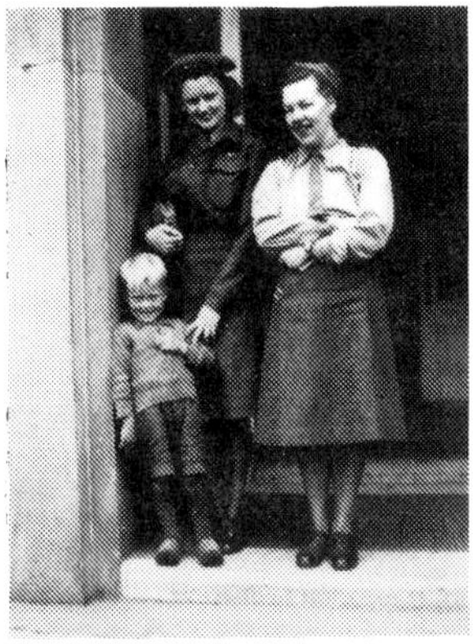

L-R: Irene Stephenson, Margaret Lutes and our little Dutch boy

In France, when the Allies crossed the Maginot line, they wouldn't believe it. Later when the Allies took the Siegfried line, the last barrier into Germany was removed. Someone strung a line and hung up some clothes on the Siegfried line with two sign one saying, *"The Siegfried line,"* and the other, *"The washing,"* in deference to the song, *"We're gonna hang up our washing on the Siegfried line."*

These German prisoners would soon be returning to a different Germany. We had seen the complete ruins of the German city of Emmerich and there were many more Emmerichs.

We soon returned to England and I had the great privilege of being in London on VJ Day. I remember the vast crowds; how the mall in front of Buckingham Palace was filled to overflowing. Vehicles carrying dignitaries up to the palace could scarcely manoeuver through. The car carrying Winston Churchill passed very close to us. I gazed with awe on the face that saved England. There was such excitement in the air. Soon the King and Queen and the two Princesses, Elizabeth and Margaret Rose, came out on the balcony and waved to the crowd. Others joined them, including Churchill. Cheers and shouts ascended. It was truly the end of the war.

After the excitement it was quite a change setting sail on a calm September day to cross again the vast Atlantic Ocean. We set sail on a ship called the *Camermia.* It was a longer journey than on the fast ship, the *Queen E.* It was exciting when we finally saw land because this land was Canada. As we sailed up the St. Lawrence, a soldier brought out his guitar and strummed the popular song.

"Gonna take a sentimental journey; gonna set my heart at ease
gonna take a sentimental journey to renew old memories

Got my hat and got my destination never more to roam
Gonna take a sentimental journey, a sentimental journey home"

The pilot came on board for the last part of the journey. We anchored off the ramparts of Quebec City. It was raining. Some dignitaries came down from Ottawa with greetings. They paraded up and down the dock with their Homburg hats and expensive coats. The final straw was when they hoisted umbrellas over their heads to ward off the few drops of rain. These returning veterans had spent years in mud and blood losing comrades before their eyes and the sight of the umbrellas was just too much! A great BOO! echoed across the water. I remembered the patient who thought he was turned to stone and of the British boy with most of his face missing begging for a cup of tea. *Boo! Boo!* echoed off the old ramparts of Quebec. I wondered, Does this happen every time a troop ship returns or is it just when it rains?

We were left on the ship overnight. Next day emotions had cooled and all were anxious to get into those big Canadian trains which would be speeding veterans home all across the great Dominion of Canada.

If possible, everyone should go back. I have been back twice. The most emotional time was going over the battlefields of Arnhem. A great sense of overwhelming sadness enveloped me. Those who died should never be forgotten. In 1980 I was at a ceremony at Groesbeek Cemetery near Nijmegen, Holland. I close now with the poem I wrote after that visit.

Groesbeek Cemetery 1980

They are Canadians yet they lie
In this distant land 'neath this distant sky.
Their place is marked by stately stone
Bearing the Maple Leaf of home
Around the base the tulips grow
Amid the green their colours glow
The soft grass bends toward the beckoning sky
Blanketing those who beneath it lie.
Fair children come to tend the graves
Of those who gave their lives for theirs
The age-ed come to shed their tears
For those who came in those bitter years.
The message had been help must come soon

The people were facing certain doom
Death and starvation stalked the land
Those were terrible times in that conquered land.
They had come from the East and from the West
All of Canada sent its best.
From mountain, valley and coastal plain
From all across the land they came.
They didn't know there was no return
That there never would be a journey home.
Here time stands still since those days of yore
When they stormed the beaches and came ashore
And crossed the rivers one by one.
And paid such a price for the victory won.
They answered the call and here they lie
Brave soldiers who were too young to die
Soldiers who gave all they had to give
Each giving his life that others might live
They gave without thought of worldly gain
Never let their sacrifice be in vain
Always remember the price they paid
Protect the freedom they died to save.

Irene Stephenson Mercier retains rights to the three poems published here but wishes them to be used in this book.

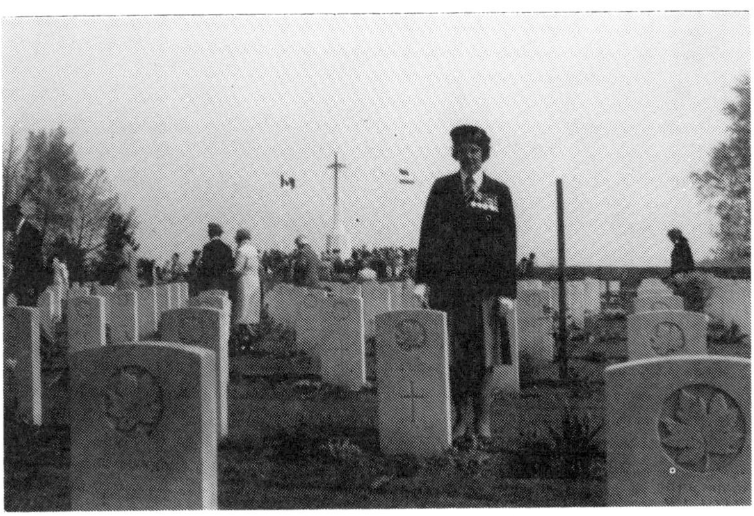

Groesbeek Cemetery, Holland

Jessie Grace Morrison

Graduated from: Winnipeg General Hospital School of Nursing. Year: 1926

Military History:

Service: RCAMC

Rank: Lt. N/S

Served: May 1941 to December 31, 1945

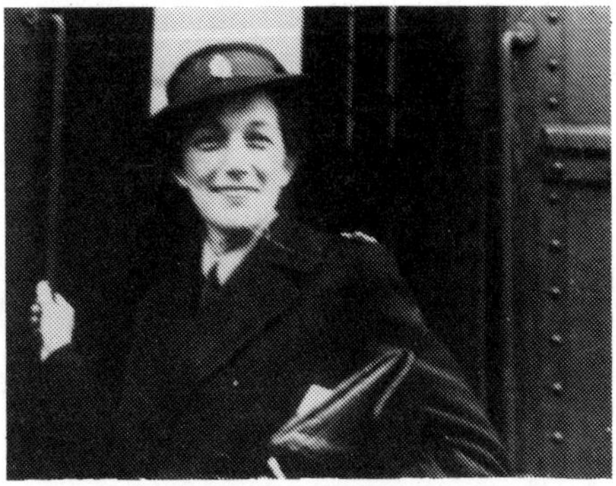

Lt. N/S Jessie Morrison, Winnipeg Station, December 1944

There was no one influence that caused me to choose a military career, it was a mixed bag. I was caught up in the fever of wartime pressures, I wished to join many of my colleagues and friends.

I joined the RCAMC in Halifax, N.S., 1941, at the old military hospital built by the Imperial Army in mid-19th century and known as "Cosgwell Street Hospital." The movement of troops from all parts of the British Commonwealth as they embarked for overseas – the assembling and movement of convoys out of Halifax Harbour – ships of every Class in the Royal Canadian Navy – casualties cared for from torpedoed ships.

Voyage overseas on the *Queen Elizabeth*, December 1941. Struck by a very severe hurricane two days out of Halifax. Posted to No. 10 Canadian General Hospital, London, Ontario, in October 1942. Served overseas with No. 10 CGH based at Leavesden, near Watford junction.

In April 1944 No. 10 CGH was posted to Scotch Corner, York, and from there to Hove, Sussex, and on to the Continent to Bayeux, Normandy, July 1944.

Experience in "The Field," in Normandy out of Bayeux from July 1944 to October 1945. We were in such close proximity to the front lines that we received casualties within a few hours of their being wounded. It was observed that most were in varying degrees of shock on arrival at the hospital. Marvellous spirit, actually, in retrospect, I can't recall any serious complaints or grumbling. I was most impressed by the smooth functioning of the organizations in the field. Of course there were bitches, but few, and minor.

Comparatively speaking, our troops were given excellent care. We (No. 10 Canadian General Hospital) with other hospital units were so close to the Front in the early weeks of the war, we really functioned on a CCS basis.

It was interesting to have had "enemy" troops as patients. I was struck by the fact that there was a great range in age – very young to late middle age. On the whole, they were grateful to be with us. It was obvious the majority disliked the SS personnel intensely. It was also noted that the only cases of gas gangrene we cared for were German troops. It seemed they were not inoculated. We had the occasional medical officer as POWs; they were most interested to learn about penicillin which was available to us at this time. The sight and sound at night of artillery fire. The strains of the "Last Post" coming to us from the burial grounds. I still become emotional at that sound.

It was a privilege to have served in HM Armed Forces, an experience like none other. We (No. 10 CGH) along with other hospitals on "Harley Street," Bayeux, were so close to the areas under fire, we felt we were sharing the bloody experience of war with our troops. They were great, despite the slanted and often untrue portrayals in *The Valour and the Horror.*

Returned to Canada in November 1944 due to length of service and age restriction. Then posted to Sydney, Cape Breton Military Hospital as nursing sister in charge, and remained there until the hospital was closed July 1945. From there moved to Windsor, N.S. Military Hospital. Terminated service with the RCAMC December 1945.

Moved to University of Alberta Hospital January to October 1946 as supervisor – Col. Mewburn and Col. Wells Pavilions. The patients were ex-servicemen.

Joined the Department of Veterans Affairs November 1946 as Matron Gr. 1, Col. Belcher Hospital, Calgary. Was assigned the task of organizing and implementing an in-service training program for nursing orderlies Gr. 1-4 by the late Agnes J. Macleod, Director of Nursing Services.

Posted for three months to Saskatoon Veterans Hospital and then as assistant to the director of the Montreal School of Nursing Aides, July 1948. Due to family reasons it was necessary to return to Alberta, July 1949. Employment with the Department of Veterans Affairs was resumed, this time as Matron Gr. 1 in charge of Veterans Home located at Government

House. Posted to Sunnybrook Hospital, Toronto, for six months – January to June 1952, to assist with newly organized school for nursing assistants. Marjorie Russell was the director. This was a DVA project.

September 1967 it was necessary to take an early retirement.

Eleanor (Robinson) Schneider

Graduated from: Victoria Hospital School of Nursing, London, Ontario. Year: 1940

Military History:

Service: RCAMC

Rank: Lt. N/S

Served: September 1942 to February 1944

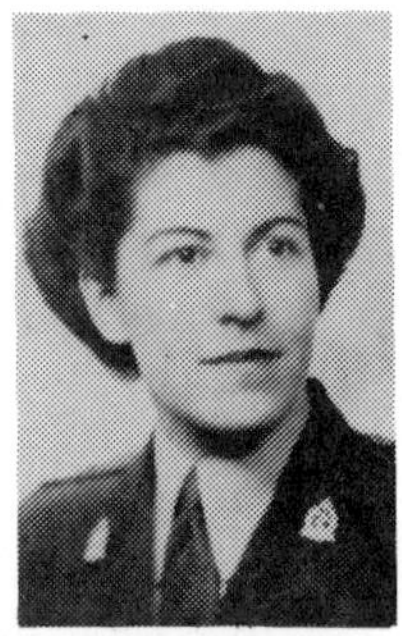

Lt. N/S Eleanor (Robinson) Schneider; No. 10 CGH, Leavesden, England 1942

The highlight of my military experience was being awarded "Mentioned in Despatches" by King George VI.

This is not amusing but more of a human interest story – on one of the wards at Leavesden a mother cat brought in her six kittens. There was a stove and the young men made sure that the mother cat and kittens had a comfortable spot near the warmth. It was touching to see how much they cared.

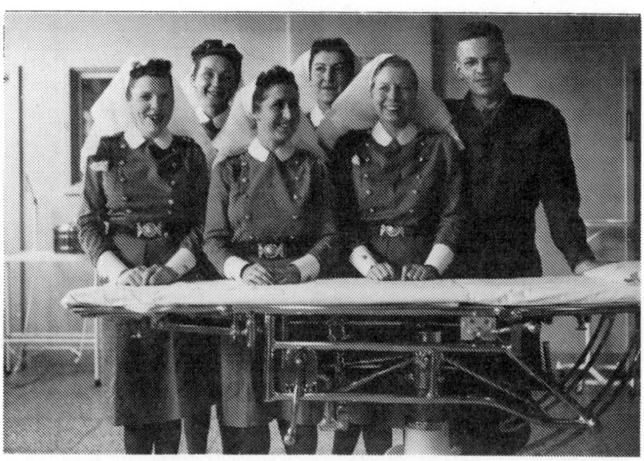

No. 10 CGH, Leavesden, England 1943 - Operating theatre No. 1; L-R: Dorothy Kersey, London, Ontario; Margaret Klasson, Kitchener; Betty Smith, St. Thomas; Eleanor Robinson, London, Ontario; Daisy Harris, London, Ontario; Major Harry Norry, Woodstock

Mary Eleanor (Winnett) Turvey

Graduated from: University of Toronto Hospital School of Nursing. Year: 1940

Military History:

Service: RCAMC

Rank: Lt./NS

Served: 1943 to 1945

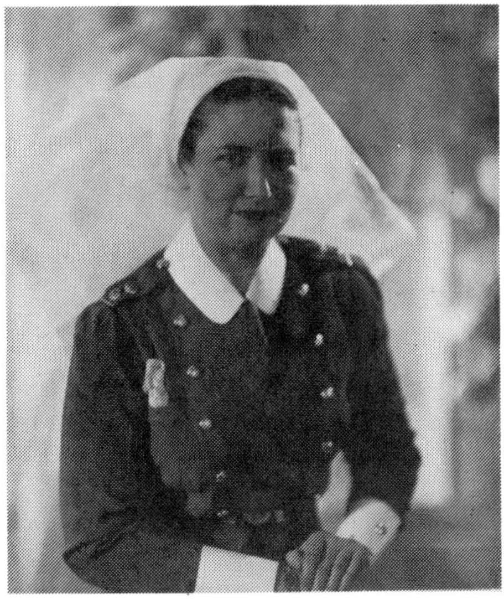

Lt. N/S Eleanor (Winnett) Turvey, No. 10 CGH

My next-door neighbour, Dr. Cec Rae (Brig.) was always asking me when I was going to join the Army so in 1943 I became a nursing sister in the RCAMC.

The first experience of Army life for nurses at Camp Borden was Parade Square, marching and drill, and then more marching around station roads and out of camp.

While stationed at Leavseden (Hertfordshire) General Hospital, we were experiencing heavy casualties as a result of the D-Day landings. There was a constant flow of wounded.

Heavy bombers were stationed at a local airfield. The nurses constantly watched the outgoing raids, keeping a count of the numbers leaving and a count of the number returning which was constantly smaller. A depressing service.

My marriage to my husband, George, a long-time friend from Toronto, (a fighter pilot), took place at Leaveseden Parish Church at the end of September 1944. A wonderful reception was held in the nurses' mess after which we left for a honeymoon in Wales.

I accompanied my husband to Buckingham Palace in early October 1944 for the Fall Investiture. George received his DFC from King George VI.

I was back at home in February 1945 stationed at Borden until September 1945 at which time I was demobilized. Our daughter arrived in November 1945.

Teresa M. (Woolsey) Weir

Graduated from: St. Mary's Hospital School of Nursing, Kitchener, Ontario. Year: 1939

Military History:

Service: RCAMC

Rank: Lt. N/S

Served: August 1943 to October 1945

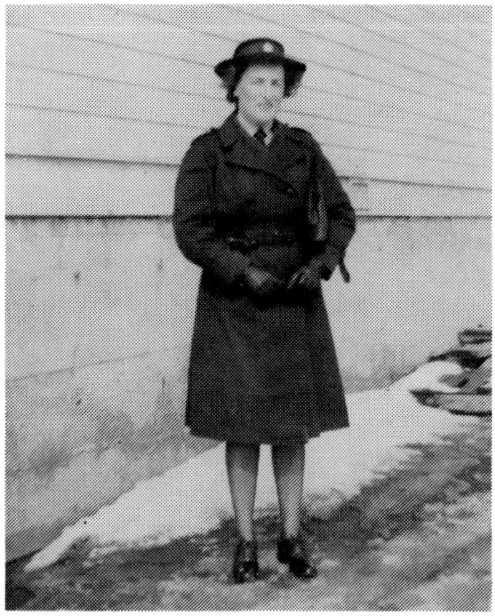

No. 10 CGH; Lt. N/S Teresa (Woolsey) Weir at Debert, NS, 1943. The face is not so hot but the legs aren't bad.

I chose a military career for nursing experience which was great, and also for adventure.

When I first joined up, I nursed at Chorley Park Military Hospital in Toronto, and then for a while at the Oakville Convalescent Military Hospital, Oakville, Ontario. From there, I went to Halifax to join a group of nurses who soon left for England, but with four others, I was delayed because of health problems (I had an ear infection). A month later the five of us sailed on the *Andes* which was loaded to the hilt with soldiers and took ten days. In England I was sent to No. 2 Canadian General Hospital in Bramshott for awhile, then to No. 10 Canadian General Hospital at Leavesden near Watford. In July 1944 I went with the No. 10 General to France, south of Bayeux.

I remember the long convoys of ambulances bringing patients in. They had wounds of all sorts; many were put into casts and flown out in a few days to England. I recall giving hundreds of shots of penicillin. We lived in bell tents, got one canvas pail of water a day for baths and laundry, ate in a mess tent carrying two fold-up square tins and a cup for meals, and we got our hot drink out of something like a boiler. As we lined up, the cook served food into our pans. The food was good. The chief cook was from Kitchener, Ontario, and I remember him running a restaurant when I was in training there. He was a real great person. We had lanterns for light. In late October, our matron,

Miss Edith Dick, got us all oil stoves, after they offered her one – she was every inch a lady and replied, *"When you come up with one for every tent, I'll have one too."* I also remember the dietitian, Alice McGuinan, whose brother was a cardinal and she was always looking for lace for his vestments.

I quite remember it being cold and muddy in Bayeux and tramping around in rubber boots. Also, the latrines were made of burlap walls and fence posts. At times, when planes flew a little low, it proved to be a good laxative.

One night when anti-aircraft artillery was noisy overhead and we heard the siren, my tent-mate Marjorie Hooper, and I crawled under our cots – the trouble was that we had lots of boxes of stuff under there (Hoop was a real pack-rat) and it was a tight squeeze, so I hollered at her, *"Do you have a can opener, in case this is for real?"* Our tent was pierced by shrapnel once.

When Jean McKenzie and I were on nights on the officers' ward, I looked after General Guy Simonds – it was rumoured that Allied bombs were dropped by mistake on our headquarters.

In the fall of 1944 we went to Turnhout, Belgium. For a while I was on a ward that was pretty well all colostomy cases; men who had been shot in the abdomen. I think we were on only a couple of days at a time and then moved to another ward and back again, as we couldn't stand the heavy duty, and most found it oppressive.

Here we were using barracks formerly occupied by Germans and the walls were white with swastikas on them as well as pictures of Hitler. Some German patients got confused as to where they were.

Once, on nights, Betty Wilson and I were in the kitchen adjoining the ward, having coffee, when I heard a motor. Looking out the window, I saw a red light moving in the sky. It was coming straight at us. Betty said, *"You look scared, Terry...* I was, and said, *"Here comes a buzz bomb!"* And she shouted, *"Open the window, let it go through!"* Well, I didn't. It sounded like a motorboat. Finally the motor stopped and we knew that someone a ways from us must have got it.

During that term of night duty we had patients from a Polish regiment and one officer gave me a pin (a white eagle on a red background) from his uniform, in appreciation of the care he got. We also had German prisoners of war, very humble and sad patients. They had been stripped when they arrived and were terribly dirty as well as lousy, but very good patients. One gave me his swastika badge – it was on the bedside table so I picked it up to look at it, then set it back. Then he picked it up, put it in my hand and kept saying, *"Ja ja schwester."* I could tell he was very frightened and wanted to be a friend. Also, the first thing they said was, *"Nichts essen, schwester,"* which I think meant "no food, sister." They were starved and some had frozen feet. We had to get them washed, and if there were any who could help we asked them to help us bath their own men. So I told one of them, *"You wash feet of that man,"* and several voices said, *"Nein, nein schwester, officer, officer."* And so I pointed to myself and said, *"officer!"* I guess he was their commander, but he obeyed my order and washed their feet. I also had a German officer who was a doctor (surgeon) and who had his right arm off at the shoulder. There were many sad cases. We had put all the lousy clothes into a big box and we used to say we expected to see the box start moving.

This is from a letter I wrote on March 26th, 1945, to a friend back home. "At the present time I am on night duty, we stay on for two weeks. I'll be very glad when my term is over as I dislike nights very much. I am a float nurse but spend some of my time on the resuscitation ward, where all the seriously and dangerously ill patients go. It is very interesting but a little depressing at times. They have three wards and can accommodate fifty-five patients. A way to describe the ward would be to say it drips with bottles and tubes. Each ward is equipped so we can give whole blood, blood plasma, oxygen, Wangensteen drainage, use of suction machine, minor surgery trays and everything you might need for resuscitating. Right next to the ward is the OR, X-ray, laboratory and dispensary, so things are very handy. We have had a lot of casualties who suffered from mine explosions. The war news seems very good these days..."

For a while in Turnhout we had an English unit with us and a couple of skin specialists on the dermatology ward. I relieved there a couple of times, and when they made rounds it was very proper.

My friend Hoop didn't like parties, said she'd rather read a good book, but we went places together and had a good time. I went out with Betty Wilson and two Americans – very nice gentlemen – to various places as well.

I still have the canvas cot issued to us, and our grandchildren sleep on it when they come; also, the wooden gray box issued to us in Belgium to keep extra things in. Our daughter

Paula refinished mine and uses it for a coffee table. I gave my khaki uniforms to the museum in Dundas, Ontario.

Though I never felt like any hero, it was the best piece of nursing I ever did!

Madge Wheaton

Military History:

Service: RCAMC

Rank: Lt. N/S

Served: March 1942 to October 1945

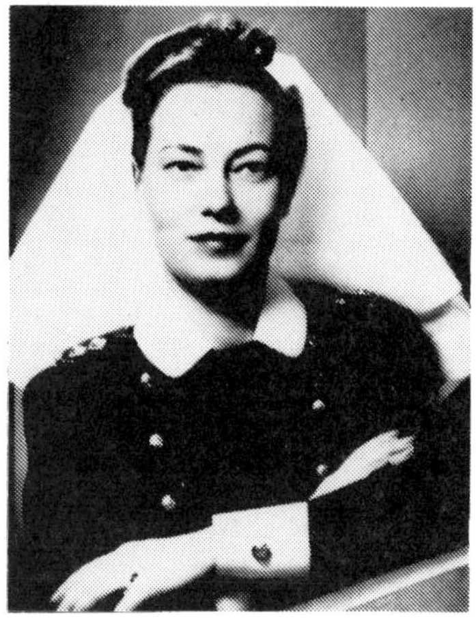

No. 10 CGH; Madge Wheaton RCAMC March 1942-October 1945

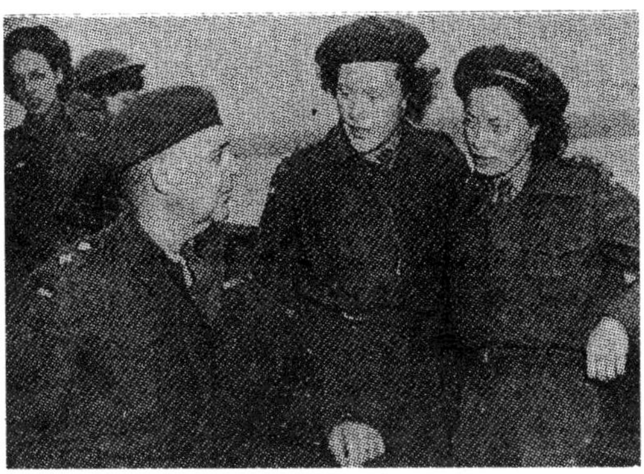

Canadian nursing sisters arrived in France recently for duty with a Canadian general hospital. L-R: Lt. Col. W.A. Kelsall, Toronto; Lt. N/S Betty Wilson, Halifax and St. John, NB, and Lt. N/S Madge Wheaton, Sackville, NB. Canadian Forces photo

Jean D. (Scrimgeour) Wilson

Graduated from: Toronto General Hospital School of Nursing.
Year: 1933

Military History:

Service: RCAMC

Rank: Lt. N/S

Served: September 1940 to August 1945

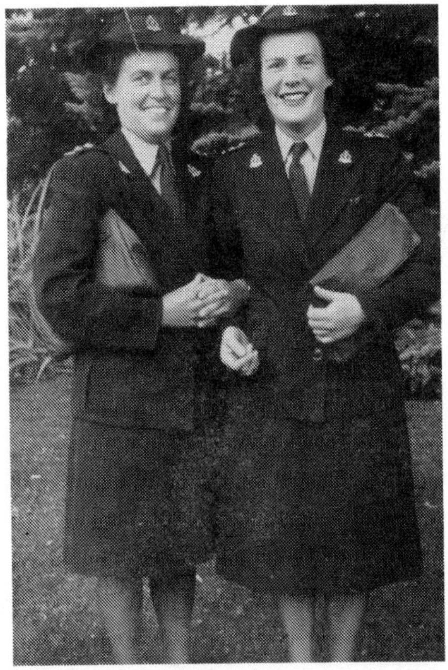

No. 10 CGH; L-R: Joyce (Chapman) Houston, Jean (Scrimgeour) Wilson

I chose a military career because of my love of adventure and I was helping to support a younger brother and sister through high school and Army pay was better than I got on civvy street. The fact of maturing and learning of life in different cultures, also learning to cope with less than basic equipment was a highlight for me.

While waiting to embark for Italy in the fall of 1943, I was the only survivor of five pedestrians hit when a passing jeep ran over a land mine. Then our ship was torpedoed and sunk in the Mediterranean. I rowed with one oar till the crew calmed and we pulled to the rescue ship and climbed up rope ladders to the deck. All our clothing, etc., sunk. I was with No. 14 Canadian General Hospital at the time.

In Europe I went over with No. 10 CGH and was on temporary loan to No. 8 CGH stationed at Antwerp. My tent mate, Joyce Chapman, and I were to be on duty Sunday but had the morning off duty, so we stayed in our tent overnight. That night a bomb demolished the corner room where we were allocated to sleep. Imagine everyone's surprise when we reported for work Sunday afternoon.

I was the first nursing sister, along with my friend Marie Cantin who spoke fluent French, to enter Paris after it was recaptured by the Allies. We had one day off duty and a British major had to get to Paris on an errand. We went AWOL and accompanied him. We said nothing for a week after a safe return. Yes, we were reprimanded, but nothing drastic occurred.

I was also one of the first nurses repatriated to Canada after VE Day. Sailed on the *Ile de France* to New York, then on by train to Toronto.

NO.11 CANADIAN GENERAL HOSPITAL

Rossalea O. (Hughes) Crowe
Margaret (Martin) Hanford
Helen (Dawson) Hurley
Violet S. Lambe
Verna (White) Lister
Mary MacDonald
Jessie (Lee) Middleton
Isabel Reinhardt
Vera Spencer
Harriet (Campbell) Stanfield
Mary (Bower) White
Helen Wilson

On 2 August 1943 Col. Hume was on his way home from overseas to organize No.11 Canadian General Hospital as a 600-bed hospital at Currie Barracks, Calgary. Mobilization date was 8 September. Matron Wilson and many nursing sisters arrived the 3rd of September.

By 13 September 1943 the unit arrived in Halifax and boarded the *Queen Elizabeth* troop ship; five days later, it anchored off Gourock, Scotland. The next day they left the ship with No. 12 General Hospital. They boarded a troop train at Gourock and arrived at their destination, Moor Park, an estate three miles from Farnham.

Since leaving the ship the nursing sisters were not with the unit. They went to No. 14 CGH at Horley and thence in small groups to various hospitals for duty.

No. 11 took over the hospital from No. 7 General at Taplow on the estate of Lady Astor and remained there until February 1946 when they ceased to function as a unit.

Rossalea O. (Hughes) Crowe

Graduated from: Medicine Hat General Hospital School of Nursing. Year: 1938

Military History:

Service: RCAMC

Rank: Lt. N/S

Served: April 20, 1942 to April 26, 1946

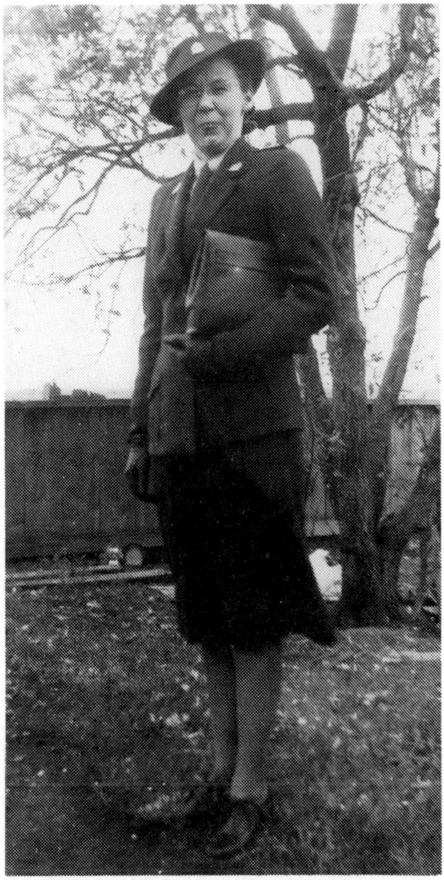

Lt. N/S Rossalea (Hughes) Crowe, No. 10 CGH and Lady Nelson *hospital ship.*

I was influenced to choose a military career by my desire to be part of the war effort, and my two brothers had also enlisted. Being a nursing sister would be challenging and exciting.

I joined the RCAMC in Calgary and was stationed at Currie Barracks. From Currie I was posted to Suffield Field Experimental Station at Suffield, Alberta. That was an interesting posting as soldiers from all the Allied forces came there for experiments and training in chemical warfare. I met many interesting people, both military and civilian.

My next posting was to the Canadian Hospital Ship, *Lady Nelson,* which was an adventure to someone raised on the Prairies. I was on the *Lady Nelson* for 15 months. During that time I made 12 complete crossings of the Atlantic. Two of the trips detoured to Italy to pick up casualties – then to England and back to Halifax. We saw ships torpedoed behind us during the Italian trips. The hospital ship was unescorted and travelled with all lights on. We were protected by the Geneva Convention – but on several occasions the war seemed too close for comfort. Strange as it may seem – I never felt afraid.

After my time on the *Lady Nelson* I was posted to England and after VE Day was posted to Germany. The ravages of war were very evident and the hostility of the German orderlies was very evident, although well controlled. They did not like Canadian nurses (women) being superior in rank to them.

I was posted back to Canada as part of the Burma Draft, but VJ came before we were to go for "Jungle Training" in Kentucky.

I am one of few nurses who was awarded the Atlantic Star.

I feel the 4 years I spent in the RCAMC was challenging and exciting.

Margarette (Martin) Hanford

Graduated from: Royal Jubilee Hospital School of Nursing, Victoria, B.C.
Year: 1941

Military History:

Service: RCAMC

Rank: Lieutenant N/S

Served: February 1943 to February 1946

I felt life in the Army would be an interesting and rewarding experience.

I started in Victoria Military Hospital, then spent a brief period in Chilliwack Military Hospital. I was sent overseas December 1943 and posted to No. 11 Canadian General Hospital. Our trip across the Atlantic was 15 rough days. Many nurses were seasick and kept the MOs busy. I was quite healthy until one morning on my usual deck walk it was quite rough and slippery; I almost went into the briny deep. Lady Luck was with me as I caught something in time. That

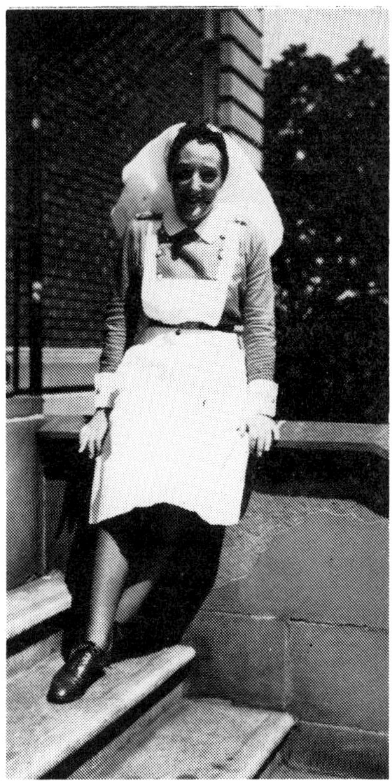

N/S Margarette Martin, Vancouver B.C., 1943, Victoria Military Hospital; (was Victoria Normal School prior to becoming Victoria Military Hospital)

was quite a lesson.

No. 11 was a very busy hospital as it was a repatriation centre. We were in a very beautiful site by the Thames River. It was on the Cliveden estate, home of Lady Astor. She loved to go through the wards in her breezy style and tell us to go out on the estate and pick daffodils for the boys.

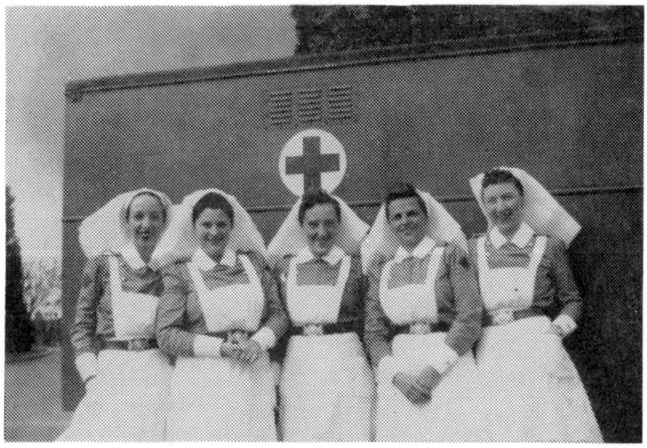

Victoria Military Hospital 1943
L-R: Nursing Sisters Erskine, Jo Rose, Margarette Martin, Helen Unsworth, Bessie Sherwin

One of our favourite off-duty pursuits was cycling around the countryside. From where we were to Windsor Castle was a nice jaunt. There was little traffic to worry about. After a 12-hour shift on the ward, a day off to cycle was most refreshing.

I was a bit harsh, sometimes, on the patients who would be playing poker. However, they usually played on the bed furthest from the nurses' station. They would see me coming and hide the money, so it was a losing battle for me.

It was hard work during my 18 months in England, but in all, a most gratifying experience and I'm thankful for the opportunity to have served and helped to do my part in the RCAMC.

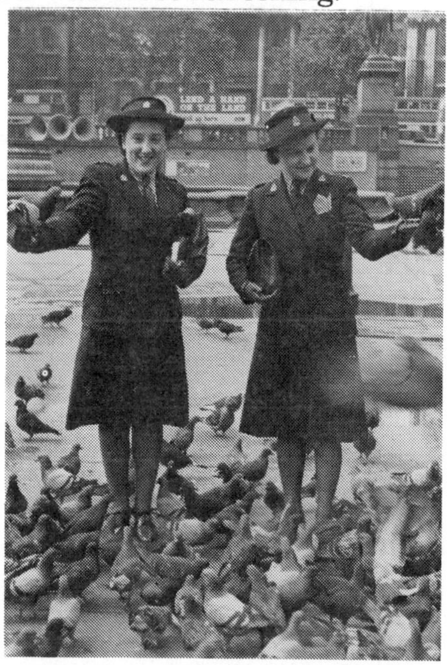

Trafalgar Square, London, England 27 June 1944. L-R: Margarette Martin, Vancouver, B.C., and Elsie Breakell, Medicine Hat, Alberta.

On my return to Canada I was on staff at Vancouver Military Hospital (Shaughnessy site) for about five months until discharge in February 1946.

I went back to visit Britain in 1990. We went to Taplow to see the hospital two weeks before it was to be demolished. An English friend took a piece of wood from a tree blown down from the windstorm on the grounds and turned it on his wood turners' machine into a lovely bowl - a great souvenir for me.

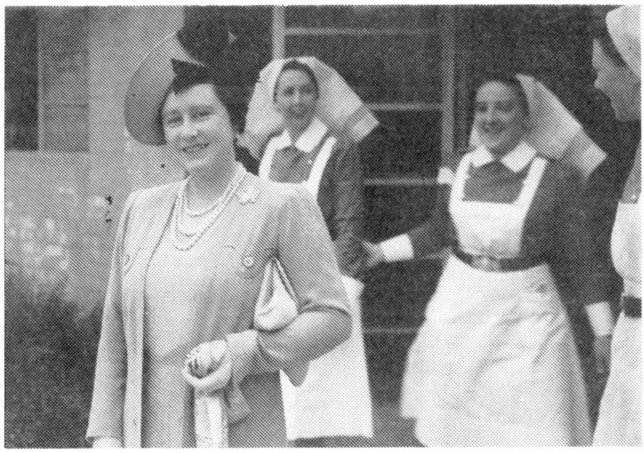

At No. 11 CGH Taplow taken just after D-Day 6 June 1944. Queen Elizabeth visited the wards at Cliveden. L-R: Queen Elizabeth, Lt. N/S Jean V. Simpson, Halifax; Lt. N/S Margarette Martin, Vancouver; Lt. N/S Owens, Toronto

After D-Day Queen Elizabeth visited our hospital. She was such a charming person. I just happened to be with her when a photographer snapped us. I will say I am proud to have this picture on the wall in my home.

Helen A. (Dawson) Hurley

Graduated from: Royal Columbian Hospital School of Nursing, New Westminster. Year: 1939

Military History:

Service: RCAMC

Rank: Lt. N/S

Served: September 1942 to April 1946

Some of the highlights of my military experience were:

The memory of wave after wave of planes passing over us on D-Day.

The speed of evacuating a hospital, remaking beds and admitting wounded from Normandy.

The kindness and appreciation of local people in England, and especially in France, of our presence.

The announcement of Armistice came while we were attending an opera in Paris. The orchestra came out on the steps and played national anthems of France, England and U.S., then lights started to come on.

The advent of penicillin, dark yellow brown in 50 or 100 cc. ampules – costly, so handled with much care. A godsend to our patients with infected wounds. When you were penicillin nurse the boys sang *"Pistol Packing Mama."*

I went overseas with No. 11 Canadian General Hospital then moved to No. 16 General. I went to Europe with No. 21 Canadian General. While in France I was again assigned to No. 16 General.

Violet Sinclair Lambe

Graduated from: Vancouver General Hospital School of Nursing. Year: 1940

Military History:

Service: RCAMC

Rank: Lt. N/S

Served: 1942 to 1946

My brothers were in the Forces; that influenced me to choose a military career.

On the Continent I was with No. 8 CGH and No. 1 General. Holland was the highlight of my experience when the buzz bombs were falling.

Verna L. (White) Lister

Graduated from: Provincial Mental Hospital and Calgary General Hospital School of Nursing. Year: 1941

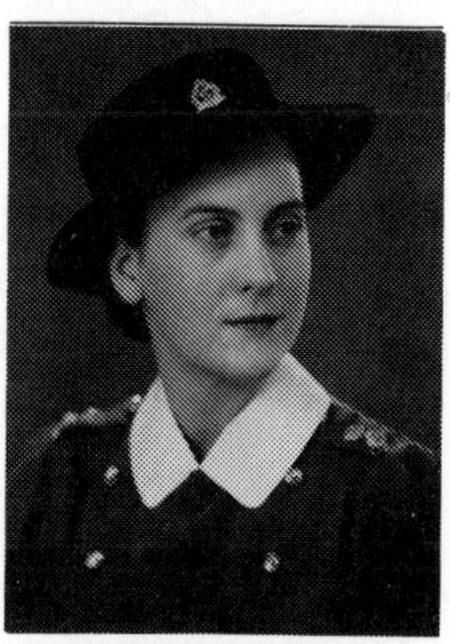

Lt. N/S Verna (White) Lister.

Military History:

Service: RCAMC

Rank: Lieutenant N/S

Served: June 1942 to June 1946

When I graduated in 1941 the military service seemed to be the best way to make use of my training and to be of service where needed. I enlisted at Currie Barracks, Calgary, Alberta, in June 1942. In September 1943 I joined No. 11 Canadian General Hospital and went to England on the *Queen Elizabeth*, arriving at Horley. From there I spent about a year at No. 16 General Hospital, Marston Green, England. In February 1945 I was sent with a small psychiatric unit to Italy and attached to No. 14 General Hospital at Caserta. Later, when No. 14 moved, the psychiatric unit was attached to No. 15 General. The psychiatric unit under tents was certainly memorable, but the numbers were soon reduced and I then worked on medical and surgical wards. The time Cassino was finally taken was probably one of the most memorable times as I was working on the chest injury ward at No. 15 General. We had a number of Polish patients who did not understand English. At the same time, we were short of staff and working long hours; patients were great and helped other patients.

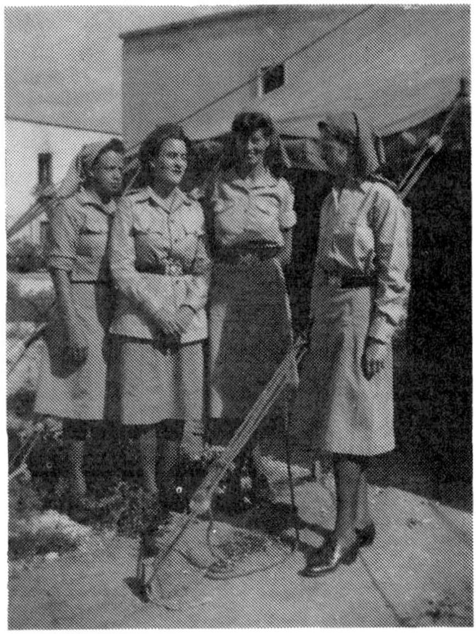

Tent Office of Neuro-Psychiatric Unit, Caserta, Italy 1944. L-R: Nursing Sisters Helen Colurn, Ontario, Verna (White) Lister, Vancouver; Mary Gamon Burke, Victoria; Buddy Galbraith, Toronto.

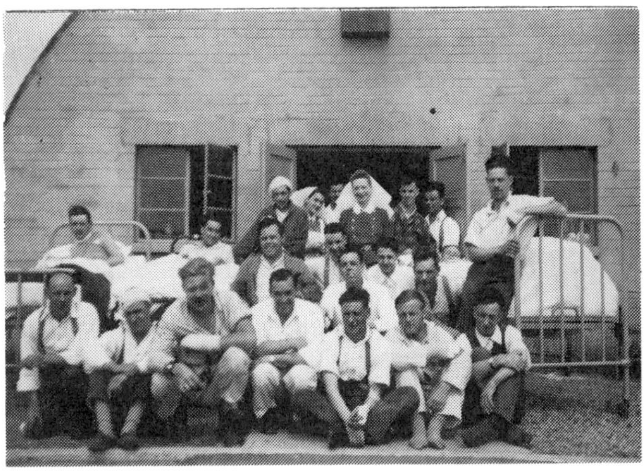

No. 1 Neurological Hospital, Basingstoke, VE Day - patients from Burn & Plastic Ward Nursing Sisters Verna White, Mona Fraser

Leaving Italy about June 1945, I went to England and was stationed at No. 1 Neurological and Plastic Surgery Hospital at

Basingstoke. This was a very memorable time also, as I worked in the burn unit which was very busy due to burns from tanks. On VE Day at Basingstoke we put as many patients as possible outside the ward for the celebration!

I remember returning from Italy to England in 1945 on a small British troop ship. I think there were only five or six nurses and we volunteered and worked in the sick bay somewhere below deck. Some of the troops were quite ill. Some had been prisoners of war and had made their way to Naples and were on their way home.

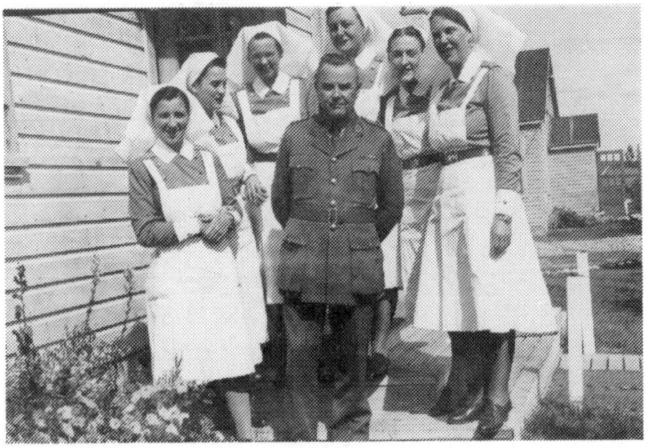

Currie Military Hospital, Calgary, 1942
L-R: Nursing Sisters Nettie Garfield, Verna White, Rossie Hughes, Mary Rose, Charlotte Langston; name unknown; Major George Clements OC

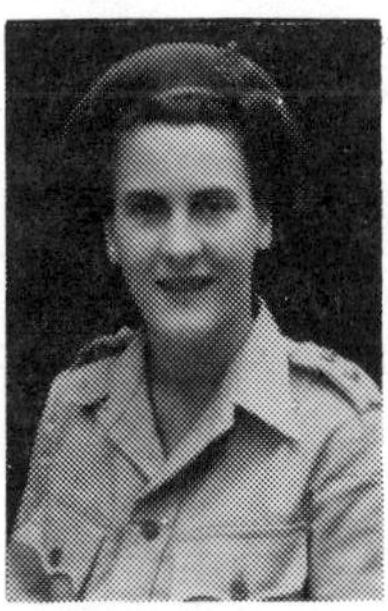

Lt. N/S Verna White wearing the ATS (Auxiliary Territorial Service) British Woman's military uniform as a Canadian nursing sister in Italy, 1944. The ship they were on was lost at sea.

Mary MacDonald

Graduated from: Misericordia Hospital School of Nursing, Edmonton, Alberta. Year: 1940

Military Service

Service: RCAMC

Rank: Lt. N/S

Served: October 1942 to June 1946

At the time war was declared in September of 1939, there was a very deep sense of duty prevalent in the Canadian population. The sentiment of the day amounted to a dedication to our country and to our cherished values. We were all imbued with rightness of being ready to defend our country and Christian principles.

In my mind, there was no question. I would become a nursing sister in the RCAMC, and the sooner the better.

The DMO (District Medical Officer) was located in Military District No. 13 at Calgary, so it was necessary to go there to be interviewed for appointment to the RCAMC. There was a delay following the interview until I was called for active duty. During that time I worked at an isolation hospital in Calgary with commonwealth military patients.

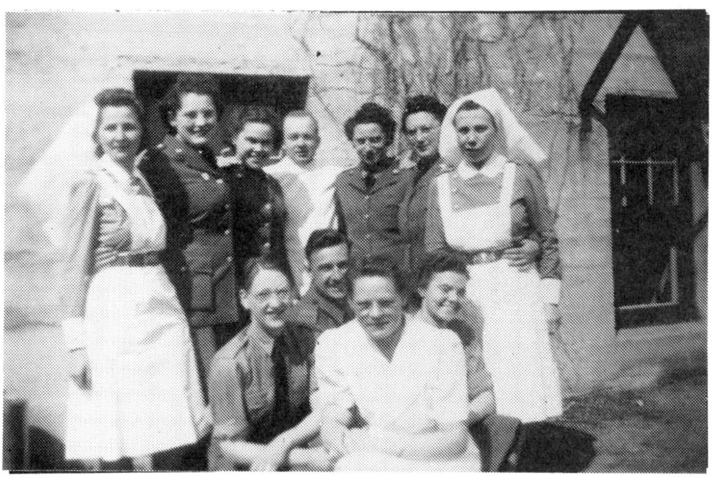

1943 Vermilion Military Hospital Staff. Left: Lt. N/S Alexandra Bury. Far right: Lt. N/S Mary MacDonald

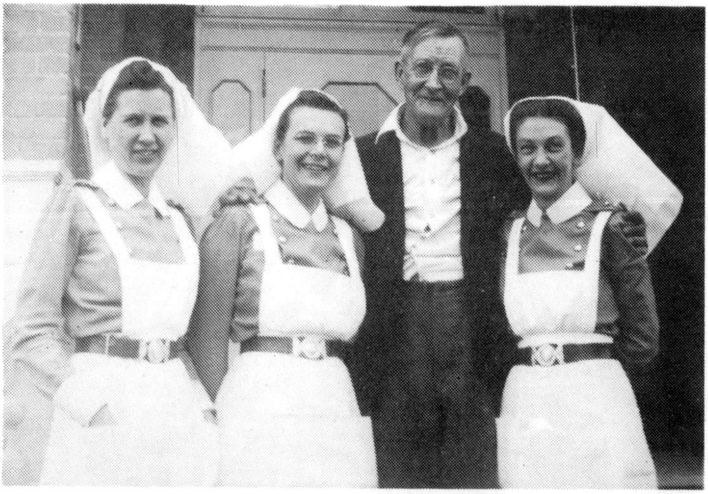

Currie Barracks 1942. L-R : Nursing Sisters Helen Hill, Lethbridge, Alberta; Betty Chinn, Edmonton, Alberta; a patient, and Doris Grinde, Rimbey, Alberta

I was called up 22 October 1942 and spent six months at the military hospital at Currie Barracks. Nettie (Garfield) Pedlar was our matron. Then Alexandra Bury and I were posted to the military hospital at the Canadian Women's Army Corps Training Centre, Vermilion, Alberta. Again, I was there for six months.

There were some very wonderful, intelligent, well educated women there. We were in the Vermilion School of Agriculture. It had been closed for years and the bathrooms were out of order. There was a sign on the board that said "Bathroom Parade 10 - 2 - 6 - 10." The truck would come and pick up the girls and take them down to the hotel bathroom at the specified hour.

It was really quite a fun place in many ways; there were concerts in which we all participated. We used to have great discussions after work – you had to be specific and have an opinion – you couldn't sit on the fence.

In August 1943, word came that I was going overseas. Nurses from all over Canada arrived in Calgary to form No. 11 Canadian General Hospital. Rossie Hughes, one of our group, was unable to go with us at that time. She presented us with a bottle of Scotch to have on our journey across Canada. It lasted for the six days of train travel. It proved to be an aid to socializing and provided us with the opportunity to talk over our fears and misgivings. There was also time for laughter and enjoyment.

In Halifax we boarded the *Queen Elizabeth* 13 September 1943 and crossed in four days and four hours. We landed in

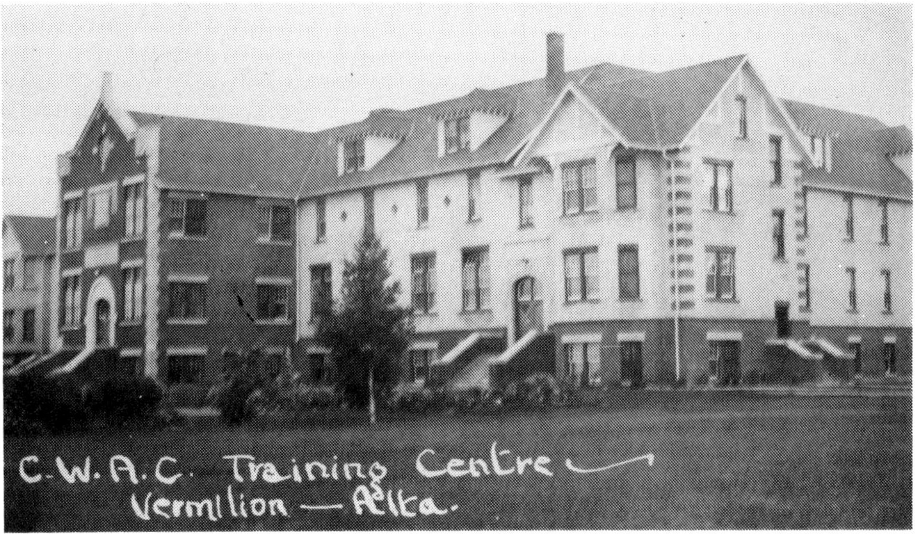

CWAC Training Centre, Vermilion, Alberta

Greenock, Scotland, and went by train to Horley, England. When we arrived, No. 14 General Hospital was preparing to go to the Continent. They were selling bicycles and all sorts of things they couldn't take with them and which we were happy to purchase.

While waiting to be located, No. 11 nurses were dispersed among a number of hospitals. Six of us were sent to No. 17 Canadian General at Crowthorne where we stayed until our unit was established at Taplow. I was on duty the night of 6 June 1944 when we heard the sound of planes overhead. Looking out the window, we realized it was an unusual sight. We immediately went out where we could see more clearly. The countless planes were in formation; it was a beautiful clear night. We were very excited because we knew there was some meaning to all this.

The following morning there was great excitement as some of our high ranking male officers were very aware of what was happening – operation D-Day had begun. Some of the first casualties came unexpectedly to our hospital at Taplow during the night. In the morning all mobile patients helped with breakfast. One young Lieutenant, on being served his tray by a brigadier, called the nurse and asked what happened. *"Did I die and go to heaven?"*

No. 11 was to remain at Taplow. Nursing sisters wishing to go to the Continent applied for transfer to another unit. I joined No. 20 Canadian General; we went to northern England to train

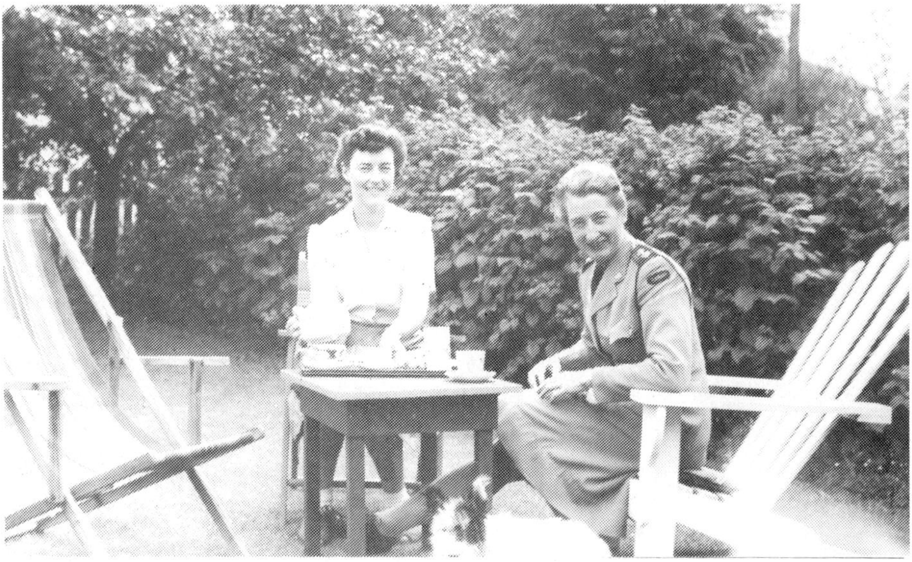

CWAC Lt. Lindrum, Victoria at Vermilion, Alberta.

until we went overseas.

Initially we set up in Antwerp. The morning of our arrival the matron informed us about a superstition in Antwerp that a bomb went off every Saturday at four o'clock and this was a Saturday at 4 o'clock.

That was the day the theatre was bombed and about a thousand people were killed. The remains of victims, service and civilian, were brought to our hospital. It was a terrible disaster. Bombs were falling every three minutes.

We were only there a few days, when on Christmas Day, 1944, CMHQ became aware of our situation and ordered us out. We were gone in four hours and off to No. 10 General at Ghent. On New Year's Eve I was supposed to go to No. 3 CCS, but as the Battle of the Bulge was on, No. 3 was inaccessible. When the fighting cleared a bit, I was sent to No. 2 CCS for a while and from there to No. 88 British General Hospital because it was in the Canadian zone caring for Canadian soldiers. I was assigned to the operating room.

I assisted Dr. Grosse, a Canadian physician from Calgary, with his eye surgery. He removed shrapnel from the eyes with a magnet. He was very good at it. Teams consisting of a surgeon, an anaesthetist, an orderly and a nursing sister were set up working 12 hours on and 12 hours off. That was a very busy time.

I left No. 88 General, went back to No. 2 CCS and finally to No. 20 at Turnhout, Belgium. There the patients were all German POWs and the guards were Belgian. The Germans would refuse their medication because they were terrified of being poisoned. The beds had a tubular frame and they would drop their pills down the hollow frame. They were all between 16 years and 83 years old.

VE Day found us still at Turnhout. Dr. Gunn from Winnipeg, our commandant, had a pipe band that went all through the hospital. The patients were terrified; I can still see them up on their elbows; they were sure they were going to be shot. However, they lived to go to their homes and soon after VE Day we closed that hospital.

When No. 20 dispersed Dr. Gunn gave a drum and a set of pipes to the townspeople. There is an interesting sequel to this event. Forty years later I witnessed a display of piping and Highland dancing at North Bay, Ontario. Pipers from Turnhout were there. In conjunction with Scottish pipers they had developed a pipe band second to none and were justly proud of their achievement.

Following the closure of the hospital, Ida Rothwell and I were sent to 2nd Echelon to look after 450 CWAC just arrived from Canada.

In December 1945 I left Echelon and came back to Canada. A lot of things stand out in my mind; to this day I feel for many of the sad cases. I remember the heroism of Canadians. I understand how these men in the Legion feel when they are criticized for their traditions.

From 1968 to 1970 I was president of the Nursing Sisters Association of Canada, and in going over the minutes, I noticed that a suggestion had been made that a book be written about nursing sisters overseas. I got in touch with Grace Johnson and Evelyn Pepper and the idea was presented at our 1970 convention. The resolution barely passed because there was concern about cost, and who we could find to take on the task. We were fortunate that Col. Nicholson did it under very difficult circumstances. The book entitled *Canada's Nursing Sisters*, was completed to our satisfaction in 1975.

Jessie A. (Lee) Middleton

Graduated from: Royal Columbian Hospital School of Nursing, New Westminster, B.C. Year: 1939

Military History:

Service: RCAMC.

Rank: Lt. N/S

Served: September 21, 1942 to November 15, 1945

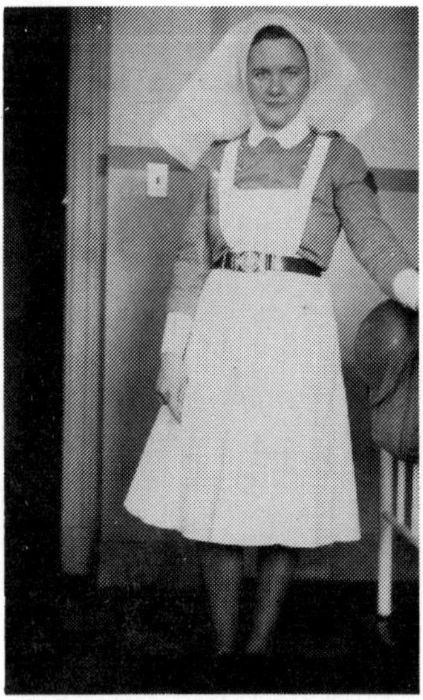

Lt. N/S Jessie (Lee) Middleton, No. 11 CGH

My two eldest brothers had been in the First World War – their stories from an early age influenced me. My friends were joining the service and I wanted to be a part of it.

I served the first year at Nanaimo and Prince Rupert. We mobilized at Camp Sarcee, Calgary, September 1943. We travelled by troop train to Halifax with No. 11 Canadian General Hospital. (300 nurses) on the *Queen Elizabeth* to Greenock in Scotland, then travelled by troop train again to Horley south of London.

I spent a great disembarkation leave with Queenie Hammell in Edingurgh. Then 10 months at Taplow on Lady Astor's estate on the Thames with No. 7 CGH.

July 31, 1944, I arrived in Italy, to Avellino; then, after 10 days' leave in Rome, north to Macerata and on the Jesi, just north of Ancona on the Adriatic. One leave in Italy, I had the opportunity to visit Florence and picnic on top of the Leaning Tower of Pisa in February, on a lovely sunny day, ("Bully Beef" sandwiches). When the Canadians left Italy, No. 1 CGH went from Naples to Marseilles by hospital ship, then were flown to Brussels. I was stationed at Nijmegen, Holland, when peace was declared. I spent two months at Oldenburg, Germany, before going back to Canada September or October on the *Rotterdam.* At Taplow the memorable event was a visit by the Queen – she visited wards in the hospital and had tea in the nurses' residence.

The parties at the Astor mansion, "Cliveden," were certainly unforgettable too. Lady Astor insisted on all ranks attending together. She could jitterbug as well as any of the young fellows!

We had already had casualties from D-Day before I left for Italy. The trip to Italy began at Liverpool on the *Volendam*, 12 days on the ship, if I remember rightly, Army food, of course, but otherwise a restful cruise.

Isabel G. Reinhardt

Graduated from: Holy Cross Hospital School of Nursing, Calgary. Year: 1940

Military History:

Service: RCAMC

Rank: Lt. N/S

Served: May 1942 to August 1945

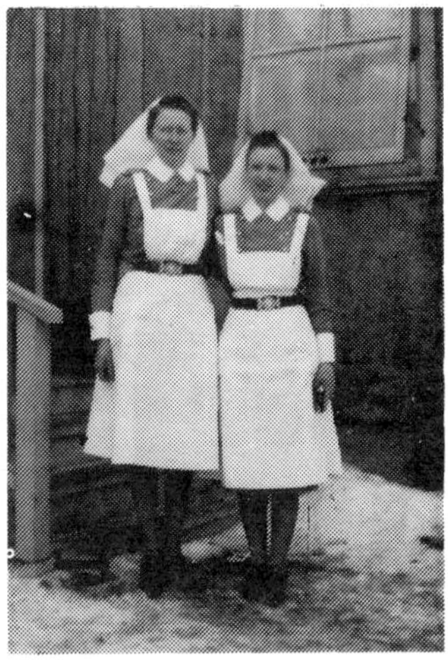

Nursing Sisters Mcleod and Isabel Reinhardt, Camrose Military Hospital, 1942.

When I chose a military career I had ideas that I would like to be of help in the war effort. Also, I was probably influenced by books I read in my early teens of Red Cross girls driving ambulances in World War I – it sounded exciting, but I wasn't aware of these immature reasons when I joined. I joined the Army in Calgary in May, 1942, and was posted to Red Deer Military Hospital until October 1942, then Camrose Military until early 1943. Again, Red Deer Military until September 1943. In September 1943, I went to England with No. 11 Canadian General Hospital and was attached to No. 7 Canadian General Hospital. I went to Normandy mid-July 1944 with No. 7 Canadian General Hospital so we were stationed near Bayeux until late in 1944. The hospital was then moved to Dieppe (about 7 miles out) until November 1944, and again moved; this time to Turnhout in Belgium until spring of 1945. At that time No. 7 was moved to Germany, not far from Bremen and I was returned to Canada, by way of England, in summer of 1945 and received my discharge in August 1945.

Vera Louise Spencer

Written by Vera's sister-in-law, Marian Marzolf

Graduated from Regina General Hospital School of Nursing. Year 1942

Military History:

Service: RCAMC

Rank: Lt. N/S

Served: 1943 to 1946

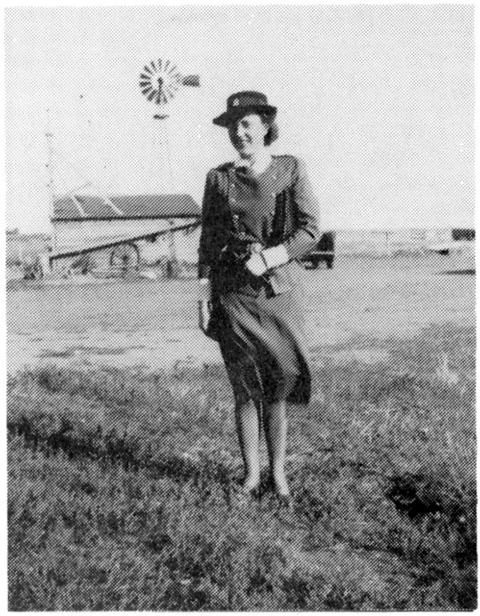

Lt. N/S Vera Louise Spencer, Moose Jaw, Saskatchewan.

Vera chose a military career because strong patriotism was instilled by her parents. She admired her servicemen brothers: Earl in Army, and Ross in Air Force.

Vera was born at the farm in the Penzance area, a small town in south central Saskatchewan. Her parents were Dr. and Mrs. Garnet Earl Spencer. He was the local veterinary surgeon. She finished high school, part by correspondence – a fine student and always an avid reader.

After graduation from Regina General with her RN, she joined the Army at Calgary, serving overseas at a Canadian General Hospital at Taplow near London. In 1946 she returned to Canada and received her discharge at Regina MD No. 12.

She spent part of 1946 and 1947 at Fort Qu'Appelle in the sanatorium as a result of nursing tuberculosis patients in England. Her lungs always gave her trouble following this.

She decided to enter the field of public health and obtained her PSCN at McGill, Montreal. She accepted a position on the staff of Saskatchewan Public Health Services as a field nurse and supervisor. In 1960 she received her Masters in Public Health at Ann Arbor Michigan. She was then made Nursing Consultant for Public Health, based in Regina. While here, she served as president of Saskatchewan Registered Nurse's

Association and was later given a life membership of Canadian Public Health.

In 1982 she retired with the early symptoms of muscle degeneration. She was given excellent care in the veteran's wing of the Wascanna Rehabilitation Centre, Regina, where she had the distinction of being the first female veteran in residence.

Vera was a person who enjoyed family and kept close to her sisters and brothers after her parents had passed away. She also played a part in the lives of her many nieces and nephews. She was dedicated to her career; her greatest luxury was her appreciation of the symphony.

We only feel so sorry that her health had denied her the pleasures retirement could have given her. She passed away 7 March 1994.

Harriet (Campbell) Stansfield

Graduated from: Victoria General Hospital School of Nursing, Halifax

Military History:

Service: RCAMC

Rank: Lt. N/S

Served: 1943 to 1945

In Memoriam – Graciously submitted by Dr. Hugh Stansfield, loving husband and best friend of Harriet.

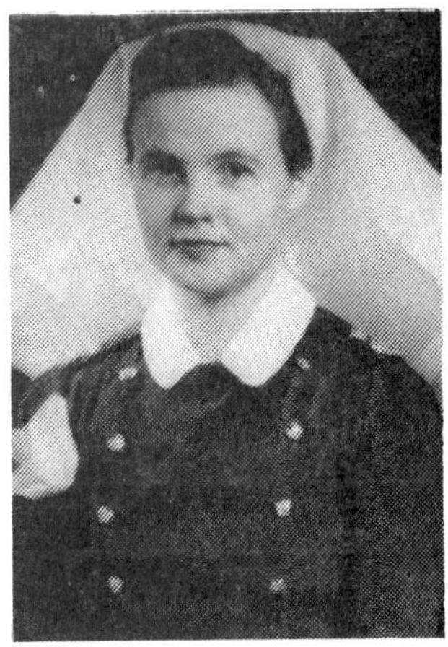

Lt. N/S Harriet (Campbell) Stansfield

Harriett Grace Campbell was born May 24, 1917, in Amherst, Nova Scotia, to Harold John Campbell and Vivian Grace Darling Rockwell Campbell. She was the eldest of four children. Maxwell (now deceased), June and Lyn. The Campbell family moved around in Nova Scotia with changes in Harold's positions with Hydro. Homes after Amherst included Bridgeport and Lunenburg and eventually, Digby, where Harriett completed high school. She had thoughts of becoming a librarian, but family finances did not permit university, and she elected instead nurses training at the Victoria General Hospital in

Halifax. Sadly, Vivian Campbell died about a year after Harriett completed her training, following which Harriett returned to Digby.

Harriett enlisted in the RCAMC in 1943, and in due course was assigned to Canadian Memorial Hospital in Taplow, England, where she was in charge of an open TB ward. There she met and became engaged to Dr. Hugh Stansfield, medical officer at Taplow. She remained at Taplow some months after VE Day, and then returned to Digby and lived with Harold and Lyn. Hugh returned to Canada August 16, 1946, and three days later they were married. They then moved to Montreal and attended McGill (Harriett for arts, and Hugh for post-graduate work).

Margaret was born in 1949. With Margaret 4 months old and Harriett 2 months pregnant with Dorothy, the family drove across the country and planted new roots in Vancouver. Dorothy's birth in 1950 was followed by Hugh Jr. in 1952 and Keith in 1956. Harriett had her hands full; parenting was a challenging full-time occupation for many years.

Marg, Dode, Hugh and Keith have rich memories of a mother who was the "glue" in the household... who could be counted on to sit with one or more of them on the kitchen floor 'til all hours solving the problems of the world... who could manage everyone else's problems and still orchestrate family gatherings or trips to Mayne Island... who could make time for volunteer service at the church, at school, in the VGH Auxiliary, for the Heart Fund, and for whomever or whatever else called upon her.

Hugh Sr. will remember a life partner who supported and enabled his professional endeavours, in addition to being lover and best friend.

It there is a single overriding impression of Harriett, it is of someone who endlessly placed the interests of others ahead of her own. For years she gave more than one might have imagined she had left to give to the care of Edgar and Marilla Stansfield, and (with June and Lyn) to her aunt, Jean Campbell.

Then in the late 1970s, just when the kids were finally on their own and possibilities of travel and relaxation should have been the order of the day, Alzheimer's Disease crept into Harriett's life. Gradually, the always competent Harriett became unable to accomplish the miraculous and, in time, could do very little. It has been a great sadness that Harriett has not been able to be an active part of the lives of the grandchildren she'd always anticipated with such joy: Jasper, Colin, Samantha, Heather,

David, Jessica, Patrick, Matthew, Rachel, and Dylan.

The cruel progression of her disease led her to Oakherst Nursing Home, to Valleyview, and to the Brock Fahrni Pavillion of Shaughnessy Hospital, where finally she was released and died peacefully July 14, 1992.

We celebrate the life of a gracious and loving wife, mother, grandmother, sister, and friend; we are mindful of, and grateful for, the spirit which remains.

Mary (Bower) White

Graduated from: Holy Cross Hospital School of Nursing, Calgary. Year: 1938

Military History

Service: RCAMC

Rank: Lt. N/S

Served: 10 June 1942 to 27 March 1945

I chose a military career because all the men in my family were killed in World War I or died as a result later. All the young men I knew were joining and being killed.

I went overseas with No. 11 but went to No. 7 Canadian General Hospital for most of my time in England. No. 7 took all the "Brass." I was ill and unable to go to France with No. 7 so stayed with No. 11 when they took over from No. 7 at Cliveden, England. I worked in the operating room, the eye ward, and on a surgical ward when the invasion started.

I have written a book, *Hello War Good-bye Sanity*, which covers my story. Published in 1992.

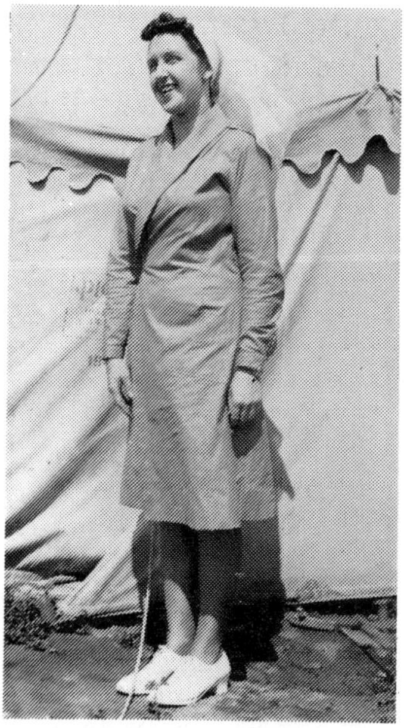

Lt. N/S Mary Bower in summer duty uniform, Red Deer Alberta

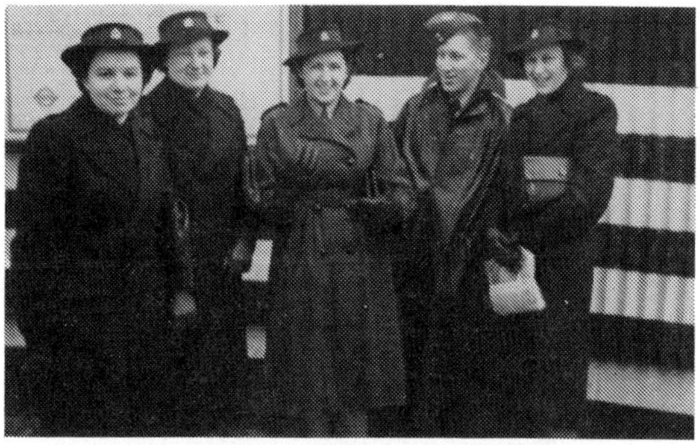

A day out at Trafalgar Square, gloves borrowed, we were frozen.
N/S Gerry Gowans, Nelson B.C.; N/S Thompson, Halifax, N/S Mary Bower, Pincher Creek, Alberta airman friend and N/S Jean Taylor McLeod, Edmonton, Alberta

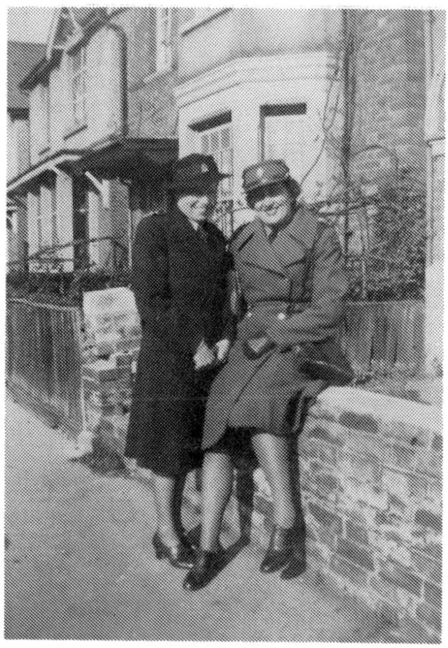

Farnborough, England
Lt. N/S Rose O'Brien RCAMC and Lt.Helen Stewart, CWAC, Edmonton, Alberta

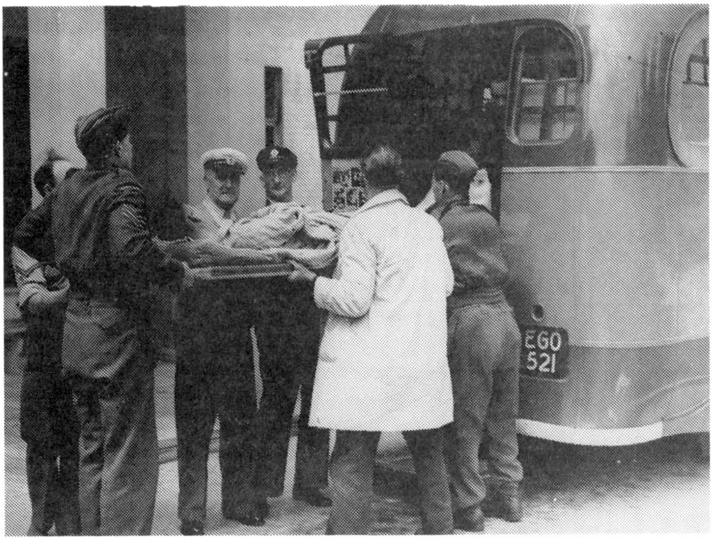

Unloading

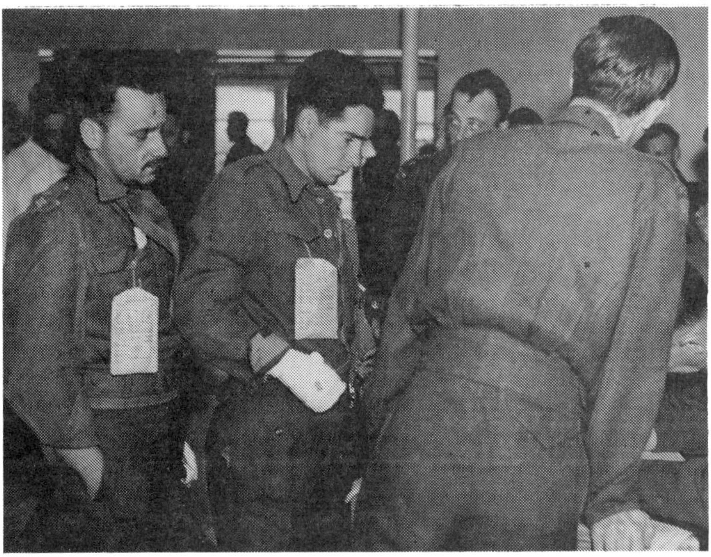

Our walking wounded with history of injury and treatment attached. They look very serious but I am sure they were soon laughing. The morale of our wounded was amazing, and one found tears of many emotions always near, in those days especially.

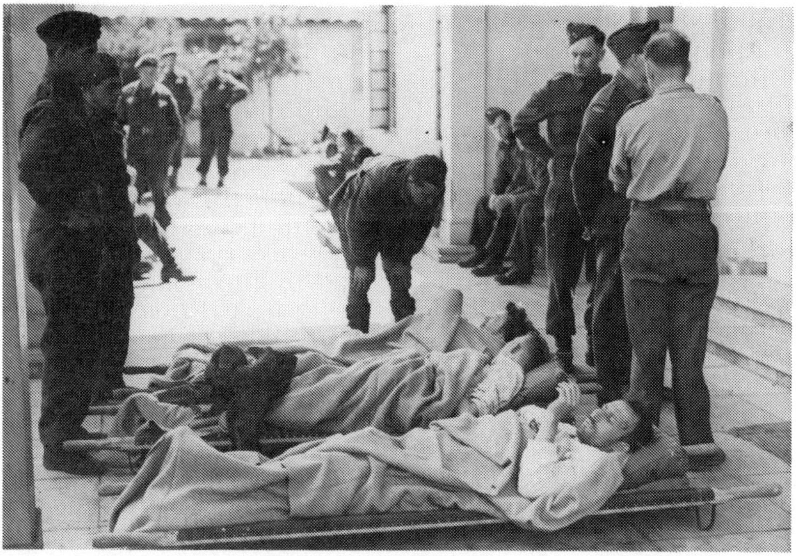

After D-Day No. 11 CGH Taplow. The most serious cases. The first words of most, "Oh Boy! A Canadian nurse; next, "a bed," where they would sleep without sedatives, exhausted from their journey.

Helen L. Wilson

Graduated from: Winnipeg General Hospital School of Nursing. Year: 1937

Military History:

Service: RCAMC

Rank: Major (Principal Matron)

Served: Early 1943 to December 1945

I joined the RCAMC in response to a letter from Col. Elizabeth Smellie asking me to consider joining. I also had a desire to serve in time of need.

My most memorable experience came from directing the nursing service in caring for the human wrecks who came to us from concentration camps in Germany, near Bremerhaven, in 1945. I also enjoyed working at RCAMC headquarters in Ottawa for six months with Lt. Col. Dorothy Warner and again for six months in London at RCAMC headquarters with Col. Agnes Neill.

NO. 12 CANADIAN GENERAL HOSPITAL

Pearl (Byers) Burns
Lorraine (Quehl) Connelly
Ethel May (Sandercock) Coulter
Anne V. (Oliver) Evans
Ann (Clark) Fraser
Esther M. (Hatfield) Gray
Edith (Biggs) Harper
Connie (Burton) Milavsky
Eva Powell

On 9 May 1943 No. 12 Canadian General Hospital was ordered to mobilize at Camp Sussex, New Brunswick, with permission to enlarge from 1200 beds if necessary.

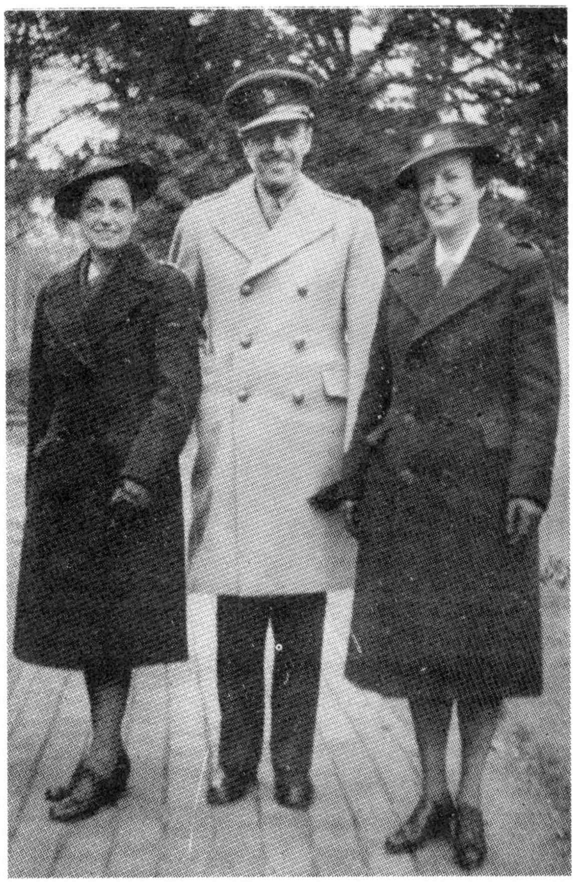

Matron M. Crawford, Colonel W. Fraser, P/Matron S. Miles

With Col.W.A. Fraser as commanding officer and P/Matron Sarah Miles as matron, the unit arrived in Halifax 12 September 1943 and boarded the *Queen Elizabeth*. They arrived in Greenock, Scotland, a week later and proceeded to Farnham, England. The nursing sisters were assigned to No. 8, No. 10 and No. 18 Canadian General Hospitals until they rejoined their unit.

With added experience gained at different places, they were reunited in October under the leadership of Colonel W.A. Fraser, P/Matron Sarah Miles and Matron Marion Crawford.

Nursing sisters took part in field exercises in July of 1944 and by mid-August embarked on the *Empire Anvil* for France. They were first assigned to No. 10 Canadian General Hospital, Littry Road, Bayeux. In late September they travelled to St. Andre near Brugge, Belgium, and received their first casualties in October.

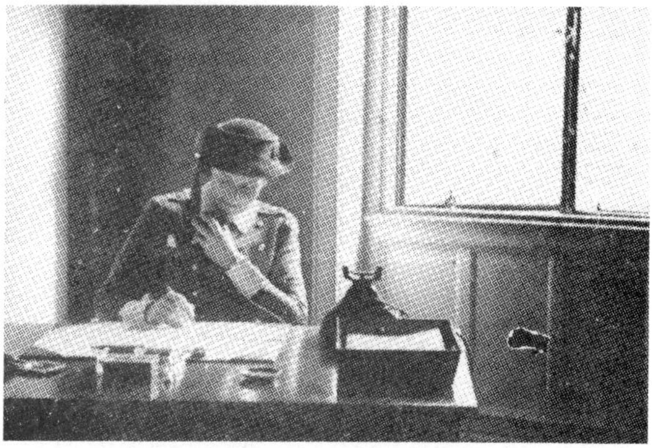

Matron-in Chief A. Neill

Major (P/M) Edna Rossiter arrived from No. 24 General at Horley to exchange with P/M Paterson 30 April 1945.

Beginning with VE Day 8 May 1945 admission of casualties ended and the hospital was quiet in July, August and September.

No. 12 General disbanded 30 November 1945 marking the end of a very active and happy unit.

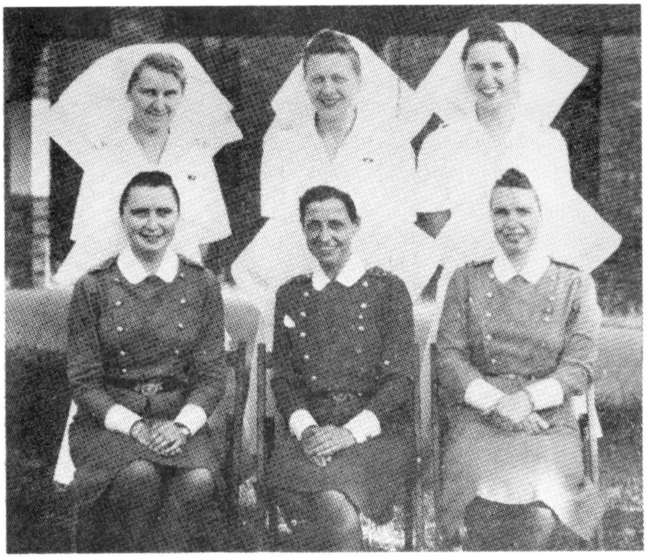

Chiefs of Departments; Standing, L-R: Jo Booth, Dietitian; Jean Amos, Home Sister; Jo Forbes, Occupational Therapist. Seated, L-R: Mary Younge, Teaching of Orderlies; Matron Marion Crawford; Stella Hayes, Operating Room; missing: Kay Jeffery, Physiotherapist.

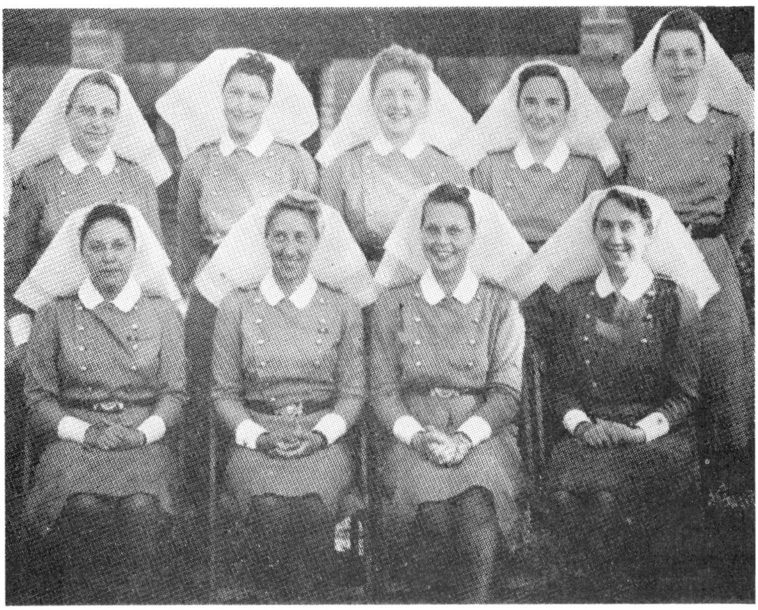

Mess Committees; Standing: Alma Kemp and Barb McQueen, Mess Secretaries; Edith Biggs, Kay Fisher and Sally Trotter, Fifth Members. Seated, L_R: Ruby Barnes, Eleanor Fleming and Mary Taylor, Mess Presidents; and Jean Haddow, Mess Secretary. Missing: Mary McNutt, Mess President; and Kay Jeffery, Mess Secretary.

Pearl (Byers) Burns

Graduated from: Chapman Memorial Hospital School of Nursing, New Brunswick Year: 1940

Military History:

Service: RCAMC

Rank: Lt. N/S
(2/Lt. for 3 mo.)

Served: November 1942 to
November 1946

I joined the RCAMC because the war was on. Marjorie, Lois Long and I went together; we were friends.

From Bayeux, Lea Lockyear and I went shopping for eggs near St. Lo. An American jeep pulled up and the soldiers asked, *"Would you like to have a turkey dinner?"* We hopped in the jeep and they took us to a U.S. mess; had our turkey dinner – we never did get the eggs.

I remember the smell (in the fall of 1944 after invasion) of animals dead, rubble everywhere. Poor little old French people were digging in rubble for things – it was so sad!

Another interesting thing – we went in trucks to Bruges. We stayed overnight in Rouen. Nancy and Ann Oliver and I went out for a walk. A British soldier asked, *"Do you want to see underground tunnels?"* He took us down. It was supposed to go all the way to the coast. They had kitchens and everything down there! Another thing funny – when we got to Rouen, people there thought we were camp followers.

Lorraine Doris (Quehl) Connelly

Graduated from: Misericordia Hospital School of Nursing, Edmonton, Alberta. Year: 1940

Military History:

Service: RCAMC

Rank: Lt. N/S

Served: September 10, 1942 to April 1945

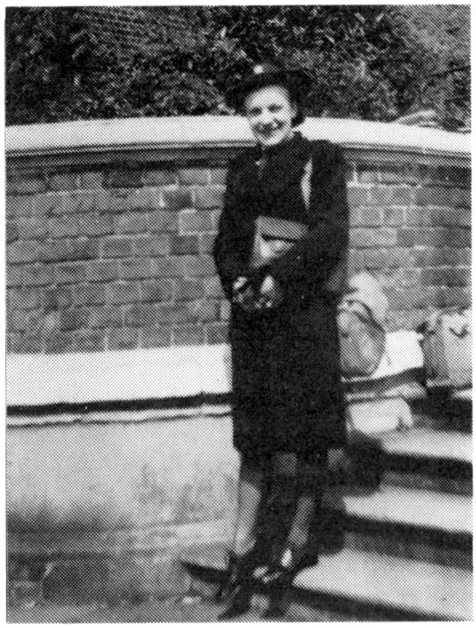

Lt. N/S Lorraine (Quehl) Connelly, No. 12 CGH

I joined the service because my brother, a doctor, and my brother-in-law, a dentist, had gone overseas. I waited on the Navy's list, then the Air Force. I walked by an Army recruiting office one day, entered, and was accepted at once.

I was so very proud to wear the Canada badges on my uniform. We were accepted and made most welcome wherever we went. I met so many wonderful people, and to this day cherish their friendship.

I met my husband in England and we married in Edinburgh. He was from Calgary and with the tank corps. We came home on the same ship. I worked with the war brides and their babies on board.

I enjoyed Sicily and Italy and returned to England on the Canadian Hospital ship, the *Lady Nelson.*

Ethel May (Sandercock) Coulter

Graduated from: Regina General Hospital School of Nursing, Saskatchewan. Year: 1941

Military History:

Service: Royal Canadian Medical Corps

Rank: Lt. N/S

Served: September 1942 to November 1946

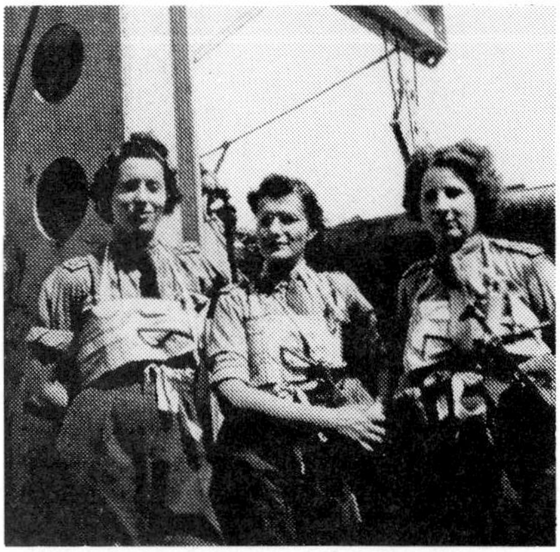

L-R: Nursing Sister Sally Trotter, May Coulter, Edna Covert Photo taken while on board the Liberty ship going to France.

When I graduated in 1941 from the Regina General Hospital I planned to take an obstetrical post-graduate course in Boston. Because of the war it was not possible for me to do so, but I did take obstetrical post-graduate courses after the war.

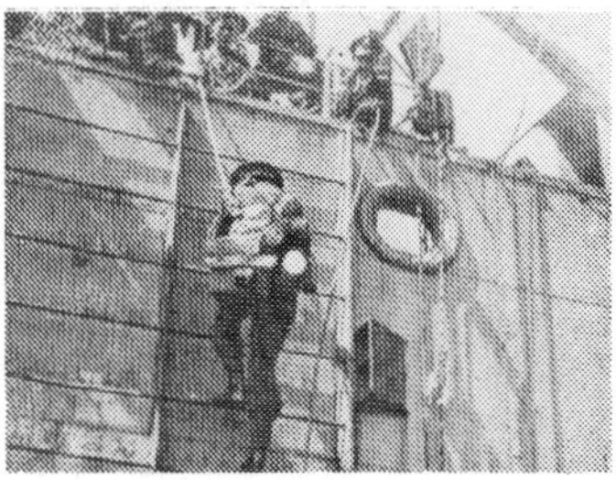

Barbara McQueen climbing down to the LCT (landing craft tank).

On I September 1942 I joined the RCAMC at Regina for patriotism and adventure, and served there and at Maple Creek, Saskatchewan. I went overseas with No. 12 Canadian General Hospital in September 1943. Our unit was at Horley, Surrey, until August 1944 when we moved to Whitby, England. It was there that we were issued kahki uniforms.

After arriving in France in September 1944 we stayed a short time with another Canadian General Hospital at Bayeux, Normandy, until we were able to advance to Bruges, Belgium, where we were stationed until the end of the war. I remained in the Army until November 1946 serving at Dundurn, Saskatchewan, and Montreal.

Waking and giving penicillin injections every three hours to wounded soldiers who came to us at Horley after D-Day remains a vivid memory. It was a new experience for us and a painful and annoying one for them.

Before leaving Belgium our unit gave us the opportunity to

visit some areas in France where Canadians fought in World War One. I appreciated seeing Vimy Ridge and the Canadian War Memorial there, also, the Menin Gate at Ypres and Canadian cemeteries.

Besides enjoying travel in Britain and on the Continent, I was able to visit my mother's family in Cornwall, England.

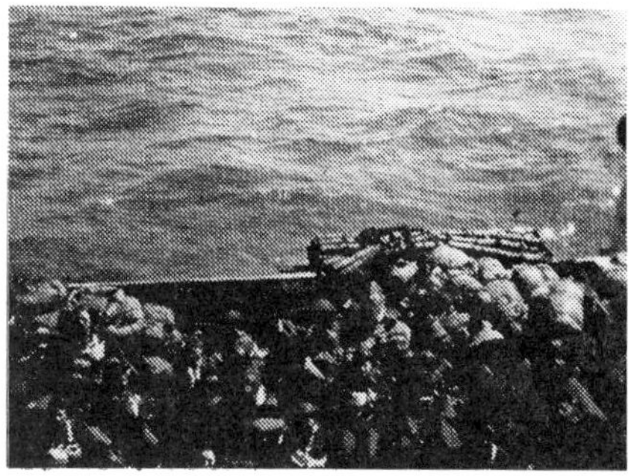

Aboard the LCT

Anne (Oliver) Evans

Graduated from: Toronto General Hospital School of Nursing Toronto, Ontario. Year: 1942

Military History:

Service: RCAMC and RCAF

Rank: Lt. N/S and Flying Officer to Flight Lieutenant

Served: 1942 to 1951

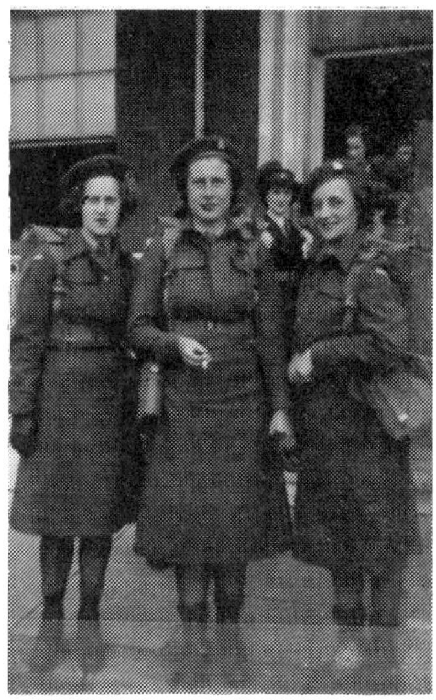

Lts. N/S Anne (Oliver) Evans, Nancy (Dunlop) Page, Pearl (Byers) Burns Ready for route march, Whitby, England, August 1944.

I was brought up in a military family. That influenced me to choose the Army. I hoped I could help as a nurse and also see some of the rest of the world.

The highlights of my military career were:

A concert put on in Horley, England.

Living under canvas in Bayeux, France.

Christmas in Bruge, Belgium, where we decorated the wards. The POW ward had the best decorations with what they had to work with.

Leaves in London, Paris, Holland and Brighton.

Getting used to English trains.

The wedding of Edie Biggs and Don Harper.

While at Horley, England, Pearl B. and I went to visit my aunt in Ashford, Kent. We missed the stop and ended up in Aldershot. We finally arrived and after two hours with Aunt Nell and three other great aunts, Aunt Nell asked me to take back to Canada to my mother, an heirloom broach. She wanted to sew it in my underwear. It took a lot of persuading to let me take it in my purse. As I told her, I wouldn't be wearing the same pants for the rest of the tour. I still have the broach.

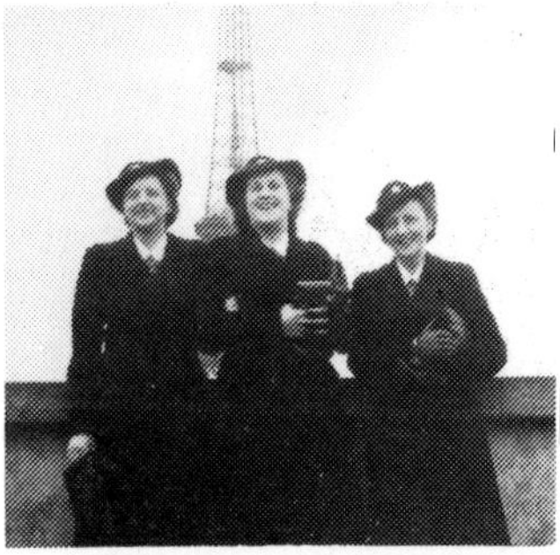

Lts. N/S Lee Lochyear, Anne (Oliver) Evans, Pearl (Byers) Burns on leave in Paris, France

On the way to Brussels, Belgium, I evidently picked up a flea or blackfly and itched all the way to Brussels. I think whatever it was that bit me died of fright or drowned in the bathtub.

Nancy and I hitchhiked to Rouen, France, to buy some perfume. We had great success getting there but getting back to camp took hours. We arrived in St. Lo at midnight. St. Lo was completely demolished and it was pitch black. We arrived back between 1 and 2 A.M. The girls were glad to see us. They didn't want to get us in trouble by reporting us missing.

When I returned to Canada I completed a course in clinical teaching and supervision in obstetrics at the University of Toronto. After finishing the course I was the head nurse on the obstetrical ward at the Ottawa Civic Hospital for two years. Some Air Force nurses who came to brush up on obstetrics finally persuaded me to join the Air Force.

I served in Rockcliffe, Ontario, and Goose Bay, Labrador, and took flight nurses course in Randolph Field, Texas. I was posted to Greenwood, N.S., as head nurse (matron).

Anne (Clark) Fraser

Military History:

Service: Medical Corps

Rank: Lieutenant N/S

Served: December 1942 to December 1945

Mother's sister from New Brunswick, Canada, was killed in France at the end of WW I while serving as a nurse with the American Medical Corps. The American government brought her remains to Arlington Cemetery. I have visited her grave site. It's very impressive with a marble statue of a nurse overlooking the designated "Nurses only" area. I believe that influenced me to become a nursing sister in the RCAMC.

It was a big thrill, at age 23 and having just become a RN, to embark from Halifax aboard a little 7000-ton Panama called the SS *Cavina*. We were 14 days crossing the Atlantic in January of 1942. The night before we disembarked at Tilsbury, I was robbed by one of the ship's stewards. As a result, when we sailed into port to be met by Matron Agnes Neil, police flags were flying and no one was allowed to leave the ship until I was questioned, along with Mary, who fortunately had come along the night before and witnessed the fact that I was robbed. As a result of all this, a month later Mary and I were detailed to appear in court in Liverpool. To make a long story short, we won our case and my money was returned to me - all 10 or 15 pounds, which was a fortune to me at that time.

We had one first meal at No. 10 Canadian General Hospital which we replaced at Horley in Surrey. We were under the direct path of the buzz bombs and V-2s going into London. So evenings were never dull.

Esther M. (Hatfield) Gray

Graduated from: Hamilton General Hospital School of Nursing. Year: 1942

Military History:

Service: RCAMC

Rank: 1st Lt.

Served: March 1943 to October 1945

With friends and family in the service I to wanted to join them. I had many interesting experiences but they are difficult for me to put into words.

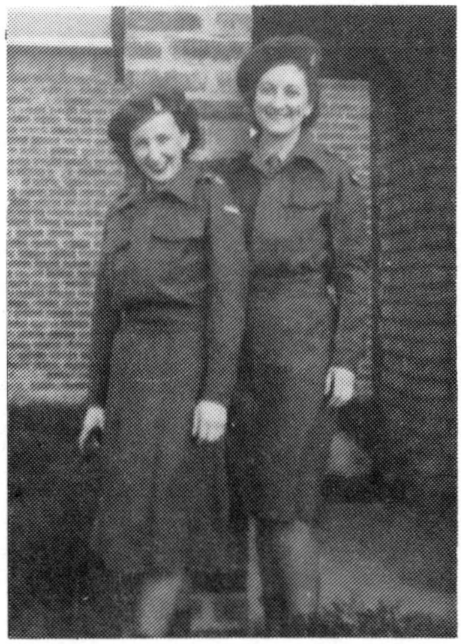

R: Esther (Hatfield) Gray, L: Anne (Clark) Fraser 12 CGH, Horley, Surrey, England in battle dress for field duty June-July 1944

Edith (Biggs) Harper

Military History:

Service: RCAMC

Rank: Lt. N/S

Served: 1942 to 1945

Patriotism influenced me to choose a military career. It was a wonderful experience. I enjoyed my leaves in England and Scotland.

I was with No. 12 Canadian General Hospital and No. 5 Casualty Clearing Station.

After our wedding 15 June 1945 we spent our honeymoon in Paris. The first night was spent in Brussels in the YMCA! There are too many amusing stories to recall. It has been a long time, but I have many fond memories.

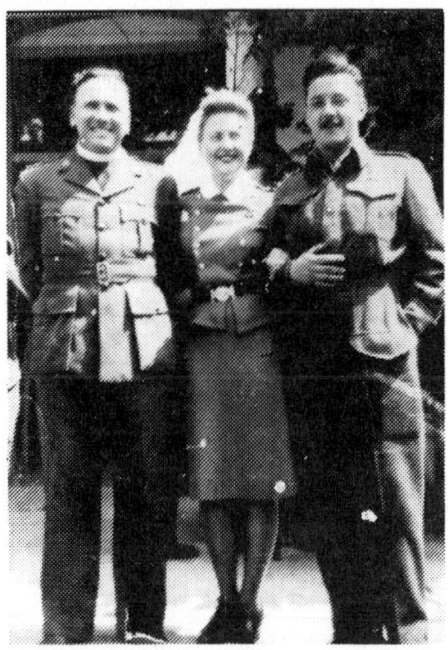

L-R: H/Capt. Vallelly, Lt. N/S Edith Biggs, Capt. Donal Harper, our wedding day 15 June 1945, Amersfoort, Netherlands.

Constance (Burton) Milavsky

Graduated from: St. Paul's Hospital School of Nursing, Saskatoon, Saskatchewan. Year: 1941

Military History:

Service: Army

Rank: Lieutenant N/S

Served: September 1, 1942 to January 17, 1945

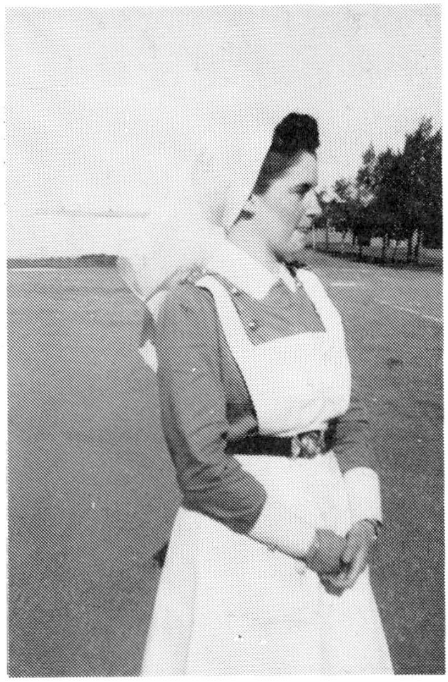

Lt. N/S Connie (Burton) Milavsky

With the war being on, there was a need for nurses. Also, the Army provided the opportunity to travel to various places. Although it was a tragic time, it was also exciting.

I joined the Army actually in Vancouver at Shaughnessy Hospital and was sent to Regina, Saskatchewan. From there I went to New Brunswick to join up with No. 12 General Hospital group. We were posted there until we went overseas to Farnborough, England, a 1600-bed hospital. I was on the surgical wards. Our hospital was hit with a bomb one night. We all had to wear hard hats while on duty. I'll never forget the black-outs – after our first night goof.

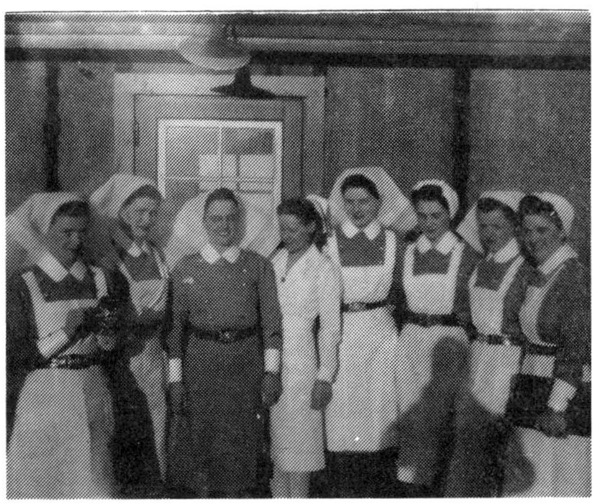

Regina Military Hospital. Nursing Sisters Parker, Schwing, Ballard, Gregg, Bissett, Meiers, Williamson, Connie (Burton) Milavsky.

Later I was married to a Canadian engineer so our dear matron-in-chief in London would not allow us further posting on the Continent; thus, I spent the rest of my time moving wherever the need was – at Basingstoke Neurological and Plastic Surgery Hospital and at Marston Green out of Birmingham with No. 16 General.

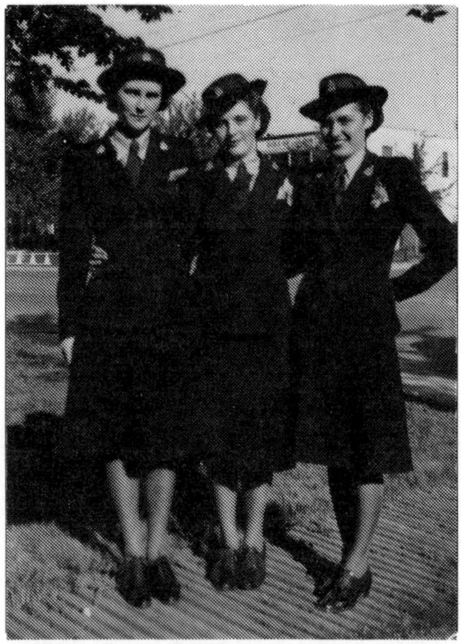

Margaret Murray, Connie (Burton) Milavsky, and Mary McKenzie, No. 12 CGH

Eva Powell

Graduated from: Moose Jaw General Hospital School of Nursing, Moose Jaw, Saskatchewan.

Military History:

Service: RCAMC

Rank: Lt. N/S

Served: World War II

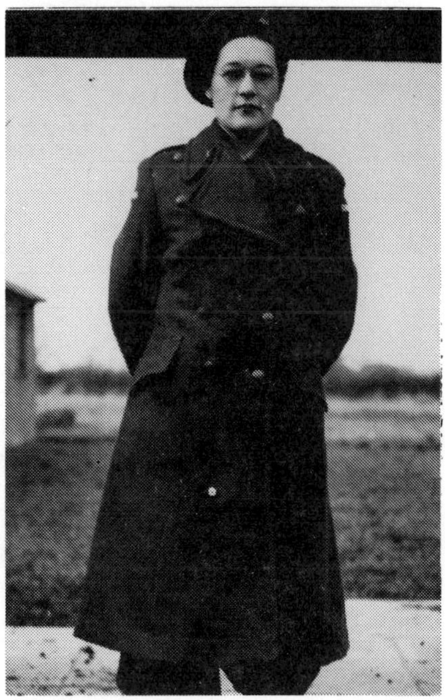

Lt. N/S Eva Powell "Stand at ease," May 1944 at No. 12 CGH, Horley, England.

Lt. N/S Eva Powell. Beside the bomb shelter outside the nursing sisters quarters at No. 12 CGH, Horley, England. Respirator drill, shows battle dress with helmet and gas mask Horley Hospital, RCAMC, 1944. Ready for route march. Some of us were on night duty and had to get up mid afternoon to route march at 4:P.M. I soon realized I could put myself into an automatic "marching mode" and doze off as I went along with our unit down the English lanes lead/accompanied by a pipe band.

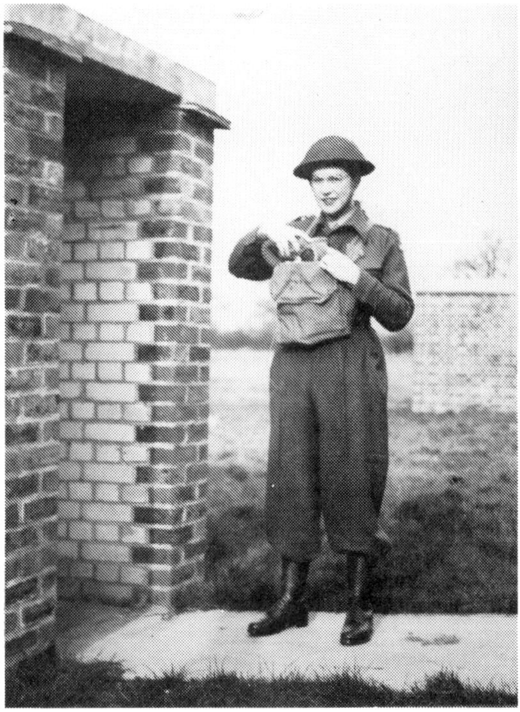

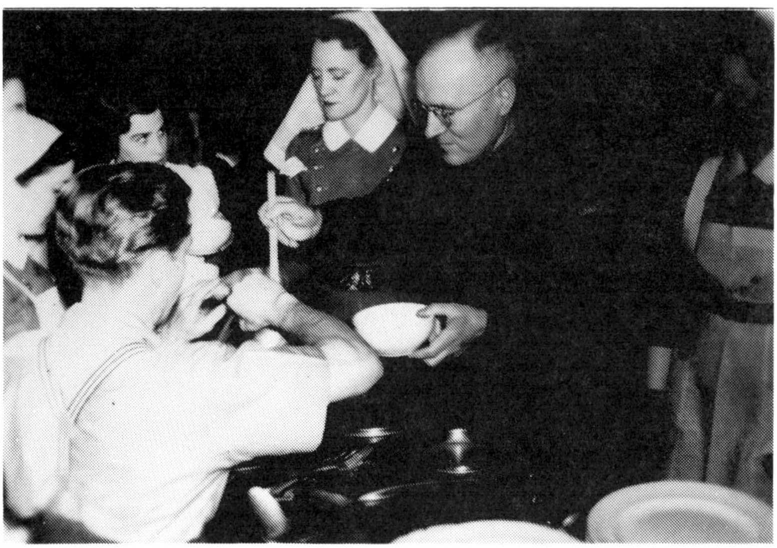

No.12 CGH,
loaned by Eva Powell
Serving Christmas dinner 1942. Matron Lunn; Capt. Caldwell; Sister Brown; Sister Meyers; Cpl. Hall.

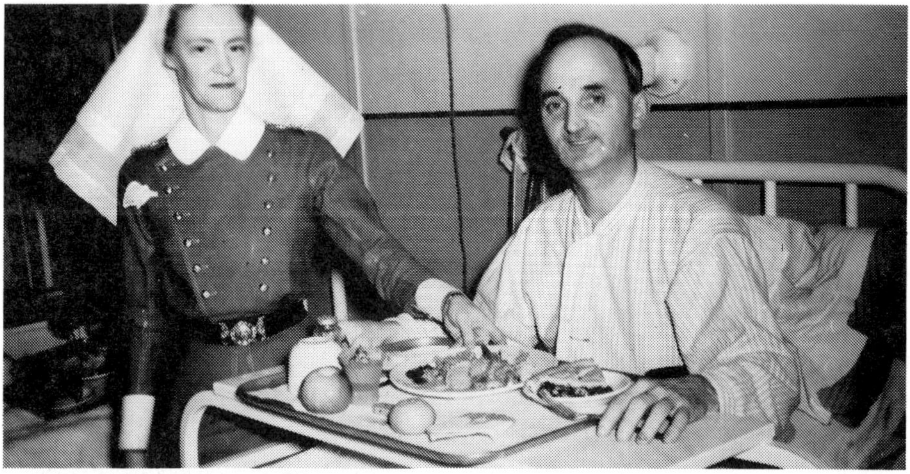

No.12 CGH, loaned by Eva Powell. A patient's Christmas dinner tray 1942. Served by Matron Lunn to Sgt. Hodgson.

NO. 13 CANADIAN GENERAL HOSPITAL

Dorothy (Van) Gonder
Marie (Pomrenk) Luke

No. 13 Canadian General Hospital was established 11 December 1942 at Hamilton, Ontario. On 1 March 1943 the unit was posted to Picton, Ontario, with Officer Commanding Col. C.E. Carr, Matron H.J. Howe and 50 nursing sisters. The unit boarded the *Queen Elizabeth* at Halifax 21 July 1943 for duty at Cuckfield, Sussex, in England.

The order to disband No. 13 General came 8 August 1945 and it was turned over to East Sussex County Council.

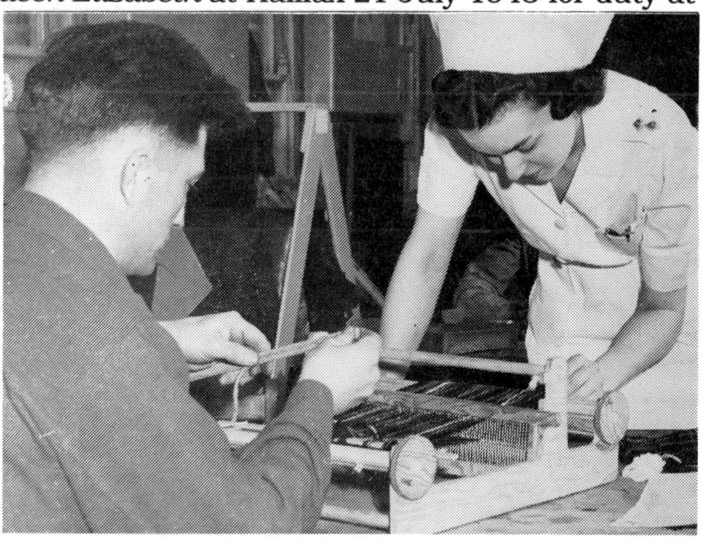

Occupational Therapy, No. 13 CGH, UK, 14 March 1945
Canadian Forces photo

Dorothy (Van) Gonder

Graduated from: Royal Jubilee Hospital School of Nursing, Victoria, B.C. Year: 1938

Military History:

Service: RCAMC

Rank: Lt. N/S

Served: February 1944 to August 9, 1945

Devotion to my Country – CANADA caused me to join the RCAMC.

I was very impressed by the fortitude of wounded Canadian service men. The efficiency and discipline of the nursing staff was a highlight of my nursing experience.

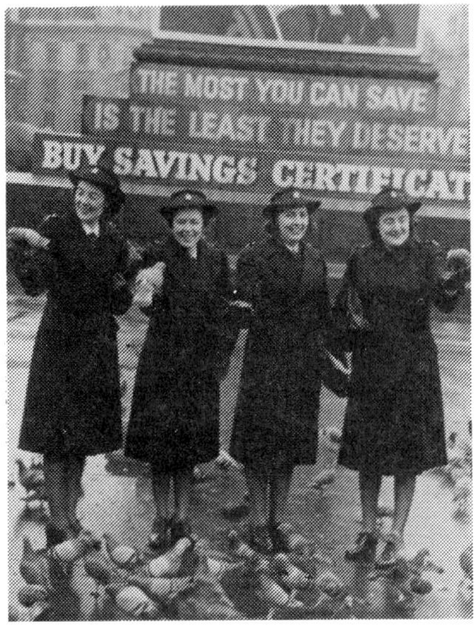
THE MOST YOU CAN SAVE
IS THE LEAST THEY DESERVE
BUY SAVINGS CERTIFICAT

Trafalgar Square 1944. Nursing sisters Dorothy (Van) Gonder, Winnie (Burwash) Ogilvie, Dottie (Marks) Kimmett, Mary Sara (Fraser) Lester. Canadian Forces photo

Marie (Pomrenk) Luke

Graduated from: Edmonton General Hospital School of Nursing, Edmonton, Alberta. Year: 1936

Military History:

Service: RCAMC

Rank: Lt. N/S

Served: January 1941 to November 1945.

Submitted by Mary White

Marie joined the RCAMC in January of 1941 and was posted to Red Deer Military Hospital. She went overseas with No. 13 Canadian General Hospital in 1942 and was stationed at Cuckfield, England. She was sent as a reinforcement to Italy in 1943 and was aboard the *Santa Elena* when it was bombed.

Just before VE Day, Marie returned to England and was repatriated to Canada in 1945 and discharged from the Army. Marie married her childhood sweetheart; they adopted two children and lived in Edmonton, Alberta. In December 1989 Marie died of a heart attack.

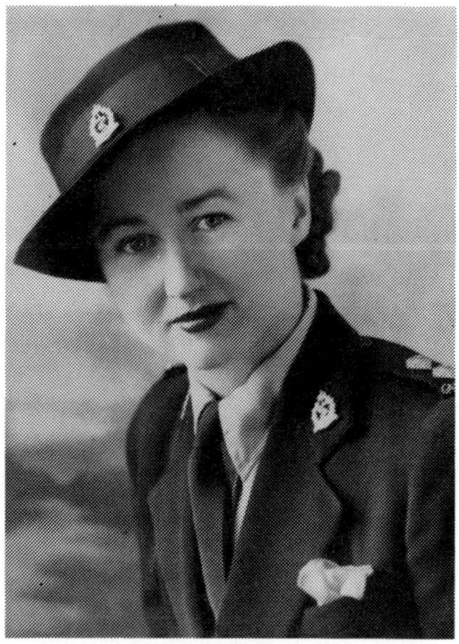

Lt. N/S Marie (Pomrenk) Luke
No. 13 CGH

NO. 14 CANADIAN GENERAL HOSPITAL

Helen (Gibson) Bell
Wendy Benson
Marie (Vermette) Doyle
Margaret (MacEachern) Frampton
Frances (Hanchet) Mitchell
Margaret Moss

No. 14 Canadian General Hospital was activated 23 June 1940 at Westmount Barracks Military District No. 4, Montreal. By 12 June 1941 the majority of nursing sisters were posted to the unit and 20 June the unit boarded the *Stirling Castle* for duty in the U.K.

Their first location was Pinewood and by November the unit located at Farnborough, near Aldershot.

In October of 1943 nursing sisters were issued with battle dress and a week later they boarded the USS *Santa Elena* of the Grace Line which formerly ran between New York and Santiago, Chile. They passed through the Strait of Gibraltar 4 November with the coast of North Africa in sight.

It was a quiet uneventful day 6 November until "Action Stations" sounded at 1811 hours and the sound of ack ack fire indicated that this was a real "Action Stations." Ten minutes later the attack was over. The main damage was a hole in the engine room; an aerial torpedo hit the engine room on the port side.

"Abandon Ship" bell sounded and nursing sisters and hospital patients got into lifeboats almost immediately. Nursing sisters helped row to either destroyers or the SS *Monterey* which stood by to pick up survivors.

The *Santa Elena* sank off Philippville harbour, North Africa the next day with the loss of medical as well as personal equipment.

No. 14 arrived in Naples harbour, disembarked and proceeded to their destination, Caserta. The nursing sisters were separated from their unit for a while; they went to No. 3 Field Dressing Station, Royal Army Medical Corps at Castella Maria until mid-November.

By the end of March 1945, the unit began preparing for their return to England and the news that the unit would be disbanded by the end of April 1945.

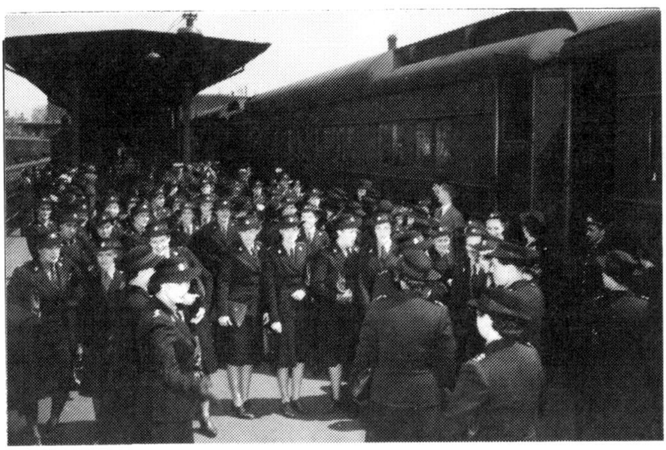

No. 14 CGH at train station, 1943

Helen Purdy (Gibson) Bell

Graduated from: University of Toronto School of Physiotherapy. Year: 1941

Military History:

Service: RCAMC

Rank: Lieutenant P/T

Served: 1941 to 1945

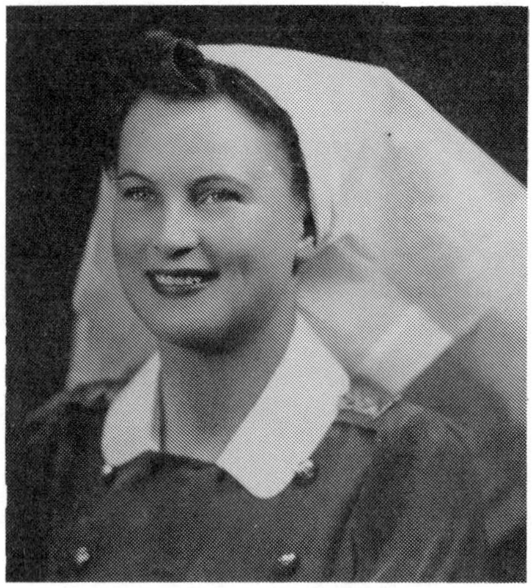

Helen Purdy (Gibson) Bell, Physiotherapist

I went overseas and remained with No. 14 Canadian General Hospital from 1941-43. After No. 14 General left for Italy, I served as a reinforcement at several general hospitals in the U.K. until 1945.

I could not go after marriage to Captain R.A. Bell in January 1943 (married Sisters were not permitted to go). I returned to Canada in 1945.

Wendy Eva Benson

Graduated from: Royal Jubilee Hospital School of Nursing, Victoria, B.C. Year: 1939

Military History:

Service: RCAMC

Rank: Lt. N/S

Served January 1942 to 1945

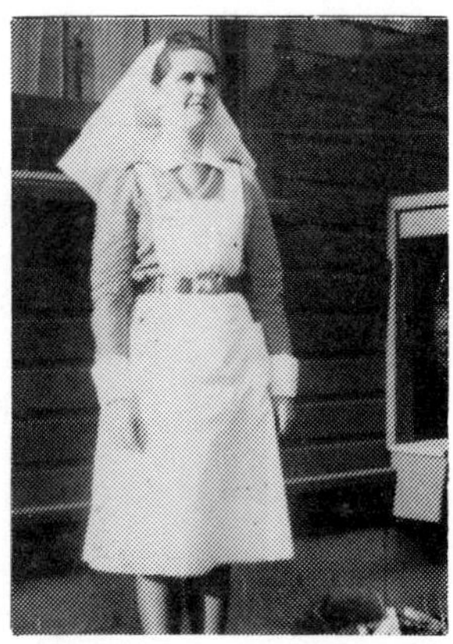

Lt. N/S Wendy Benson

Units served with: No. 1 Neurological and Plastic Surgery Hospital at Basingstoke. No. 14 General Hospital from Montreal – ship torpedoed on the way to Italy. No. 9 General (Horsham, Hanks). We were in a convoy consisting of 29 ships

(American) on November 6, 1943. We sailed through the Strait of Gibraltar at sunset and could see people on the shores of Spain. (We should have waited until it was dark.) On November 6 at about the same time three aeroplanes flew over and dropped magnetic torpedoes – one hit our ship in the stern and another one hit one of the destroyers escorting us. A gunner on top of our ship was killed. We were taken off in lifeboats. I was in a group of 30 who were picked up by a destroyer (the matron, Miss Herman, was with our group). The next morning we were dropped at Philippville in North Africa and lived in one huge tent attached to No. 15 General Hospital which was stationed there. We were there 2 weeks before being taken to Naples. The remaining survivors were picked up by the *Monterey* – another troop ship which also stayed behind to help.

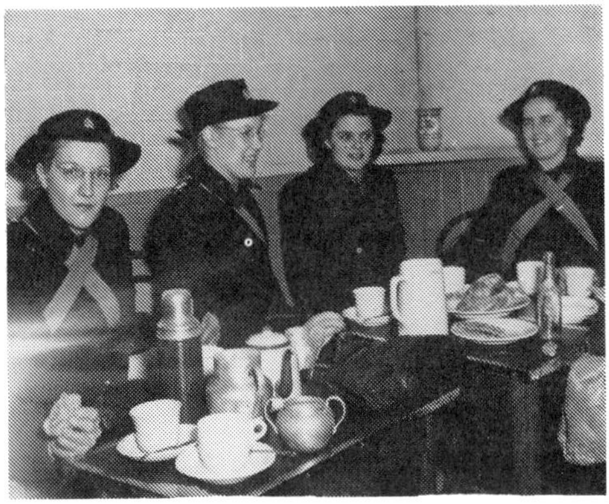

Lts N/S Wendy Benson, Gladys Foster, Felicity Hyde, name unknown

The *Santa Elena* sank next morning while being towed to shore. This was viewed very sadly from the *Monterey*, which then carried on to Naples, where, I might add, Vesuvius was erupting.

Marie Albina (Vermette) Doyle

Graduated from: Grey Nuns' Hospital School of Nursing, Regina Saskatchewan. Year: 1940

Military History:

Service: RCAMC

Rank: Lt. N/S

Served: April 1942 to November 1945

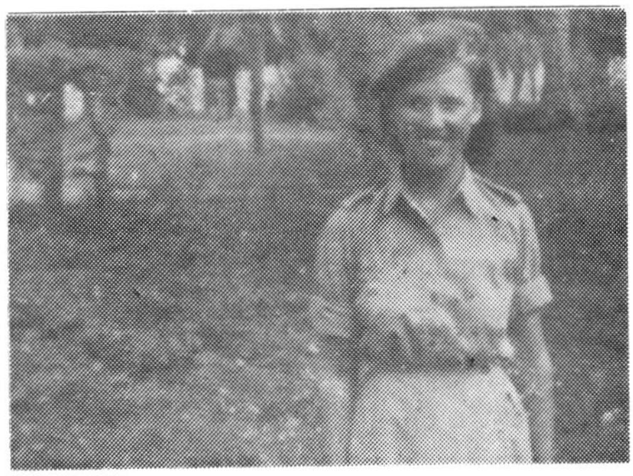

Lt. N/S Marie Albina Vermette, Caserta, Italy, summer of 1944

My country in its time of need was reason enough for me to join the RCAMC. The following is a list of postings during my military career overseas:

No. 10 CGH.	U.K.	4/4/43 - 15/4/43
Alton Convalescent Hospital U.K.		30/9/43 to 30/9/43
No. 18 CGH	U.K.	1/11/43 to 3/11/43
No. 5 CGH	Catania Sicily	13/11/43 to 25/1/44
No. 1 CGH	Italy	1/27/44 to 2/1/44
No. 14 CGH	Caserta, Sicily	2/2/44 to 7/26/44
No. 1 CGH	U.K.	8/13/44 to 8/14/44
No. 22 CGH	U.K.	8/14/44 to 8/16/44
No. 4 CGH	U.K.	8/16/44 to 4/12/45

One of the highlights of my military career was my posting to Canadian Field Hospital No. 14 CGH, Caserta, Italy, not too far from the front (No. 15 was across the square from No. 14). We were able to tend to the soldiers soon after they were wounded. Our hours were long and we had to make do with what was available. There would be a lull for maybe a day, or even hours, then there would be a battle and the wounded started to pour in. I was also sent to Bari on the Adriatic Coast to help out for a short period.

Another highlight was meeting my future husband, a Spitfire fighter pilot, F/O Jack Doyle, in Italy. We have been married 47 years.

One more amusing highlight was in a visit to a U.S. air base. I was offered a ride in a Spitfire. The pilot altered the Spitfire by removing the header gas tank and substituting a seat. It was quite thrilling, but when I told my future husband about it, he wasn't amused – explaining it was a risky thing to do and he was quite annoyed at the American pilot.

After my tour overseas, I was sent back to Canada and discharged because of loss of weight and general debility. I was sent to Harrison Hot Springs, B.C., for a few months for rehabilitation.

In 1952 I joined my husband who was stationed with 421 Squadron as a jet fighter pilot in Grostenquin, France. The military hospital was short of nurses so I served as a civilian nurse. We took care of the wives and children of military personnel. There were many babies born while I was there; approximately 60 were born on the base, including a set of twins. The mother was a French girl from St. Avalde; the father an airman from Canada. This birth caused quite a stir as it was the first twin birth in 90 years.

H. Margaret (McEachern) Frampton

Graduated from: Prince Edward Island Hospital School of Nursing. Year: 1938

Military History:

Service: RCAMC

Rank: Lieutenant N/S

Served: February 1941 to May 1946

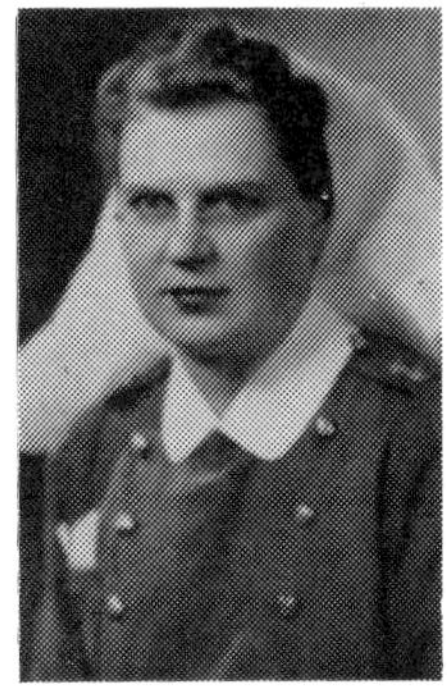

N/S Margaret (McEachern) Frampton

These five years will never be forgotten; they were truly a learning experience. One unpleasant highlight took place on November 6, 1943, when our troopship, the SS *Santa Elena*, en route from England to Italy, was bombed and damaged. All persons on board the *Santa Elena* were rescued, the majority by the SS *Monterey*, the others by a destroyer. Our hospital unit was No. 14 Canadian General Hospital.

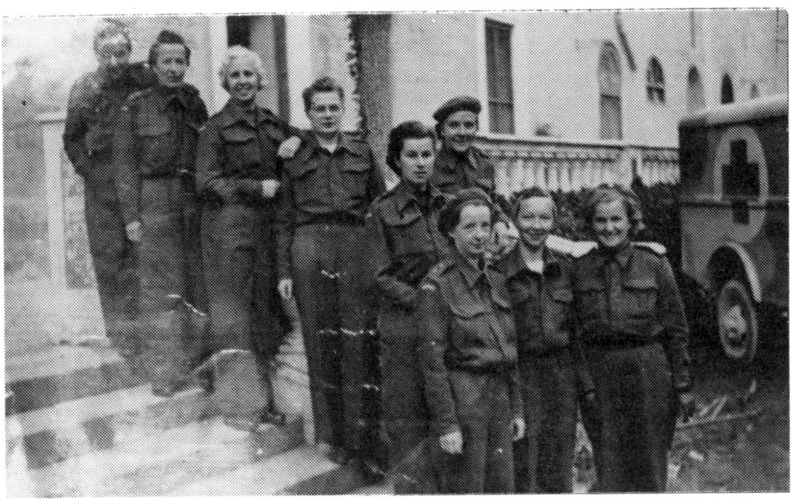

CANADIAN NURSES SURVIVE TORPEDOING
Shown here are some Canadian nursing sisters who were aboard a troopship which was torpedoed while enroute to the Mediterranean recently. This picture was taken shortly after they had arrived in Italy. Left to right: Lieuts. J. Stewart, Montreal; J.A. Smeaton, Montreal; T. McDonald, Alexandria; H.M. MacEachern, Charlottetown; P. Cox, Westmount, Quebec; R. Chuse, Chippewa; Frances Hanchet, Ottawa; E. Tullock, Montreal; and A. Cooney, Shomberg. Canadian Forces photo 26547-N

Frances (Howard Hanchet) Mitchell

Graduated from: Montreal General Hospital School of Nursing

Military History:

Service: RCAMC

Rank: Lt. N/S

Served: 1941 to 1945

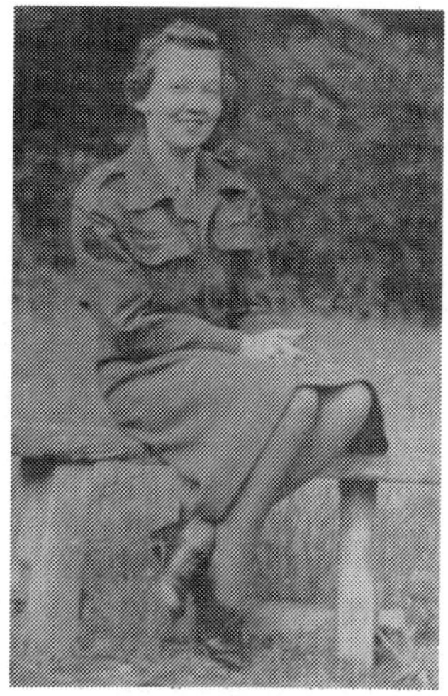

Lt. N/S Frances (Hanchet) Mitchell, No. 14 CGH

I was attached to the Canadian General Hospitals No. 14 and No. 6 for four years, two years with each. No. 14 CGH departed for Britain July 1941. After zigging and zagging in convoy across the Atlantic we arrived at the Scottish port. The troops aboard our ship put on a concert; it happened to be Dominion Day as it was known then.

Our hospital in England was not ready for occupancy so we were farmed out to other facilities. Some of us went to the Taplow estate of Lady Astor. She brought around George Bernard Shaw and Winston Churchill. She wanted to show them how untidy Canadian nurses were; we lived in tiny rooms and our possessions were packed into this small space. These famous people could not have cared less.

Our first Christmas in Britain was spent in one of the old Crimean vintage hospitals. Our next residence was a series of Nissen huts in Horley, Surrey, on the south shore of Great Britain. Horley was a nice place and the country club treated us very well. After another Christmas in Horley we were uprooted again and were soon on our way to Italy.

After a peaceful trip through the Strait of Gibraltar we were torpedoed by a lone German plane which sent us very quickly to the lifeboats. We were picked up later by an American boat, the SS *Monterey*. An American destroyer bustled up beside us and asked if there were any casualties. When we said *no*, they said *okay, push off*, and told us to get climbing. Have you ever had to climb up the side of a ship with a scramble net clutching a bottle of Chanel No. 5? That was the one item I did not want to give up. When our ship was sunk we were on deck. Suddenly one of the nurses announced at the top of her lungs, *"Look a balloon."* It floated past us and we could read prophylactic, or condom as they are known today.

Bond Street is a very wonderful street in London; if you buy something on Bond Street you get something good. I had bought the five guineas pair of pyjamas which at that time was worth $25.00, 25 pounds or whatever, and I put the pyjamas in my Elizabeth Arden train make-up case. Why I was taking them out to Italy I will never know. The next day after our boat was sunk all I could think of was my silk pyjamas and my make-up kit. I never did use any of it.

There went my camera and everything. I had a comb, the only one among 90 nurses, and a lipstick which I didn't admit to having, I did not want other people using my lipstick and that was it. When we got to Naples after being torpedoed, we didn't have anything, just the things we stood up in. So the head of the Canadians in Italy – I don't know who he was at the time – appealed to the head of the American Army, who went right to the top, to let the girls go to the PX in the morning to pick up combs, toilettries and personal items. They still would not let us! They used to sit in their coke factory and drink coke and never even offer us one. They were awful! After we got to Naples there were a number of items we had to find – sanitary pads topped the list, everybody needed them. After tramping all over Naples we located the pads in a shoe store.

Before going to our Army hospital we spent time in a castle overlooking the Bay of Naples. We were nearly eaten alive by bed-bugs and a very vicious type of flea. We were glad to get to our hospital but we found that the Germans had beat us to it and had thrown cement down the drains and toilets. The windows had also been smashed, and to make matters worse, it was the coldest winter they had ever had in Italy. Most of us didn't take off our PJs for months.

We arrived at the Caserta Hospital; it was an Army barracks with 150 patients and only one hurricane lamp – a seeing eye dog would have been more useful. I was on night duty from 7 P.M. to 7 A.M. and I saw very little of the orderly during my lone session. I went to the ward kitchen and was accosted by a soldier wielding a large butcher knife. First he looked at me and said I looked like Hitler and he was going to slit my throat, then he had a mood swing and said I reminded him of his mother and gave me a big hug. Finally, a couple of burly privates carted him off to the psychiatric ward. Someone had neglected to lock the door. I don't suppose this event was ever recorded for posterity, my son and I were the only ones particularly interested. He takes a great interest in these events.

Because I was bilingual I was asked to return to England for D-Day which turned out to be 6 June 1944. At this time I was attached to No. 6 CGH which originated in Quebec City. We were then sent to Ling Field to await final embarkation to France. We stayed at Ford Manor. The people who owned the manor were relatives of royalty. Enclosed find a picture of me sitting on a rustic bench in a garden. I was told by the owner that Queen Elizabeth and King George often sat there; in fact, they became engaged on that very bench – believe it or not. My husband and I even got engaged there. He was in the RCAF; we met on the boat on the way home from Italy. We were married when we got back to Canada.

Once our Canadian Hospital was established in Normandy the staff followed. Our next hospital was in France just outside Caen, which was a pile of rubble. The nurses were put in an apple orchard, part of the convent behind a wall 10 feet high with broken glass sprinkled all over the top. A sentry was posted outside the wall and the door was locked with a long heavy key from 7 P.M. to 7 A.M. I had a call from the operating room one night and when I was ready to go back I was locked out with no way of getting back in, so I had no option but to walk two miles down a dark road to the front door of the convent. Mother Superior opened the door eventually and not very graciously. The next day she told the colonel she preferred Germans to Canadian nurses. Our tents were put in a field of rotting cabbages – our home away from home.

Antwerp was a great city, our hospital was there in a seminary. We took pets to Antwerp from England. They soon disappeared; we were told they were eaten by the Belgians who were very hungry – the same as the Dutch who ate tulip bulbs.

Antwerp was another attraction in war time, mainly a zoo. Only people in uniform could go in. We were greeted as a bunch of bawd, raucous women. Some of the women there were collaborators who had shared the bed with Germans. The spectators were pelting the women with ripe tomatoes and other goodies. These women were locked in the lions' cage and nobody seemed particularly sorry for them.

Near Boulogne we didn't set up our hospital so we had a few

days to explore the neighbourhood. Deep in the woods we found a V-1 still on its launch pad. These are unmanned missiles. Then there was a V-2, otherwise known as a flying telegraph pole. Hitler thought these were going to win the war at the last minute, but he missed by a mile. War is a terrible waste, but in spite of all the dangers and discomforts I would not have missed it for the world. When we went overseas we were like a bunch of high school kids, but when we came home we were very grown up.

Lady Astor trusted all the nurses to go into her special garden. She didn't know what she was doing because we used to pick the strawberries, peaches, pears, anything we could get our hands on and stuff them inside our battle dress. I took one of her beautiful carnations back and put it on the table. I guess she came in soon after that, she used to fly into the wards, and she said, *"Where did you get that carnation? I have much better ones than that."* Well the guys in the beds nearby nearly fell out. *"You never told us you picked that in her garden." "You just shut-up,"* I said, *"or you'll get me in trouble."*

When I was in Caserta, some of the people could speak English. This old guy used to wander in, and if you were lucky to be on duty at seven in the morning, that's when this old guy came in with flowers. One day as I took them and shoved them into water, something pricked my hand – it was wire. I said to Tony, *"What in the name of God is that?"* They were all wired and must have come from the cemetery which was just across the road from the hospital. So I asked Tony, *"Where did you get these flowers?"* He used to bring them on Mondays since Sunday was visiting day at the cemetery. I said, *"Did you get them there?"* He said, *"Yes, you people here, people over there are dead, over here they'll do you more good."* And that was that.

The opera singer was a young fellow who had worked his way down from the Rome Opera House and he picked a pair of beautiful leather boots off some German; they were beautiful things. He could not understand a word of English and the guys tried to teach him English. He came up to me and saluted and said, *"Sister get up them stairs."* I said, *"Tony, do you know what you are saying?"* He said, *"Yeah."* The guys in the beds nearby almost fell out laughing. I said, *"Did you people teach him that?"* They answered, *"Oh there's nothing to that."* I replied, *"Well he thinks there is."* I don't know what else they taught him, but whenever he saw me he saluted and said, *"Get up them stairs."*

At night he had no where to go so he used to come back; he really was an opera singer.

Princess Mary was supposed to come for a visit at ten o'clock in the morning – she's dead now, she looked just like Princess Anne. These Royal visits were a pain, spit and polish, we had all the guys sitting out in their wheelchairs, covered up, and they were there waiting, I said, *"I guess I'll have to go and get your lunch, she will be coming after lunch."* She never showed up. Five o'clock the dinner trays came out. We said, *"Go ahead and eat your dinner."* She never did show up.

We had batteries for the lights on our bikes, there were no cars anyway. Every now and again the batteries used to run out. We came home from the movies one night and our lights kept going out, there were these two young cops, I don't know why they were not in the Army, anyway. *"Come on there, aye there where's your light?"* I said, *"Oh the batteries have run out." "Oh you got to walk."* I said, *"It's another two miles home, never mind."* So they got on their bikes and rode off. As soon as they were off we were on our bikes again, they came back. *"Now girls, we told you not to do that, you're not afraid of the walk are you? Well then we'll walk with you."* They walked with us, I could have killed them. All the street signs had been taken down in case the Germans invaded so they would not know where they were, if you asked a farmer what town is this, he would say sorry, I can't tell you and they wouldn't give me any information whatsoever. I said, *"Well I'm not the enemy,"* he said, *"can't tell you, I don't know that."*

We had Nissen huts; at Christmas we had this great big tree in it and one of the doctors said to me we're all like a big family – bet you can't go up. I ripped my dress going up the ladder. Oh it was very high, about 15 feet to the ceiling. I lay down on this thing and stuck my feet in the air to make a mark on the ceiling. I said, *"This won't make a mark on the ceiling."* So they said, *"Hold on, hold on."* They went and got soot from the kitchen and put in on the bottom of my shoes, I lay there on the ladder and put my feet up on the ceiling. They said, *"We do this every Christmas."*

Lord Beaverbrook's sister did voluntary work taking around tins of Canadian juice to the surgical wards where they had no juice, but had lots of solids. I went up to this cart – we had nothing – and asked for three cans of juice. She said; *"What do you want three cans for, isn't this enough for you?"* I said, *"It's not for me, its for the boys who don't have any drinks at all."* She said, *"Oh, I know you girls."* I replied, *"I take exception to that. Are you accusing us of stealing from our own troops? We bring this stuff over ourselves and that stuff is for the Red Cross."* I went to the matron before this old bag did. She didn't do it much longer. She was so bossy.

Lord Beaverbrook was a horrible old man, he was a Canadian who rose very high in England.

The Lions Club used to send me, I think it was about 5000 cigarettes a month. I wrote a letter to my mother once, it wasn't for publication, but she put it in the paper, the *Ottawa Citizen*, that nobody was bothering with the guys in the wars at all. They would not get parcels or mail. We then got letters saying, *"Send me a list of 20 kids who don't get mail,"* and they posted them around the Lions Club and they used to put my name down as an alternative address. I met this kid in London one day and he said, *"God, you got drag around here,"* and he told me he got this parcel and the other one he got had my name on it, "How did you get your name on it?" I told him that I work through the Lions Club; they send me cigarettes and things, we work back and forth with them, they wouldn't know anybody else so I dole them out myself, I think I got 5000 cigarettes a month. Some of the kids who had not had any letters, they all got letters now. Some of them showed us the letters, it was very successful and the material passed on and on. Many people got involved. I only wrote that one letter!

I was sent back to Ottawa, Canada, just before the war ended in Europe. I was accompanied by 900 war brides and their kids. Enough said!

Margaret Moss

Graduated from: Montreal General Hospital School of Nursing, Quebec. Year: 1935

Other: B.A., Manitoba University, 1928

Military History:

Service: RCAMC

Rank: Lt. Nursing Sister

Served: 1942 to 1945

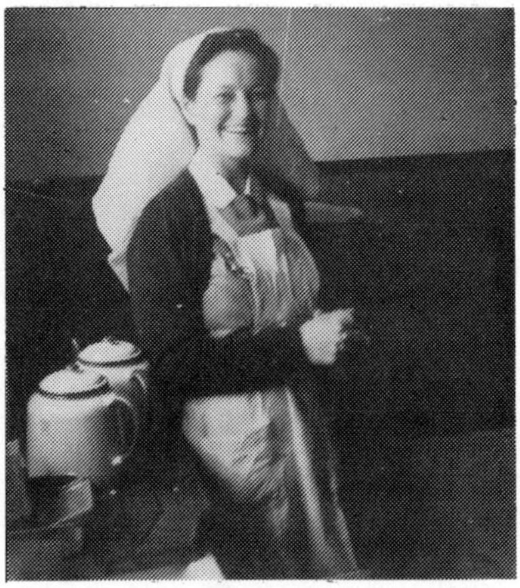

Lt. N/S Peggy Moss, Horley, England, 1943

In the fall of 1942 I joined the RCAMC in England, having transferred from the British WAAFs and was sent to unit No. 14 Canadian General Hospital. It was well managed and had excellent doctors. We were moved from Pinewood to Farnborough and then to Horley. This last move we really enjoyed as the surrounding country was beautiful. Most of us acquired bicycles and did a lot of exploring with our white veils streaming behind us. We must have looked rather like a group of "Flying Nuns." I had a pet name for mine (bicycle) and when we left sold it with regret, even though there was a small profit in the transaction. By then any mode of gasless transport was at a premium.

I must say a word about the wonderful courage of the soldiers. There was a sergeant in the hospital from the tank brigade. He had been very badly burned and was in saline baths continually. When he recovered, and in spite of his experience, he was determined to return to the tanks. One night on the officers' ward I was settling the patients for the night. I came to one man and asked him if he would like to have his back rubbed. He gave me a cheery, *"Yes,"* grabbed hold of the bar at the head of his bed doing a half somersault to turn over, and it was only then that I realized that he was a double leg amputee. I was silently crying all through the back rub. Later, I heard that he was returned to Canada and became a member of a provincial legislature.

Our journey to Italy had an inauspicious beginning. We were to go from Horley to our port of embarkment, which was Colchester, by train. It was a long day's trip and someone had forgotten to include any lunch for us. When we arrived at Colchester, in a rather weary state, we discovered that our luggage had been moved to a different ship from the one we were expecting and we eventually sailed on the *Santa Elena.* It was manned by the American Merchant Navy – a motley crew of men who were not trained for warfare.

As the convoy was passing Gibraltar the *St. Elena* was hit by aerial torpedoes and it was decided to "abandon ship!" We'd just finished dinner, grabbed what we could in the way of possessions and hurried up on deck. There was no panic but we huddled in what shelter there was as we could hear random strafing hitting various parts of the ship, (luckily they were poor shots). A small number of the nursing sisters were rescued by a British destroyer and taken to North Africa. The rest of us had to climb an enormous rope ladder let down over the side of the *Monterey,* our rescue ship. We had to roll up the slacks of our battle dress and rely on our monkey ancestry to make the climb. I had been clutching my trench coat but had to let it go halfway up, however at the top I insisted on stopping and rolling down my pant legs so that I could "preserve my dignity" in front of the cheering soldiers. Since we had lost all our luggage, the men were very kind to us and gave us some of their underwear, toothpaste, and soap. Because of the extra numbers on board we slept on the floor. The captain was forced to reduce the meals to two a day – but were quite good and we didn't suffer.

We landed at Naples and were billeted in the palace of an 'absentee' duke and were thrilled at the prospect of real beds and white sheets. It wasn't long before we discovered one good reason why the duke was an absentee. One by one we sat up in bed scratching madly and found that we had been attacked by bedbugs. We had to get the British Army in to exterminate them.

While in Naples each of us had an opportunity to visit the Roman Baths and we were each allotted twenty minutes to wash ourselves, our hair, and our underwear. It was an occasion for real celebration. It was also in Naples where we washed our few clothes and put them on the roof to dry and I had my pants stolen. I was lucky to have had a sister in Winnipeg who sent me "Care Parcels." Finally, the Canadian government caught up with us and reimbursed all the torpedo victims $500.00 each.

After a short time we went to Conchella where we established No. 14 in tents. It was two nursing sisters to a tent and we had Gurkhas from the British Army as orderlies. We were given a canvas folding bath, a real treat, and the water was brought in in large cans. One day the two of us were bathing in the nude when who should enter the tent but our Gurkha with more hot water. It was a toss up as to who was the most astonished.

There was a scarcity of food until military supplies caught up with us and no evidence of any pasta in the region. In the officers' mess we had Italian prisoners of war as waiters and one day they came to the table singing opera arias and balancing large plates aloft. This was the antipasto, one large delicious olive on each plate. Our mess cook was really talented and claimed that he could produce the M & V in 50 different ways.

I forgot to say that after the torpedoing other medical units were generous in sending us underwear and toilet articles. I was not lucky at this distribution and only got a cake of soap. However, I did find a lipstick in my pocket that had somehow survived the rope ladder and this we used sparingly.

At the time *Monte Cassino* was captured, the news gave all the credit to the Americans. This was NOT true as it had been a joint effort of the Poles and the Canadians that won the battle. There was quite an uproar and the Canadian Army gave all its personnel five days' leave. Most of us went to Rome and were able to have an audience with the Pope. Our various leaves sent us to the Isle of Capri, Rome and Florence. Italy was a marvellous place to be. I enjoyed the heat after the English cold. The Italian cooking used a great deal of olive oil and we were so unused to it that we were glad to get back to the 'brussel sprout.'

The unit moved to Perugia, halfway between Florence and Rome. Here we lived in huts with two to a room. We had been asked to a big party and were getting ready when the heating stove exploded, no one was hurt but we were covered with fine powdered ash from head to foot; however, we shook ourselves and went anyway. In December of 1944 we were still stationed in Perugia so we all decided that we would have a real Canadian Christmas. We formed a decorating committee and two or three of the nursing sisters, myself included, went out with our men to gather up evergreen trees. There was to be a tree on each ward and one in each mess. We found a likely looking field and came back laden with greenery and were told that we had been in a minefield! There was very little decorative material to buy in the local shops so we settled down to make our own. There was lots of talent in the unit and among the patients. They painted Christmas posters and place cards, made little candy baskets, decorated candles from our Army store, and painted the candle holders made by our unit carpenter. Everyone saved their silver cigarette paper for tree icicles and unit members gave gifts from their Canadian parcels including Christmas paper and ribbon. We also hung all the brightly coloured animals that the patients were making in their therapy classes on the trees. The tables were covered with white sheets and decorated with evergreen branches. It was wonderful therapy for all of us and everyone remarked that it was indeed a very Merry Christmas.

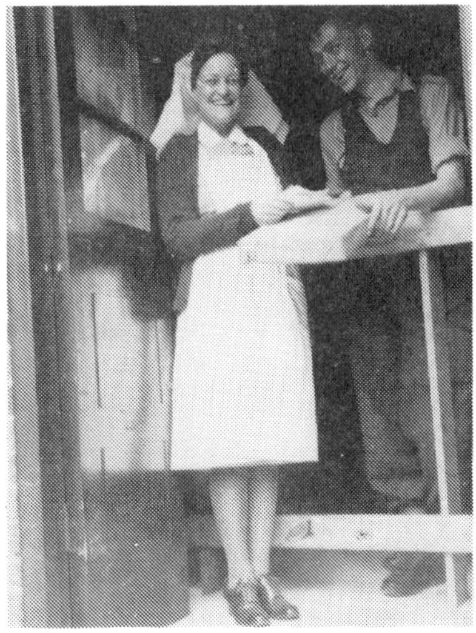

Peggy Moss and patient, Horley, England, 1945

In 1945 the war was quietening down and we were posted back to England in small groups and the unit was disbanded. For quite a few years after there was an annual reunion party in November in Montreal to talk about all our experiences. I long for my diary which the mermaids are probably reading and I hope no one else!

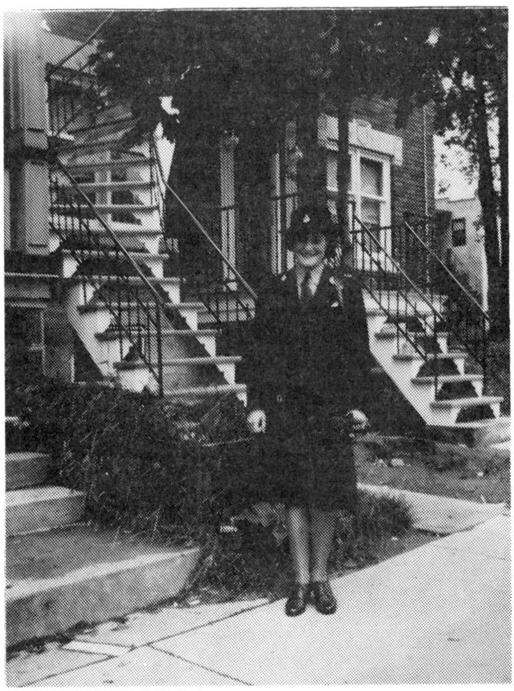

Lt. N/S Peggy Moss, Montreal, 1945

NO. 15 CANADIAN GENERAL HOSPITAL

Florence Evelyn (Richardson) Cooke
Margaret Kellough
Dorothy Macham
Elizabeth (Pense) Neil
Bernice Seeds

No. 15 Canadian General Hospital was mobilized 1 September 1939 at Toronto with Col. C.A. Rae as CO.

By 24 January 1940 all nursing sisters on strength with No. 15 General were posted for duty with Toronto Military Hospital.

The unit embarked aboard the *Empress of Britain* at Halifax 29 January 1940 for overseas duty. They arrived a week later. In July 1940 they were assigned to Bramshott until the end of June 1943 when the unit embarked on the SS *Nea Hellas* bound for El Arrouch, Algeria. The nursing sisters arrived 22 July and remained in North Africa until the unit moved to Caserta near Naples in January 1944.

At the end of April 1944 arrangments were made to move and the unit returned to Bramshott. On 12 May 1945 the administrative order came to disband the unit. Personnel were struck off strength to their various holding units.

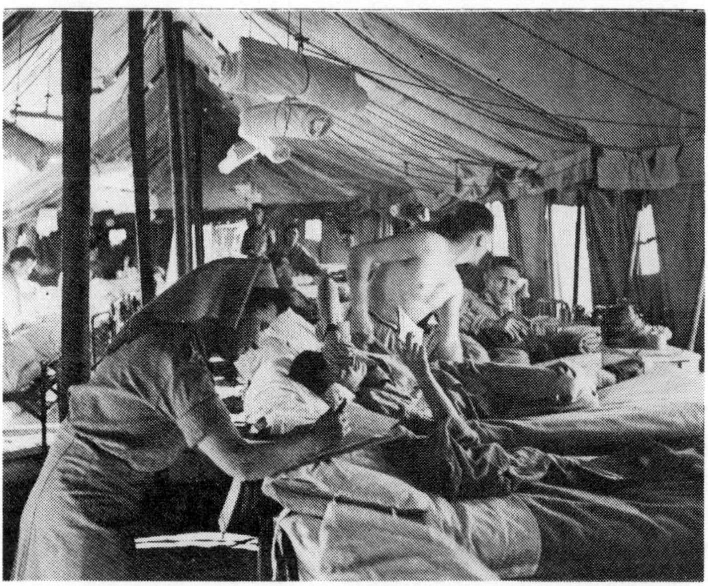

N/S Irene Mick at a tent ward, No. 15 CGH at El Arrouch, Algiers, North Africa 1943
Canadian Forces photo 22911

Florence Evelyn (Richardson) Cooke

Graduated from: Mack School of Nursing, St. Catharines Ontario. Year: 1935

Military History:

Service: RCAMC

Rank: Lt. N/S

Served: December 28, 1939 to August 22, 1945

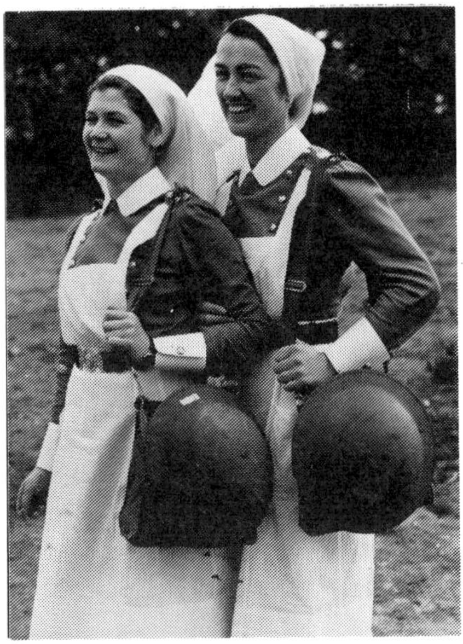

No. 15 CGH, Bramshott, Hants, England June 1940. L-R: Florence (Richardson) Cooke and Sally Eade

Both my parents were born in Great Britain, I think that was one reason I wanted to become a nursing sister in the RCAMC. On joining No. 15 Canadian General Hospital, I worked at old Grace Hospital in Toronto until Lt. N/S Kay Scott (now Harries) and I were posted to RCAF Trenton in May 1940. We were the only two female service personnel on base so accommodation was provided in downtown Trenton. We were called back to Toronto in early June 1940 to proceed overseas, arriving in Bramshott, Hants, 21 June 1940. In 1943 I met and married my husband, Colonel Donald N. Cooke, RCEME. Three weeks after our wedding, 15th General was sent to North Africa to support the invasion of Sicily. I was posted back to England in December 1943 and did not see my husband again until Christmas 1944 when he passed through London on a flight from Italy to Germany. We were reunited in March 1945 and I returned to Canada in July of 1945. We have 3 children, Richard J. Cooke B.Sc., Ph.D., Elizabeth A. Wicary B.Sc. Nursing, and Donald W. Cooke, B.Sc., MD.

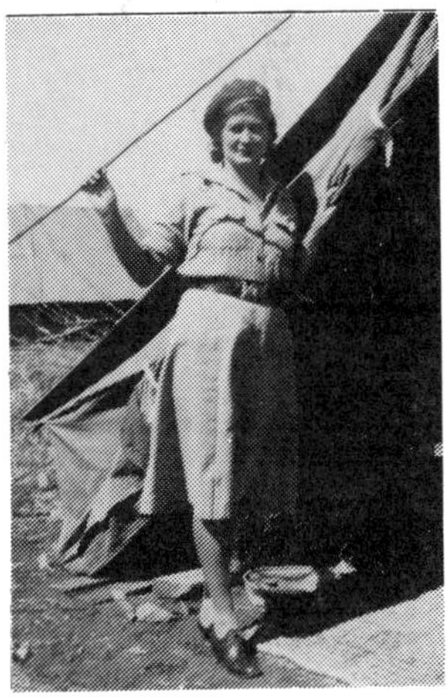

Lt. N/S Florence (Richardson) Cooke July 1943 El Arrouch, Algeria with No. 15 CGH

Margaret H. Kellough

Graduated from: Toronto General Hospital School of Nursing

Military History:

Service: RCAMC

Rank: Captain A/Matron

Served: 10 September 1939
to May 1946

I was among the nursing sisters of No. 15 Canadian General Hospital (1200 beds) Toronto and 50 nursing sisters of No. 5 Canadian General Hospital to board the train 7 June 1940 for Halifax where we joined a military convoy of ships and three destroyers to proceed overseas.

We had heard we were headed for Dieppe but while we were on the Atlantic, France capitulated and we landed at Liverpool, England. From there we located at Bramshott Military Camp (Nissen huts), Surrey, England.

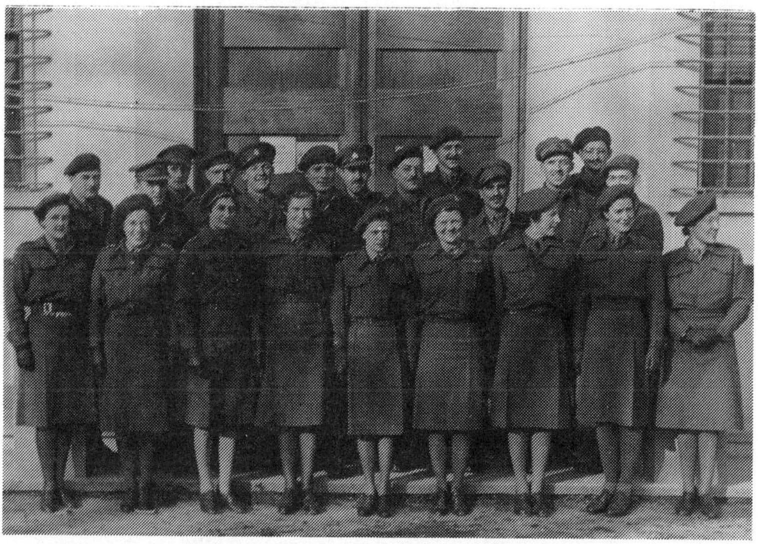

*Officers of No. 5 CCS: BACK ROW:
Bob Meiklejohn, 'Rusty' Wilkes, Mickey Korman, Homer Eskov, Bob Myers, L. Boulter, Frank Edward, Ed Shaw, Al Contway, John Handley, Joe Vallely, Gordon Cook, Fred Cowan.
FRONT ROW LEFT- RIGHT
Nursing Sisters Muriel Archer, Ruth Fleming, Olive Stewart, Betty Pense, Eire Galbraith, Margaret Kellough, Annette Beauchamp, Anna Cran, Helen Craig*

During the Dieppe raid, August 1942, we admitted many casualties as we were on the Portsmouth Road.

I was made assistant matron in 1942 while in England. Later we went by ship June 1943 to North Africa – inland in Algeria. We had been issued khaki uniforms and cotton veils and took mepacrine pills to ward off malaria. We arrived at a small village, El Arrouch, a very dirty, mountainous region. We lived in tents with no electricity except in the operating rooms. We used hurricane lanterns and flashlights. Hot! Oh, boy, it sure was. We had flying locusts, centipedes and chameleon lizards. Our instructions, if bitten by any of these which could be poisonous, was to have someone suck out the poison. On siesta one day, I was hot, but felt hotter when bitten on the rear. I jumped up to find a long centipede. I didn't like to ask anyone to suck out the poison and decided to wait to see what happened, telling no one. Nothing happened and I survived.

While there we had a Sirocco, a violent rain storm which broke some tent poles; patients had to be removed to safety. Also unknown to us while I was in charge one evening – there was a complete eclipse of the moon. During this time we took casualties from Sicily, being the only Canadian hospital there; an American hospital was there too. We proceeded to Caserta, Southern Italy, near Naples and admitted 200 casualties per day from Hitler and Gothic lines with field dressings on only. Our count went up to 1700 patients. To get 200 patients in we had to discharge 200 patients. Our operating room staff worked eight hours on and eight hours off.

I was sent as matron from captain (assistant matron) to No. 5 Canadian Casualty Station behind the front lines five to seven miles from Germans and kept only dangerously injured patients. No. 4 CCS was there, too, and we leap-frogged over them when they were filled up.

We were situated at various places ending up at Ravenna, the only Canadian medical unit there. We left there in 1944 and went by ship to Marseilles, France, a very stormy trip. We flew to Belgium and eventually arrived as Oss, Holland. We were billeted with the Dutch people, our hospital was in a different spot.

One night during almost a black fog, the Germans were coming across the canal and we were gathered at 4:00 A.M. from our billets and taken to the CCS. However, the Germans didn't get to the town. Later, on account of my mother's illness, I came home after VE Day. I had been away about five years.

Dorothy A. Macham

Graduate of: Women's College Hospital School of Nursing, Toronto. Year: 1932 and Psychiatric Nursing and Unit Administration at Ontario Hospital School of Nursing 1933

Military History:

Service: RCAMC

Rank: Lt. N/S to Captain/Matron to Major P/M

Served: September 10, 1939 to November 1945

I enlisted on September 10, 1939, in the RCAMC as a Lieutenant (nursing sister). My OR experience over the past $3^1/_2$ years at the Women's College Hospital, Toronto had considerable bearing on my future.

Following some weeks of training in Army organization and lectures on associated medical subjects, our unit No. 15 Canadian General Hospital was set up in what had been the old Grace Hospital building on College Street. During the winter of 1939-40 many of the soldiers suffered acute chest diseases. These men were housed in the Horse Palace at the exhibition grounds which were very dusty and contributed to the problem. The male officers and other ranks of No. 15 CGH left for England in January 1940, we remained on staff of what became the Toronto Military Hospital until we left for England June 6, 1940. We arrived at our unit, No. 15 CGH on June 21, 1940. The hospital was located at Bramshott Chase. It had a capacity for 1200 beds.

I was assigned to the operating room as very few of the total nursing establishment (80 altogether) had had OR experience. Many of the surgical cases were fractures but there were also the surgical needs found in a population of relatively young men. Included were some cases requiring plastic or restorative surgery. One surgeon whose specialty was plastic surgery obtained permission in the fall of 1941 to establish a plastic surgery unit in association with a plastic surgery unit of a large British Emergency Medical Services complex located at what had

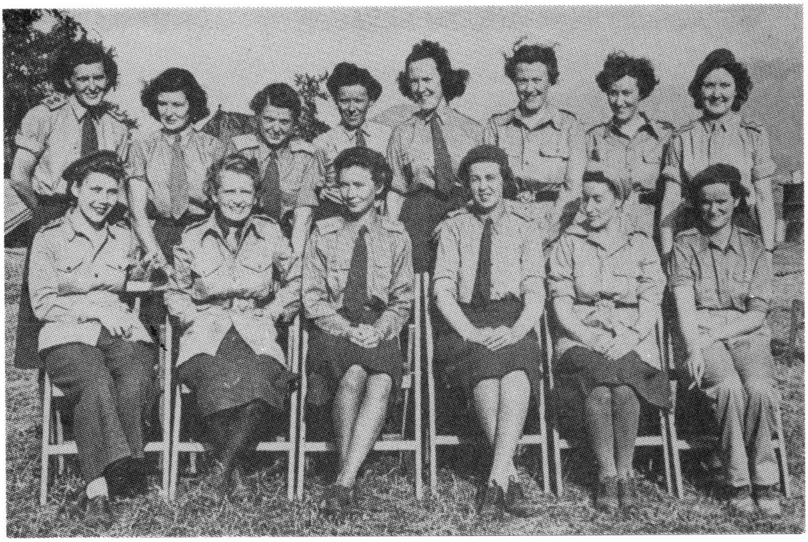

Canadian nursing sisters stationed at No. 5 Canadian Casualty Clearing Station, Italy. Front row, left to right: Lieut. (N/S) A. Halbuza, Willowbrook, Sask.; Lieut. (N/S) Dorothy Dent, Ottawa; Capt. (N/S) Dorothy Macham, Toronto; Capt. (N/S) Constance Winter, Ottawa; Lieut. (N/S) Elizabeth Cleland, Toronto; Lieut. (N/S) Bernice Bigley, Montreal; Back Row, left to right: Lieut. (N/S) Audrey Auger, Toronto; Lieut. (N/S) Irene Henderson, Quebec; Lieut. (N/S) Evelyn Galbraith, Renfrew, Ontario; Lieut. (N/S) Mary MacDonald, Saint John, N.B.; Lieut. (N/S) Mary Angus, Victoria, B.C.; Lieut. (N/S) Evelyn Pepper, Ottawa; Lieut. (N/S) Elizabeth Crothers, Kingston, Ontario; Lieut. (N/S) Maxine Fuller, Edmonton
Courtesy Canada's Weekly No. 3190 Vol. CXX111, 26 MAY 1944

been a mental institution near the town of Basingstoke, Hants. Four London hospitals had relocated there due to the severe bombing in London (leaving skeleton staffs in London). The Westminster Hospital was responsible for the plastic surgery building with Sir Harold Gillies (the pioneer of plastic surgery) as the chief surgeon. He came frequently from London to operate and consult. I had had experience working with the Plastic Surgery Unit at No. 15 and was asked if I would transfer to the Plastic Surgery Unit as nursing sister-in-charge. This meant leaving many good friends but I agreed to the transfer. Fortunately, one other nursing sister of No. 15 CGH transferred too. This helped make the transition from a large unit to a small unit within a very large establishment. We started with 20 beds, five nursing sisters, and two medical orderlies. There was, in addition to the surgeon, an anesthetist and a dentist. This proved to be a most interesting experience. We were on civilian rations – each week we were doled out individual shares of sugar, margarine, etc. We ate in what was a huge auditorium – there was a very large number of people located in these buildings – those London hospitals with nursing schools had their students there as well. Sometimes our rations were stolen from our table. We Canadians were so much better off than the English as we received parcels from home to supplement our diet.

Many of our patients had fractured jaws caused mainly in motorcycle accidents – their teeth and jaws were wired together. It was difficult to obtain sufficient nourishing food – eggs in particular. These men were very enterprising – they soon learned how to push food through their teeth. We treated burns necessitating skin grafts – in some cases ears and noses were rebuilt. A saline burn bath was built while we were with the British. We became quite attached to our British friends although we worked quite independently of them.

Eventually we obtained 30 beds and our nursing establishment was increased to eight. In February 1943 our Plastic and Jaw Surgery Unit (the word *Jaw* had been added to the name) was moved to the other side of Basingstoke and incorporated into No. 1 Canadian Neurological Hospital. This was located on Lord Camrose's estate; huts had been built at the rear of the mansion to accommodate the patients. I was still the nursing sister-in-charge of the plastic & jaw section but we were now under the general orders or administration of the officer commanding the No. 1 Neurological Hospital. In the spring of 1943 Matron-in-Chief (Lt/Col.) Agnes Neill visited the hospital. I took the opportunity to ask for a transfer to a hospital where I might get back into operating room work. I felt I couldn't remove the nursing sister I had assigned to our OR.

Rather than transferring me in accordance with my request, I was transferred in June 1943 to No. 5 Casualty Clearing Station located at Copthorne, and promoted to captain (matron). My predecessor had been transferred to a General Hospital. The nursing establishment of the CCS was a total of eight with several medical orderlies. The patients were accommodated in what had been the classrooms of a private boys' school. Minor illnesses and minor surgical problems were taken care of – serious cases were transferred or sent to a General Hospital located at Horsham. I very quickly felt quite at home and comfortable with this group. The nursing sisters appeared to quite readily accept me.

In October 1943 all personnel in the unit were issued equipment and uniforms for service out of England. The nursing sisters received khaki uniforms for daily wear rather than our blue uniforms. We embarked at Liverpool on an American ship, the *Argentina*, carrying some 7000 troops. No. 4 CCS was also on this ship so altogether there were just 16 women on board. While on the trip I had the privilege of having a conducted tour through the galley – the one thing still vivid in my mind were the large bins of eggs – after over three years in England where powdered egg was almost the only egg available, I was almost overcome. Two meals a day were served while on board. It was not until some place mid-Atlantic that we were told of our destination.

The convoy consisted of over thirty ships plus three or four destroyers accompanying it. When going through the Strait of Gibraltar the flag-ship dropped anchor to one side of the strait while the remaining ships sailed through in single file. This was an awesome sight as it was at sundown and the Rock glowed red – later that evening the convoy was attacked from the air. One ship in the convoy was hit but all troops were safely removed including 80 Lts. (nursing sisters) of a Canadian General Hospital. The ship was lost. In the morning the convoy had completely dispersed – later that day we disembarked at Augusta, Sicily – this was during the first week of November 1943. For about 4 or 5 days we remained in Catania and then all the nursing sisters and two of the medical doctors were posted to a British Field Hospital at Messina. The building had been an Italian TB hospital facing right on to the Strait of Messina. The rest of our unit set up in a schoolhouse with a limited number of beds. On one occasion about 14 soldiers were admitted with ptomaine poisoning – these men were desperately ill. Mosquito nets had to be used during the day to keep flies off and mosquitoes at night, but nothing could keep fleas and bedbugs off.

It was on New Year's Day 1944 that our officer commanding announced that word had been received that I had been awarded the Associate Royal Red Cross. This came as a complete surprise. I never did know the reason for it unless it was in recognition of our plastic surgery nursing staff pioneering in that service. It was many months before I was able to attend an investiture at Buckingham Palace.

In mid-January 1944 our unit, No. 5 CCS, moved to Corato on the Adriatic side of Italy not far from Bari. We nurses were flown from Catania, Sicily, to Bari. This was my first plane trip –

it was an American transport plane with benches along both sides of the body of the plane. The pilot invited we gals (there were five of us on this plane with about seven or eight British ground crew) to the cockpit one at a time and gave each of us the opportunity to pilot the plane. We were flying, if I remember correctly, at 5000 feet and from the cockpit had a wonderful view of the country. My inclination was to go higher – the pilot would say, *"Bring it down."*

Our unit again set up in a school – the nursing sisters lived in a small house out of the town (we were told the population of the town was 50,000). It was always an interesting experience to walk to and from work. In a letter home I wrote, "I have started to wear my high top boots as we have a five minute walk between where we live and where we work and the streets are filthy as well as rough. The people throw all their slop into the gutter. They sweep all their dirt from their houses onto the street. They may have a couple of hens in crates on the sidewalk outside their front doors and maybe a goat or two tied there too. On wash day the clothes are hung on clothes lines propped up on the centre of the sidewalk. There are many children – at first they followed us like a bunch of cats but the novelty is wearing off a bit. You see them running to tell the rest of their families to come and look at the Signorina Englese or Canadese."

In another letter I report, "We have found a place to have a bath. It is in connection with a bakery in town. It is for public use. There are six or seven baths – the water is heated by the fire used to bake the bread. We have made the acquaintance of the baker's daughter. She came to visit. We were trying to brush up on Italian and she is quite anxious to learn English."

From Corato we moved north close to Ortona where the Canadians fought a tough battle. The CCS was set up in a tobacco factory – a big barn of a place with shell holes in the roof – in the town of Lanciano. This being the month of February there was snow on the ground and shelling at night which all provided a miserable situation. After a few weeks in this location we moved south but into the hills to a place called Casacalenda. A school was again used to accommodate the patients. In four weeks' time we moved to the west side of Italy to a place called Telese – this time we occupied a hotel with patients on the first and second floors – we nursing sisters on the third floor.

The weather was improving and the Allied forces were making preparations for the spring offensive. Early in May we moved once again but this time under canvas, in a staging area, in preparation for the move north. It was here I learned that I was being posted back to England. I did see the beginning of the big offensive toward Mt. Cassino – we had heard that midnight was set for a tremendous barrage of shelling – we were able to see the flashes, the sky was really lit up. In the early morning, about 6 A.M., many bombers flew over. I pulled my cot out of my tent and lay there and watched wave after wave of planes go over.

I regretted leaving the unit very much. I was transported to one of the General Hospitals in Caserta where I stayed a couple of days and then to Naples from which I embarked on the *Empress of Australia.* (I am a little vague now as to which ship it was.) There were some twenty-four nursing sisters returning to England; many of the troops on board were British who had been for many months and years in the Middle East and north Africa. The ship was packed – there was no place to sit except on one's bunk or on the deck floor. The ship's doctor, a Scot, was most kind to we gals and allowed us the use of his cabin during the day, also part of the ship's infirmary. We docked at Gurock, Scotland, May 30, 1944, but could not disembark until the following day as there was not sufficient transportation (trains) to take us to our various destinations – it was that evening that we saw the battleship *Rodney* and two cruisers leave port – we believe these battleships were on the way to the channel in preparation for D-Day.

On my return to England from Italy in early June 1944, I was posted to No. 8 Canadian General Hospital. No. 8 CGH was a 600-bed hospital which had originated in Saskatchewan. The unit had arrived in England on March 24, 1942. It was located at Pinewood Hospital until May 20-25, 1942, when it was relocated to the Aldershot Hospital at Farnborough. The personnel had been recruited in Saskatchewan and were very pro the West – even though by the time I arrived the OC as well as the major (P/M) were from Ontario. The major suggested that I avoid saying I was from Toronto when asked, so I began by saying I was from Corn Hill – this was actually the small community where I was born, near Barrie, but no one knew whether it was in Saskatchewan or Ontario.

Just prior to my joining the unit it had been sent to Yorkshire for field training in preparation for the invasion of Europe. The personnel learned to pitch tents and live under those conditions. A field kit was issued which included the following: a water bottle, canvas pail, canvas tub and wash basin (the tub took a canvas pail of water), khaki tams, jackets, skirts, slacks and shirts, heavy boots, sleeping bag and folding camp bed.

Following field training we were transported by train overnight to London and then on to Hove on the south coast of England where we were billeted in houses, after which we were moved to a staging unit somewhere close to Southampton. The staging area was concealed in a forest (probably part of the New Forest near Eastbourne).

During our time in Hove the buzz bombs (V-1) were frequent disturbances – they were quite noisy and were mainly directed at London and were generally sent over during the night hours.

As there was double daylight saving in Britain it was not really dark in July until near midnight – although we were loaded onto a ILC (Infantry Landing Craft) in daylight we did not leave Southampton until close to midnight of July 18, 1944. The 60 nursing sisters were assigned to one of the holds with stacks of bunks four deep. There were not sufficient bunks to accommodate all 60 and, although narrow, in more than one instance two people tried resting on one bunk. About 3 A.M. our ILC either ran into an object (we were told it was on oil tanker) or was run into. The engines immediately stopped. I was resting on the third level of the bunks but below me on the lowest level there were two girls trying to sleep. Prior to lying down someone had left a canvas pail of water right beside the lowest bunk – with the jolt of hitting the tanker the canvas pail of water upset. The nursing sister on the outside of the lowest bunk, which was about 6 inches from the floor, put her hand out into the water. She jumped to her feet and tore up the ladder to the deck yelling, *"Girls we'll have to swim for it."* This incident prevented further sleep. There was one toilet off the hold – thank goodness we had been issued with vomit bags.

Mid-morning of July 19, 1944, (my birthday) we docked at Arromanches on the coast of France. A temporary harbour and dock had been made at this location by towing sunken ships into position. The British were in charge on dock and the good old British Tommys had tea brewing on the open dock and offered us some. We were carrying our own mugs.

We were loaded into lorries and transported to our hospital site which was in a field about three or four miles east of Bayeux. I remember there were Canadian soldiers – Engineer Corp. I think – working on the roads and cheering us as we went by.

No. 7 CGH had preceded No. 8 CGH to France by four days and already had some of their tents, hospital extending, erected in the field next to us. We were given accommodation in one of the big tents for 2 or 3 nights before our equipment was located and established.

The nursing sisters' tents were pitched in an apple orchard. In this location the latrine had been dug behind a hedge. There were canvas walls to give privacy but no cover. I always felt that the guys in the little reconnaissance planes flew low over the hospital area and could see us in it. It was quite essential to have flashlights in order to go to the latrine during the dark hours.

By July 26th, 1944, our hospital was in operation – the surgical teams were able to operate during the night by light provided by a generator. Hurricane lanterns were used in patients' tents.

The nights were disturbed by the ack ack guns; shrapnel fell around, some cutting through our tents. As we had not obtained all our expanding hospital canvas we had extra beds and mattresses which the OC had issued to the nursing sisters so that we were able to sleep in our bedrolls on the ground under the beds.

The weather was good the first three or four weeks in France – in a letter of August 11, 1944 I say, "The roads are terribly dusty. Today was really hot and the poor lads with chest wounds seemed to suffer with it quite a good deal."

Shortly before September 5, 1955, No. 8 CGH was moved closer to the front lines – again we were set up under canvas near the village of St. Andre-Sur-Cailly which is just north of Rouen. To reach this location the convoy crossed the Orne River via a railway bridge which had had planks laid so that lorries could cross – this was a very slow process. I recall a couple of dead horses that apparently had been caught in the attempt to escape. The stench was horrible.

Casualties were heavy. I usually worked in the triage area. I vividly recall one patient who had a great gash in the left side of his abdomen – when I removed the field dressing it appeared as though someone had stuffed a cloth in the wound; much to my chagrin it was his liver protruding. He was clearly conscious but died soon after admission. I recall a young German lad, about 16 or 17 years old, who had a bullet in his back. The bullet had entered on one side of his chest and slid right over his rib cage to the other side of his chest. There were great tears rolling down his cheeks – the MO made a little slit and just slipped the bullet out. I recall another young German who was completely unmanageable; after a couple of days the MO on the ward gave him a green apple to eat and he almost immediately became quiet.

On September 12, 1944, I wrote home that it had been dry for a few days so the ground had dried out. We were thankful for our rubber boots during the wet times. The night staff found it miserably cold. We wore everything woollen we had.

I write that one of the nursing sisters and I had gone into the village to see if we could find anyone to do our shirts, sheets, towels and pyjamas; we were directed to the mayor's house for information. The mayor's wife took us to a home and made arrangements for us. We had to supply soap as the French had none and we had to be very careful with what we had sent from home.

Quote from a letter dated September 24, 1944: "We have to laugh at the natives here. It seems that Sunday is the day for strolling out. They come to the hospital grounds (even today and it was raining) and go around peering into the tents and even going in if they can get away with it. About ten boys ranging from 8 to 14 years of age came to our office tent; all shook hands with me when they entered and when they left. The one question I understood was whether I was English. I put them straight on that and made them pronounce Canadian correctly."

I made comment in a letter to my sister re rulers and erasers she had sent, that the nursing sisters on the wards were most grateful for them. Sept. 24, 1944, I indicated in a letter that we were waiting for a move and that it would hopefully be to a building. My comment relative to the patients was that they were so tired, dirty and most were without possessions. "We have three Red Cross workers attached to our unit. They are grand girls and certainly work hard. Nothing is too much trouble for them. They write letters for the patients, give them reading material, make tea and give all the necessities that the Red Cross supply. These are all the little things the nursing sisters haven't time for and yet are so important.

"There are three of us writing letters on the one table in the mess tent under the one lamp and one gal shakes the table when she is writing that it is very difficult to write."

It was just down the road from our hospital that we discovered a V-1 launching site, the main framework was still there concealed in a woods; tree limbs had been interlaced over top of it so that it could not be seen from the air. We had experienced these noisy bombs in England; at least one could hear them coming where as the V-2s were not heard until they exploded. The V-2s were more devastating too.

In a letter dated October 12, 1944, I indicated that we were already settled into Antwerp (of course I could not say where we were). The lorry in which I travel led from St. Andre-Sur-Cailly to Antwerp along with one other lorry got separated from the rest of the convoy. We had left with the whole convoy very early in the A.M. I have no idea where the driver went wrong but the day wore on and it became late and very dark; the road we were travelling had a great deal of heavy equipment on it, tanks, guns and lorries. I felt we were getting very close to the front lines – about 10 P.M. the lorry I was in broke down. Enquiries were made and it was discovered we were some distance from Antwerp – those of us in the broken-down lorry transferred to the other one and retraced some of the miles we had gone. We finally arrived at the hospital in Antwerp around midnight. We were hungry and tired. Our superiors were most concerned for our welfare. I often have wondered about the poor guy with the broken-down lorry.

Our hospital occupied what had been a Belgian military hospital, then taken over by the Germans. We inherited some German patients and both black and white Belgians. A token number of German nurses and orderlies had been left behind to care for their patients but were not retained as helpers very long. They were sent off to a POW camp.

The hospital was quite a large complex – several buildings with connecting corridors which had windows interspersed – windows were quite often blown in when V-2s exploded. One Sunday A.M. the Maj. (P/M) had decided to take a few hours off but a V-2 landed quite close to our residence. She came to the hospital and said, *"I decided to come to the hospital, I don't want to die alone over there!"* There was an R.C. convent associated with the hospital. The R.C. sisters came each day at noon to collect food from our kitchen. I never knew whether they had had the same service from the Germans.

A comment in a letter home stated that there seemed to be much more to attend to in buildings. The Belgians also liked to visit the hospital; they always shook hands on arriving and departing. I noted in a letter of October 16, 1944, that we didn't receive as many Belgian francs for the British pound as we had for the French franc – so things were more expensive. I never thought of dollars and cents anymore – just convert to pounds.

The nursing sisters were housed in different buildings – one very large house had been occupied by German nurses. It was evident they had left in a great hurry, the dirty dishes were still on the table from their last meal.

The only thing I can remember about our food was the tinned M & V (meat and vegetable) but of course parcels from home were very important and greatly appreciated. We rationed the goodies to make them last as long as possible. In Antwerp we saw farmers bringing produce to market on their bicycles and one item which we were able to buy was grapes – I had never seen such beautiful green and blue grapes – they were almost the size of plums.

Quote: "I got quite a kick out of the letter you sent me written by a nursing sister over here. I do not know her but it just goes to show how silly they sound when in print. She said the carts were pulled by dogs. That is a rare sight. I have seen one or two but the dog is hitched onto the side of the cart and helps to pull it."

During our stay in Antwerp the V-2 bombs were particularly troublesome. One fell on a busy intersection of the city. A large number of patients was admitted to our hospital – both civilians and Armed Forces; some fifty were brought to our morgue for identification and preparation for burial. One was a British nursing sister who had come into Antwerp for the day. It fell to the Maj. (P/M) and myself to escort the British matron to the morgue to identify the body. The morgue was a sight never to be forgotten. I had great sympathy for the Sgt. in charge.

It was understood that the German Forces had not been entirely cleared from east Antwerp when we arrived in that city.

Our hospital operated at a high occupancy rate but the care given to patients was improved over what was possible when under canvas. It was wonderful to have running water. A comment in a letter dated October 21, 1944, was that we were still pretty busy but had had a few extra nursing sisters assigned to our unit which would help. "The wounded almost make your heart ache at times – they are grand patients."

The Belgians were really kind people, at least the majority. They brought a lot of fruit and flowers to the patients; as an example, one man brought in a beautiful tray of grapes, they tray being approximately 1 x 2 feet in size. On November 8,

1944, I wrote to the effect that we could still buy tomatoes for lunch on our way from the hospital to our house.

There were occasions when we had an opportunity to get away for a few hours. I wrote on November 21, 1944, telling that Miss Maclaren and I had gone to the opera. We saw the Tales of Hoffman which was very enjoyable except that I was so sleepy I had dozed off. I must have slept through a lot of it because 50 years later I have no recollection of attending the performance.

In a letter dated December 3, 1944, I indicated that Miss Maclaren, Maj. (P/M) had gone to another unit and that I had been promoted to Maj. (P/M). In a letter of December 12, 1944, I told that my assistant had arrived; that she was Janet Wallace from the Neurological Unit at Basingstoke and that she was three years younger than me. One of the nursing sisters had said to me, *"Do you think you two are old enough to look after all of us?"* I said, *"If I don't look old enough now then I will in a few weeks time as I probably will have more gray hairs by then."*

Most of the time during our stay on the Continent we had a neurosurgical team attached to our unit. I had great admiration for the nursing sisters and orderlies who cared for these patients with severe head wounds. The patients were noisy and very difficult to control.

In the book, *The Canadian Medical Services*, written by Dr. W. R. Feasby, on page 270 he has stated that No. 6 CGH and No. 8 CGH moved to St. Michielsgestel late in December 1944 due to the persistent rocket attacks on Antwerp. I question this statement as our OC, Col. E. Hume, was always keen for the hospital to be as close to the front lines as possible. However, be that as it may, another CGH was being moved into our Antwerp site. We had packed our medical and surgical panniers ready for the move when a V-2 hit a movie theatre in the city centre. The nursing sisters and other staff members did a tremendous job of setting up again in order to care for the many casualties resulting from this catastrophe. Patients, both civilian and Army, were covered with plaster dust which made them all look in deep shock.

In a few days following this disaster we did move to St. Michielsgestel near 'S Hertogenbosch in Holland. We occupied an R.C. seminary which had been used by the Germans to hold political prisoners. The large classrooms made good wards and there were suitable rooms in separate buildings for unit personnel. On arriving in Holland it seemed to me there was water everywhere.

We did not immediately open to receive patients – the OC advised us on Christmas Eve that there was rumour of a German parachute jump in our area and that we might have to be evacuated. He warned anyone who might have a revolver to by no means use it if we were surrounded by the Germans, that we were protected by the Geneva Red Cross Agreement. To my knowledge there was no attempted paratroops invasion; nevertheless, we didn't admit patients until January 7, 1945. The chapel was stripped of its pews to make a reception area for triage purposes.

In a letter of December 28, 1944, I wrote of our activities over Christmas. We somehow or other gathered sufficient articles which enabled us to give a stocking to each of the 'other ranks.' The Col. played Santa Claus. When one of the boys who had been paraded before the Col. a couple of times came to receive his Christmas stocking the Col. said to him, *"I don't know who would knit you a pair of socks."*

On Christmas Day we helped serve Christmas dinner to the other ranks. We were able to use the patients' plates and utensils. A number of us will always remember the Dutch children who gathered at the windows of the mess hall. When the men finished eating we let the children in to finish off anything there might have been left on the plates. A commentary made by a Sgt. (who was with the unit) many years later, *"I think I'll never forget the drawn and thin faces of the children, and I prayed that my children would never have to live under the conditions that these children had lived for 5 years."* I believe the other ranks quite frequently gave food to the children.

We engaged some civilians to work with us. They wore wooden shoes and make a great clatter when they arrived in the morning (on the tile floors). During the first weeks the casualties were light but we received many medically ill – a large percentage of these were diagnosed possible diphtheria, there being diphtheria in the Dutch civilian population. On occasion we had as many as 80 patients quarantined – it was difficult to carry out proper isolation technique.

January 9, 1945: "We have had a little snow; the bells on the horses and carts sound more natural with snow on the ground."

January 14, 1945: "Jan and I went for a long walk yesterday. We don't often get out. We called into a Dutchman's place. They had us go in and sit by the fire – there were seven children and they were all present. We had quite a chat – we talked in our language and they talked in theirs and we all got along fine."

January 22, 1945: "I went to Brussels but it wasn't a very satisfactory day. I really went to get some khaki shirts for the nursing sisters but by the time I fooled around getting money changed (gelders to francs), etc., it was time to come home. It is too long a trip for one day. We ran into a bad storm coming home and I wondered if the driver and I might be stranded on the road for the night but we made it safe and sound."

January 31, 1945: "We don't have to use lanterns or candles now but did at first. Occasionally our lights fail but on the whole are pretty good." We had a generator which operated the OR lights 24 hours a day. Those of us who had our sleeping quarters facing onto the area where the generator was located had to get used to the continual noise.

February 3, 1945: "We go to church service every Sunday A.M.; last Sunday we had quite a good attendance as we seemed to have quite a number of up-patients who were able to attend."

I recall the death of one of our patients who had a younger brother in a regiment located not very far from the hospital. Word was dispatched to the younger brother who was permitted to come to the hospital. The burial service was to be held quite close by and because the younger brother was present the padre thought I should accompany them. We travelled in what we always referred to as a 'passion buggy.' It was a vehicle with a seat beside the driver and seats to accommodate six or eight people along each side with space in the centre. The padre, younger brother, driver and myself with the body on a stretcher in the centre, proceeded to the place where graves had been dug. This being in Holland there was a good deal of water in the grave. The body was lowered in a blanket into the grave and the padre performed the service. We took the young brother back to our mess and gave him a cup of tea and some cookies from home and sent him off to his unit. I have often thought of him and what he must have felt; it must have been a very lonely trek back to his unit.

During early February 1945 the average admission and discharge rate was 300 patients per day. Around February 18 the rate dropped to 177 and the official unit diary called admissions slow at 160 per day, but by February 21 we were back up to 300. The highest total for one day was 426 admissions. This represented a tremendous turnover and there was no way patients could be given anything other than the most essential care. Penicillin by this time was in general use and had frequently been started at a Field Dressing Station. It was essential that each patient's field card be checked for what had been administered, and if penicillin had been given, to have it immediately repeated. At that time it had to be given every three to four hours.

I recall telling one of the nursing sisters on one of the large wards to at least try to have the patient's feet washed if nothing else could be managed.

February 18, 1945: "This is Sunday A.M. and I have been pretty well around the hospital and think everyone has enough help to contend with their particular needs but even at that I could do with more. We have been really busy. I think this 'do' has topped the lot for us although each one has been a little different.

I can't give any particulars but I think I am returning to England shortly. I guess I have had my 'fightin'. I will be sorry to go but I really think I am beginning to take these moves with a little less concern... they are beginning to bring people over who have been sitting in England all during the show or since they came over. Seeing as how I have had a couple of trips, Italy and here, I am one of the first to go back."

March 1, 1945: "I am very much behind in writing but have a good excuse. I have had a 48-hour leave in Paris. Isn't that something! Of course, it took as long to get there and get back as we had to stay but it was certainly worth it. Miss Laclaren and I went, got special permission seeing as how I am supposed to be going to the U.K. soon. She is now the senior (P/M) at HQ here. Paris is certainly a lovely city and has been practically untouched. Things are awfully expensive but it is nice to look at the shops anyway. We drove along the Champs Elysees, saw and drove under the Eiffel Tower, were through Notre Dame Cathedral which is rather drab. They removed the stained glass windows in 1939. We were through the Paris mosque although we didn't get into the harem!

Rode on the underground and managed not to get lost, saw the windows and streets lighted at night. It was wonderful not to have to use a flashlight, stayed at the YWCA which was really comfortable, visited Elizabeth Arden's which was just as you would imagine a posh setup like that might be. I had my hair and nails done at Antoines which was an education in itself, seeing all kinds and sorts getting all kinds and sorts of things done to their hair while having their toe nails manicured."

"We were in Napoleon's tomb which is like a cathedral, all the other Napoleons are buried there too. The building has a dome which is decorated with gold leaf costing about $17,000. The city is beautifully planned and is easy to find your way around."

That trip was by train from Brussels to Paris, travelled by night both going and returning. A unit diary in early March 1945 noted that the number of admissions dropped and that the number of V-2 bombs were lessening.

On approximately March 10, 1945, I returned to England, travelled by air from Brussels to London in a small Anson plane. There were three passengers. We sat on our luggage in the body of the plane. The pilot explained that he had to be careful not to fly over a small pocket of Germans on the coast at Dunkirk. We landed on a grass landing strip on the south coast of England in order that the pilot could telephone London to get the weather report. We were able to proceed to Heathrow where it was necessary to go through customs. At the same time another small plane carrying three Canadian nursing sisters landed on the coast. We had been allowed to get out of the plane I was travelling in, and as I walked around, I noticed that the other plane had a bird cage hanging in the cockpit. I didn't particularly wonder about it until I was being interviewed by one of the customs men (as I recall, I seemed to be the only person in this large customs room) when one of the men said to the other one, *"What have we got over there?"* I looked to see and lo and behold one of the nursing sisters from the other plane was carrying the bird cage.

As we were being picked up by a lorry driver to be taken into London there was delay as the bird (budgie I think) had to be examined by the custom's medical officer. The MO was not available so the bird had to be left at customs. Finally, we were all settled in the lorry ready to go when this nursing sister remembered she had not left any bird seed for the budgie and had to dash back into the building with it.

I was in no way responsible for these three nursing sisters and they were dispatched to different hospitals in England. I was given a few days' leave in London and before I left I was contacted by customs to say that the budgie could not be admitted to England and wanted to know what they should do with it. I said,

"Send it to Miss Maclaren in Brussels." It was years later that I asked her if she had ever received it. She said, *"I wondered who was responsible for that."* I don't know if the nursing sister who had brought the budgie to England ever knew what happened to it.

I was posted to No. 18 CGH located near Colchester, Essex.

On my posting back to England in mid-March 1945, I joined the No. 18 Canadian General Hospital as major (P/M), a 600-bed hospital located just outside Colchester, Essex. It was while at No. 18 CGH that VE Day occurred. I happened to be in London on May 6th when it was first learned that Germany had surrendered. There was great rejoicing and when the surrender papers were signed on May 8th there were further celebrations. Once the war was over there was an immediate effort to close some hospitals. Our patient numbers were gradually reduced and No. 18 was closed. It was while at Colchester that the OC and I were invited to participate in the St. George's Day celebrations. We gathered in the mayor's parlours and marched to a church.

All the civic folk were there: judges with their wigs, the ex-mayors, the councillors, Girl Guides, St. John's Ambulance representatives, etc. The procession was led by a band and the Services were all represented. After the church service we returned to the town hall and had a cup of coffee and few speeches. In one of my letters home I tell of having been invited to tea at an elderly lady's home – another nurse and I cycled to her home. Her husband was present and was a retired brigadier general. He entertained us with his stories of experiences in Burma 50 years ago as well as the South African War. He told me I was much too young to be a matron. I felt like telling him some of the British matrons were far too old. He started to criticize Canada's conscription policy and his wife had a problem trying to get him to shut up.

While at No. 18 CGH there was a continual movement of nursing sisters, some being posted to the Continent; some arriving from the Continent and others returning to Canada. I felt that I could have taken charge of a moving company. In early June 1945 all the patients had either been transferred to other hospitals or discharged to their units and the hospital was closed. I was then posted to No. 13 Canadian General Hospital. This hospital was located at Cuckfield, Sussex. The previous matron had returned to Canada on compassionate grounds. We went through the same process as at No. 18 CGH and the hospital was closed in early July. It was while I was at No. 13 CGH that a British general election took place. On my way to the hospital on the morning of the election I met the English carpenter, employed at the hospital, on his way to vote. I said, *"Who are you voting for?"* his reply was, *"Labour."* I was non-plussed when the results came in that Winston Churchill had been defeated and that the Labour party had come into power.

My next posting took me to No. 22 General Hospital located at Bramshott Chase – the same location at which I was first stationed in England. There were about 1000 patients; this was being used as a holding hospital – patients were being transferred from hospitals being closed. It was while at No. 22 CGH that I was invited to attend an investiture at Buckingham Palace. I had once before been invited to attend between the time I returned from Italy and went to Normandy. On that occasion it had had to be cancelled due to bomb damage to the palace. The investiture was quite an interesting and exciting experience. I was able to have two guests attend. As I recall now the only women receiving a decoration were three Canadian nursing sisters. There were some 200 altogether, Army, Navy and Air Force. We women were at the tail end. My guests were Lt. (N/S) Marjorie (Cambon) Quail; she had been with me at the Plastic Surgery Unit and Major Hoyle Campbell who was also with the Plastic Surgery Unit. When we women arrived at the palace we were shown into what appeared to be a billiard room. This is where we changed from our street hats to our veils. We then assembled in a large lounge and were lined up in the order in which we would be presented. From this room we could see into the gardens at the rear of the palace. A door led into an auditorium. It was here that we were presented to King George VI who pinned on our medals. We were instructed to step close to him so that he didn't have to reach too far. We were also instructed to give a half curtsy and on leaving the platform to take three steps back before turning to walk down the steps. Major Campbell told me later that the King's face lit up when he saw we three women appear. His face lit up probably because we were at the end of the line. King George made some comment to me to the effect that I had been in Italy and Europe; he could tell this by the ribbons I was wearing. Following the ceremony, which was in the morning, my two guests and I had lunch at the Dorchester Hotel.

Twice during the past three months I had had communications from the Board of Governors of Women's College Hospital,

Toronto, asking me to consider taking the position of superintendent. While still in England the idea seemed quite remote so after the second communication I decided to request that I be sent home. In October 1945 I arrived home after 5 years and 4 months overseas.

After visiting with my family I made an appointment with the Executive Committee of the Board of Governors of Women' s College Hospital and agreed to accept the position of superintendent of the hospital to commence January 1, 1946. This was the beginning of almost thirty years as superintendent, administrator, and latterly, executive director of Women's College Hospital.

Elizabeth B. (Pense) Neil

Graduate of: Hamilton General Hospital School of Nursing, Hamilton, Ontario. Year: 1933

Military History:

Service: RCAMC

Rank: Major

Served: Regular Force

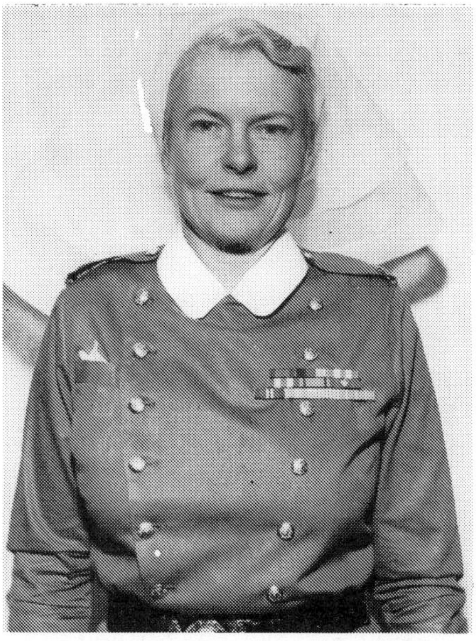

Major Elizabeth Pense, 1960

Prior to World War II, I lived in Kingston and did part-time work at Kingston Military Hospital. In those days most of the small military hospitals were staffed by one medical officer (doctor), one nursing sister and a number of NCOs (non-commissioned officers). When there were any seriously ill patients, special nurses were employed. That is how I got started. The reason for such a staff was that in preparation for war it was essential to have a nucleus of well-trained medical assistants (NCOs). There would be no problem getting nursing sisters.

I applied for the RCAMC but there were no vacancies, so I went to Toronto and took a course in public health nursing at the University of Toronto. I was just finishing the course in the summer of 1939 when I was called by the Army to report to the military hospital at St. Jean's, Quebec. The sister there was getting married. I worked with her for the month of July and alone in August while she went on leave. She returned and got her discharge on September 1st. I was sworn in on the 2nd, and war was declared on the 3rd, so I just made it. No new appointments were made during the war (to the Regular Army). Of course, we were very busy from then on and many hundreds of nursing sisters were taken on, but not in the Regular Army.

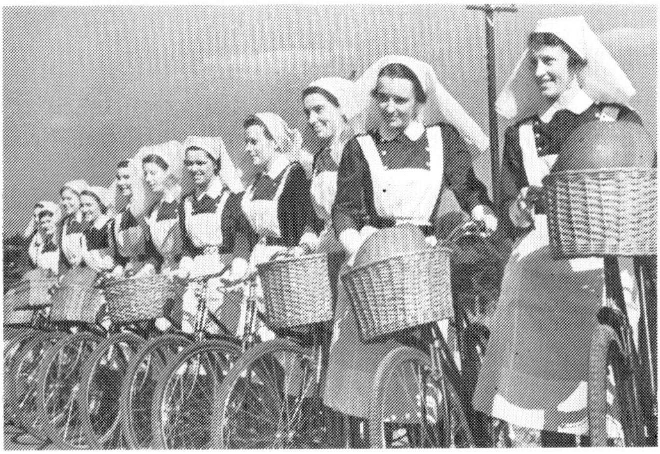

Transport was scarce so we all bought bicycles, Bramshott, Surrey, England 1941
Canadian Forces photo. Photographer: Audrain 23-16

In the spring of 1940 I was posted to the Toronto Military Hospital and a few weeks later we (now officially No. 15 Canadian General Hospital) sailed for England. We heard rumours that No. 5 General from Winnipeg was in the convoy and after a day or two, with the help of binoculars, I saw nursing sisters on another ship.

For three years we served at Bramshott in Surrey, an area where Canadians were serving.

In the spring of 1943 the two senior hospitals (No. 15 with 1200 beds and No. 5 with 600) left England and sailed for the Mediterranean. No. 5 went to Sicily and we set up in Algeria. It was entirely in tents – the wards and our living quarters.

When Italy was invaded, the two hospitals moved forward. No. 15 was set up in Caserta. As we advanced up beyond Rome, I left No. 15 and joined a Casualty Clearing Station, No. 5 CCS – a small mobile hospital. Number 5 and 4 CCS worked together. One would set up as close as was safe and fill up with casualties. Then, as the Army advanced, the other CCS would leap-frog ahead and give the first a chance to deal with its patients.

When Italy was pretty well cleared, the two CCSs moved to Holland and that is where I "finished" the war. By the time it was all over, we were on our way back to England. I spent VE Day as orderly officer in the transit camp in England and, of course, I was annoyed.

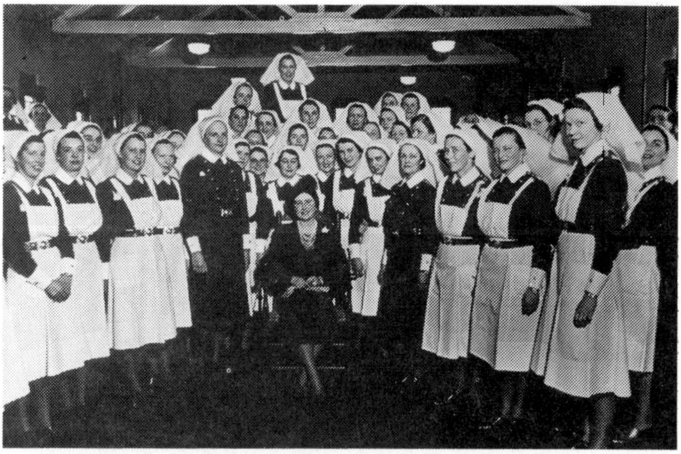

In the Nursing Sister's Mess - a visit from the Queen
No. 15 Candian General Hospital
Canadian Forces photo, 15833

On returning to Canada as many as possible of the nursing sisters were posted to or near their homes, so I had a year in Kingston. (Of course, the majority were released.)

In 1946 I was posted to Winnipeg and promoted to captain (matron). I had about a year at the Winnipeg Military Hospital and then it was closed and the patients were sent to the DVA (Veteran's) hospital. Our staff (NCOs and nurses) went with them but still lived with the Army. However, there was no position for a matron and I was taken on the staff of the (Prairie) Command Medical Officer as command matron. I learned a lot there. I made regular visits to the other military hospitals in Prairie Command – at Shilo, Rivers and Churchill.

During the three years I was there it was decided that some nursing sisters should train for survival in arctic conditions which were available at Churchill on Hudson's Bay. I was put in charge and we ran two courses with five nurses in each. The Americans were interested and sent two of the U.S. Army nurses (the U.S. Army nurses were Frances Thorp and Ruth Schultz) to take the course. We slept in tents (five to a tent) and in a snow hut (igloo). We were taught how to build an igloo – but two of our nurses were small, and even I found the 40-pound blocks of snow very tiring. We never got a top on ours. The temperature was 40 degrees F.

After three years in Prairie Command, I was posted to Whitehorse in the Yukon Territories where I spent a year as matron of the military hospital.

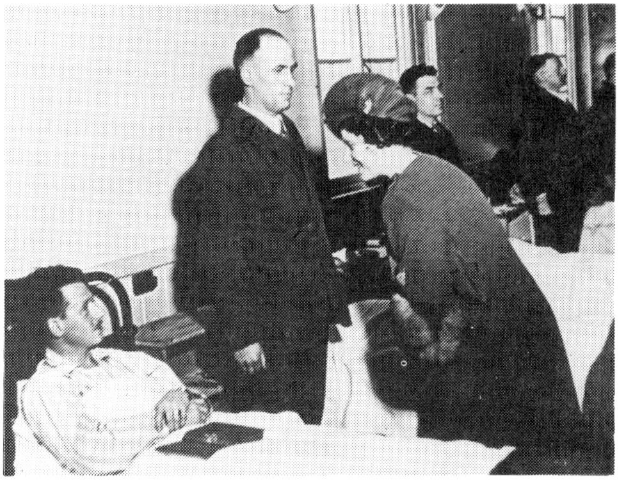

1941 The Queen visited the hospital and all the wards (20 of them)
No. 15 Canadian General Hospital in Surrey

Next I was posted as matron to the Toronto Military Hospital and served there until the start of the second year of the Korean War. In Japan they had a British Commonwealth Military Hospital – Captain Margaret Dodderidge was the Canadian matron for the first year. The British and Australians had nursing sisters there, too, but there were only the American nurses in Korea.

About the time I arrived in Japan it was decided that they must have a Commonwealth hospital in Korea in order to cut down the time lost by soldiers sent to Japan for minor surgery or medical reasons. Then probably to a convalescent centre and perhaps, on leave. Therefore, I was sent over with five other nursing sisters (two British, two Australian and one other Canadian). Illness and minor surgery could then be looked after in Korea and the men returned to duty without long delays.

Several months later the Canadian Field Dressing Station was enlarged and the Canadian nurses were posted there leaving the British and Australians at the Commonwealth hospital. The war was less mobile by this time and most surgery could be done at the FDS. More Canadians were sent over from Japan. I was the matron.

When the Korean War ended, I was on my way home (my year being up). It was disappointing.

After a year as matron at Kingston Military Hospital I was posted to the RCAMC School at Camp Borden. There I was put in charge of the medical training company where we ran courses for RCAMC personnel – new entry soldiers (after their basic training), more advanced ones, and nursing sisters. I was at Borden for six years, and then reached retirement age – and was replaced by Major (later Lt./Colonel) Hallie Sloan. She went on from there to become matron-in-chief in Ottawa.

After retirement I met, again, a New Zealand retired officer whom I had known in Italy, and to everyone's surprise, I married him and moved to New Zealand. There we had a very happy life living in a small town on the Coast. He died a few years ago, and now I am in a very pleasant retirement home.

Bernice Seeds

Graduated from: Toronto Western Hospital School of Nursing.
Year: 1938

Military History:

Service: RCAMC

Rank: Lt. N/S

Served: 10 September, 1939
to 10 August, 1945

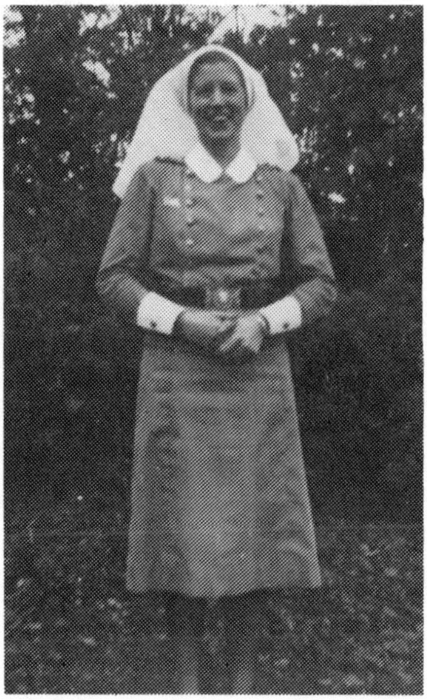

Lt. N/S Bernice Seeds

I was asked to join the 15th Canadian General Hospital by my superintendent of nurses, and I was pleased to do so. I left for England in June of 1940.

I served in Canada, England, North Africa, and Italy with the No. 15 Canadian General Hospital. Our hospital was broken up in Italy and I returned to a hospital in England in December 1944. From there I returned to Canada (Chorly Park) in May 1945 where I remained until my discharge in August 1945. I spent five years overseas. Our first casualties were from Dieppe and this was our introduction to the wastefulness of young lives. War is no solution to problems.

NO. 16 CANADIAN GENERAL HOSPITAL

Alyce Baines
Elspeth (Monteith) Beckett
Muriel (Archer) Gilchrist
Mae (Cartwright) McKay

No. 16 Canadian General Hospital, Vancouver, B.C., received orders to mobilize on 27 December 1941; they were to replace No. 8 General Hospital at Debert, Nova Scotia. Matron Mary E. Minor interviewed prospective nursing sisters – they were not to mobilize at present.

The unit boarded the train 10 June 1942, the first hospital unit to leave British Columbia. They boarded the HMT (Hospital Motor Transport) *Letitia* 15 June 1942 at Halifax and a week later arrived in Scotland. After a brief stay at Minley Manor, they located at Cuckfield until June 1942 when the unit moved to Marston Green, Warwickshire, England.

In May 1944 nursing sisters were sent to various hospitals as the unit prepared for field training. Major P/M P.J. Nelson replaced P/M M.E. Mills who married and was assigned to No. 9 General Hospital.

With Matron Nelson and 22 nursing sisters at camp "C" near Southampton the unit prepared to move. On 30 August 1944 the No. 16 General arrived at Bayeux in France. Nursing sisters were taken over by hospital ship *Lady Mann* and were across the road from No. 10 General on Littry Road, known as "Harley Street." As with most Canadian medical units that followed the advance of the Allied troops, No. 16 moved from France through Belgium to Holland. In August of 1945, No. 16 was located at Sogel, Germany, in the old hunting lodge of the Duke of Arenburg.

The end of March 1946 the unit left Cuxhaven, Germany, for the Repatriation Depot in England and No. 16 General ceased to be a unit in the Canadian Army.

Alyce Baines

Information provided for Alyce Baines by Jean Gagnon.

Graduate of: University of British Columbia, B.A., X-ray Technician

Military History:

Service: RCAMC

Rank: 2nd Lt. Home Sister

Served: 1942 to 1946

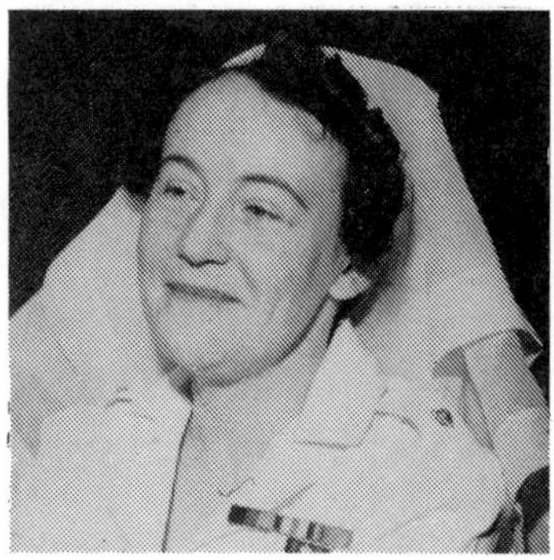

2/Lt. Home Sister Alyce Baines 1942

No. 16 Canadian General Hospital was indeed fortunate to have Alyce as our "home sister." She made a home away from home for us. She managed even with rationing to have the cooks turn out excellent meals – with the help of some scrounging and our parcels. As a hostess she was beyond compare – our parties were always a great success. These things might sound trivial but we were a very happy unit thanks to Alyce!

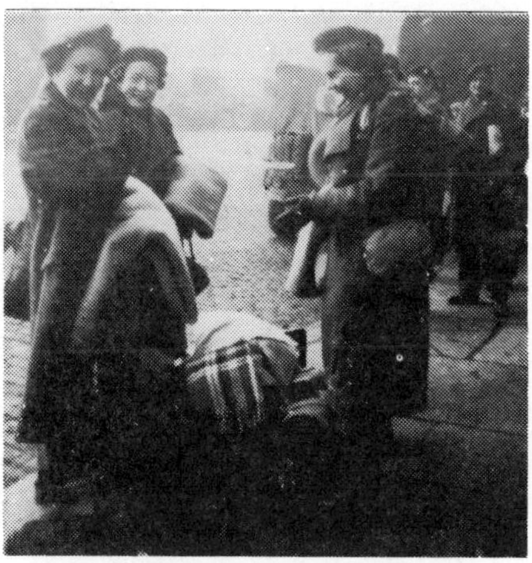

N/S Muriel Burnes, H/S Alyce Baines, Isobet McAstock
Iso, Alyce and Muriel looking like refugees. It was cold as ice.

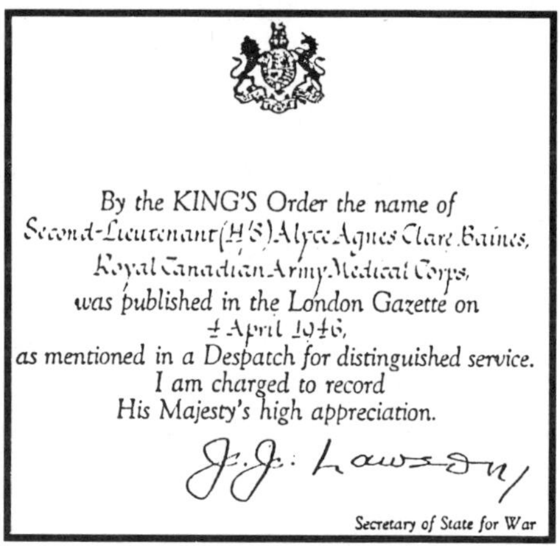

By the KING'S Order the name of
Second-Lieutenant (H/S) Alyce Agnes Clare Baines,
Royal Canadian Army Medical Corps,
was published in the London Gazette on
4 April 1946,
as mentioned in a Despatch for distinguished service.
I am charged to record
His Majesty's high appreciation.

J. J. Lawson

Secretary of State for War

Mentioned in Despatches

V.E. (Elspeth [Bette] Monteith) Beckett

Graduated from: Vancouver General Hospital School of Nursing. Year: 1936

Military History:

Service: RCAMC

Rank: Lt. N/S

Served: May 1940 to April 1942

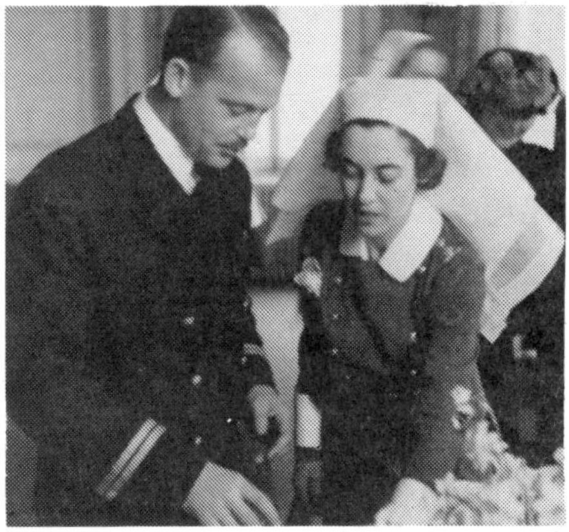

Wedding reception in the Lodge, No. 5 CGH. I was an hour late as I got my discharge that day. We were married in Taplow Anglican Church April 1942

I worked at Vancouver General from 1936, mostly nights at first, till applying for the Army in November 1939. I wanted a change as I was doing head nurse and assistant and was tired after six months. Also, my father had been in World War One and was badly wounded, so, of course, I was interested in becoming a member of the RCAMC.

I was accepted in the Canadian Army in May 1940 and posted to MD No. 11 at Work Point Military Hospital, Victoria, B.C. We were five nursing sisters – two from the First World War. They later formed No. 16 Canadian General and went overseas in 1942. I went with matron in May 1941. We left Montreal on the *Vancouver Island* , formerly a German supply ship, the *Weser*, captured by Commander Beard in the Gulf of Mexico. Fourteen nursing sisters boarded with a crew of about six to eight. A fast ship we

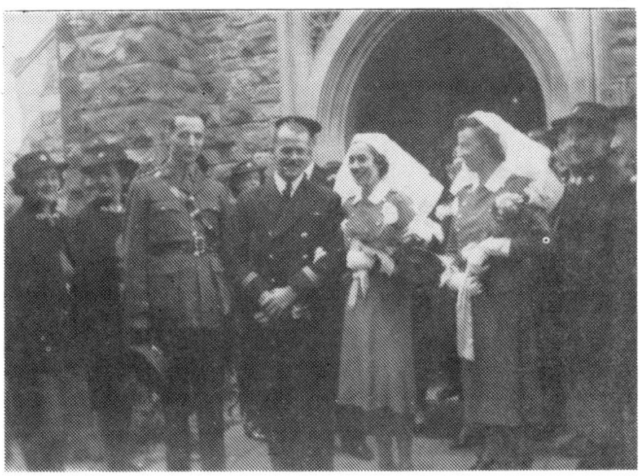

Wedding to Fred Beckett, Imperial Airways, Taplow church, 21 April 1942. Best man - Harvey McNicol, MD; bridesmaid - Dorothy Richardson, No. 5 CGH The nursing sisters were mainly Winnipeg General Hospital graduates.

were told, so no convoy. We were attacked by submarine and shelled on surface mid-Atlantic and chased for one and a half hours. They left us and we went back to our route but engines were damaged. We kept our clothes on all the way and proceeded slowly on to Greenoch. We had radio silence on ship so did not know who Hess was. The train track ahead of us was bombed so we were dirty and late getting into London. We were met by head staff of nursing sisters and given nine days' leave. The *Weser* was sunk with all hands on the return trip: having women aboard saved us, probably!

Muriel (Archer) Gilchrist

Graduated from: Vancouver General Hospital School of Nursing. Year: 1940

Military History:

Service: RCAMC

Rank: Lt. N/S

Served: May 1942 to March 1946

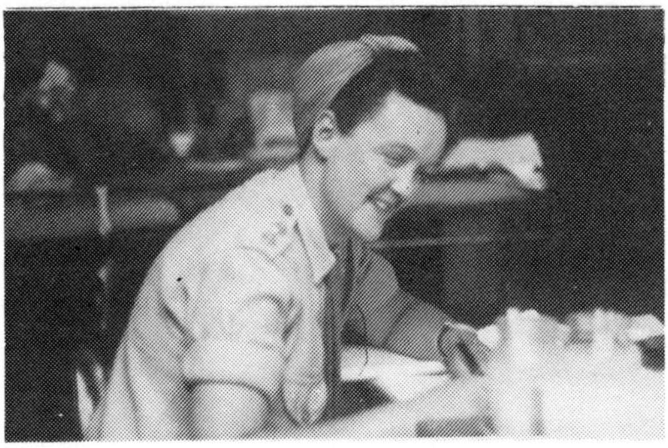

Lt. N/S Muriel (Archer) Gilchrist, July 1945

I had been on the Reserve list for over a year when I was appointed to No. 16 Canadian General Hospital in May 1942. In June of that year, the unit travelled by train to Halifax, thence sailing in a small convoy to Scotland.

No installation being ready for the hospital, the nursing sisters were quartered in buildings adjacent to No. 15 CGH at Bramshott, Surrey. In August Evelyn Johnstone and I were temporarily attached to No. 2 CCS on an estate near Cranleigh. On 19 August the unfortunate raid on Dieppe occurred and we received some of the less serious casualties. Work was not arduous so there was plenty of time to ride our bikes around the lovely countryside, to swim in the pool or play tennis, and we enjoyed, too, the company of the friendly members of the unit and the mess dinners in the former nursery.

It was October before we returned to No. 16 which was set up now at Cuckfield, Sussex, near Hayward's Heath. The unit took part in the "Sawbones" scheme (exercise) in early November, but it was later in the month before we finally moved to Marston Green, near Birmingham – a different sort of place altogether. No more quick trips to London or dances and parties at other units. On 31 July Evelyn Johnstone was married in the village church and I was her bridesmaid. Several of our nurses had been wed in the past year.

In October, Ruth F. and I were sent to No. 5 CCS at Copthorne, Sussex, for an "indefinite period of training in the field," which turned out to be more than ten days. There were many changes in personnel and even more rumours in the air at that time.

Finally, in January 1944, Ruth and I were back at Bramshott, part of a group going to Italy as increment and reinforcements. Assembling the proper kit and changing into khaki as well as drilling and marching kept us busy. Blues, civvies and other items were put into kit storage. After 14 days at sea on board *Almanzora* we reached Naples and went out to No. 14 CGH at Caserta, March 1944. There we nursed more seriously wounded and dreadful burn cases from tank brew-ups. In July the hospital was packed up and the move on, but a gradual process, so that it was late in

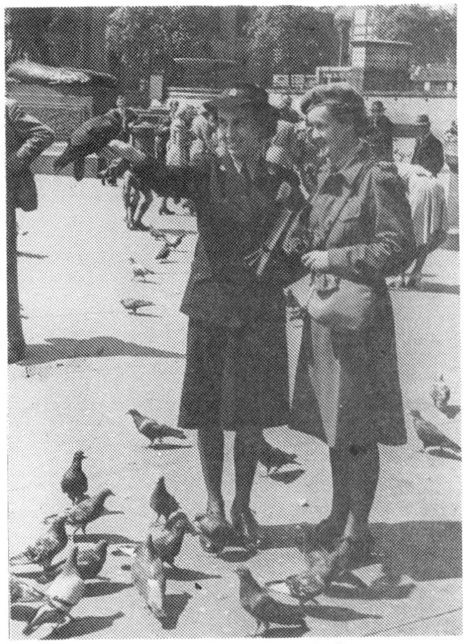

Trafalgar Square 4 August 1945
L: Norah (Mallandaine) Noiles
R: Muriel (Archer)

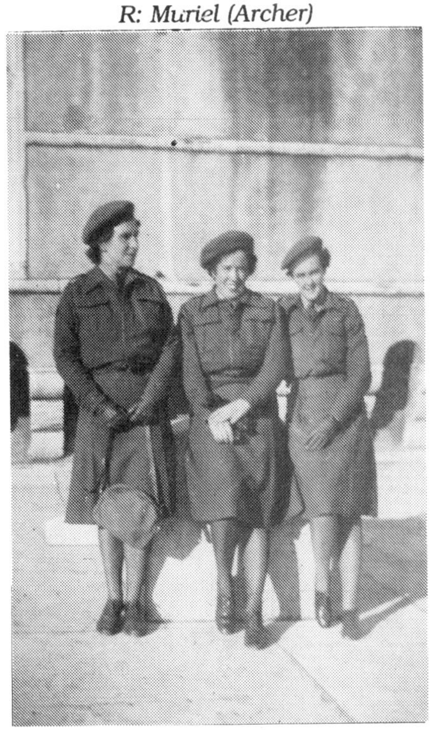

L-R: Lt. Allison, Dietitian, Lt. N/S Ruth Fleming, Lt. N/S Muriel Archer at Castel San Angelo Rome 1944

August when we reached Perugia. Immediately a dozen of us were sent off to No. 1 CGH at Iesi on the Adriatic. A week there only, followed by a move up the coast to Cattolica, the hospital in a former hotel right on the sandy beach. Mmmm.

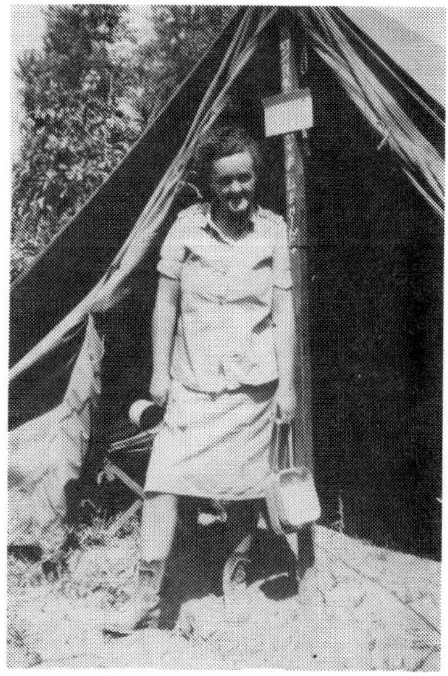

"Dust Bowl" Cancello, Italy July 1944 No. 14 Cdn. General Hospital. Lt. N/S Muriel Archer.

In early December, Ruth and I spent a week at No. 1 FDS on a quiet country estate, sleeping in the tiny chapel (toilet in the confessional). From there to 2 FDS at Russi within shooting distance of "the other side." I did not get to 5 CCS at Ravenna for Christmas dinner, but had a meal out of cans with a friend on lone duty at his ack-ack battery. I had attended a carol service in the gunners' mess Christmas Eve and found the simple service and decorations and the sincerity of the men moving. We rejoined 5 CCS at Ravenna in January 1945 and in March the big move was on. We nursing sisters sailed from Naples to Marseilles, overnighted at an American hospital (real butter and ice cream were among the tasty foods that were a treat to us, but not to the U.S. nurses). Next, we flew in a small plane ranged on either side on metal seats with our backs to the windows. From Ghent we all had a nine-day leave in England and then joined the rest of the unit at Oss, Holland, where we were billeted in private homes in pairs.

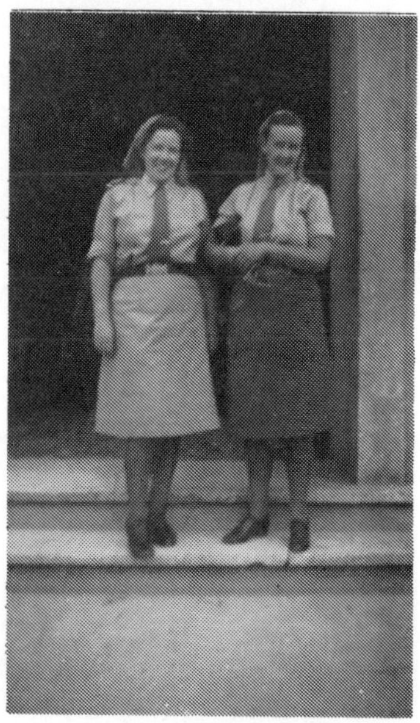

L: Ruth Fleming
R: Muriel (Archer) Gilchrist

In the ensuing months 5 CCS moved several times around Holland, and I had the occasional short tour of duty at 4 CCS, No. 1 CGH, etc. Finally, in July, I left Holland and reached Winnipeg in September.

After a few months at Fort

Osborne I was discharged in March.

While I was unhappy at leaving No. 16 which I always felt was my unit, I am grateful for the experience in Italy and Holland, not to mention that I would never have otherwise met my husband.

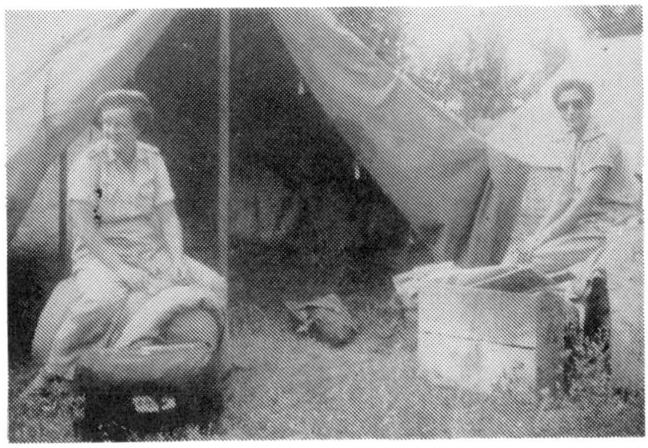

Monday PM, 11 September 1944, waiting for an ambulance to take us to Catallica. L: Muriel Archer R: Olive Stewart

---

Mary [May] (Cartwright) McKay

Graduated from: Royal Jubilee Hospital School of Nursing, Victoria, B.C. Year: 1931

Military History:

Service: RCAMC

Rank: Lt. N/S

Served: June 1941 to October 1944

The fall of Poland and European countries convinced me I should join the Army.

My military experience began in June 1941 at Nanaimo Military Hospital. From there I went overseas with No. 16 Canadian General Hospital. I was with No. 16 at Cuckfield and Marston Green 1942-1943, then went to No. 2 CCS, No. 22 CGH, No. 9 CGH (Horsham).

Finally, I was in charge of the Rehabilitation Centre, near Bramshott

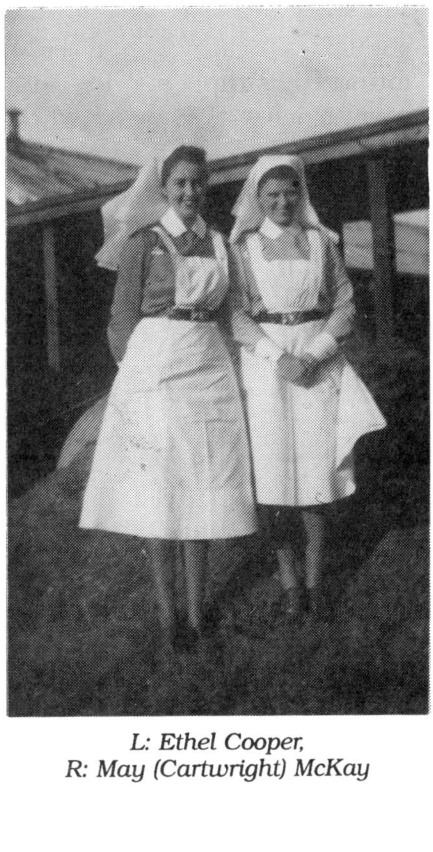

L: Ethel Cooper, R: May (Cartwright) McKay

NO. 17 CANADIAN GENERAL HOSPITAL

Irene (Shantz) Lescom
Gaetane (LaBonte) Kerr

No. 17 Canadian General Hospital mobilized at Montreal. In the fall of 1942, No. 17 General left Halifax for overseas duty in a convoy of fifty-seven ships. They first arrived at Crowthorne, then were assigned to Pinewood in February of 1943. The matron was Suzanne Giroux.

No. 17 General remained a fixed installation in the U.K. and prepared for casualties coming from Normandy. In May of 1944 the unit began preparations for D-Day; their patients were evacuated to No. 11 General at Taplow and No. 20 General at Leavesden.

The unit closed in December of 1945.

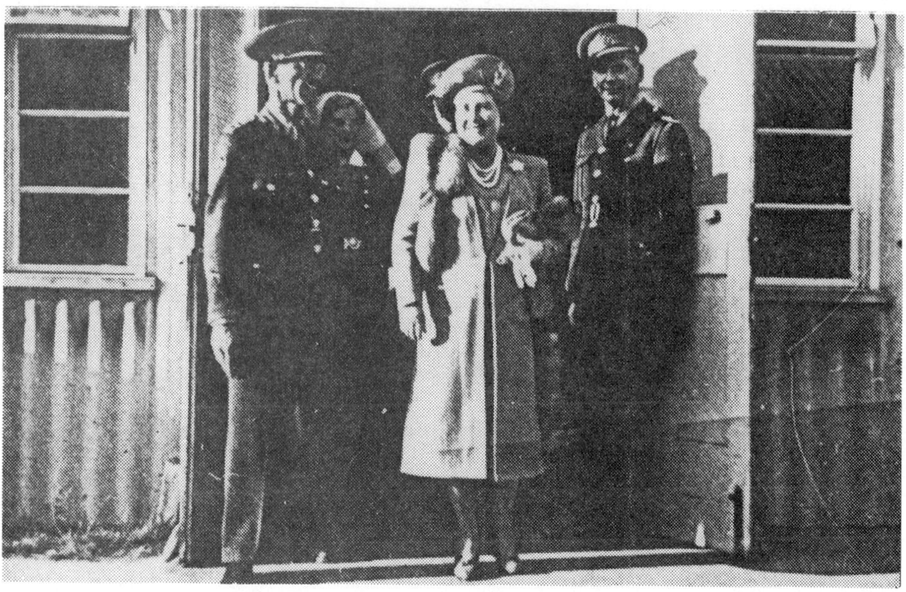

Queen Elizabeth visited No. 17 CGH, Pinewood 23 March 1945

Irene (Shantz) Lescom

Graduated from: Kitchener-Waterloo Hospital School of Nursing. Year: 1940

Military History:

Service: RCAMC

Rank: Lieutenant N/S.

Served: 1940 to 1942

Written by her daughter, Mrs. Cheryl Lescom Shubat.

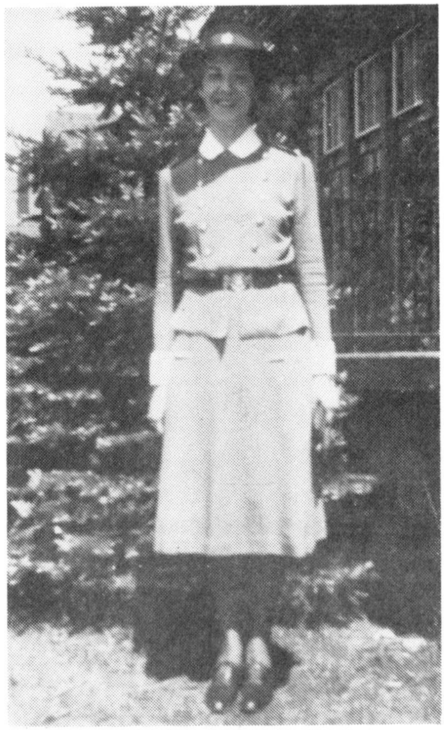

Lt. N/S Irene Shantz

My mother passed away 17 March 1993. I am her only daughter and I would like to have her mentioned in the book about Canadian military nurses.

She often talked about her war years and as I grew older I learned to enjoy the memories she shared with me.

When I asked her why she chose the Army she always said she joined the Service because cigarettes were a penny apiece. She went overseas with No. 17 Canadian General Hospital in 1942. She fondly remembered her companions from her time in the RCAMC.

Gaetane (LaBonte) Kerr

Graduated from: St. Jean de Dieu Psychiatric Hospital School of Nursing, Montreal, Quebec. Year: 1940

Military History:

Service: RCAMC

Rank: Lieut. N/S

Served: August 1942 to May 1947

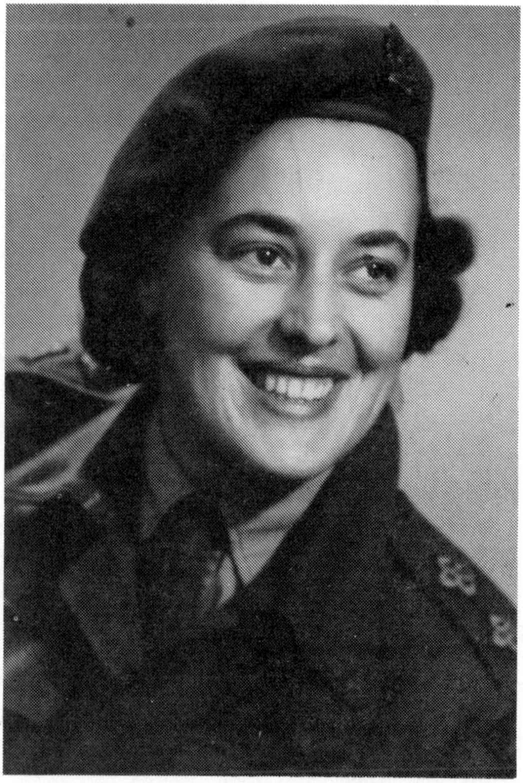

Lieut. N/S Gaetane LaBonte Kerr, May 1945

When I graduated in Public Health, I was working in Montreal doing mental tests. I missed bedside care very much – that was my reason for joining the Service.

No. 17 Canadian General Hospital, which I joined in the summer of 1942, sailed for overseas duties almost immediately after our military training of two months in the old Kingston Military Hospital. We thought the worst was over, as we had been transplanted very suddenly from our cosy French milieu to a completely different world in English. Matron Goodeve told us we had all passed with flying colours and congratulated us. She seemed to enjoy our joie de vivre (when not studying) and had us sing in French. I was soon called "All Wet" because she would order me to sing that thing of a song that my generation never sang: *Allouette*.

Our convoy of 75 ships was the largest one to date. It all seemed like a rather pleasant adventure at first, until we repeatedly had to dive down into the dark womb of our beautiful ship because of the numerous alerts. The large patches of oil on the sea often reminded us of the seriousness of the hour.

In England, one hour away from London, Pinewood was our

new location, in the beautiful English countryside, for the next three years. The Nissen huts harbouring the bombs alongside the road, the multiple alerts, the majestic sight of the searchlights criss-crossing the sky every night were to remind us of the reason why we were over there.

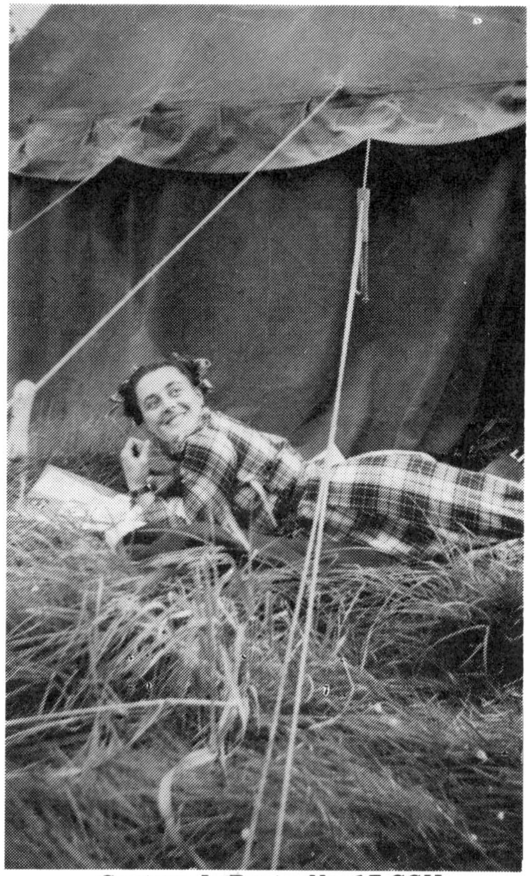

Gaetane LaBonte, No. 17 CGH

Although our hospital was kept busy, it did not seem all that different from a general hospital except for the young patients all about the same age group. We treated, for the most part, the common illnesses and the surgery did not deal with any unusual cases except during a routine training exercise where accidents did occur. The patients helped us a great deal in correcting us in English, when the lack of current language experience got us into trouble. They especially marvelled at the fact that all of us unconsciously reverted to French when counting for the dreadful Monday inventory.

When bombings were reactivated, we were confined to a five or six mile zone for travelling. We then used our beloved bicycles, went horseback riding, and admired the countryside, beautiful in every season.

Our Hospital Anniversary Shows were very colourful and really entertaining. It also revealed hidden or earlier talents in some of us. Ruth McKinnon, our Physiotherapist (from Lake Qu'appelle), took three months of her spare time once, to organize a "Gay Paree" number. I was asked to practise with the boys (10 orderlies) who were really good at kicking – oh la la la... The day before the great opening, they informed me that they were not going to go on the stage if I did not go on myself. Well what could I do – I was given a tutu, a bit longer than theirs, and I hear that it was a great success.

When the invasion finally came, some of us were bicycling as usual for a night fling just before D-Day, a deafening sound growing louder and louder had us call the rest of the nurses outside where we witnessed the great formation of the gliders circling overhead. The Americans, stationed near us in Reading, were taking their hundreds and hundreds of parachutists over.

Only three days afterwards did we receive our first convoy of patients. What a ridiculous war, I thought, as I was surprised to see a German helping a Tommy and visa versa. A day before they would have shot each other. The Canadians came to us two or three days later, much to our concern.

Soon after, anxious to get closer to action, I joined No. 20 CGH but only managed to cross the Channel three months later after learning to be a real soldier, or at least to be more efficient in the field.

My few months in Antwerp where the Jerries had vowed to flatten that big harbour by January were certainly the worst of my war. One big bombing of an ENSA (recreational) house on Saturday brought us about 500 casualties. As we entered our wards, we were greeted by incessant moaning, growing louder when the buzz bombs renewed their activities. Just before Christmas, the hospital, in a too-dangerous zone, was evacuated.

Poor No. 20 CGH again disbanded. I was sent to 88 British General in Tilburg, Holland. It was a very dour surrounding. Holland, so hurt, was very sad then, the nurses were also very tired as they had endured since Bayeux. They would go to their little camp cot bed after work to rest or read. The dormitories in the old convent had one ration of heating oil at 4:00 P.M. No one bothered to fetch it.

Because I spoke French I was often invited into homes where this generation spoke French as a second language. Nothing to eat but oysters in the good months. We all appreciated the ancestors' wine. We occasionally provided Spam or sardines.

The flying bombs were still going at night, but flying overhead to Belgium, probably.

Back to Belgium and I am posted to 10 CGH in the

Resuscitation Ward. My three weeks there topped all previous war experience. We cared for the very ill of all nationalities, Allied or prisoner. I was so often overwhelmed in witnessing the sense of abnegation and generosity in those so badly wounded. Lepke, this fierçe looking man sitting on a bed, head and neck bandaged, body cast, arm extended, his eyes following my every move. When my failing courage took me to his side, I offered my help. He said to me in good French *"Canayin Sister, if you sit here for five minutes to rest your feet, it will do me more good than any prescription you have to offer."* He was one of the few "La Chaudiere Regt." who had fought in Italy earlier.

Other times you would feel totally useless, helpless, short of words. In the next bed was a Tommy, blinded in a recent encounter. He was suffering to the point where no sedation had taken effect. Trying to comfort him, I pointed out that after sunrise, often pains subside a little. He shouted at me *"How can you be so cruel as to remind me of sunrise, when you know that I'll never see the sun again?"*

In spite of it all – on top of it all – Victory came about. No. 20 CGH, a whole unit again, had been caring for POWs. Our Canadians, for the most part, were now way ahead of Turnhout, which meant that rejoicing for Victory was rather limited. I quickly joined my adopted Belgian family hoping to laugh and let go, only to be met in the great marble hall by five solemn little grandchildren. They were dressed with their "official" little sailor suits, like in the Von Trapp family. One at a time they kissed my hand, congratulated me. I was, they said, a Liberator.

NO. 18 CANADIAN GENERAL HOSPITAL

No. 18 Canadian General Hospital was formed in Toronto in November 1942 and moved to Kingston 1 January 1943 with Lt. Col. Abbott as commanding officer. The unit moved to Coburg, Ontario, in February of 1943, then to New Brunswick in July of 1943. From there the unit proceeded overseas to Bramshott, England, then to Cherry Tree Hospital, Colchester.

The following letter describing Christmas 1944 in No. 18 Canadian General Hospital at Colchester, England, was sent by Nursing Sister Margaret Middleton to her parents in Clinton, Ontario.

"Happy New Year to all, here's hoping I will be home before next one comes along. Well, Christmas is over and I think we all had a very nice one under present conditions. We worked so hard making it a good one for the boys in hospital that we completely forgot ourselves which was a good thing. Right now we are so tired we can hardly keep going.

"We decorated each ward with holly which is very plentiful and lovely over here. We saved all cellophane and silver paper for past months and were able to make icicles for the trees, also cellophane wreaths with a bit of red and holly tied on them. We had some red and green streamers which we put up around the ward.

"The occupational therapy girls and Red Cross have worked since November 1st painting Santa faces, candy sticks, stars and small things for the trees. Each ward had a pine tree. My boys gathered acorns from the bush and painted them red and hung them on the trees. We also used a lot of white cotton wool with Epsom Salts on it for snow. It is marvelous what you can do when you try.

"We set up tables with sheets on them for all up patients. Each patient had one orange and two eggs for breakfast. Christmas dinner they had soup, chicken and goose, dressing, potatoes, gravy, carrots, peas, celery, pickles, rolls, Christmas pudding, coffee, candy, nuts, a Mac apple and cigarettes. They really had a marvelous Christmas; everyone said they had been here four years and this was the best since they left home.

"The sisters of our ward had enough of their own stuff to wrap either soap and cigarettes, chocolate bars and gum, or cigarettes and gum for each patient. We did up 90 small gifts. Then there were 16 boys who had never received parcels since coming overseas and we packed a box for each of them. There are only ten nursing sisters on our ward so we thought we did very well. Then the Red Cross gave each patient in hospital one pair of socks and a handkerchief, one package of cigarettes, shaving cream, candy and a pencil which certainly meant a lot to the boys. I thought you would be interested in what the Red Cross gave.

"We had the mess – ours and the officers' – to decorate which made a lot of work. We had our dinner Christmas Eve in order that we might spend all day Christmas in the ward with the boys. Our dinner was just the same as the one the patients had the next day. The tables looked lovely with holly, candles in holders made from tin cans cut and curled. We had dinner at six then the Army show was here to put on a concert. Then at midnight fifty of us went to church. We went in ambulances. On the way, we sang hymns and carols. We were all rather homesick. I thought of last year, all the family at church on Christmas day.

"Here we are so far away, Canadians and Americans in an English church. Figuring the time, it would be just seven o'clock at home. No one said a word, but everyone's mind was away off to the things each held dear at Christmas."

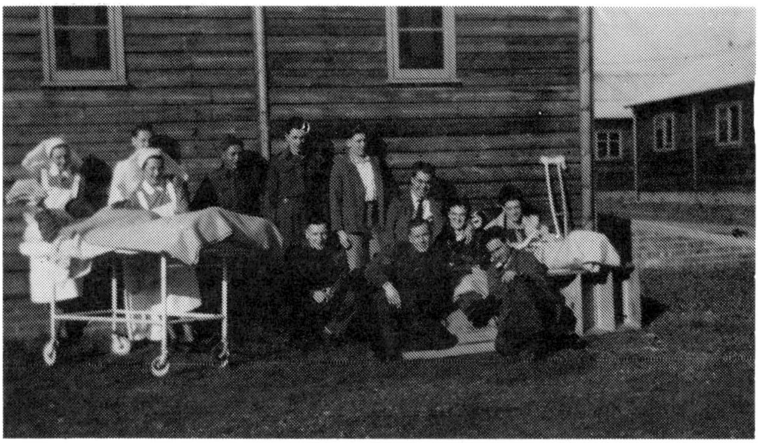

No. 18 CGH, Colchester, England
L: N/S Bambi Morton, N/S Margaret (Middleton) Counter with patients outside Spider C

NO. 19 CANADIAN GENERAL HOSPITAL

Anne (Gair) Evans
Gertrude James
Elsie McIntyre
Florence (Taylor) Mellway
Helen Mussallem
Edith Schofield
Angela Marie (La Croix) Smith

No. 19 Canadian General Hospital left Sussex, New Brunswick, for Halifax on 3 May 1944. The unit sailed on the *Empress of Scotland* two days later, zigzagging across the Atlantic until they reached Liverpool. They were assigned to Marston Green, Warwickshire, England with Matron Major Foster and Captain Assistant Matron C.T. Lunn. No. 19 was one of the last group of hospitals to go overseas and remained in the U.K. to accept casualties from the Continent.

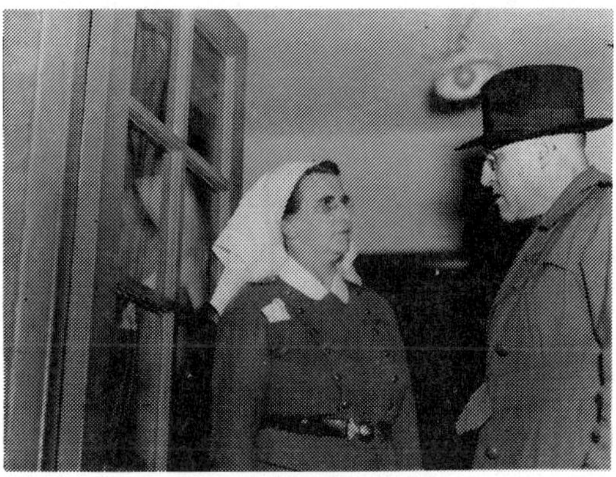

No. 19 CGH Marston Green, 15 October 1944
Colonel the Honourable J.L. Ralston, Canada's Minister of National Defence chatting with Chief Matron A/Major Ann Foster, Berwick, NS in a Canadian hospital in England.
Canadian Forces photo

Anne A. (Gair) Evans

Graduated from: University of Alberta Faculty of Nursing, Edmonton, Alberta. Year: 1941

Military History:

Service: RCAMC

Rank: Lieut. N/S

Served: January 11, 1943 to April 26,1946

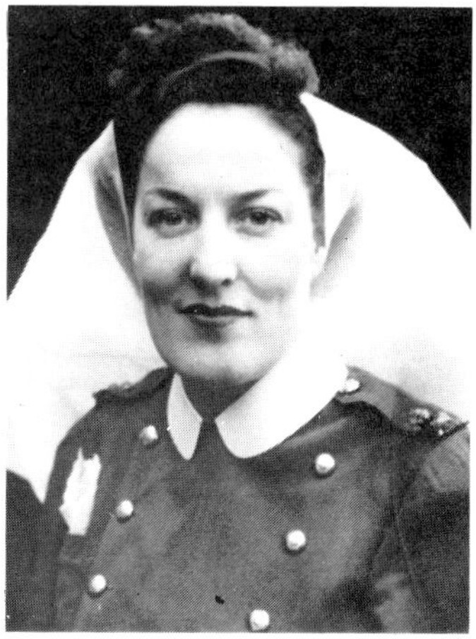

Lt. N/S Anne (Gair) Evans

I graduated from the University of Alberta hospital in 1941. After working in a small country hospital, a sanatorium and a crippled children's hospital I wanted to move on and try something that would give me adventure and something entirely different. I joined the RCAMC in Calgary and was called to duty on January 11th, 1943, and posted to the Currie Military Hospital in that city. After a short period there I was sent to the Suffield Military Hospital in southern Alberta, which was a mustard gas experimental station and had a chemical warfare station close by. I was jokingly told I must have done something awful to be sent to a desert area in such isolation. It turned out to be one of my more interesting experiences in military nursing.

The nursing care at this hospital was very different than I had experienced anywhere at that time. Young men who had volunteered for service at this camp were treated for severe burns from mustard gas, and until then I had never seen such extensive burns. One day when they were on

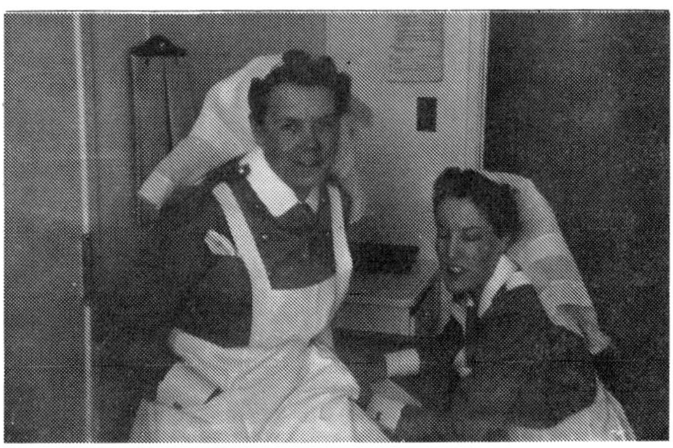

L: Margaret Hodson R: Anne Gair on duty, Suffield, Alberta 1943

a manoeuvre, the wind changed direction and the troops were caught unaware and 24 hours later were admitted with badly burned eyes. This required careful treatment and was something that was not common to nurses usually. Other nursing sisters I knew there were: Margaret Hodson, Rossie Hughes, Jean Boychuk and Elsie Smith.

Due to family circumstances I was on compassionate leave so my departure for overseas was delayed. I was posted to the Edmonton Military Hospital for a short time and in the spring of 1944 went to Sussex, New Brunswick, for basic training, route marches, map reading, etc. I went overseas with No. 19 CGH which consisted of nurses from all across Canada. After a few route marches some of us found we didn't have proper fitting boots.

In May of 1944 we arrived in England and were stationed at Marston Green, near Birmingham. It wasn't long until we started sending patients home to make way for the casualties we expected as D-Day was approaching. In the early hours of June 6th we heard the drone of many planes going over our camp and my pal, Nursing Sister Lu McComb, whispered to me to see if I was awake. We knew the day had arrived and we went to the mess for coffee. Gradually other nurses joined us. Very little was said and we weren't quite sure what to expect next.

It was not long before our hospital was full of the casualties we expected, and we were very busy for weeks. All being young men, most our own age, it was sad to see what some of them had suffered through, particularly those with amputations and loss of vision. However, most of them were happy patients as many knew their time of serving was over and they would be going home.

In July 1944 five sisters were chosen to go to No. 15 CGH in Italy. Sisters Skelton, Margaret Chisholm, Lu McComb, one called Jessie, and me – Anne Gair, left on the 12-day journey. This hospital was near Naples and many nurses there had served in Africa. The first thing we noticed was how yellow their skins were and it wasn't long before we were the same, as we had to take a medication to ward off malaria and it had a discolouring effect on the skin.

Here we had wounds of all kinds, some severe and some not. There were a number of amputations of limbs, some internal injuries and many malarial patients. The malaria patients suffered a lot with the repetitive relapses of shaking chills, fever and sweats. Again, I found many patients happy and glad to be in a hospital and have a bed to sleep in. They were happy to know their duties were finished and they said it was nice for them to be able to talk to girls who could understand them. One patient I had had a large part of his back that had lost its pigmentation. He was a man I had nursed in the mustard gas station in Alberta.

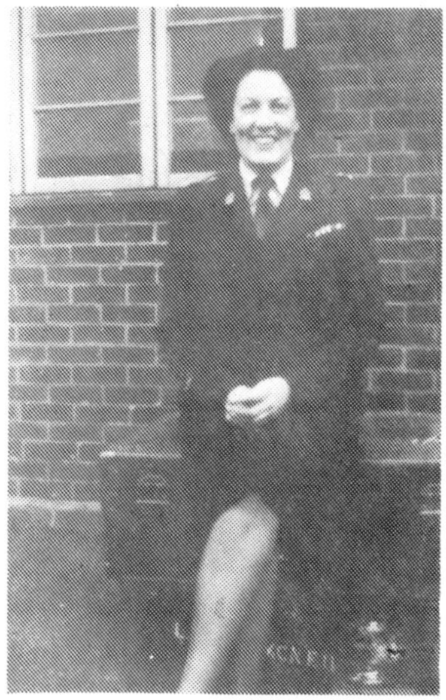

Anne Gair ready to leave England 1946 waiting for pickup of trunks

A number of patients were insecure and wondered how they would fit in to life at home with what injuries they had. Some wondered if their girlfriends would still want to marry them. I feel we could have helped them more if we had more time to spend with them, and in some cases, had more psychological training. Sisters at this hospital I remember were: June Plummer, Maxine Llewellyn, Queena Esdale, Roz Turner, Sally Turnbull, Verna White, and Betty Pense.

I remember being very cold in the winter and hot in the summer. We had little heat in our living quarters – a small coal oil heater that didn't warm you unless you were right bedside it. When we washed our underclothing and stockings we put them on a few days later and they were still damp. On night duty the only skin showing was our face and hands as we had to be protected against malarial mosquitoes, and it was very hot to be dressed like that.

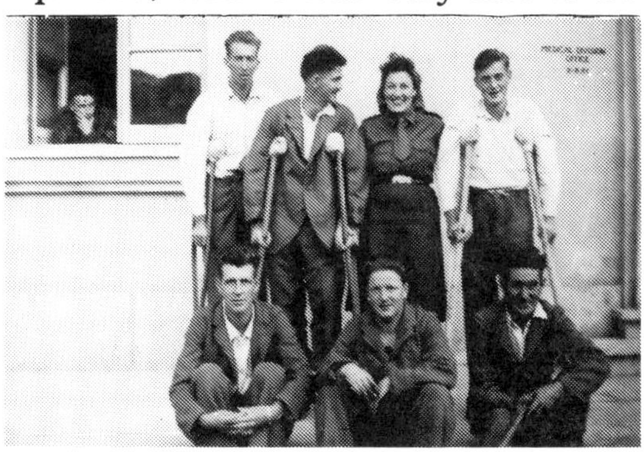

Anne Gair with patients at No. 15 CGH, Caserta, Italy, 1945

When we closed down No. 15 CGH and returned to No. 23 in England which was near Watford. My stay there wasn't long and I was transferred to No. 4 CGH at Farnborough. It was here my friend Lu McComb was sent to Germany for the duration and I missed her a great deal.

When the war ended in May 1945 we were confined to barracks. This was understood and accepted. After being a nurse in training there were no restrictions or discipline imposed on me that I would ever find a worry to me. I remained at No. 4 CGH until my departure to Canada in April 1946.

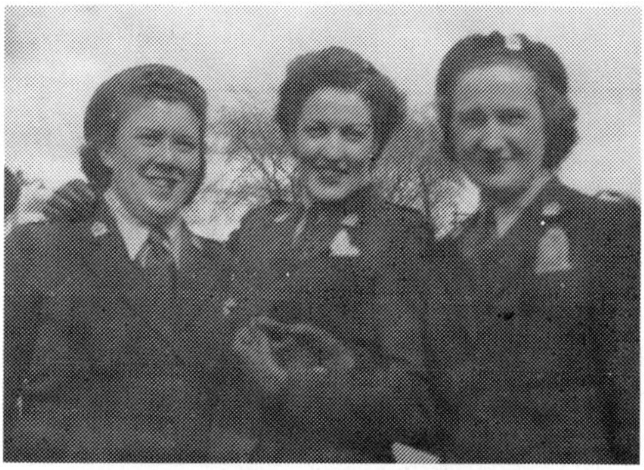

L-R: Lu McComb, Anne Gair, Jeannie Fontana, Sussex, NB, 1994

After my return home and having time with my family and a good rest, I felt lonely and found I missed my Army friends very much and I missed the active life I had had. I did special nursing for the summer in Calgary, but decided to return for studies in public health. I went back to the University of Alberta and following graduation I accepted work as a Public Health nurse for the City of Vancouver. I remained there for six years during which time I married and we adopted our son, and I was happy to spend some time at home. I took courses in interior design and took a course in scouting. I was a leader of a pack of cubs for a few years until arthritis forced me to restrict my activities. I now enjoy my son and two grandsons and feel I have had a very full and happy life.

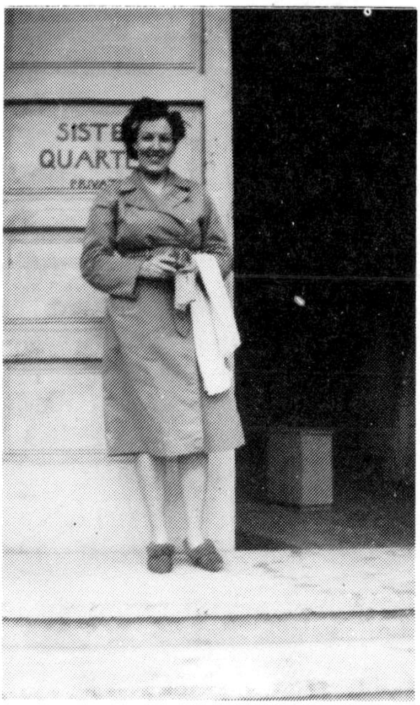

On the dusty road to the only shower house, Anne Gair, No. 15 CGH Caserta, Italy, 1944

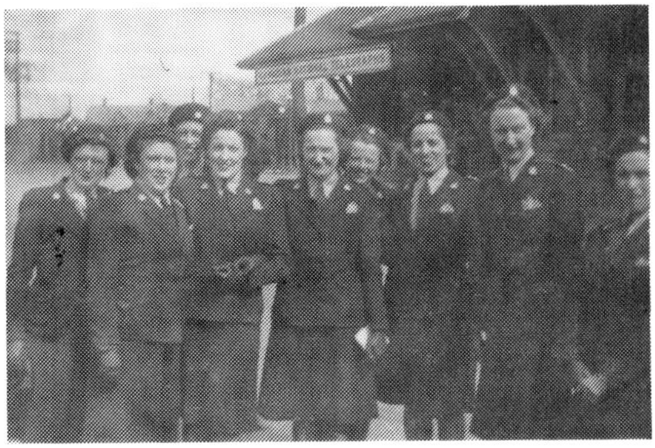

Nursing Sisters, Sussex, New Brunswick, 1944. Front: Alice Bush, Lu McComb, Anne Gair, Jean Fontana, Helen Mussallem Back: Phyllis Slater

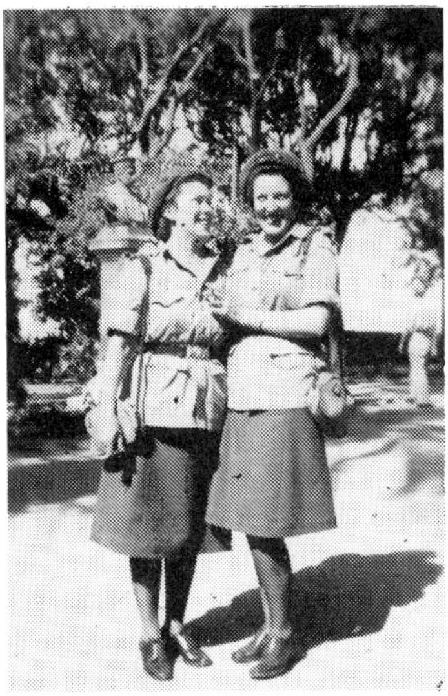

L: Lu McComb, R: Anne Gair, Sorrento, Italy 1944

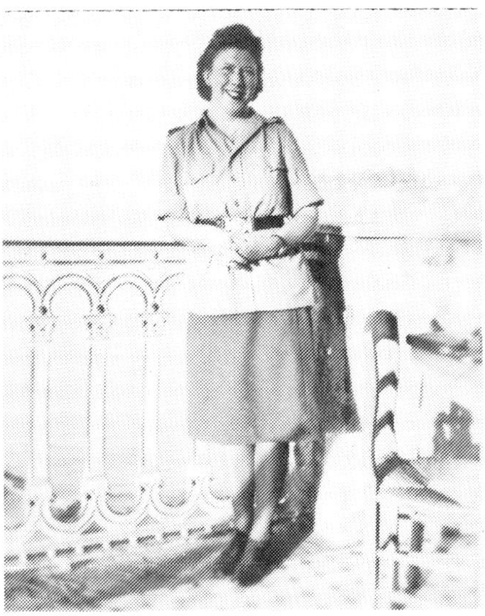

My Army pal now deceased, Lu McComb, Sorrento, Italy, 1944

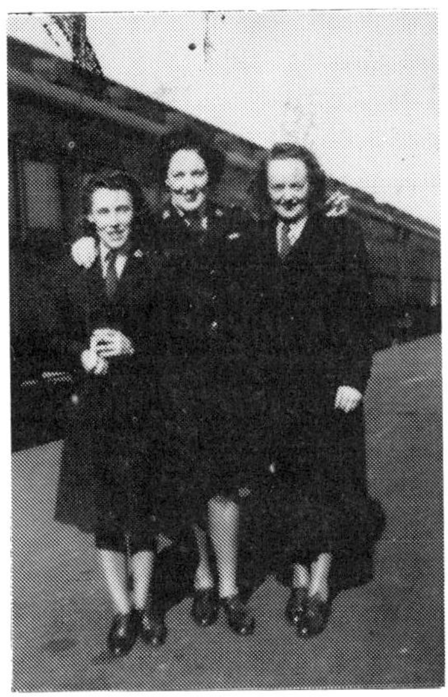

Montreal, returning from overseas 1946. L: Phyllis Lamme, Anne Gair, June Plummer

Gertrude M. James

Graduated from: Royal Alexandra Hospital School of Nursing, Edmonton, Alberta. Year: 1942

Military History:

Service: RCAMC

Rank: 1st Lt.

Served: 1944 to 1946

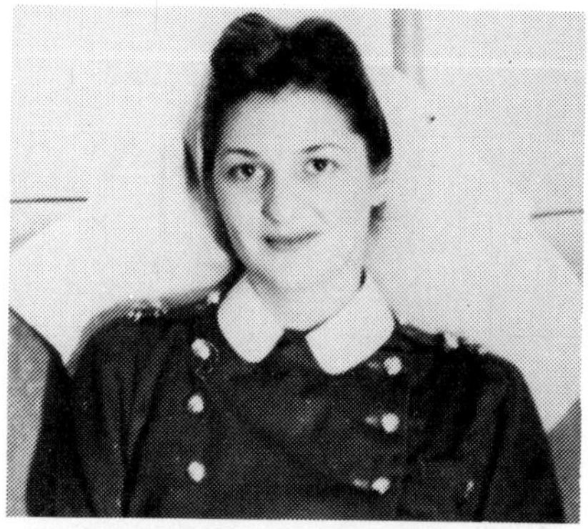

Lt. N/S Gertrude James at No. 19 CGH Marston Green, England

I thought the Army would be an interesting experience. It was! I was first assigned to Vernon Military Hospital, then transferred to Chilliwack, and sent to England within a few months. In England I was stationed at No. 19 Canadian General Hospital at Marston Green (near Birmingham). During that time I had the honour of being one of the nurses to represent Canadian nurses at an Empire Day Festival. We paraded before the Royal Family at Albert Hall in London. When No. 19 closed after VE Day, I was transferred to Horsham or Horley (can't remember which).

After VJ Day, I applied and was accepted at Khaki University of Canada which was located at Watford. During the first semester I studied chemistry and mathematics. During the second semester I became a member of the faculty assisting in the chemistry lab. I was honored to be the only woman on the faculty. During a tour by King George and Queen Elizabeth I was fortunate to speak to both of them.

In 1946 I returned to Canada on the *Ile de France*. As they needed nurses during the changeover of the Montreal Military Hospital to the Queen Mary Veterans Hospital, I was assigned there for a short time before my discharge.

After my discharge, I obtained my B.N. and M.A. and have taught and been an administrator in schools of nursing. In 1959 I joined the American Red Cross as a nursing consultant and later Director of Nursing of the Minneapolis Area Chapter. After leaving Red Cross, I was in administration at the County Public Health agency. I retired nine years ago but continue to work part time for the Public Health Nursing Agency.

Elsie MacIntyre

Graduate from: Moncton General Hospital School of Nursing. Year: 1939

Military History:

Service: RCAMC

Rank: Lt N/S

Served: September 1943 to February 1946

The Army needed nurses and that was why I joined up.

The day I was posted overseas was the highlight of my career! I went overseas with No. 19 Canadian General Hospital in 1944. I was posted with No. 1 General in 1945.

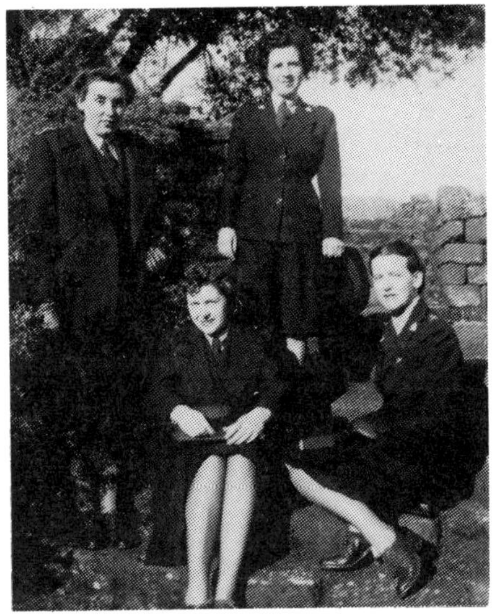

On leave in Torquay, England
Upper left - Helen Christian,
R: Florence (Mellway) Taylor
Lower left - Elsie McIntyre,
R: Eileen Ingram

Florence (Taylor) Mellway

Graduated from: Royal Victoria Hospital School of Nursing, Montreal. Year: 1942

Military History:

Service: RCAMC

Rank: Lieutenant N/S

Served: February 1944 to April 1946

I joined the military because of my desire to serve and also hoped to be nearer to a brother and two nephews who were in the Service. I enlisted in Montreal and took basic training in Kingston, Ontario, then went to Sussex, N.B. We sailed from Halifax, May 1944. No. 19 Canadian General Hospital was located at Marston Green, England. I loved England and was grateful to be able to care for our wonderful Canadian boys. No. 19 was a Repatriation Hospital so it was a happy place most of the time.

On 15 April 1945 I arrived at No. 1 Canadian General Hospital in Nijmegen, Holland. I was assigned to the Neurological Unit since I had worked at Montreal Neurological Institute after graduation. It was an exciting time – hard work, but rewarding.

We also had great leaves. I was able to visit my brother's grave near Caen, while on a Cultural Educational Course in Paris, in August 1945.

We sailed from England in February 1946. A few of us staffed the Hospital on the *Cythia*, a small ship with war brides and babies. It was offered to us as an early trip home. Hectic at the best, with seasickness and storms, but I was happy to be home.

I was discharged in Montreal April 1946. In November 1946 I was married in Toronto to a Navy man, an ex-patient I met at No. 19 CGH. We are still together and happy.

Helen K. Mussallem

Graduated from: Vancouver General Hospital School of Nursing

Military History:

Service: RCAMC

Rank: Lt. N/S

Served: 1943 to 2 April 1946

I joined the Army because Canada was at war and I wished to offer my services.

No. 19 Canadian General Hospital mobilized as a 600-bed hospital at Camp Sussex, New Brunswick, in April of 1944 and by 10 April all the nursing sisters had reported with the exception of the assistant matron.

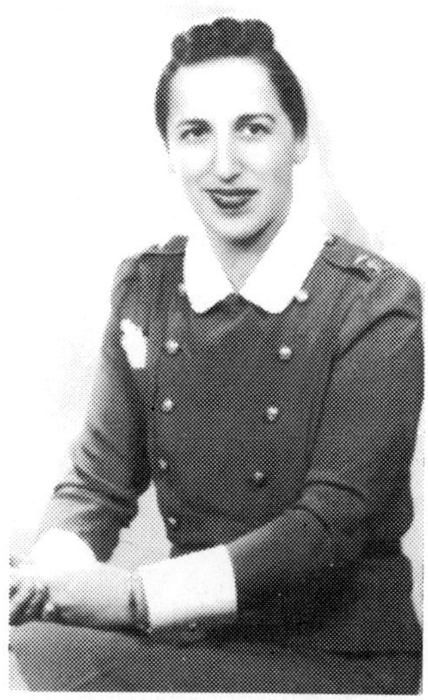

Lt. N/S Helen Mussallem, No. 19 CGH

We arrived in England 10 May 1944 to be met by Matron McNeil and Col.

Winfield from CMHQ. Marston Green was to be the home of No. 19 General. No. 16 General was in the process of moving out. Some few hundred patients remained in the hospital so we immediately started to work. I was the operating room supervisor at No. 19.

Edith Schofield

Graduated from: Victoria General Hospital School of Nursing, Winnipeg, Manitoba. Year: 1942

Other: Certified Registered Nurse Anaesthetist.

Military History:

Service: RCAMC

Rank: Lieutenant N/S

Served: 25 August 1943 to 13 September 1945

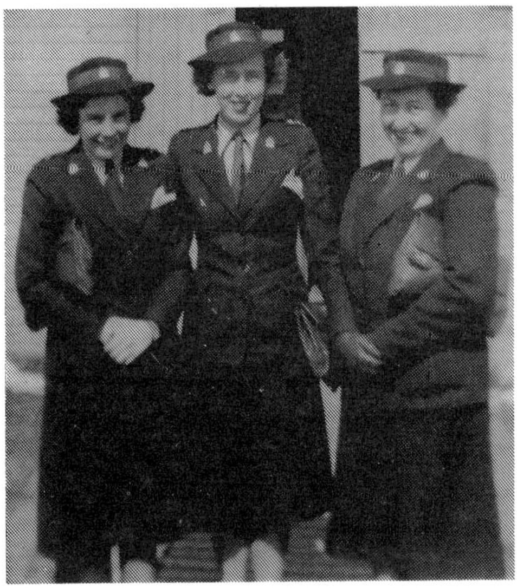

Martson Green near Birmingham, England.
L-R: N/S Taylor, N/S Schofield, N/S Rhoda Howting

Nurses were needed and I offered my services to be a part of caring for our soldiers. My joining the RCAMC was not a mistake. It was the best experience of my nursing career. I came in contact with so many courageous young men whose lives were changed forever. They were superb patients; I take my hat off to them! May they never be forgotten!

Once when I was on E Ward at No. 19 General, the men wanted to know my first name and I wouldn't tell them. They went through all the Es and guessed Elizabeth; they made up a board with "Aunt Lizzie's Boarding House" on it. When the colonel came to inspect the ward they had to scramble to hide it.

I saved that board; I put it under my mattress. When I came back from leave my mattress was rolled up and all my belongings were piled up on my bed – my board was gone.

Angela M. (La Croix) Smith

Graduated from: Misericordia Hospital School of Nursing, Winnipeg, Manitoba. Year: 1935

Military History:

Service: SAMNS & RCAMC

Rank: Lt. & Captain

Served: November 1941 to December 1945

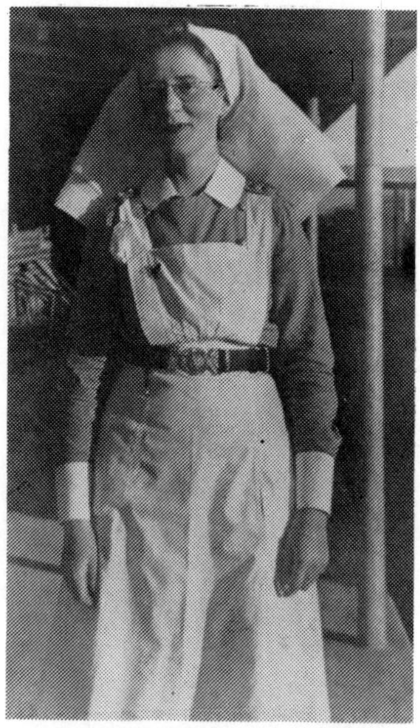

Angela Marie (LaCroix) Smith at Oribi Military Hospital, Pietermaritzburg, Natal, South Africa, 1942

Nursing experience and spirit of adventure are why I joined the Army.

The highlight of my military experience was nursing in South Africa. South Africa in those days seemed like going to the end of the world. I found it interesting stopping at Trinidad, and going ashore, as well as stopping at Pernambuco in Brazil. We docked in Capetown on Christmas Day, but only disembarked on Boxing Day.

We travelled by train to Durban, where we were welcomed by the South African matron and were assigned to the various Military Hospitals of our choice. I never knew one from another, but two of my friends and I decided we would volunteer for service at Oribi Military Hospital in Pietermaritzburg, Natal. It was a 3000-bed hospital with 100 patients on each ward, divided into four sections.

I was assigned to Ward 21 and Sister Mavis Marwick, a South African nursing sister, was in charge. Captain Jack Jankovitz was the medical officer in charge. Sister Marwick was so kind and helpful so I adjusted very easily to military nursing. After some months of experience I was made night supervisor, and a captain, and my salary was increased to 12 pounds a month.

I decided to return to Winnipeg after our one year contract was completed for financial reasons, as my mother was a widow.

I returned to Winnipeg on February 23 and I joined the RCAMC on March 2nd, 1943, as a 2nd Lieutenant.

I was stationed at Fort Osborne Military Hospital, and later at Brandon Military Hospital.

In early 1944 I was sent to Sussex, New Brunswick, and after several weeks we sailed for Halifax for the United Kingdom and docked at Liverpool on May 5th. Our unit was No. 19 Canadian General Hospital, and Colonel Kenner was in charge of our unit. Our principal matron was Anne Foster.

On my leave, September 4th, I travelled with Nursing Sister Margo Laird to Belfast and Dublin. On February 1945 I sailed from Tillbury to Ostend and spent two weeks with No. 7 Canadian General Hospital at Turnout, Belgium.

On March 5th I was sent to No. 3 CCS in Bedburg, Germany, then to No. 21 FDS in Emmerrich, and later No. 5 FDS at Bielen, Holland, then back to No. 3 CCS at Meppen, Germany, and the war was over May 5th, 1945.

On June 1945 I had a 72-hour pass and I went to Paris, Cambrai, St. Vaast-en Auge near Caen, and visited my brother's grave.

On August 1945 I had seven days' leave. I flew from Apeldoorn to Brussels and took the night train to Paris. I met a British nursing sister, Ray Harkness, she was alone so we travelled together and visited all the places of interest.

September 20th, 1945, we sailed from Calais on the SS *Daffodil* and docked at Dover. On October 15th, I sailed on the *Ile de France* and docked at Halifax, October 20th, 1945.

I arrived home in Winnipeg in October and I obtained my discharge from the Army on December 8th, 1945.

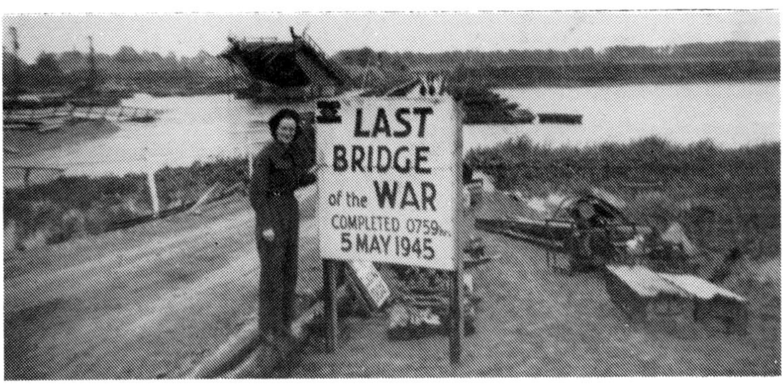

Angela Marie (LaCroix) Smith on the way to Oldenburg, Germany shortly after peace was declared May 1945.

NO. 20 CANADIAN GENERAL HOSPITAL

Kay (Dickie) Allen
Jean Gilroy

Authorization to form No. 20 Canadian General Hospital was issued in December 1943. Both No. 20 and No. 21 were to be formed at Listowel, Ontario.

No. 20 Canadian General Hospital moved to Sussex, New Brunswick, in February 1944.

The unit sailed 3 May 1944 on the *Ile de France* and arrived in Liverpool, England, a week later. There were three hospital units on that ship, Nos. 19, 20 and 21. No. 20 went to Watford, England.

On 16 December 1944 the unit sailed with a large convoy for Europe. Two days later the unit set up in Antwerp, Belgium. The nursing sisters went to other units. Three months later they moved to Turnhout, Belgium, and remained there until disbanded in September1945.

10 September 1945 No. 20 General was considered closed.

Kathleen (Dickey) Allan

Graduated from: Ontario Hospital School of Nursing, Hamilton, Ontario – first two years, Psychiatric Training: Brantford General Hospital School of Nursing, third year – general nursing. Year: 1941

Military History:

Service: RCAMC

Rank: Lt. N/S

Served: 1943 to 1946

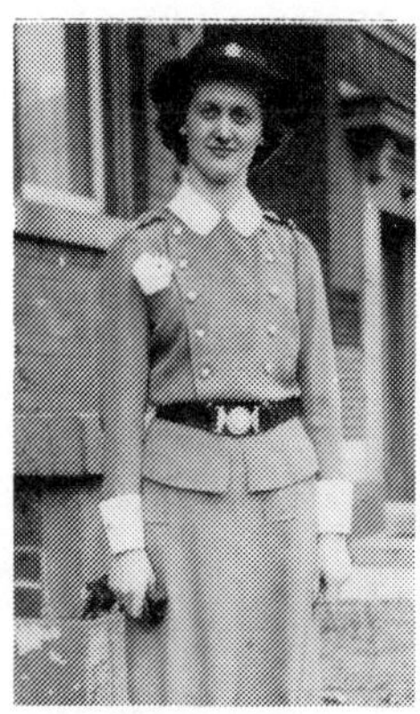

Lt. N/S Kathleen (Dickey) Allen No. 20 CGH, 1943

Two years ago, Matron Boyd at Camp Borden asked me, *"Have you got a military size trunk yet?"* When I replied, *"No,"* she said, *"Well you better get one immediately, as there are hospital units being formed for overseas and you had better be ready."* Everyone was so excited and enthused. Wondering what unit we were going with – who was going together and who the matron and colonel were. These questions were the highlight of all conversation.

The next thing I knew I was on my way west for a 48-hour embarkation leave. The word embarkation wasn't used very often at that time as it broke security. So to my folks, I said I was being posted to Windsor, Nova Scotia, and was allowed home for forty-eight hours before leaving for Camp Borden.

Reported back to camp about first week in April and found there were eight of us altogether leaving the next day. The matrons, Miss Tennant and Miss Fair had both left, and an MO, Major Middleboro, would be in charge of us. He was a grey-haired, elderly man and got quite a kick out of his responsibilities of eight females on his hands.

Leaving camp was an ordeal we will never forget. Matron Boyd had been overseas in World War I and envied seeing us going and leaving her behind. She came into Toronto to see us off. Said at least she could go that far. Everyone in camp took a great interest in seeing the sisters off at the trains. They took pictures of us with our respirators and haversacks over our shoulders and loaded down with luggage. So help me, you would think we were going to the end of the earth forever and a day. We soon learned to travel light as the longest I stayed in one place while I was overseas was four and a half months. The trip didn't seem long nor monotonous as it was new territory for most of us. And with eight women and one man, there wasn't a silent moment. Major Middleboro, I am sure, was glad when we all settled down for the night. The next day we learned there were several more nursing sisters on the train belonging to Number 20 Canadian General Hospital. We were a group of ninety from all across Canada. On arriving at Windsor we were met by the matrons and MOs. The excitement was great as the camp there was comparatively new and we were the first females to arrive. I think the civilians of Windsor wondered just what was taking place. After we were transported to our quarters which were a good mile from the town, the matron took us to the mess where we had coffee and cookies.

Our quarters were temporary buildings set up for the purpose of accommodating troops as they passed through. Therefore, they only had mere essentials, no modern conveniences, so we thought, but found out accommodations could be and were less modern once we left Canada. Our quarters were referred to as huts. Hut sixty-three wasn't large enough, so some of us were put in hut fifty. Our mess where we ate and the lounge, so to speak, were in hut sixty-four. Hut sixty-four was most popular because of the notice board, matron's office, dining hall and where we collected our mail and entertained friends. Mail, food and the notice board were three things uppermost in our minds.

The matron now realized she had ninety nurses whom she was responsible for and knew only eight of them. However, she didn't lose any time in getting acquainted. She interviewed each one and made a note of everything a matron should know regarding address of next of kin, type of work we were interested in, and also asked of our hobbies.

One of the first things we did was organize a mess committee. It was a bit difficult because we hardly knew one another.

After about two days' grace we began a training program. The matron spoke to us, telling us the men of our unit had been there training for a few weeks and the colonel was very proud of their military accomplishments and that it was our responsibility to quickly learn, take this training seriously and not spoil the show for the sake of the men. So at 9 A.M. every morning after that we were into blue slacks, tin helmets, and with respirators over our shoulders, we boldly marched up to the north drill hall to learn squad drill. One of the things we found most difficult was how we could blow our noses when we were suppose to stand at attention! I don't know how the boys managed. To step out of line was inexcusable. The officers who were training us had been through these ropes years back and, as the Army says, knew the score. I might say they were very keen to get a look at the nursing sisters in training for soldiers.

At this point most of us realized we were marching to war and often wondered just what part a nursing sister did play in the Army. As for nursing, we were learning nothing. When we asked questions concerning it; the answer was obviously, *"This is the Army – Mrs. Jones. You asked for it. And if you don't like it, now is the time to say so."* Needless to say, no one would be called a quitter so one we went merrily to squad drill, lectures, movies on gas and war events. To wind up the day we had a little PT thrown in. All this summed up was suppose to toughen us and keep us in condition for grim times ahead we were about to face. This to us was a joke. After all the lecturing and preaching we got in training about rest, care, not being exposed to rainy weather, but let me tell you, in the Army the principles of good health are the opposite. However, we had time off for recreation. One Saturday afternoon our group of twenty-five went on a hike, carrying our lunch in haversacks, we set out to explore the country. We travelled up and down large hills, passing many small lakes.

It was the time in spring when the grass was beginning to become green and the sun was plenty hot when it was shinning. We returned in the evening, more tired than from squad drill. I can say that, now that the matron isn't here to hear me.

During our short stay in Windsor we were inspected by what we called Brass Hats. This was always a great ordeal for us. As usual, they could never make up their minds whether the nurses should wear tin helmets or berets. If it was windy our hats would blow off. Berets were uniform but we usually ended up wearing tin helmets, with the strap just under the chin and the buckle on the left side or else you had it on back to front. It wasn't only windy, but very often snowing and raining. The inspecting officials were to arrive at a certain hour and we would all fall in and march on the parade square in order with the pipe band on the lead. Without fail they were late, and we were so stiff from standing at attention for so long we could hardly turn left or right for the grand march. We were divided into two platoons in alphabetic order, the matrons being as sergeant majors. They shouted the orders and took the salutes while we had our eyes to the right and kept in step and in line. After our show the inspectors spoke to us and congratulated us on our fine show, whether it was good or not. Then the colonel gave us the order to remove head-dress and give three cheers, but with three cheers under our breath, glad that they had gone. This ordeal took place at least three times. Finally, things began happening. A notice on the board appeared to the effect all personnel including officers and nursing sisters to parade to the First United Church in Windsor at ten o'clock Sunday morning. We all had our suspicions as to what it was all about but would anyone give! Oh, no. That would be breaking security. This church parade made quite an impression on the civilians in Windsor. They suspected what we were about to do and all the churches wanted to entertain us. Our matron faced quite a problem, telling these kind ladies tactfully we couldn't accept and not telling the real reason.

There were three hundred all totalled in the unit. With two hundred in khaki and one hundred in blue, all proudly marching down the crooked road as fully trained soldiers. We thought it was quite a sight. We thought it was best our folks weren't around to see.

The minister opened his sermon by saying he had been asked to speak to us on our last Sunday here. This really let the cat out of the bag. We didn't have to surmise any longer and were greatly amused at the break in security. Before he finished talking to us, he had us feeling we were really going across the ocean, leaving our loved ones and our friends, never to return. However, he did say he hoped to be on deck to welcome us back.

The next couple of days more queer things happened. We had QM parades, blankets parades, pay parades, signing over half our pay to be left in Canada. But the pay-off was when the boys came to our huts and took our mattresses. Immediately we jumped to the conclusion we must be leaving in the middle of the night. How well I remember one of the girls, Dotty Marshall, saying, *"The dirty beggars just like the Army."* Mother always told me there would be days like this. About ten o'clock that evening, Matron Tennant called us to the mess, told us we were all confined to barracks from now on. We will rise at 0400 hours, strip our beds, quarter master parade at five, and breakfast at six, at permanent mess number thirty-eight. After that she would give us further instructions.

It happened not to be raining that morning but we wore rubbers, nevertheless, as they were easier than carried; and besides, we hadn't any place to pack them. I had cartons of everything imaginable that I knew I couldn't get over there – books to read on the train, etc.

We wore trench coats, hats, and rubbers. We carried suitcase, haversack with tin helmets attached and respirators. We discovered we could carry chocolate bars and such things to eat conveniently in our tin helmets, unbeknown to the matron. We were surprised to find she had done exactly the same thing!

Finally, we boarded the train after a march of half a mile to the end of camp. We were headed for Halifax to sail on what boat we didn't know, but were all very curious. Our colonel was the only one who knew. He told us it was neither of the Queens but one which we would like just as well. The *Empress of Scotland* was the larger liner sitting in the dock as our train pulled in.

The next thing was the mad scramble to get off the train with all our luggage, line up in our usual platoons, march down to the dock where we received our embarkation and cabin tickets. We were warned that if we lost these we were as good as sunk, because without it we couldn't march up the gangplank. This was quite a thrill. Like myself, many of us had never been on such a liner before in our lives. We were directed to the female quarters, fourteen to a cabin, hardly room to squeeze in, let alone turn around and all wash in one sink with soft water for only a couple of hours a day. Here we found our water bottles and thermoses very useful, if they weren't already full. Which reminds me of an medical officer who was going to do a kind act for one of his cabin mates and refill his water bottles with fresh water; later discovered he had poured real Canadian Scotch whiskey down the sink. We soon cleared out and got up on deck to take a look around.

Many of the girls met up with their best friends, each not knowing the other would be sailing on the same ship. We received our meal tickets telling us fourth sitting was at 8:30 P.M. and breakfast at 10:30 A.M. Two meals a day! To those who fed the fish, it couldn't matter less, but to us who enjoyed retaining our food, ate heartily and asked for more, it was disappointing. The food was good. Instead of bread, we had home-made buns that were handy to have about 1:00 P.M. for noon snack.

In England the expression was any gum chum, but on the boat it was any buns chum? There were about 7000 on the ship. You ask me what we did to put in time. Well, there were 200 nursing sisters and about 700 officers, so figure it out for yourself. We were soon given our life belts with a little red light on each one. They were attached so they could be easily detected if we should have to swim the ocean. They proved very troublesome and every time you forgot to take it with you, about three or four MPs were always on their guard and never hesitated to tell you. We sailed from Halifax at 0700 hours, on May 4th, 1944. During the trip across, five of Number 20's boys came down with the mumps. We also had a funeral at sea. A colonel and his wife died here in Canada and it was their wishes to be cremated and the ashes thrown in the sea on the coast of England. This the padres took care of, but we were all stretching our necks to see the performance.

We had boat drill every morning. Everyone had to learn the respective decks and know where they were to assemble and get there the shortest possible way. Whatever we did, whether we were lost or not, was to keep moving – don't hold up traffic. The ship commandant inspected us, seeing that we wore our life belts correctly. The sisters wore slacks, trench coats, berets and as many warm clothes as they had with them, as it was mighty cold out there in the middle of the Atlantic even though it was May.

We got full benefit of all sea breezes from all sides. The ship was controlled by the Air Force who for some unknown reason took a dim view of females being aboard. One took every opportunity he could, to criticize us. He received a complaint that one of the nursing sisters was seen out on deck after blackout. Blackout hour was announced every evening over the loud speaker which meant everyone to their cabins, much to our disgust. But we didn't dare be spotted at this stage of the game as we were travelling without convoy.

The ship's commandant called all three matrons to his office and asked if they knew about this. Matron Tennant said she was sure it wasn't one of the Number 20's girls, and if it was, more power to her – wish I knew how she passed the MPs to get that far. Incidentally, we never did find out either. As I believe, there was a double staff of MPs put on guard duty. We as Army personnel got a kick out of seeing the Air Force doing the work instead of the Army. Usually there is strife between the two and to see one working and not the other, the feeling is more noticeable on board ship.

On May 10th, we docked at Liverpool at 1600 hours. That day at noon, we picked up Air Force navigators who knew the course well, and knew how to avoid submarines. We were allowed to be out on deck to watch the ship dock and to see as much of Liverpool as possible. It looked old, dirty, smoky and badly bombed. There was a large Air Force band playing many welcome happy sing-songs. The music really put a frog in my throat. But just couldn't do anything but stare and wonder just what I had let myself in for. Matron Tennant was making her second trip over. She was over at the time of Dieppe and was a great help to us. People were waving to us from their upstairs windows. Men in uniforms – what did Canada look like when you left? – Cheers – you line-up, take a look at this group of Canadians – even Canadian nursing sisters. Angels from heaven have arrived to help us.

Chief Matron Agnes Neill was there with Colonel White from CMHQ London to greet us. No sooner had the boat stopped than the unloading started. The men in the docks began unloading the bags and bags and bags of luggage. Matron Neill came on board and welcomed us, told each of the hospital units where they were going. Number 20 was going to Watford, in Hartsford, fifteen miles north of London. We were thrilled to learn that London was within the twenty-mile band as at that time we thought London was the place to see in England.

Number 20 didn't disembark until 9 o'clock the next morning, so the previous evening our colonel got our famous three-piece band, who had only played about three times together, up to the lounge for a dance. By this time everyone was in a very gay mood; even the stewards joined in and whirled us nearly off our feet.

Walking down the gangplank wasn't nearly as thrilling as marching up although most of us were glad to see land. We assembled in our platoons and marched up to a special train that took us right to Watford. There we were met by Miss Dick from Number 10 Canadian General Hospital. The Army Service Corps delivered us and our luggage safely to Leavesden Military Hospital, about four miles from Watford. This was about 2:30 in the afternoon. It was a very warm sunny day, and England really looked nice – the flowers you can hardly visualize, particularly the red, yellow and white roses.

Number 10 Canadian General Hospital was going to France, but at that time they were going out under canvas. They were all in khaki and did we envy them. Miss Dick had her girls moved to an empty ward in the hospital so we could occupy the quarters on arrival. Our quarters were called villas. Each accommodated about thirty; they were called Oak Villa and Fur Villa. They were long, narrow one-storey buildings. For doors, curtains were supplied – heavy material called blackout curtains. There was an orderly officer responsible for drawing blackout curtains every night. Miss Dick warned us to keep our money locked, as someone who apparently knew the grounds well would come into the villas in the night and take our purses. Next morning we would find all the purses on the back doorstep, everything intact except all money would be gone. Number 20 soon put an end to that. They put guards on each villa and all around the hospital area. We even had to identify ourselves to get in. It often proved difficult if we were in civilian clothes and didn't have our identification cards with us.

The following day after our arrival we were free and most of the girls went to London. Then we were to begin working half days as we had only a very few patients. But that lasted one day and convoys started pouring in on us. We didn't know the score, and in the Army, particularly when it was so near D-Day, explanations were omitted. Later we learned that a certain area in southern England was being cleared and restricted to the combat troops for the invasion only.

The hospitals within this area were cleared of all their patients by sending them to us so they could prepare for the D-Day casualties. Most of these patients were from Italy and they hadn't remained in any one hospital long enough to have their casts changed or much surgery done. So our OR and plaster room worked day and night, because as soon as the boys were fixed up, they had to be documented and sent to Canada for further convalescence. That in itself was a big job. We had convoys going out during the night and new casualties pouring in during the day. Sometimes the patients were transported by huge buses from the boat in southern England. The drivers very often got lost and would be hours late and we would find ourselves with convoys pouring out and coming in at the same time. The admitting and discharging department worked day and night. Anyone who thinks the boys in the RCAMC who did clerical work – and all of them privates – didn't do their part in the war is sadly mistaken. The orderlies did their part too. They were from all walks of life, and most of them were pushed into medical corps very much against their wishes because they were physically unfit for combat duty. They learned to carry stretchers, sweep and scrub floors, help with the meals, feed helpless patients, cut hair and all manner of things. We just couldn't have managed without them.

They very often won the confidence of the patient, and they would tell the orderlies things they wouldn't report to us.

Two weeks of this and I was put on night duty. The reason I mention night duty is that it was very much different in England than in Canada. In the first place, we had to be always conscious of the blackout, never went on duty without flashlights and tin helmets. We wore tin helmets when going from one building to the other as our white veils, they thought, were easily detected and at that time there were still enemy planes flying over our heads. Near us was an underground factory where airplane parts were made. It was always thought the enemy was trying to bomb it, and had they, we would likely be bombed too.

Buzz bombs (we called them doodle bugs) or V-1s were very numerous at that time. They were the jet controlled airplanes with a red flare on the tail and this was considered a last resource for the Germans who had to continue their bombing on London. Their Air Force was practically nil except for that on their home front. We were warned to stay away from open windows during an alert, but after we became accustomed to the different sounds and felt the danger had passed overhead, curiosity got the better of us as we were greatly intrigued by the powerful search lights. I always felt the ones controlling these lights must have been highly trained to know when and when not to flash the flares.

My first night off I went into London, stayed at the Canadian Sisters Club. Watford is a suburb of London, which meant we took an underground train into Waterloo station, where we changed to an Inner Circle to Gloucer Road.

The club was about two blocks, or as the English would say, a five-minute walk and you can't miss it. In the evening we decided to go for a walk. The streets were wide and everything looked strange, old, dirty and gloomy. We walked toward South High Kensington and there saw the Royal Albert Hall. It is a huge round-shaped building with sandbags placed neatly all around. Many of the windows were broken and boarded up. Across from there was a beautiful park, South Kensington Park. The hedges, flowers, trees and walks all looked so well cared for, you wonder who had the time, as in England everyone worked and worked hard for very little pay. Every inch of land was cultivated. People always appeared in such a rush; they always ran or walked up and down the escalators, never rode as we Canucks did.

Sometimes a well dressed Englishman wearing a derby and carrying a cane, after one look at us, would know we were lost and would say, *"Can I be of any help to you, Madame?"* There were very few people on the street after dark. Everyone had to carry tin helmets when travelling in London for protection from falling bricks and window panes. The civilians were trained in protection the same as those in uniform. That night I didn't sleep well. I still hadn't learned the difference between the noise the ack-ack guns made and the doodle bugs. They sounded to me like huge hail stones hitting on the roof. I expected the ceilings and walls to come in anytime.

Next day, when I came downstairs, everyone seemed in such a dither. I wondered if we really had been hit, when one of the Red Cross girls said, *"Don't you know the invasion is on?"* Our divisions went in early this morning; so far no reports have been broadcast. At this point, I didn't know whether I wanted to spend the rest of the day touring around London or return to the hospital. Finally decided to go back while going was good.

The patients were all very excited and would say, *"I was to be in on this, been over here training for three years and here I am in hospital with a black eye received from bumping into the door of the corner pub in the blackout."* Instead of being happy they were disappointed. I have heard others say, *"I have waited a long time for this opportunity to crack back at those Germans for what they did to us here during the Blitz."* Many of the boys who were in England during the Blitz were very nervous of the doodle bugs, and if they could walk at all, would always go to the shelter during an alert.

For the next three weeks our work was very heavy. It was during this time we learned the different kinds of bullet wounds and how to care and dress them. We ran a penicillin ward – everyone on penicillin, and nearly everyone was, at least all fresh casualties were, was admitted to Ward 30. It took one nurse to give the penicillin q3h. After I saw the results I didn't mind giving it, but before that I dreaded it as much as the patient. I remember one asking me if I thought he was a dart board.

Alas! The Army is full of weird and wonderful surprises. Number 20 was going out under canvas, and Number 23 had arrived overseas and were taking over our establishment at Watford. I remember telling the matron I wanted to be one of the first to leave. Thought we were going to France the next day.

Little did I know, now when I look back, it's just as well I didn't. Number 23 were placed in a transient camp in Helmsly in Yorkshire, an all-day train ride from us. They moved down in groups and we moved up there in groups. The matrons remained behind to help the new matrons get acquainted, which meant the first group of us who went to this camp were five jack-of-all trades. An MO was in charge who didn't know half the time what or where we were. This transient camp consisted of Nissen huts situated on a hill back in the trees well out of sight. An ideal spot for further training in squad drill. We knew as soon as our ambitious matron arrived that our holiday would be over, so we made good use of our time. We visited Whitby, Scarborough and Darlington. There were other hospital units at these places, and usually someone had friends in each unit.

One day Colonel Gunn informed us our holiday was over and that we would begin route marches at nine o'clock in the morning, lectures on gas and equipment at ten thirty, OCs parade at one thirty in the afternoon, in full marching order for inspection. Remainder of the afternoon would be spent at organized sports. If we didn't play soft ball, we had to go on a hike. This continued for nearly five weeks when an order came from headquarters for a detail inspection. It was really the first movement order; that is, they intended to finally let us cross the Channel. This inspection meant we had to pack our trunks and bed rolls so as not to exceed one hundred and sixty-eight pounds. This I found very difficult, as the day previous to the inspection our trunks were weighed and I found myself removing nine pounds – on the side of a hill in front of many male spectators.

The day for this final inspection we had with us only what we could carry in our packs. The rest of our luggage was loaded in trucks. Everyone in the unit marched out on the parade square as we had done so many times before and everyone had to be identified and accounted for. We were identified by our dog tags we had around our necks and our Army identification card. Then we had to march down the road a mile to prove our strength and endurance for the job ahead. It was a long mile, and with fifty or sixty pounds on your back, I thought I would die. And if anyone shouted gas, I would gladly have been gassed. However, we survived and were relieved when the inspectors told us we could remove our equipment and sit down, but no smoking. This was no hardship for us for we hadn't breath to smoke anyway. We came through at the top. The nurses were the least criticized, and we were told if the men looked after their equipment as well, we would, no doubt, have little or no trouble.

After all this, when time came for the final push off, Number 21 received the order to go to France. Were we angry and disappointed. The reasons for this were many, but I don't expect we will ever know the truth of the matter.

We were a very disgruntled group. We hadn't the courage to carry on with further training if our efforts were in vain. The next we knew half of us were posted to work in hospitals in England. I went to Number 4 at Farnborough near Aldershot. Patients would say to us, *"Sister! are you going or coming? I hope you aren't going to Europe, It isn't fit for our Canadian nurses."* We were dressed in khaki and they knew we were either going or had just arrived back. After working there for about three weeks we were all called back to camp. Immediately we thought, *"This is it, we surely are going this time."* The matron met us at York. York was a city about twenty-five miles from camp. She told us we were all going on a forty-eight. Even though it was our first forty-eight since we had arrived overseas, we still would rather be going over where the fight was taking place. Three other girls and I went to Edinburgh. It took practically a whole day on the train which didn't leave us much time to see the city. We spent most of the time looking for a place to eat and sleep. We went on conducted tours of the castle. Hostess from the King George Queen Elizabeth Club went with us. Edinburgh is much like a Canadian city. Streets are wide. People are very friendly. In stores or on the street they would speak to us and ask if there was anything they could help us with in regard to seeing the best in Edinburgh. Some would say, *"Canadians!! Welcome to Edinburgh. I had a brother go to Canada many years ago. I think he lives somewhere in Upper Canada – know where that is? Do you know how big Canada is? Well, I know it is bigger than our country. Like to go to Canada sometime."*

We had to stand in a very long queue for about two hours to get on the train to return to camp. Arrived back about supper, very tired, wonder if there was any exciting news awaiting us, only to find nothing new or different except some appreciated mail from Canada.

A few days later we learned we had to move in convoy to Scotch Corners. Our camp was going to be used for other training purposes. More troops had arrived from Canada and they were taking over our happy hunting ground. This didn't please us as we were by now very tired of this useless life. Scotch Corners was a hotel seven miles from Darlington, last bus at 9 P.M. Life was very grim there. Although we had a forty-eight every weekend, we were so far from places of interest it was pointless to try to travel.

The matrons, Colonel Gunn and padres racked their brains trying to find things of interest to bide our time. We continued to route march, weather permitting. We had shows and parties and were entertained at different RCAF stations nearby. Sometimes we went forty miles. We went on tours in a sixty cwt. to Barnard Castle, and Lake District in Carlisle.

Finally, Colonel Gunn succeeded in getting us a nine-day principal leave. Being our first, everyone decided to ask for permission to proceed to Ireland. As too many had asked, none were granted. Four took off for London and Torquay district. In spite the fact it was cold, windy, and raining we enjoyed most of the leave except the crowded trains. Torquay, a summer resort and this being November, wasn't the time to see it at its best. However, where we went we always found Canadians who appreciated the opportunity of meeting and entertaining Canadian girls. We went pub crawling one night in the blackout and in the rain. Returning, we got lost and, so help me, I have never route marched as far as we walked that night. The people of the lodge where we stayed figured we got lost so remained up until we got in. They were very nice to us and the food was the best I had ever eaten in England.

On return we found we were being posted. Again we were disappointed and sad – began wondering if we would ever get to Europe. Only bright spot was mail which always helped to keep up our morale. This time I went to Number 18 CGH at Colchester – about two hour trip west of London. On arriving, we were greeted and met by Matron Harvey and fed a hot supper – two eggs each. We thought we would line up again – first time we had tasted fresh eggs in England. This hospital was laid out in spiders. It had been a training camp in World War 1. I worked in D Spider – six wards, forty patients in each and busy. Had several convoys of boys just back from the fighting zone which was in Belgium at that time. Again, the patients asked me if I was coming or going. I remember one saying to me, *"Sister you should see Antwerp. It is just like New York."* It may have been then, but certainly wasn't when I saw it.

I spent three weeks of trying to make fracture cases comfortable, dressing wounds and burns and trying to cheer up boys who had lost an eye, one or both legs, arms or hands, when we were called back to camp. This time it was surely the real thing. Sure enough, we packed, had a farewell party and left Scotch Corners December 13, 1944. The night before we left we were confined to barracks and had roll call at 10 P.M. Our matron told us she would announce next day on the train what part we were leaving from. Next day we got on the train, not ever thinking where we were embarking. We were so thrilled to really be going this time. The men and the MO had left several days ahead of us with luggage and hospital equipment. We were ninety-six females marching to war and don't think we were just a little bit proud.

We arrived in Southampton late that night and stayed in a transient camp run by ATS. There we had our money changed to

Belgian francs. We were so thrilled, we couldn't control our excitement, as this meant we weren't going to be so far behind the troops. Incidentally, Number 21 CGH, even though they had reached the shores of Normandy ahead of us, was situated at St. Omer near Dieppe which was a long way behind us. At the transit camp we had a hot supper, served cafeteria style, and we ate off long bare tables with benches to sit on. Really Army style. Then we had a show and crawled into upper and lower deck beds. In the morning we were called at 7:00. We washed, dressed and had breakfast. Then we stripped our beds and handed in our blankets. Large Army trucks came for us to transport us to the boat. We, by this time, were in full marching order and had to be accounted for. Really think if many of us were missing, it would have been less worry for the Matron.

We were all very anxious to see and know what boat was taking us across the channel. We were rather disappointed as the *Lady of Man* was about as dirty as any boat could get. We sailed from Southampton at four P.M. Had several stops for an hour each time and soon learned we were docking at Ostende. Disembarking from this boat we could lose no time. Besides being unpleasant, as so many were seasick, we had to be off the ship so it could be reloaded so it could go out with the tide. At Ostende, we saw much destruction and poverty. We marched from the port to another transit camp for our dinner.

This camp was more or less in the making, as it wasn't anywhere near being completed. However, some Belgium cooks in white and long black coats served us up a fairly good dinner. We weren't to leave here until four P.M. when we were to take a train to Brussels. So we walked around to see Ostende even though the MPs warned us it wasn't altogether safe as there were still a few loose Jerrys in hiding around. The people of Ostende were not exactly happy at the time, as they were given to understand as soon as the Allies came and freed them of the looting enemy, there wouldn't be any black market and that food would be plentiful. Food was still scarce and they were on the verge of loosing faith in the Allies.

Again, we were called together and marched to what was left of the bombed station and got on a European train. They are much the same as the English trains but could see they were being badly used. We arrived in Brussels late that night and were met by Colonel White and Chief Matron Shaffner. We were all divided up in groups and billeted at several hotels. Again we were fed and went to bed. The hotels at one time had been the best, but at this time lacked heat and had very little warm water. Next morning we again were gathered together in usual manner and marched to the station where we got a train to Antwerp. This was only a short trip, but at one place had to get off train and walk across a bridge and get on another train. The Germans had blown the bridge as they were retreating from Belgium.

The MOs of our advanced party met us at Antwerp. We were no sooner off the train at Antwerp when we heard the old familiar sound, the air alert. Anyone who asked us where we were going, was horrified to hear us say Antwerp. *"That awful place, do you want to get killed?"* We were taken to our hospital in ambulances. This building had been a German hospital and when Number 8 Canadian General Hospital moved in, the German Medical Corps were still there. Many of the German orderlies stayed and worked for us. They didn't seem to mind wheeling in our casualties from their bombs. One of them looked after the bathrooms; they were the only ones that had hot water. The MOs said if we wanted a bath there was a good German over there and he will look after things. He sure did. He was used to waiting on you hand and foot while you had your bath. Not being able to speak the language, we had quite the bath.

That afternoon at four o'clock a buzz bomb hit the Allied theatre killing and wounding hundreds of Canadians, British, and Americans who were there on leave. Antwerp was a leave centre, also an important port. The Germans were making every effort to destroy the port and were hitting everything else but the docks. By the next day the nurses were all posted out to other hospitals situated in safer spots than Antwerp. I went to Number 7 Canadian General Hospital at Turnhout. It was about twenty-five miles, or forty kilometres, as the Belgians would say. It was about one week before Christmas and Number 7 accepted us like lost orphans and made Christmas one of the happiest for us possible. For the first time in my life I slept on a bed without a mattress. Our luggage hadn't arrived with us and didn't until one week later which meant we worked in our battle dress – had only what we wore and carried with us for a whole week.

I never felt so crummy in all my life. Our big laced boots with the cobble nails and steel lifts made plenty of noise on cement floors. Christmas Eve we had a Christmas tree in the dining room and one of the MOs was Santa Claus and everyone got a gift. The evening was spent nearest to what a Christmas Eve could be so far away from home. Christmas Day was Christmas for the patients and the other ranks. The nursing sisters and all officers waited and served them their dinner plus all the champagne anyone could drink. Next day the other ranks served us our dinner. We had three long tables, nicely decorated, mostly with champagne bottles. They had place cards so Number 20 wouldn't all click and sit together. The turkey and cranberry sauce was canned products sent to us by our faithful home folk. The pre-usual Christmas parties followed in like manner until after New Years. Not until then did I really realize I had spent Christmas in a foreign land so far from Canada.

All was quiet on the Western Front except a few paratroopers (German) who had been picked up near us wearing American uniforms. We were not allowed out day or night unless an armed officer was with us. We had to wear our Red Cross band on the left sleeve of our coats. The Canadian divisions were situated mainly in Holland around Nijmegen, south of Arnhem. The German troops were in Arnhem and to the north. The dykes were all blown up and the country was flooded. The Germans had slides placed just north of Arnhem where they sent off their buzz bombs. The Canadian and British Artillery were too close to them to shoot them down, so they went flying on over us to Antwerp. There was very little shelling in January. The troops lived in mud, water and fear of the buzz bombs. In February things started to move and across the Rhine we went. Germans were really surprised as they never thought the Allies would ever get through the Reichwald forest to the other side of the Rhine River. Holland was completely liberated. To them, a load as big as the earth had risen off their shoulders.

Then, one bright sunny day in May, came that long looked for VE Day. The people of Europe celebrated for a whole week, parades, street dancing and such goings on, one could never name or describe. This was the end of the war and the end of Number 20, as we were to close our hospital and be posted to other units until our turn according to the point system came to return to Canada. This time I went to Number 2 Canadian General Hospital. There we lived in a very luxurious hotel but our hospital was one and a half miles out of the town Bruges. We were taken to and from work in the ration truck. There I spent June to October. Life was dull in the port, as we were the only Canadians in Belgium at that time. Bruges was a very quaint old town with many points of interest. Our hotel faced the town square. On our right was a Belfry with chimes that rang every fifteen minutes.

There were many old cathedrals, bridges and canals. Streets were very narrow and roads were cobblestones. A great deal of lace was made in Bruges. The older women sat at their doors by the street spinning lace. People of Belgium weren't richly dressed. They wore shoes – sandals with high heels looked very uncomfortable and of poor quality. Black was one of their favourite colors. The widows wore all black. Black hats with long black veils. Belgians are very crafty, shrewd people and when the Germans were there they made it a point to get along with them thinking that opposing them, they would suffer more. The country was not damaged so much as Holland, and the Belgian people showed their appreciation for what the Allies had done to free them of the Germans. And they were truer than the Dutch. The Dutch were extremely happy to be liberated but as soon as the war ended and Queen Wilhelmina returned from England, they wanted to be free of the Canadians too. I spent a nine-day leave in Holland in August, during which time VJ Day arrived. I saw Amsterdam, The Hague, Rotterdam, a cheese factory, The Islands, Volendam and Marken. Amsterdam is the capital of Holland, because it is where the queens are crowned. But The Hague is also considered the capital because all the government buildings are there. Amsterdam gets its name from the location of the city. It surrounds a long canal shaped like a half-moon and has many bridges. There was a great deal of destruction there, both by the Germans and the RAF when they planted their bombs on the Germans there. Also, you could see it had been one of their thriving industrial cities. In The Hague there was no industry and it had really been battered. Queen Wilhelmina's summer home was there and wasn't damaged. The Germans had very strong fortifications on the coast of the North Sea. There was also the National Court of Justice to which every country in the world has donated to. The islands were of great interest. The real old-fashioned Dutch live there.

Finally, one day I saw my name posted along with seventeen others to return to Canada. We left Bruges at six o'clock on Tuesday evening and drove to Calais – six-hour trip in the back of an Army sixty cwt. Here we stayed overnight in a transient camp (once again). Got our money changed back to English currency. Climbed the gang plank and set sail across the channel for Dover. On our way across we were able to take snaps of the

White Cliffs. We were two hours crossing. Were met at Dover by Miss Reid; had our dinner and drove for another 6 hours to Bramshott. This time we stayed at a reception centre. Next day Miss Reid interviewed us individually. This is when I learned I had been returned to England to work, wasn't on Canada draft at all. I didn't take this very badly, and was ever so happy when at the end of four and half weeks I had made a Canada draft and was to sail on the *Queen Elizabeth* on December 2nd. I was docking at New York on December 7, 1945 – Pearl Harbour Anniversary. At last! Canada! My home and native land. Nevermore do I want to roam to any other country. Canada looks so bright and cheerful, no debris, no destruction. People don't go without shoes and stockings or go picking up cigarette butts or begging for cigarettes for mama and papa.

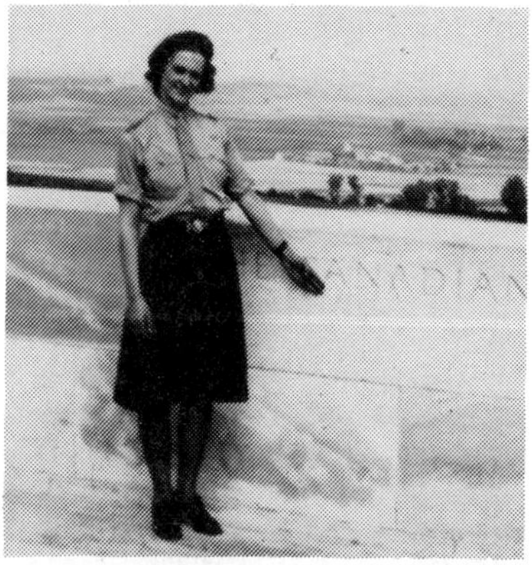

Lt. N/S Kathleen (Dickey) Allen No. 20 CGH at Vimy Ridge

Jean Gilroy

Graduate from: University of Toronto School for Physiotherapy, Ontario. Year: 1943 Diploma: Physiotherapy

Military History:

Service: RCAMC

Rank: Lt. P/A

Served: September 1943 to March 1946

After living in a small town the excitement of finally becoming a member of the RCAMC is something I still remember.

In May 1944 went overseas on the *Empress of Scotland* – 14 in a cabin for two.

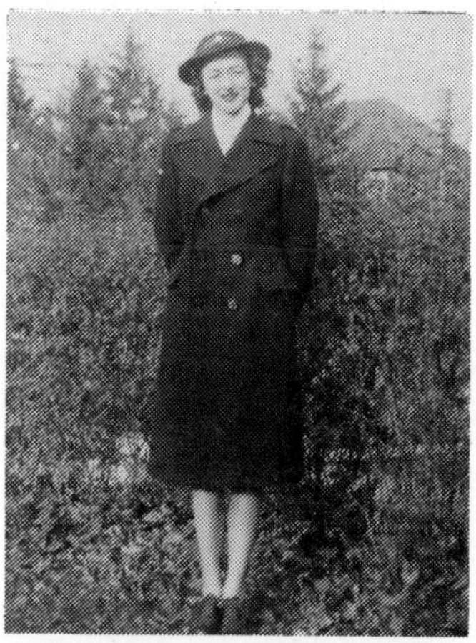

Lt. N/S Jean Gilroy, Mt. Forest, Ontario, No. 20 CGH

Several experiences stand out in

my mind as highlights of the time I spent in the Army.

My first leave was to the Scilly Isles. It was also my first plane ride as the ocean was too rough for a ferry boat, so we were transported in a tiny plane.

My second leave was in Ireland. I stood in front of the German embassy in Dublin.

My third leave was in Scotland. I spent VE Day in Glasgow.

I saw the Queen and the two young Princesses on the back platform of a train going to Brighton.

NO. 21 CANADIAN GENERAL HOSPITAL

Grace (Canning) Clarke
Irene (Poole) Lavallee
Ruth (Hunter) Percival
Eileen (Robinson) Shaw
Caroline (Livingstone) Stacey

No. 21 Canadian General Hospital formed at Bennett Barracks, Listowel, Ontario 15 December 1943. By June 1944 the unit arrived in Halifax and prepared to proceed overseas

22 May 1944 nursing sisters were interviewed for duty with the unit and 44 of them embarked on the *Lady Nelson* 1 June 1944 arriving in Liverpool, England, 10 June. The unit was assigned to Horley in Surrey.

15 September 1944 the unit boarded three LCIs and landed at Arromanches, France. The nursing sisters arrived 3 October after landing at Dieppe. They travelled to Mesnieres-en-Bray where No. 21 took over an ancient chateau. In January 1945 the unit moved to St.Omer and took over a former German hospital.

No. 21 General was disbanded 10 September, 1945.

Grace (Canning) Clarke

Graduated from: Moose Jaw Hospital School of Nursing, Moose Jaw, Saskatchewan. Year: 1941

Military History:

Service: Royal Canadian Army Canadian Medical Corps

Rank: Lt. N/S

Served: 7 January 1943 to February 1946

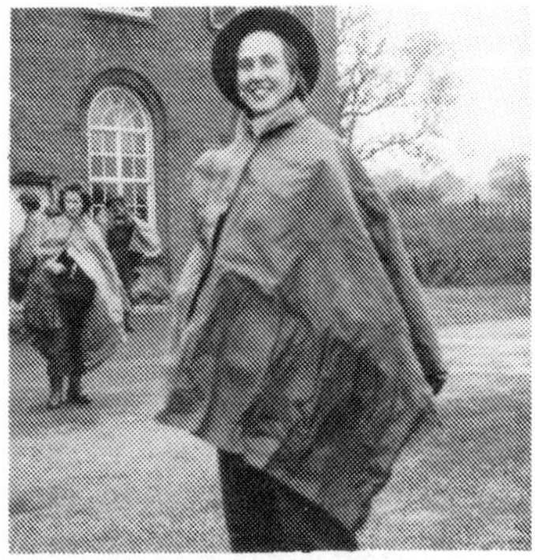

Grace Canning wearing gas cape. We used this cape as a ground sheet when we slept in tents. This is what we wore when we boarded trucks to travel. This was everything we had.

Every one in my family and all the boys I went to school with were in the Forces. It seemed natural for me to join the Army.

We lived in tents when we first arrived in France in 1944. It was January 1945, just before we moved to St.Omer, that we lived in huts. Our tents were heated by pot bellied stoves. Our food was terrible; we used to say the cabbage was made from boiling our gas capes. We got our bread from England. To make it more edible we slapped slabs of it against the side of the stove to toast it.

One of the units gave a great Christmas party at Dieppe. We were invited as well as U.S. personnel whose ship was in the harbour. Afterwards they visited us at Mesnières-en-Bray. We invited them for supper and they brought us some fresh oranges they had. They were horrified at our primitive living conditions; they couldn't believe we lived in tents.

On 7 January 1945 we moved to St.Omer, there we lived in an old convent. The hospital was taken over from the Germans. It was a proper hospital, quite well equipped. There were still German patients there that had been left behind. We asked them if they were afraid of us. They said they weren't afraid because they had been told by the departing Germans that Canadians were coming.

There is an interesting story about this hospital. RAF pilot Douglas Bader had escaped from this hospital He had artificial legs from a 1931 aircraft crash but was able to talk his way into the RAF. He commanded the 242nd Squadron which was manned by Canadians. He had been shot down and escaped twice. At this hospital, while it was in German hands, they took his artificial limbs away from him so he couldn't escape again.

I was discharged from the Army at Winnipeg in 1946. We had as patients men from the Winnipeg Grenadiers. They had been prisoners of war of the Japanese at Hong Kong. They required a tremendous amount of rehabilitation and reconstructive surgery.

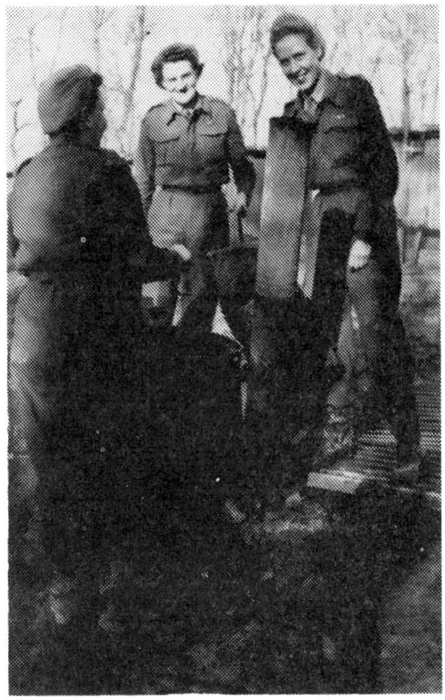

L-R: Margaret Mitchell, Wilma Bergman, Grace Canning. The water hole. One canvas bucket of hot water for our tent. This one was for washing. Note the duck boards and rubber boots because of mud.

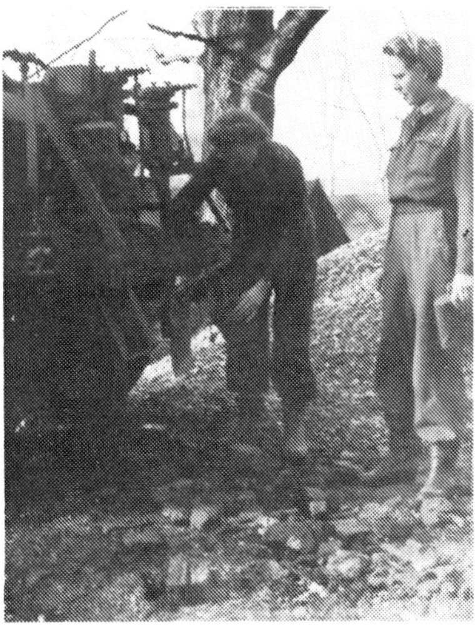

L-R: Wilma Bergman, Saskatchewan; Grace Canning, Moose Jaw Saskatchewan. Mesnières-en-Bray, France 1944. Filling our water bottles with drinking water. We were allowed one bottle per day.

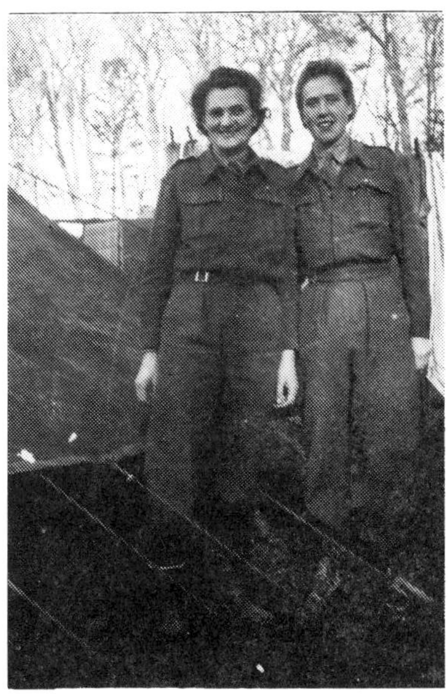

Wilma (Bergman) Morin and Grace Canning Our home in France 1944

Irene (Poole) Lavallee

Graduated from: Regina General Hospital School of Nursing. Year: 1941

Military History:

Service: RCAMC

Rank: Lieutenant N/S

Served: 18 December 1942 to 16 November 1945

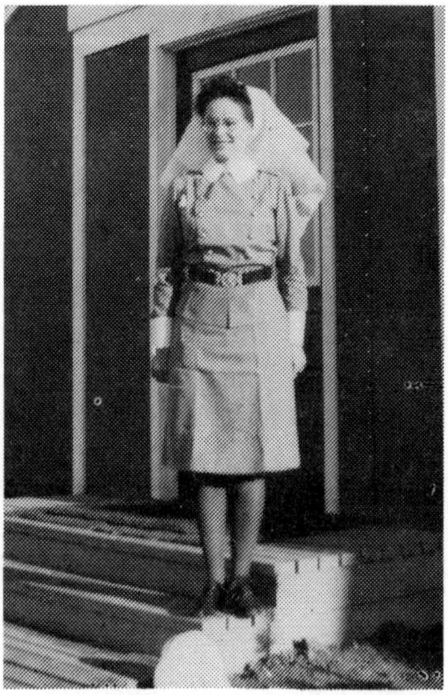

Lt. N/S Irene (Poole) Lavallee Maple Creek 1943

Friends and co-workers were joining the service and I wanted to be a part of it. Some things stand out in my mind as I recollect my experiences in the Army: Most important was making new friends in No. 21 General Military Hospital. Of great importance, also, was hearing news of the D-Day invasion while on a troop ship crossing the Atlantic. Being in England for the first time and then seeing parts of France was a highlight for me. Most important of all – my reason for being in the service – meeting and caring for our Canadian troops.

Ruth (Hunter) Percival

Graduate from: Brantford General Hospital School of Nursing. Year: 1941

Military History:

Service: RCAMC

Rank: Lt. N/S

Served: August 27, 1943 to January 12, 1946

My brother Lloyd was badly injured during military training exercises at Brockville, Ontario. He suffered a leg wound, chest wound and eye wound. He lost the ends of all his fingers of the right hand from distal joints, his thumb joint was destroyed. If I needed a reason to join the service this did influence me.

When Christmas approached in 1944, we decided we would have a special Christmas party in our own shacks. There were five of us. Three of that number had shared a tent when we first arrived in France, and we had also been together for a time when at Hamilton Military Hospital and so were the other two who joined us. Remember, on Christmas Day nursing sisters served dinner to our orderlies, etc. So our little party probably was not on Christmas Day.

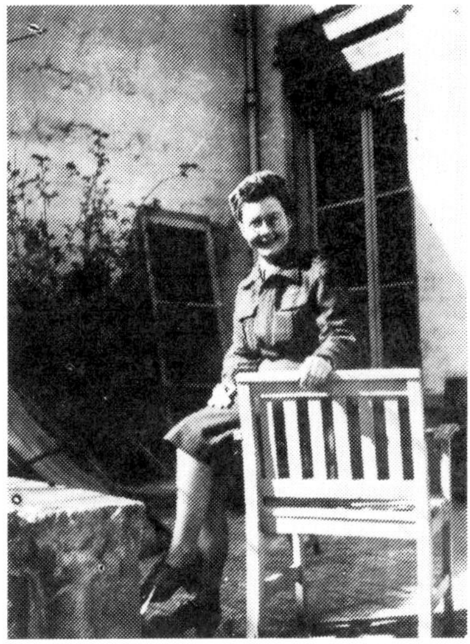

Ruth (Hunter) Percival, No. 21 CGH at St. Omer, France. I was stationed there from mid-January to after V-E Day 1945 when I went to Sogel, Germany.

Two of the nurses had arranged to have a turkey cooked for us in the village, so we prepared all the other items. I think our table was probably the top of someone's trunk. Turkey was brought from the village (Mesnieres-en-Bray) but the two deliverers seemed to have lost their appetite. The rest of us enjoyed our meal, but were glad the girls had kept their news to themselves. Their news was that the turkey, cooked without stuffing, was cooked with its head on, and they had stopped on their way to cut it off with a pocket knife which one of them had.

Another anecdote happened that fall, 1944. The building our hospital was in what had been a Catholic boys' school, complete with church, moat and in the middle, a Calvados still. Out of bounds to us of course. The moat and bridge over it faced a country lane, and up this lane one afternoon came a padre, who was white-haired and somewhat elderly looking. He had a long stick, a branch of something, and before him he was herding four, I think, Germans who had surrendered to him – because they were starving – they said!

When we crossed the channel we expected to see France any minute, but our trip was delayed several times. We were on a hospital ship and it was too large to land unless the tide was just

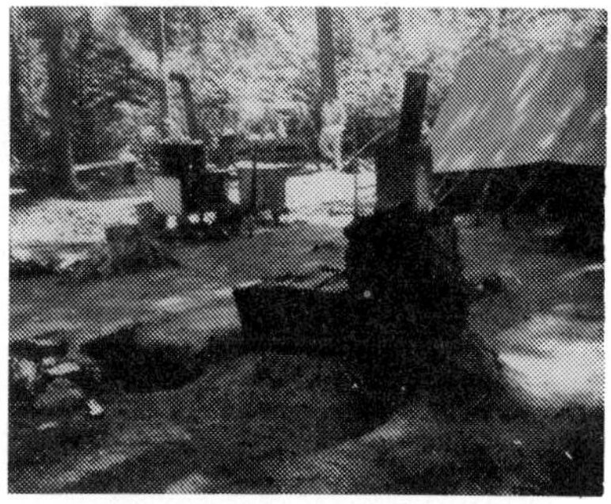

Pit fire for heating water

right. It took us five days. By the third day food supplies ran out, and we were served semolina pudding (Cream of Wheat porridge to us) and Naafi tea. I think at that time we just laughed it off. Some of the nurses added a bit of chocolate to improve the pudding. We had all packed chocolate bars (our idea of emergency food). Also, we landed in "full pack."

Then there was a period when, for some reason, our food supplies were carrots, hard tack biscuits, corned beef and that dreadful Naafi tea. It was all sweetened, you know, and tasted dreadful. The water was not all it should have been, which we expected, as we were all allowed only one water bottle of water a day (that included for washing ourselves too). Also, we had heard about "the Normandy glide," a nasty diarrhea which was very hard to get rid of. Possibly because the French believed in watering their gardens with "night soil."

After VE Day, we all felt that we would soon be going home, but of course, there were many nurses with more points than we had.

We were still at St. Omer waiting for the Germans in Dunkirk to be brought out. Their commanding officer would not surrender, and finally committed suicide. Many of the patients were up patients, and of the bed patients, many were so frail that they soon died. I suppose the move was just too much for them. Among them there were a few Russians, an occasional Czech or whatever. There were also Hitler Youth, Nazis, whatever. They refused to admit defeat and were a problem. These were soon sent to POW Camps. Many of these patients were in body casts – very debilitated. Many had wounds that had healed by "first intention" which left very bad scars. These men each had jars of cooked meat and other supplies. Apparently they had not expected the care we could give them. They were also given cigarettes, which they seemed to enjoy.

Since our hospital then included parts of a school; there were smaller areas that were harder to cover. I recall a diphtheria patient, isolated with a resulting paralysis of the palate, and I was on my way to check on him. I had to go through a group of young Russians who were fighting over cigarettes (Red Cross) they had been given. I don't mean arguing, one had lost a tooth, one had a bloody nose, and so on. So I was taking the cigarettes away from them when the medical officer came in. It was hard to tell if he was angrier at the patients for causing trouble, or at me for acting so impulsively! Anyway, they stopped fighting.

We soon learned that No. 21 was splitting up and we were to be separated. No. 21 was a 1200-bed unit and No. 16 was 600 beds. I don't recall whether we knew we were to nurse Russians or not, but I doubt it. No. 16 was brought to Germany some months before we arrived there. You may remember that during and immediately after the war there were many sectors, not just the Russians and the Allies, which people now know were the arrangements during the occupation period.

The area where No. 16 was situated was in the Polish sector, and the Poles did not have hospital units in the field, so we Canadians got the job. It was near a small village named Sogel which had been reduced to rubble. The only building standing was a brick house that had been a nun's residence, and that was where we nurse's were quartered. Our area and the field across the road were both surrounded by barbed wire. We were not to go anywhere without an armed guard. The song, *Don't Fence Me In*, was popular just then, and we really thought it might have been written by one of us!

The hospital itself was planned around a fine, ordinary looking two-storied brick house which had been the Duke of Oldenburg's hunting lodge. We were told some of the medical officers had gone hunting for wild boar, but we never saw any results of such. The houses were used by the central supply, drug store, dental office and other facilities. All our patients were considered to be tubercular, and most of them were.

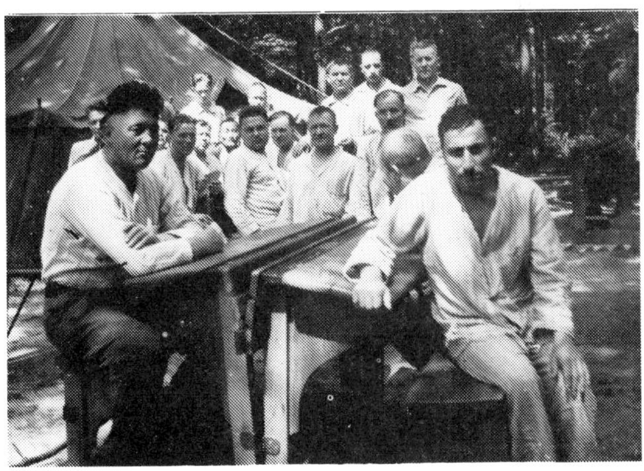

Russian patients at Sogel (ex POWs) June 1945 Germany, they considered their cotton housecoats quite a prize and seldom wore them; they would not exercise but loved the sunshine.

Surgery patients were kept

in one tent, considered, "the clean ward." Operations consisted mainly of removal of a kidney, part of a lung, and other things resulting from tuberculosis. A couple of us did not have a positive IC test, so were nursing on this ward. Approximately one-half to two-thirds of our patients on surgery were confined to bed. Trees had been removed in swatches between the houses. Each cleared area held two long rows of canvas, set end to end.

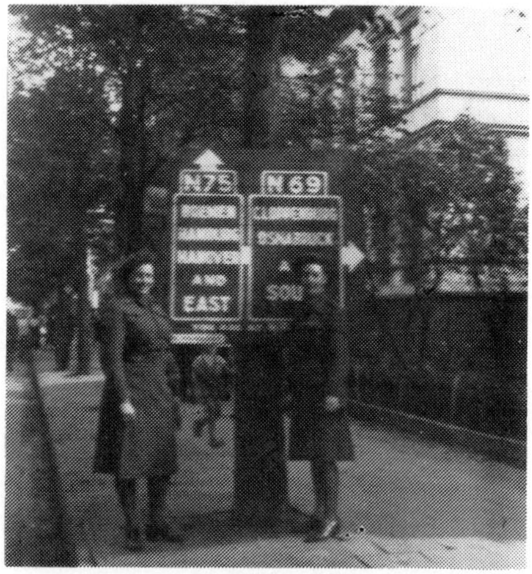

L-R: Gladys (West) Bartholomew, Ruth (Hunter) Percival, at Oldenburg, Germany, We used to take pictures of sign posts as a means of telling our family where we were.

The ward end-to-end with our clean ward was all "up patients," and these were some of the men who had been making "hooch" and had brought bottles of same back to their beds. Around midnight they started making considerable noise, and suddenly someone shouted, *"Fire!"* The sisters on duty in that ward left in a hurry. Since all those patients were able to walk there was none hurt. It really scared us old "21ers" as we lost our mess tent to fire just before Christmas in France. It only took 11 minutes to finish our tent in the fire! Two or three nights after the fire, one of my up patients arrived back at the tent with a bottle of hooch. I called the Sgt. on duty, and asked him to take it away from the men. He refused, saying that would be foolish. All I could think of was not being able to move the patients in a hurry; in a fire we would not be able to get them out. I had worked on that ward for some weeks, and felt I had given good post-operation care. So I held out my hand to get him to give up his bottle where upon the Sgt. turned quickly and left. The man said something that I think was "please," but I dumped it out. As long as I live, I don't want to ever consider doing such a foolish thing, but our tent wasn't burnt down, and the patients stopped bringing their liquor to bed!

The meals for our Russians was of good supply. I think the ex-POW diet was to be 2600 calories. They were served five meals a day, the three regular, mid-afternoon tea with bread and jam or juices and the same in the evening. Not so the nursing staff, no milk or butter for us, as there was no pasteurization, we had dehydrated vegetables, powdered milk and black bread. Dehydrated turnips are the closest thing to sawdust I've ever seen. There wasn't much fuss when the move was made to send all our patients to the Russian zone. A few of the original No. 16 nurses went ahead to Oldenburg – we soon packed up. A convoy arrived to take the patients. Some of them seemed very loathe to go, but were sent on. The hospital in Oldenburg was a well-built and attractive place. There was a very large physiotherapy department and operating theatres with lots of green ceramic tiles.

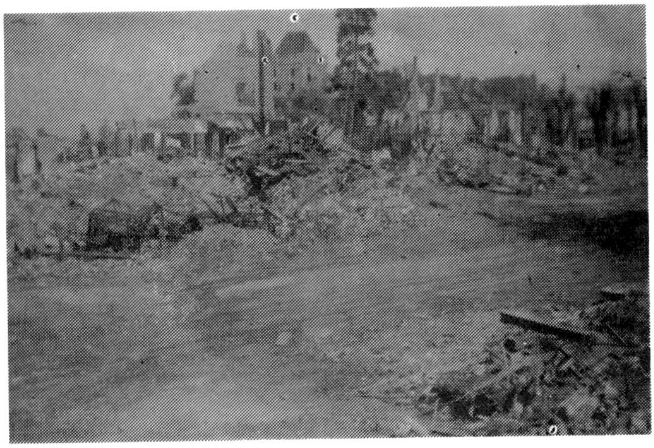

All that's left of the village of Sogel, Germany, July 1945. No. 16 CGH was near here.

I haven't mentioned the arrangement for 48-hour leaves. These were arranged for all nurses every two weeks, approximately, to give us a rest from the tuberculosis threat. We were sent to Amsterdam, Holland for these.

The nuclear bomb was dropped on Nagasaki and Hiroshima, Japan. We were told we had too many points to stay to run the occupation hospital and staff of nurses, many straight from Canada, were to replace us. The "no fraternizing" rule was dropped and we started back to England.

The truck that I was travelling in was near the border with Holland when we were side-swiped by a Polish truck. Our truck then crossed the road and tipped back onto its right side. There were twelve to fourteen nurses and about four other ranks. We were taken to No. 6 CCS at Almelo, Holland; a few went on. There were two nurses with broken legs, several others with cracked ribs, pulled tendons and so on. One nurse with a fractured skull and two with broken legs were flown to England. The rest of us went first to No. 2 General at Ghent, then to No. 3 at Bruges. This meant, of course, that we had lost our chance to be off home. From late August until the end of October was very boring for me. We received some physiotherapy at Ghent; then when we arrived at Bruges we were put straight on the wards, which was not good, but that is another story.

I have enclosed a snap taken of Lt. N/S MacDonell putting flowers on Laliberte's grave. This boy was one of our orderlies from No. 21. Because he spoke French he was employed in admitting to translate. He was in an accident that should never have happened, as accidents so often are. When he died, a group of us from No. 21 was his guard of honour, and he was buried in the corner of a wheat field in Germany. The reason for including other POWs is because we always seemed to have them after we arrived in France, and they were bedded and cared for just like our own. Any other way would just not have been possible.

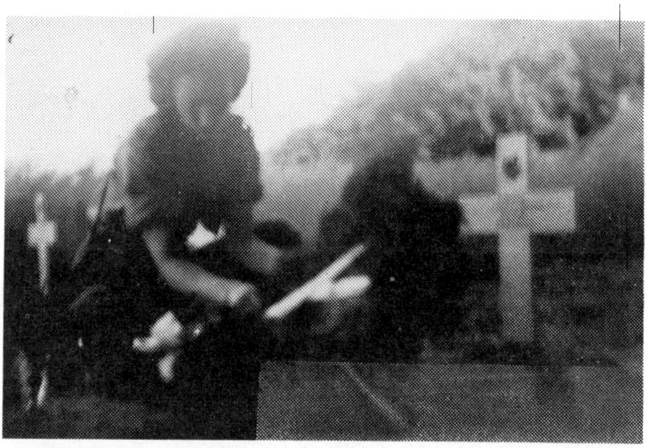

Lt. N/S MacDonnell at Laliberte's grave, July 1945

Eileen (Robinson) Shaw

Graduated from: St. Joseph's Hospital School of Nursing, Victoria, B.C. Year: 1936

Military History:

Service: RCAMC

Rank: Lt. N/S

Served: World War Two

No. 21 Canadian General Hospital as well as 22 and 24 General were made up for D-Day; that is, personnel came from every military district in Canada to make up these units. Nos. 21 and 22 went overseas on the *Andes* and the *Lady Nelson*, half of each unit went on

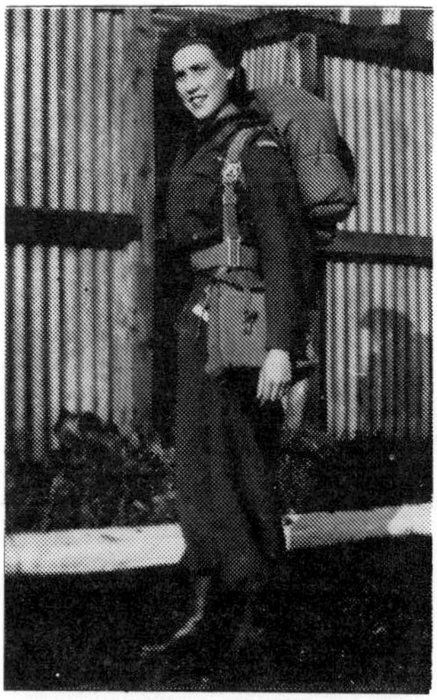

No. 21 CGH. Eileen (Robinson) Shaw, 1944

each ship so if one ship were lost the whole unit would not be lost.

I was stationed at Prince Rupert and was in charge of the operating room after I finished basic training in Victoria. In early May 1944 we went by troop train to Windsor, Nova Scotia, and embarked at Halifax for overseas duty 1 June 1944. Twelve days later we docked at Liverpool and travelled by train to Whitby on the Yorkshire coast. We were the first of our unit to arrive, the others followed a few days later.

We next moved to Horley in Surrey and from there to Scotch Corners in Yorkshire. From there, we moved to a transit camp – all of this moving took most of September.

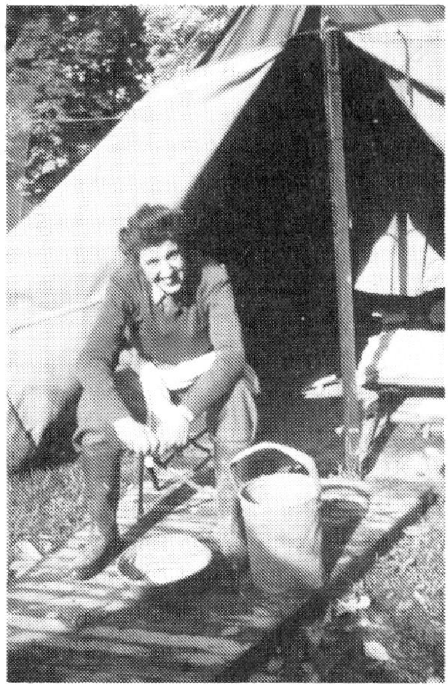

Eileen Robinson, France, 1944. The water bucket outside our tent. Three or four of us lived in one tent.

Lt. N/S Eileen Robinson summer of 1944 in England before going to the Continent. In gas cape with all my belongings. We were allowed one extra kit bag.

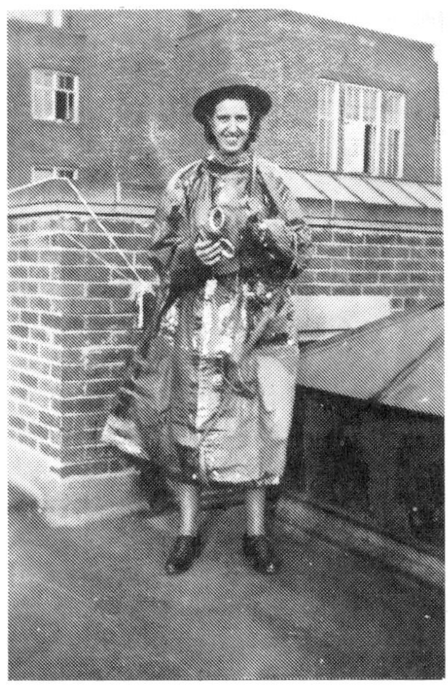

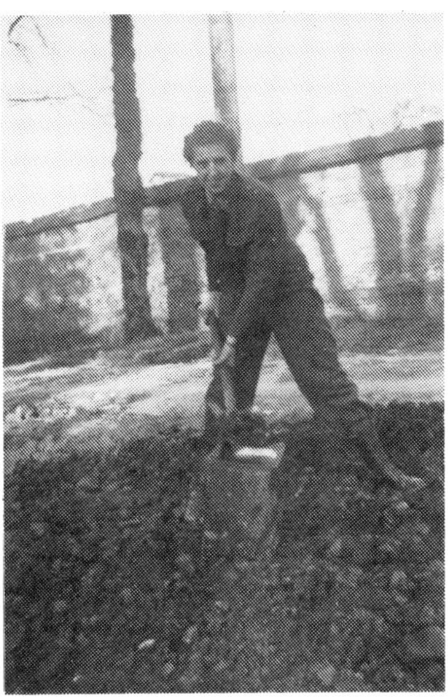

Eileen Robinson digging coal from the dump in Mesnières. We needed coal for the pot bellied stoves. We had them in our huts but we never had anything to burn in them.

At the end of September we embarked for the Continent and landed at Dieppe. We travelled by truck to Mesnieres-en-Bray where No. 21 General was located in an ancient chateau.

We were a 1200-bed hospital with a great staff, good medical officers – easy to work with – we all got along very well. We had good equipment and supplies. I was in charge of our operating room and set it up in tents. We moved to St. Omer in early January 1945. There were regular autoclaves in this hospital that had only recently been occupied by the Germans.

I was with No. 21 General until it disbanded in September of 1945.

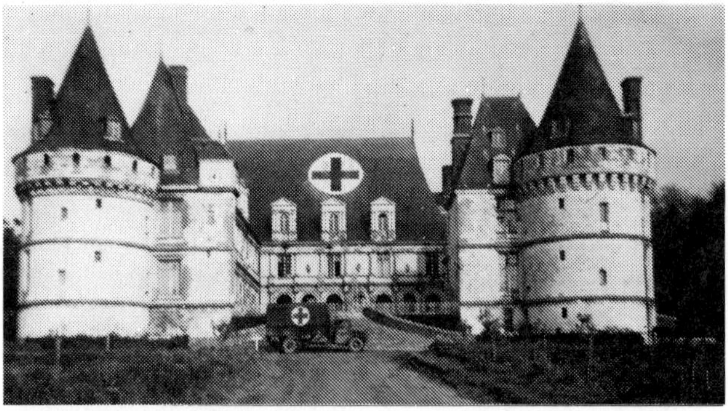

Our hospital, No. 21 General was in the Chateau Mesnières-en-Bray. The Red Cross was put on by Germans when they occupied it to keep the Allies from bombing it. It was their ammunition dump.

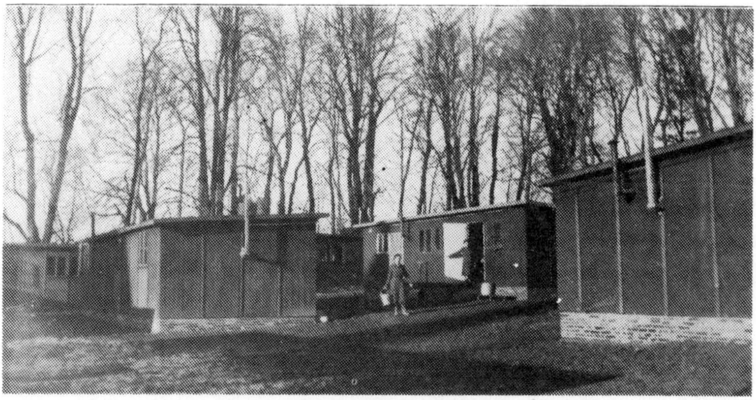

France January 1945
We had graduated to the luxury of huts.
Our abode is the one with the door open.

Caroline (Livingstone) Stacey

Graduated from: St. Paul's Hospital School of Nursing, Vancouver B.C. Year: 1943

Military History:

Branch of Service: RCAMC

Rank: Lt. N/S

Served: February 1944 to May 1946

My mother, Edith Esther Clarke, was a WW I volunteer. She graduated in 1917 from Newton Hospital School of Nursing in Newton, Mass. U.S.A. She returned to Canada on a Red Cross special train from Boston to nurse victims of the Halifax explosion December 7, 1917. She enlisted in the CAMC early in 1918. She was stationed at Shornecliff Military Hospital near Dover, England. She returned to Halifax late in 1918 after the Armistice and was on staff at Camp Hill Military Hospital until her marriage October 1919.

We are the only known mother- daughter military nurse combination in the Canadian Armed Forces.

My father was a WW I Infantry volunteer who had much experience in Army hospitals having had five wound stripes and an MC and Bar.

My brother Grant was in the Army and a war amputee; he lost his right hand. My sister Kathleen was in the navy, WRCNS.

Our family were all patriotic Nova Scotians for 200 years and not types to shirk our duties. I grew up in the old garrison town, oldest settlement, first capital of Nova Scotia, Annapolis Royal. I was a volunteer in WW II; for me it was not a career. My service was overseas with No. 21 Canadian General Hospital

NO. 22 CANADIAN GENERAL HOSPITAL

Claire (Murray) Bowman
Florence (Kirkpatrick) Dougherty
Evelyn (Brown) Furnajieff
Shirley (Gooding) Garrioch
Lydia Last
Bertha (Jones) Rudow
Joan (Gore) Spring
Marion Rhae (Nichols) Stewart

No. 22 Canadian General Hospital mobilized at Stratford, Ontario, 20 February 1944. Col. W.A. Jones was appointed CO and on 5 April N/S Tavener was appointed matron. Nursing sisters arrived 15 April and by the end of May they embarked at Halifax for duty in the U.K. By 28 June all No. 22 General nursing sisters had reported for duty at Bramshott. The hospital remained at this permanent installation in England and served as a base hospital for casualties arriving from the Continent. By 1 August 1946 the hospital ceased admitting patients as No. 22 General was to close mid-September 1946. No. 22 was the last Canadian General Hospital to occupy the site at Bramshott.

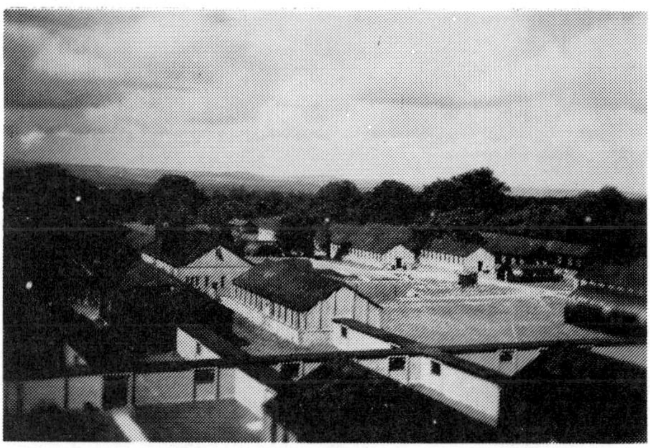

Bramshott Military Hospital showing the compound between medical and surgical sides

Claire (Murray) Bowman

Graduated from: Winnipeg General Hospital School of Nursing. Year: 1942

Military History:

Served: RCAMC

Rank: Lt. N/S

Served: 24 January 1944 to May 1946

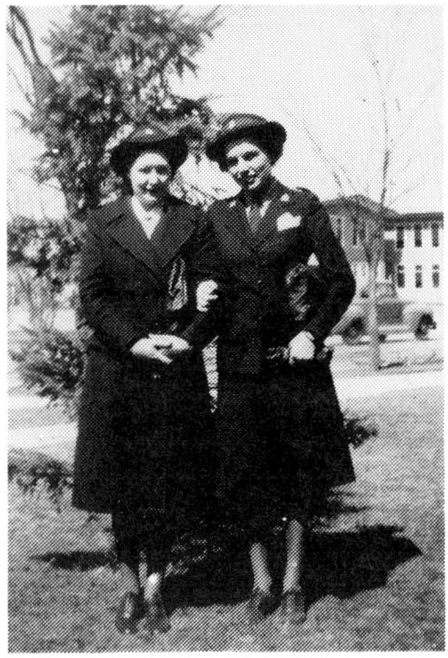

L-R: Ruth Jack; Claire Murray at Fort Osborne Military Hospital, Winnipeg, Manitoba, April, 1944.

I decided to become a nursing sister after seeing countless train-loads of young people take off from Winnipeg while we were training. Among these were my brother and five cousins – none of whom returned.

I enlisted at Fort Osborne Military Hospital, Winnipeg, Manitoba, and left in April for Stratford, Ontario.

I did not have any moments that called for great courage or incredible skill or that brought honours in any specific area. My experience in the Army was relatively straightforward, and probably does not offer what you might consider highlights, though the whole experience was a highlight in my life. In fact, it was exciting first to get into the Army, even though I was advised on enlisting that I would never get out of Canada. There were plenty ahead of me with more experience waiting to get into the Army and others in line to go overseas. Nevertheless, I was accepted in January of 1944, two weeks after I applied, and went overseas in June. We sailed on the *Andes*, and were on the water for D-Day, arriving in Liverpool 8 June 1944.

We were posted to Bramshott where I spent my entire overseas time as a member of our surgical group, except for the last two months, which I spent on a surgical ward.

Our surgical group consisted of 12 nursing sisters, with at least one from each province. It was interesting how quickly we became a team.

Upon arrival in England we were sent by train across the country to Whitby on the coast of the North Sea for a week before heading to Bramshott. Here we were billeted in what had been a grand old hotel. It had suffered from the bombing in the earlier years of the war, and a good part of it was destroyed. The rooms we had were damaged; there were cracked basins, fireplace mantles, and windows. But the hotel provided us with shelter, bed and breakfast, a marvellous old pub, (quite undamaged!) and lots of laughs. I mention breakfast especially because there we had our first experience with English sausage. We did also have lunch and dinner.

Three of us from Manitoba shared one room with a cot each and three grey blankets... one cot had a broken leg, so we placed it in between the other two, in an attempt to prop it up, and took turns sleeping in it. It never failed but that it collapsed during efforts to get in and then frequently throughout the night when the user made the mistake of turning over.

We travelled by train from Whitby to London where we were to change trains in Waterloo Station. When we arrived in Waterloo there was considerable activity and concern. One train load of our unit had already left, and word had come in that the tracks on which they were to travel had been bombed. At that time, it was not clear whether the train was beyond the blast or in it. As it turned out, they had passed through safely, ahead of the bomb. We were herded up to a Salvation Army canteen to wait until the tracks were repaired. As we headed for the stairs there was the sound of an alert, the first of many we were to hear. A cleaning lady on the stairs grabbed up her bucket and dashed on up the stairs, saying, *"Blimey, it's thim divils again,"* whereupon the tension among our group was relieved with a good laugh.

Our unit, No. 22 CGH, served as Casualty Clearing for several weeks until units were able to move on to the Continent. During this period our patients were flown across from the battlefield in Normandy and brought by convoy to our unit where they proceeded from admitting to surgery where we carried out what was called "wound toilette and debridement." Their wounds were cleansed, loose tissue trimmed and fresh dressing applied. Then those who were fit to travel were sent on to other hospitals for further treatment and care. Those whose injuries required more attention, or who were not ready for further travel, remained with us for needed repair and until they were considered fit to travel.

From time to time a V-1 that had overshot London would pass over our unit, travelling the whole length of our hospital, which stretched along for a mile. In spite of the speed at which these missiles travelled, it seemed to take a long time before it was out of range. At those times we were always pleased to have the noise of the V-1 continue.

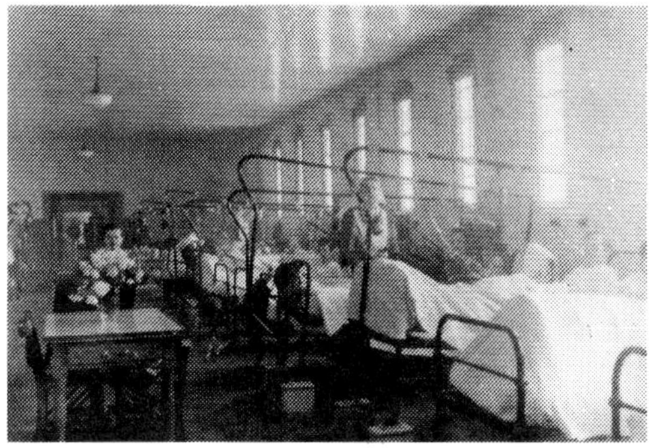

A view of a surgical ward at No. 22 CGH, Bramshott 1945

Although we were to have a week's leave every three months, we did not count on getting leave until there was a bit of a break in the number of casualties coming in. We did spend one leave in Scotland, one in Devon, one in Northern Ireland, and one in Cornwall – each a rare experience.

It was interesting to note the attitude of some of the English people towards our profession of nursing. It did not rate very high in the opinion of some. I rode in a carriage on a train one day and was queried by a very fine looking lady as to the nature of my uniform and as to my purpose in being there. When I told her we were nurses in the Canadian Army she became somewhat cool. She said, *"But you wouldn't be doing this when you are at home, would you?"* When I replied that I would, she immediately stiffened and there was no further conversation. Obviously it was not considered to be a suitable occupation.

At one time we had an English civilian in hospital as a patient since he had been knocked down by a Canadian Army vehicle. He was very uneasy, though his injuries were not severe. It turned out that he was afraid of us, being 'colonials'. He did not really expect to find us civilized. In due time he turned out to be a very pleasant, cooperative patient and he did laugh at his initial concern.

There were, of course, many who undertook to make our stay in England as pleasant as could be under the circumstances. One family, a Lord and Lady, invited us to make use of their tennis court if ever we had free time. We went many times and enjoyed their lovely gardens as well as the game. They never came out while we were there until one evening they came to make the grand announcement that the war was over. Victory in

Europe had been won. They had just heard the good news.

Our trip back to Canada in March of 1946 aboard the *Ile de France* took much longer than our trip over, since we were no longer dodging U-boats. I remember on that trip that we had two nursing sisters who became dreadfully ill on our second day out. They went to bed and stayed there, barely eating, until the day came that an announcement was made over the PA system that we would be docking in Halifax the following day. They immediately climbed down from their bunks, pinned up their hair, packed what they had scattered around and in due time came down to dinner, just as though they had never had an ill moment. The power of "Homecoming!"

Florence (Kirkpatrick) Dougherty

Graduated from: St. Boniface School of Nursing at St. Boniface, Manitoba. Year: 1938

Military History:

Service: RCAMC

Rank: Lt. N/S

Served: July 1943 to January 1946

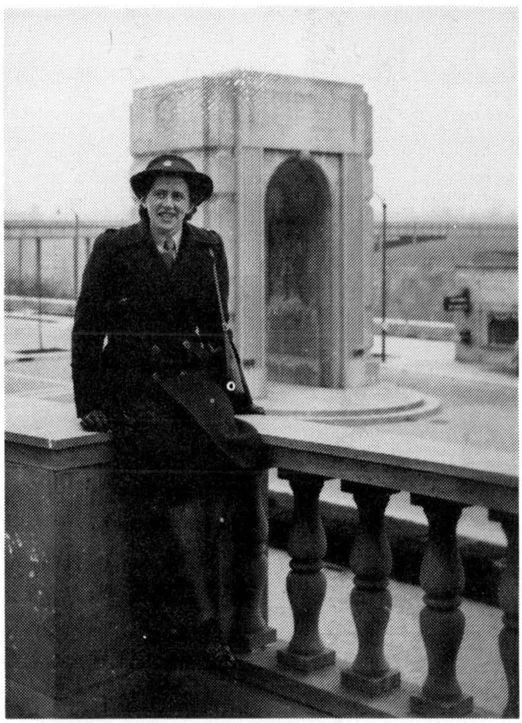

Lt. N/S (Kirkpatrick) Dougherty at Niagara Falls on the way overseas

My memories of No. 22 Canadian General Hospital at Bramshott (June 1944 - April 1945) are still vivid. How busy we were, a 1200-bed hospital. We often had more than that number; even up to 1600, as we were used as a casualty clearing station. We admitted casualties flown directly from the battlefields to be assessed, cleaned up and often moved on to another hospital to meet their particular needs. What wonderful patients they were – never complaining – just grateful to have a clean bed and good food – real "crackleberries" instead of dried eggs. Their wounds were so varied and severe, but they bore their suffering stoically. I remember one patient particularly who had a shattered shoulder and had an aeroplane splint on it. One morning when I was with him, he looked desperate and blurted out, *"Sister, I have maggots."* Sure enough, there were maggots wriggling around the edges of the cast and in his bed. The MO left things as they were, as the maggots cleaned up the inflected flesh. We didn't have the many antibiotics we have today – only a limited supply of penicillin.

At this time there were hundreds of buzz bombs directed toward London, many of them passing right over us. Often, during the night when the alert would sound and we heard the bomb overhead, some of the patients would throw themselves under their beds and not be aware that they had done so.

Another vivid memory is of the time spent with No. 16 General the summer of 1945. We were stationed at Sogel in northwest Germany. The village had been pretty well bombed out and there was bitter hostility evident in the faces of the villagers. The nursing sisters were quartered in a convent school which had been damaged. No glass was left in the windows and many slats were missing from the roof with consequent leaks when it rained, which was often; no heat and no plumbing, as the German troops had poured concrete into all water facilities. The hospital was set up on the Duke of Arenburg's hunting estate on the edge of the village. The brick lodge and guest houses were used for the operating room, X-ray, pharmacy stores, etc. Tents were set up in clearings in the forest, arranged as the spokes of a wheel, with the hub being the solid buildings. Our patients were Russian and Polish POWs brought in from surrounding prison camps – those judged most likely to survive. Many of them had TB of the bones, and all suffered from malnutrition. We fed them well, and gave them a "tonic." They each had a tablespoon and would hold it out to us as we went around with our big bottle of tonic and say "Schnapps Sistra!"

They had been deprived of freedom for so long, that now that they could move around, we had a hard time keeping track of them. They would get up in the morning wearing only pyjama bottoms and a rag of some kind around their head and wash themselves at the washing stands, and after breakfast, wander off through the woods, often to raid the villagers' gardens, bringing back handfuls of vegetable greens and the odd egg. Even the most ill patients would be up and around, although some of them would be dead the next day.

We had only one interpreter, so it was difficult to communicate with the patients, but they didn't seem to mind. I remember one early morning going to a patient who was to have surgery that day. The interpreter had told him he was to go to the OR in the morning and that he was not to have breakfast. I stood beside his cot and saw movements under the blanket that had been pulled up over his head, and I heard munching sounds. So I lifted the blanket off his face, and there he was with a big handful of fresh garlic, busily chewing it up! Needless to say, he didn't have his surgery that day.

After about four months, arrangements were made to return the patients to their home areas. I shall never forget the excitement there was as these men were loaded into trucks and started off to homes they hadn't seen for a long time, and indeed most of them didn't know if they had homes to go to. There was eagerness and hope on their faces and they sang with exuberance, as only Russians can, as they left the hospital camp. We could only hope they would be reunited with their families and friends.

After this brief period in Sogel, we moved to Oldenburg, where our first patient was General Montgomery. I chose to be returned to England, then home to Canada, rather than face another winter in the cold.

I feel that the experience of wartime nursing was the best any nurse could wish for.

M. Evelyn Mary (Brown) Furnadjieff

Graduated from: Royal Columbian Hospital School of Nursing. Year: 1943

Other: Psychiatric Graduate 1940 (PMH), Post graduate, Montreal Neurological Institute

Military History:

Service: RCAMC

Rank: Lieut. N/S Active - Captain Matron (R)

Served: 14 February 1944 to 29 April 1946. Struck Off Strength. Promoted to Capt. (M) E. M. Furnadjieff (Reserve); remained in Reserve

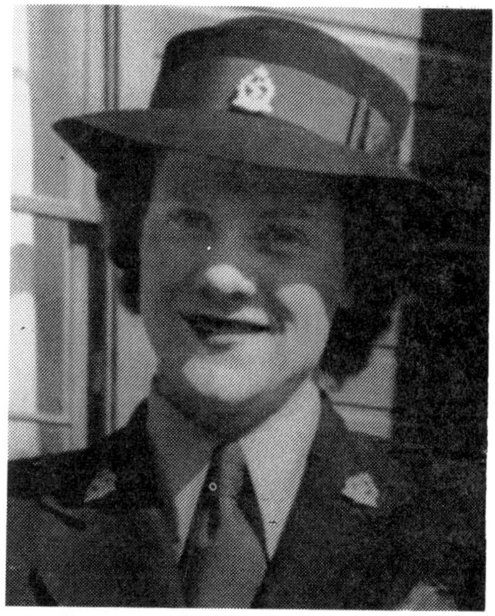

Captain Matron Evelyn (Brown) Furnadjieff, No. 24 Medical Company, RCAMC (R) Vancouver 1947

My first assignment before I went overseas was organizing the Tent Operating Room in the new training camp hospital in Wainwright, Alberta, May 1944. As live ammunition was used by the Army units training there, serious accidents often occurred requiring ambulances, intravenous in the field etc. – all intensive training for a recent graduate nurse. I learned to cope and the memories of these valuable experiences have remained with me to this day!

Those people in Alberta have a great sense of humour and they were very good to us. I was in the operating room – I was the one they called out to set up for emergency surgery. I would put my boots on and wade through the mud to get there, then I would have to clean the mud off before I could start work.

The civilian hospital autoclaved our supplies. The local people invited us to great dinners. I wish the people here were more like that; they couldn't do enough for us. The beer parlours were something else, though. At camp we practically lived in each others armpits, then men and women had to separate when we went to the beer parlours in Calgary.

I was posted to Great Britain in 1944 and served in the operating room of the 22nd Canadian General Hospital, Bramshott, Surrey, until my return to Canada on the *Ile de France* in 1946. At Bramshott our wounded arrived in long lines of trucks marked with large red crosses; two walking wounded and four stretcher cases per truck. These convoys usually came from Dover. Even after a long and wearisome trip, "our boys" had smiles for "their sisters." We loved them all!

A highlight in my military career occurred when, as Captain Matron E. Furnadjieff, Reserve, I received orders to join Commanding Officer Colonel Leeson, RCAMC (R) in forming the No. 24 Medical Company, RCAMC, 968 West 27th Avenue, Vancouver, B.C. My responsibilities in this were to recruit registered nurses and to train them as nursing sisters in the military reserves.

This company was formed of 2 units – 1 field company and 1 field hospital. The 24th Company in successive years took part in the national championship field trials and were victorious, winning 3 Ryerson and 2 Shillington trophies.

My pride in the personnel knew no bounds and then to be rewarded Her Majesty's Coronation Award on their behalf was indeed a highlight in my military career!

The following is reproduced by permission of the Queen.

Olive Wilkinson and I were returning from Harrowgate, Yorkshire, where we had stayed with Olive's aunt for a weekend. We were in a hurry to get back to London in time for duty. We caught the first train we saw, and it was full. Not only was it full, but by now it was locked at both ends, and we couldn't get off. We walked up and down the aisle looking for empty compartments but there were none. Wilks said, *"We're just going to have to throw our kit bag on the floor."* At this point, the door to a compartment opened and we heard someone say, *"There are two seats in here if you ladies would care to use them."* Wilks said, *"Oh, thanks very much"*; threw her kit on the shelf overhead, propped her hat over her face, and promptly went to sleep. I sat down and attempted to make conversation.

By this time I knew we had made a mistake in getting on this carriage as we had third class tickets and now the train was locked at both ends. The lady who had invited us in to her compartment was writing in a beautiful leather bound case. She said, *"I'm writing to my son, he's a POW you know."* At this point the train lurched and the case slid off her knees. We knocked heads together as we both bent down to pick up the writing case. I got quite a blow on the head and my hat fell backwards but I read the inscription of the writing case. It read, "Princess Royal Harewood House Leeds." By this time I realized the compartment was occupied by the Princess Royal and her husband, the Earl of Harewood. I'll try to explain what a beautiful, kind person she was. She wore a British military uniform, I think she was a general. I felt very grubby and here was this gorgeous creature. What could I do? I said, *"Excuse me, I must tidy up, we nearly missed the train and it wouldn't do to be late for duty." "No, it certainly wouldn't,"* she said. I found a lavatory and a clean blue shirt. When I came back she said, *"My, you look very nice in your uniform."* Wilks woke up from her sleep and, not knowing we were sharing the Royal compartment, said, *"Brownie, I'm hungry."* Her aunt had made packages of anchovy paste sandwiches. She hauled down her kit bag, took out two packages of sandwiches wrapped in newspaper and handed me one package. The whole compartment soon smelled of fish. I closed up my package and stuffed it in my kit bag.

The Princess Royal said to her lady-in-waiting, *"We should have lunch now."* They placed a beautiful picnic basket on the floor. It had rows of watercress sandwiches in it. The Princess Royal insisted that we share their lunch. The Earl of Harewood offered me a cigarette. It was embossed with a gold crest and I wanted to save it; however, I smoked it and saved the stub end. It eventually disintegrated, but I did want to keep it. The Princess Royal asked many questions about our province. British Columbia had sent them 30 evergreen trees as a wedding present. She described them by their Latin name and said they were very pleased with their gift. The trees lined the driveway at Harewood House in Leeds and by now they were 30 feet high. Wilks piped up to say, *"Oh, they grow higher than that in B.C."*

Princess Royal asked us many questions about our duties and our unit. She wanted to know what nursing sisters did and if they had a specialty. She said it was wonderful that young Canadian women took such a great part in the war effort. For me, there was that strain of knowing she was thc Princess Royal and that the train was non-stop to London.

When the train did stop, a conductor materialized. If a man can curtsy, he almost curtsied to the Princess Royal and addressed her as "Ma'am." He turned to us and with a straight, stern English face, asked for our tickets. He was shocked, of course. He told us in pounds and pence how much we owed and I paid him the amount he requested. The Princess Royal sat there with a smile on her face, understanding all the while what was going on.

At the end of the journey we were off first. People in the station seemed surprised to see us step off the train. Apparently, the Princess Royal had made a note of our names and addresses, for the next day a large box of books arrived for our mess at No. 22 Canadian General Hospital. Wilks received inscribed, leather bound volumes of Shakespeare. I had carried on quite a discussion of Shakespeare on the train. I received a leather bound, inscribed volume of *India Recalled.*

She wrote a letter to the director of our hospital saying she was privileged to have met two nursing sisters. When it was read out in the mess, the matron stood up and asked who these two nursing sisters were. When I stood up, she thanked me. Then Wilks stood up and said, *"I was the other one. Did you know that my father worked on the estate of Harewood. After he lost his leg, they retired him early and he went to Canada."* I couldn't understand why she hadn't told them this on the train, but Wilks said that was not the sort of thing she would do.

I've never forgotten this experience with the Princess Royal; I enjoyed it. I knew she loved the trees by the way she described how they lined their driveway; the graciousness of her in writing to our matron, and the books – they were wonderful. She was interested in everything we said. There is so much sadness in war, and yet there is a goodness too.

A soldier wrote this poem and slipped it into my pocket:

Nurses

Nurses have hearts that are golden
Nurses have love near divine
If it isn't so; then it ought to be
For the work they are doing's sublime
Not sublime from an earthly standpoint
For that certainly cannot be so
But someone looks on as they linger
He too walks about to and fro
He sees all the kind little touches
For which they never are paid
Except when a poor tired patient
Says; "Thank you, dear nurse, for your aid."
G.W.P.

Shirley (Gooding) Garrioch

Graduated from: Royal Jubilee Hospital School of Nursing.
Year: 1942

Military History:

Service: RCAMC

Rank: Lt. N/S

Served: August 1943 to August 1945

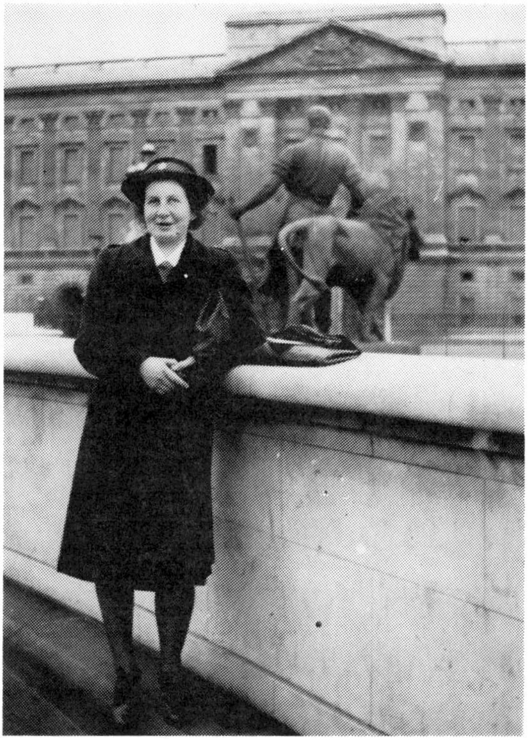

Lt. N/S Shirley (Gooding) Garriock, No. 22 CGH, London 1944

My first assignment was Army training at Nanaimo Military Hospital August 1943. In April of 1944 I had a few months' duty at Harrison Hot Springs which was the hotel itself. Then, on to Stratford, Ontario in May of 1944 and training at Sussex, New Brunswick, before going overseas.

We went overseas on the hospital ship *Lady Nelson*. We docked at Liverpool, travelled by train to Whitby, Yorkshire, where we stayed for a couple of weeks before finally arriving at No. 22 Canadian General Hospital at Bramshott. There I remained until July 1945 when I returned home to Canada.

Lydia Harriet Last

Graduated from: St. Mary's General Hospital School of Nursing, Timmins, Ontario. Year: 1937

Military History:

Service: RCAMC

Rank: Lt. N/S

Served: 22 September 1943 to 27 August 1946 Canadian Army Militia 1950 to 1954

Written by her niece, Connie Dube

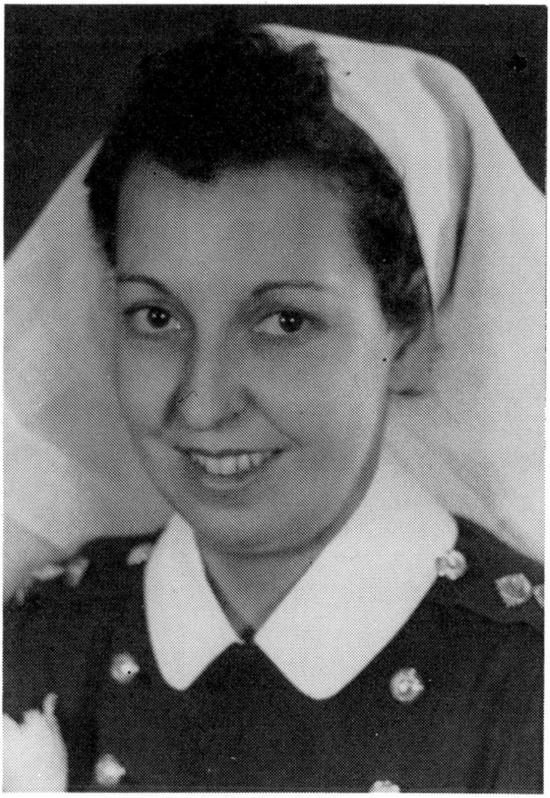

Lt. N/S Lydia Last

Enlisting in September 1943, Lydia Last served with the RCAMC in Canada for six months and then approximately two and a half years as operating room nurse in England at No. 22 CGH and with the Army of Occupation in Germany, until August 1946.

Following discharge, she was employed at the Neurological Institute, Montreal and the Queen Mary's Veteran's Hospital, Montreal, Quebec, as well as Shaughnessy DVA Hospital, Vancouver, BC. She also served in the Canadian Army Militia, completing her annual training for the years 1950 through 1954.

Bertha R. (Jones) Rudow

Graduated from: Kitchener Waterloo Hospital School of Nursing, King St., Kitchener, Ontario.
Year: 1941

Military History:

Service: RCAMC

Rank: Lieut. N/S

Served: 7 February 1944 to 29 May 1946

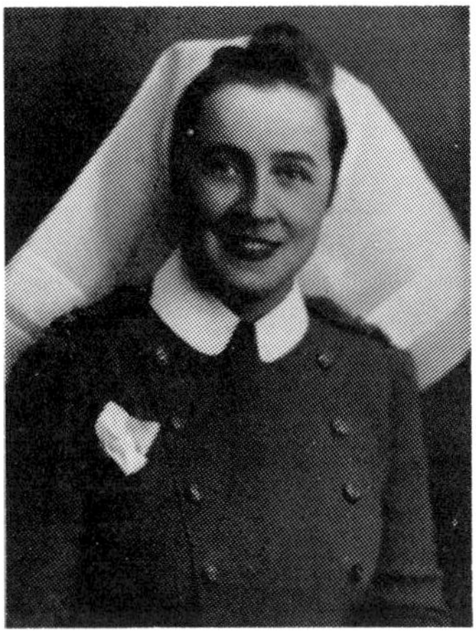

Lt. N/S Bertha (Jones) Rudow 1944

We were still living in nurses' residence when we were asked to wear our civvy capes and take part in a Victory Bond parade. A great many of the population were of German descent so there were mixed feelings. They also enrolled many of us in Civil Defence. I must not have made it, as I still have the card. No. 10 CGH was formed in Kitchener. We were required to be 25 years of age and pay for our uniforms. I was 20 when I graduated so had to wait a while. The age was lowered soon.

I often think of the procedures we were asked to do for which we had not been trained, like having all blood samples taken and in the right tubes with their requisition, while it was still dark out. No. 22 CGH had very patient teachers.

In England learning to ride a bicycle was a must. The person who taught me rode across a narrow stream and I followed. I must have been heavier, as the wheels sank and I fell in. We tried to light a fire to get me dried off, since I had to be on duty in half an hour. No luck. We had a special fence to crawl through and to the hut where there was a drying room for our personal laundry.

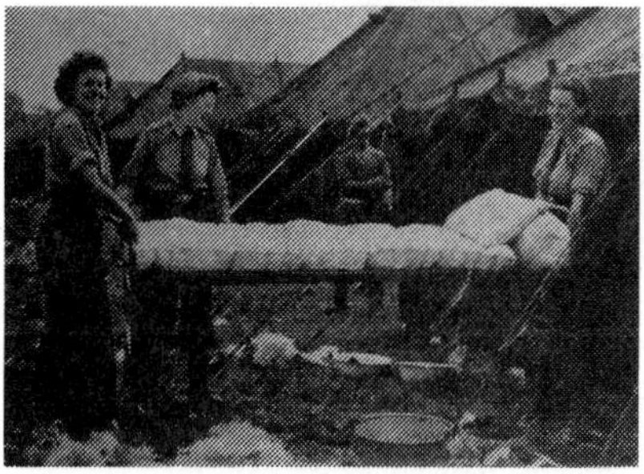

REMEMBER WHEN
All was not a bed of roses for Canadian nurses when they followed up the D-day landings in Normandy during World War II. Here Canadian nursing sisters are shown "on fatigue" carrying beds into one of the wards after a Canadian General Hospital was set up under canvas. Lt N/S Irene (Stephenson) Mercier second from left. From Royal Canadian Legion Magazine January, 1972

After D-Day 1944 No. 22 CGH Several wounded are in each of these vehicles, waiting to be taken care of at Admitting. There each was bathed and ready for a bed with clean sheets. If they had a yellow card fastened to their uniform it would mean they needed penicillin which was yellow then.

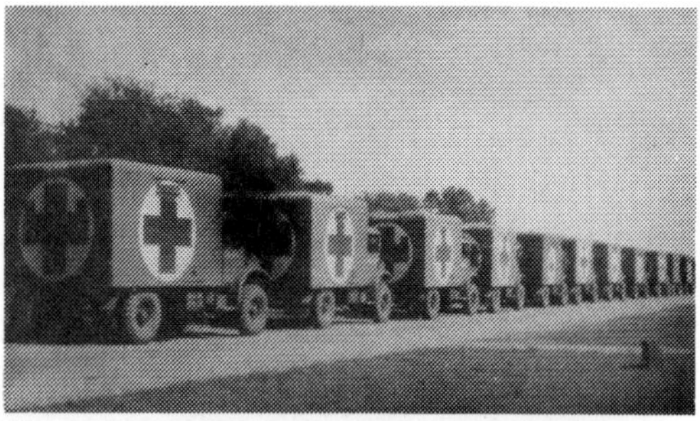

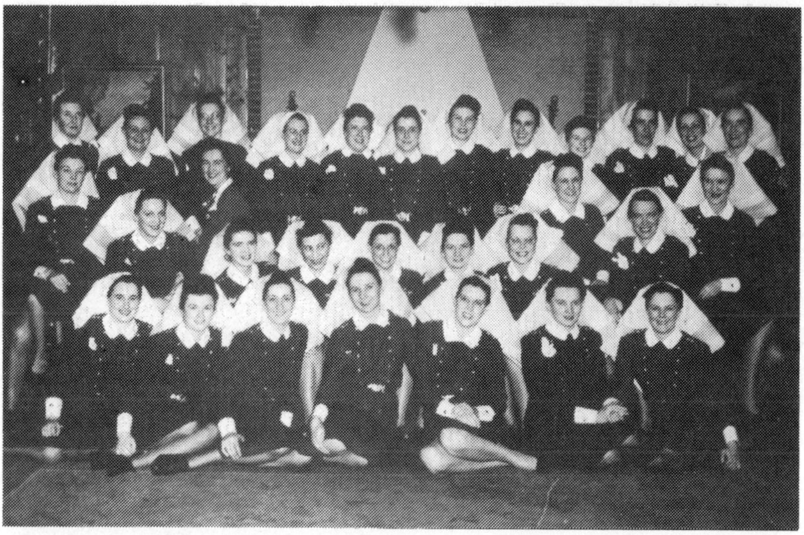

No. 16 CGH Oldenburg, Germany, Canadian Occupation Forces
L-R: FRONT ROW: Murodena Morrison, Mary Froesch, Jean Doerr, Evelyn Johnson, Kay Hart, Grace Knisley, Betty Stevens
MIDDLE ROW: Eve King, Clarissa Steeves, Joan Ward - Red Cross, Betty McLean, Kay Fiesel, Marian Barr - matron, Janet Dunn, Mary Taylor, L. Ritchie, Peg Parker - Home Sister, Mary Jo McDonald
THIRD ROW: Mary Williams, Myrtle Stibnicki, Peg Egerton, Ruth Blackwood, Lou McComb, Bertha Jones, Olive Wilkinson, Dorothy Burton, Connie Dingman, Connie Spall, Rita Ferguson, Kay Paris
Names courtesy Grace (Knisely) White, Olds, Alberta

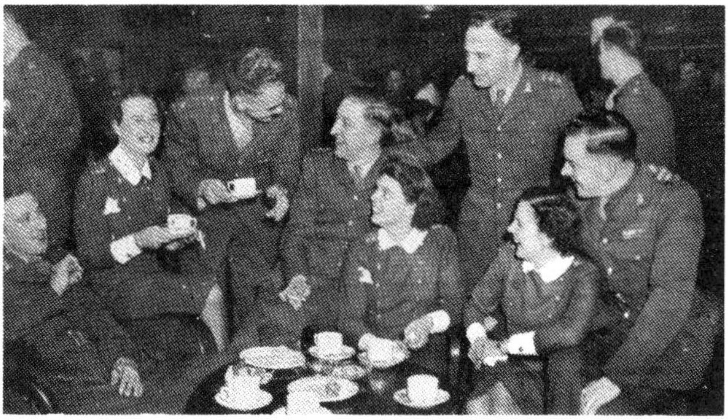

A group at the opening of the nursing sister's mess at No. 16 Canadian General Hospital at Oldenburg including Lieut. W. J. Panagapho (Dauphin, Man.), Lieut. N/S Ruth Blackwood, Prince Albert, Sask., Major G.F. Richardson, Lardner Lake, Ont., Capt. G.H. Hodgkiss, London, Ont., Lieut. N/S Olive Wilkinson, Port Alberni, BC, Capt. D.T.K. Reid, Mimico, Ont., Lieut. N/S Betty Stephens, Brockville, Ont., and Major L.M. Fourney, Lancaster, Ont.

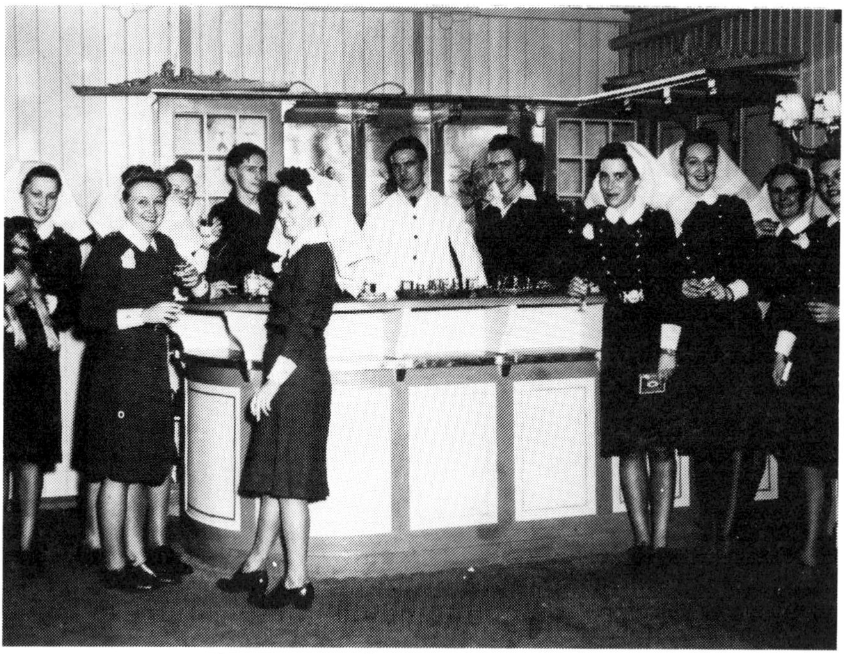

A group at the opening of the nursing sister's mess at No. 16 Canadian General Hospital at Oldenburg, this was a German facility taken over by our Allies, third from right - L. Ritchie, far right - Olive Wilkinson, next- Betty Stevens, fourth from right - Bertha Jones.

THE WOUNDED GET ALL THE BEST

The following article was loaned by Bertha (Jones) Rudow, No. 16 and No. 22 C.G.H. It is excerpted from an English newspaper published in July, 1944. The hospital was not named, according to wartime directives, but the reader may be able to determine the hospital and it's nurses by the content of the photos. – Ed.

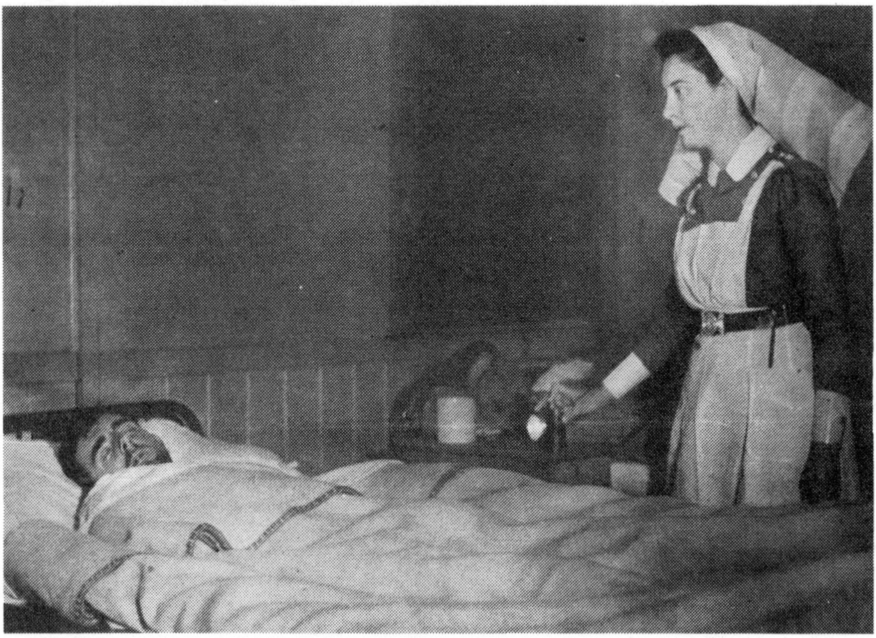

"THE WOUNDED GET ALL THE BEST" ILLUSTRATED - July 29,1944, London, England.

Photos by Lawrence Earl

Lawrence Earl's camera shows modern science aiding the injured fighting men in a Canadian Transit Hospital

PICTURES SHOW A CANADIAN TRANSIT HOSPITAL IN SOUTHERN ENGLAND, CLEARING HOUSE FOR WOUNDED FROM FRANCE;

Sister Marirose MacDonald at one of the 1600 beds.

Casualties of this period of the war are getting the best possible medical attention. If any one dear to you has been wounded, you may console yourself with this certainty: all that can be done for him is being done.

These pictures tell only part of the story, but it is a very important part. They depict what used to be just another Canadian military base hospital in the South of England, but what is now known as a Transit hospital.

And the name is eloquent because it tells of speed – the utmost possible swiftness in the handling of casualties, speed in placing at their service all the available resources of contemporary science (penicillin for instance, is always available for the fighting men): speed in distributing them to base hospitals far away to the north, remote from the memory of the smell of battle.

During the weeks before D-day this Canadian hospital underwent a veritable transformation scene. It's twelve hundred beds were increased to sixteen hundred. Tents and other temporary structures went up, completely equipped as hospital wards. Staffs were expanded. The place became a clearing station; and everything worked without a hitch.

Seven-eighths of the cases handled by this Canadian set-up are British troops (there are British hospitals handling mostly Canadian cases). Seven out of ten arrivals – they come by ship, by hospital train, by ambulance convoy – are moved on within twenty-four hours. Says Nursing Sister Mary Ryan, from Nova Scotia: "This place is intended to make the wounded man feel better, to set his mind as well as his body at rest. He's weary when he gets here. The journey has been long, there will have been bumpy travel despite the utmost care. Maybe he's hungry, in pain. First thing we feed him, then give him cigarettes, tasty chocolate. Then into bed he goes, into snow white linen, clean, comfortable. Now the tension is relieved. Worry fades away. 'Ah' he murmurs ever so contentedly, 'now I may relax'."

But things will have been happening even before our friend gets as far as the Transit Hospital. The best of treatment will have been at his disposal from immediately behind the front line near Caen or St. Lo. On his way he will have been given, if his case demanded it sulpha drugs or penicillin.

When the penicillin treatment is completed the tag bearing the records of its administration is forwarded to the Medical Research Council for examination.

Soon after he arrives at the Transit Hospital our casualty has his wounds redressed, if they need redressing. He is operated on, if he needs operating on. Otherwise he is allowed to sleep. "Sleep," the boys will tell you, "is just bliss." Once when H.M. the Queen was on a surprise visit she stopped at a bed and chatted with its wakeful occupant. In the next bed a soldier lay asleep; then, as the Queen turned to him, he opened his eyes dreamily for a moment. "You're the Queen aren't you? Or am I dreaming?" His eyelids dropped and he fell again into a deep slumber.

Food? Transit Hospital has a dietician atta_hed to its staff – a girl responsible for the food the casualties get. She plans the diet weeks ahead, works out special individual diets where they are needed. As for stories, well , there is no end of them. Every casualty has his narrative, though not all the men are communicative – and some men are better narrators than others.

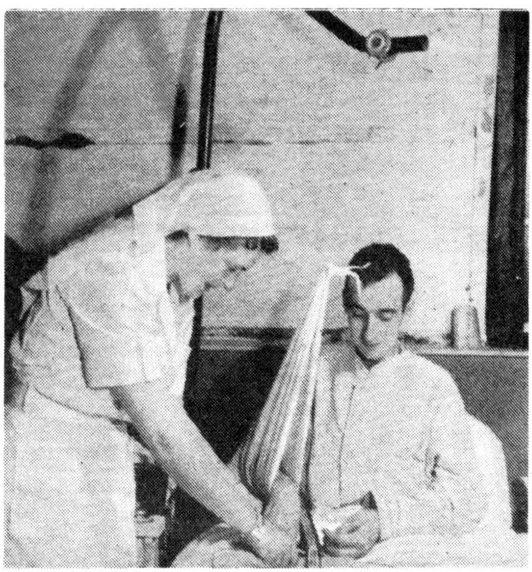

Occupational therapist Anna Culley aids him to restore use of his fingers. In tiiis way many men are made fit again for pre-war jobs.

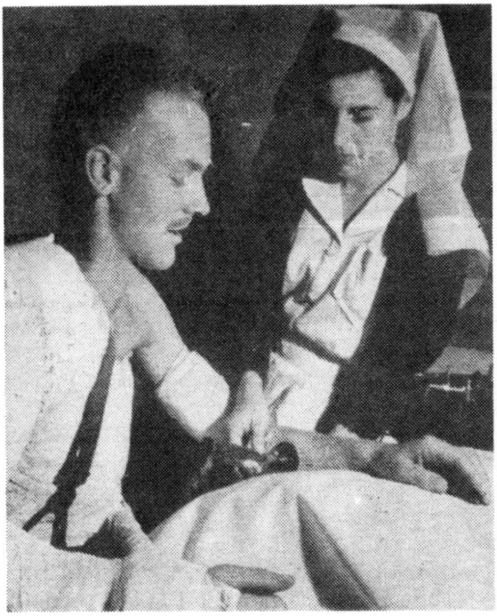

Electrical cure applied by the skilled hands of Lieut. Elizabeth Carroll restores arm nerves and muscles crushed in a bad motorcycle crash.

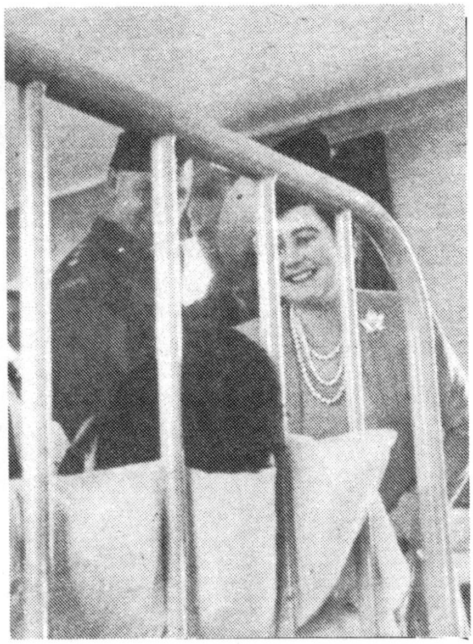

The Queen calls at the hospital and exchanges greetings with wounded men, many of whom in former wars would not have survived in the absence of modern drugs and treatment.

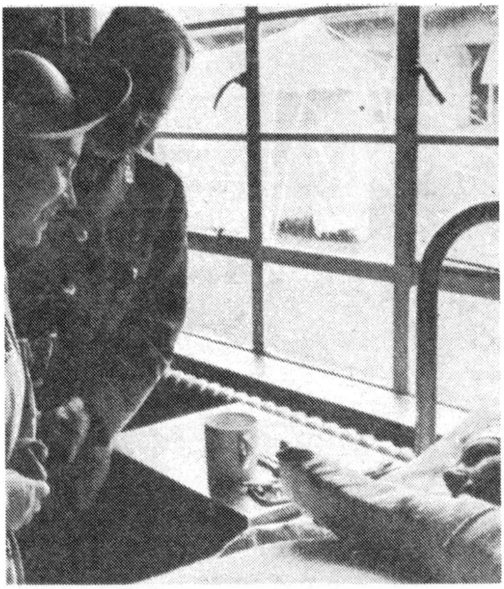

Modern surgery with its limb restoring and life-saving achievements impresses Her Majesty, who finds that the beneficiaries of these miracles are highly appreciative.

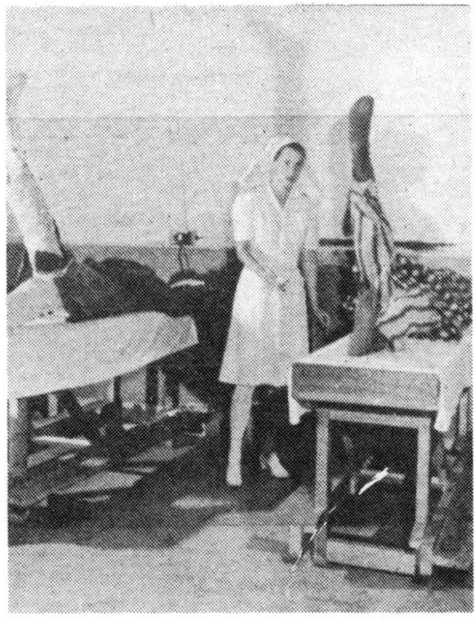

Physiotherapy directed by Lieut. Jean Johnson, is used in post-operative knee cases and when casts are removed from legs. The exercise restores normal muscular action.

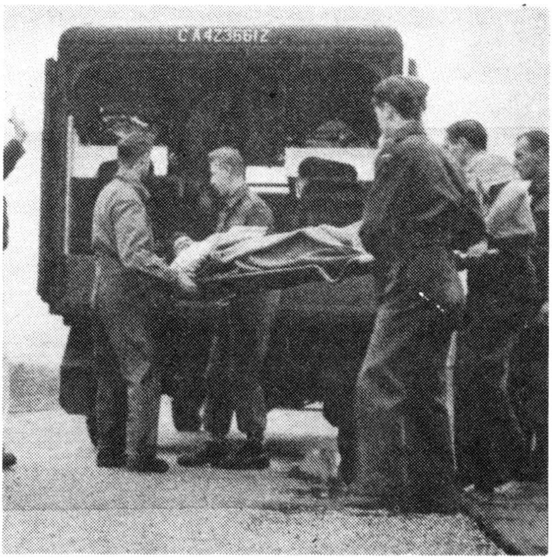

Northward Ho! Soon the transit hospital is only a happy memory, and the casualties, for whom medical science has done everything possible, are en route for base hospitals.

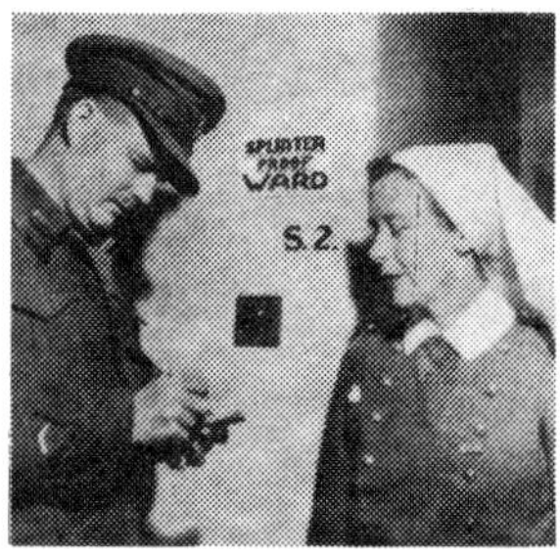

In command is Col. W.A. Jones of Kingston, talking here with his Principal Matron, Constance Tavener from Toronto.

ILLUSTRATED, 29 July 1944, London, England. Photos by Lawrence Earl, London, England

Joan M. (Gore) Spring

Graduated from: Toronto Sick Children's Hospital School of Nursing. Year :1931

Military History:

Service: RCAMC

Rank: Lt. N/S

Served: February 2, 1944 to November 13, 1946

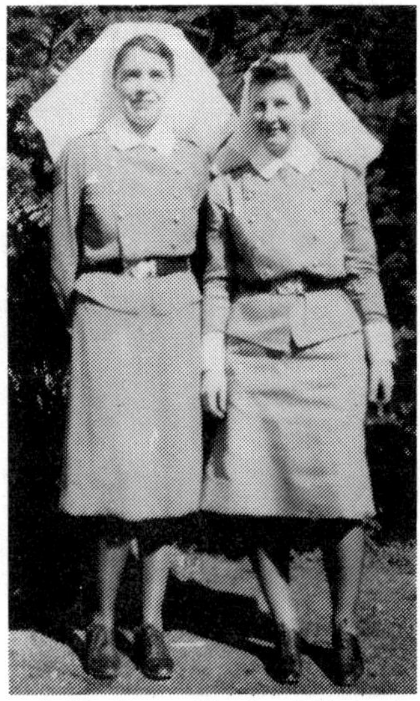

L-R: Joan (Spring) Gore, Shirley (Gooding) Garriock

The Army provided a chance to travel – a chance to help soldiers who were wounded. I met new and interesting men and women in basic training. We travelled from Kelowna, B.C., to an England at war. I had never crossed the ocean before. There were cheers as we travelled through Scotland to London, England. My mother and father were born and married in England, then came to Canada to live.

Marion Rhae (Nichols) Stewart

Graduated from: University of Toronto School of Occupational Therapy, Ontario. Year: 1940
Occupational Therapist.

Military History:

Service: RCAMC

Rank: Lt. O/T

Served: January 1943 to January 1946

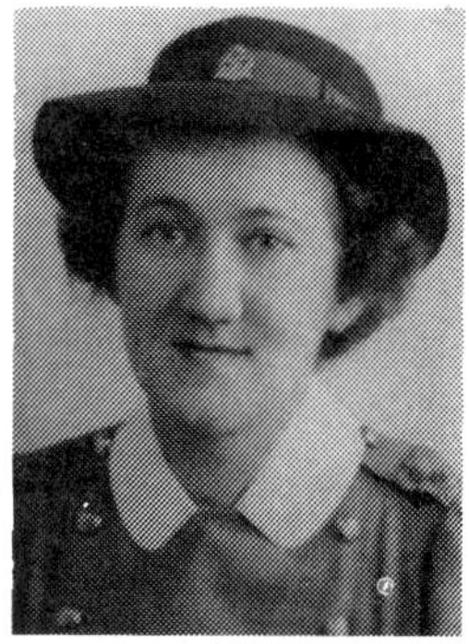

Lt. O/T Marian Rhae (Nichols) Stewart

I needed a change in my life and joining the Army was a spur of the moment decision.

Highlights of days in the Army were:
My friends from the Maritimes.
My leave in Scotland in the Trossachs.
My honeymoon on the Isle of Wight.

Our hospital unit docked at Liverpool June 9, 1944. We went by train to Whitby, Yorkshire, where we were billeted in an old hotel facing the north sea. We arrived early on Sunday morning to the consternation of the kitchen staff. We had no mess tins and they had no dishes or cutlery. Eventually the problem was solved; we had sausage on a piece of bread. Dishes and cutlery arrived later in the day.

After breakfast our padre decided to have a communion service – several of us went. In the midst of serving wine the shore batteries were shot off – practice, we found out later! We thought we were being attacked and were some scared!

We did not have five-star accommodation – sagging cots and grey blankets. We eventually took over No. 22 Canadian General Hospital at Bramshott in the south of England. On arrival, I had a hot bath and crawled between lovely white sheets. The alert went – I rolled over and said, *"I am too tired to move,"* and went to sleep. We found out later we got all the London alerts.

NO. 23 CANADIAN GENERAL HOSPITAL

Dorothy (Grainger) Anderson
Patricia (Porter) (Hall)Hedley
Kathleen (Walker) McCabe

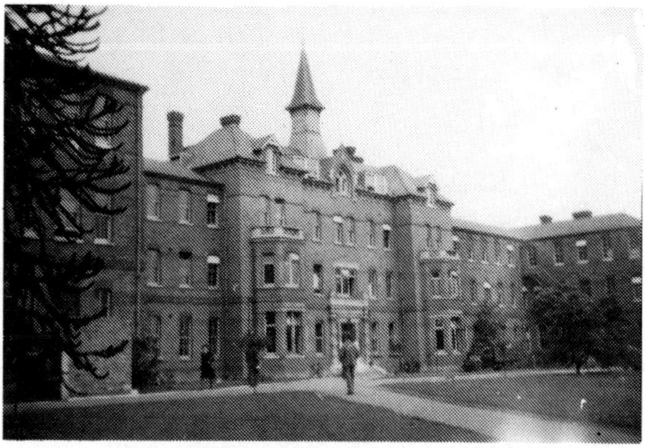

Front of No. 23 CGH in England, a landmark to many patients and nurses.

No. 23 Canadian General Hospital was mobilized at Stratford, Ontario, in conjunction with No. 22 General. Both were 1200-bed units. Col. A.A. James was CO. Nurses came from every military district in Canada and Newfoundland to form the nursing service for No. 23 General.

Matron Patterson, 78 nursing sisters, one dietitian, one home sister, one physiotherapist and three occupational therapists were billeted throughout the city.

The unit embarked on the *Empress of Scotland* at Halifax 16 June 1944 to arrive in Scotland 23 June. They disembarked and travelled to Helmsley, York. No. 23 General remained as a permanent installation in England; it served as a base for the casualties evacuated from the Continent.

The unit disbanded 31 July 1945.

Dorothy M. (Grainger) Anderson

Graduated from: Royal Alexandra Hospital School of Nursing, Edmonton, Alberta. Year: 1942

Military History:

Service: RCAMC

Rank: 1st Lieut. N/S

Served: October 1943 to June 1945

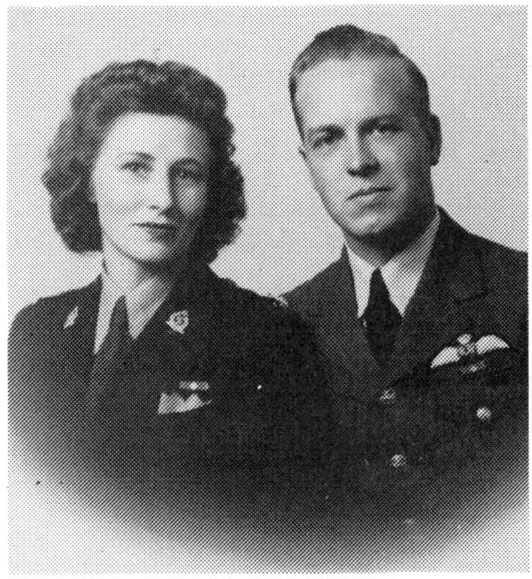

Dorothy (Grainger) and Frank Anderson

For me, the Army provided a chance to travel and experience other cultures. My parents came from Yorkshire, England, and I had a chance to meet relatives for the first time. Military nursing was appealing.

After graduation I entered private duty nursing to initiate myself into the role of registered nurse. Business was slow in Calgary so I combined a labourer's job with private nursing. The Col. Belcher Hospital was being built near my home, and the builders were desperate for workers. I applied and was soon on the job learning the skill of laying steel re-enforcements for concrete. Blueprints were easy to read and my male boss was impressed with my progress. Wages were much higher than the $5.00 offered RNs for a twelve-hour shift. Cold autumn mornings encouraged me to accept ward nursing at the Baker TB Sanitarium. My isolation training under Miss Jenner was invaluable here. We worked in teams and gave patients top quality bedside nursing care. The staff was pleasant to work with, and the board and room excellent. Nearby was Bowness Park, ideal for skating, and snowy hills provided good ski runs.

My brother was stationed at Gordon Head, B.C., with the Army. He had heard of an urgent need for nurses at Garden Bay Anglican Mission Hospital, fifty miles north of Vancouver. Spring time on the shores of the Pacific Ocean and the thrill of a new adventure were irresistible. The Union Steamship boat dropped me off at the hospital dock April 1st, 1943. Dr. Pierce, his wife and four children greeted me. The family came direct from China where Dr. Pierce had served as a medical missionary. Now we served the Indians, fishermen and loggers in this remote region. Home visits were made via an outboard motorboat. The hospital was blacked out each night due to the threat of Japanese invasion. The staff had to be multi-skilled and resourceful as help from Vancouver came on board the Union Steamship once a week. Hours off duty were spent hiking, boating and swimming. Living was easy.

The RCAMC was trying to attract registered nurses to enlist. I applied to Currie Barracks, Calgary. My call-up came 1 October 1943. Soon, I was learning the basic requirements of a nursing sister in a military hospital. Suffield Research Centre needed a relief nurse for December/January, 1944. I volunteered and entered a world of scientists preparing for biological warfare. I learned gas mask protection and the care of victims of the gas warfare experiments. A barracks full of CWACs made me aware of the vital roles women were playing in the war effort. In May, a troop train took me to Stratford, Ontario, where No. 23 Canadian General Hospital was being mobilized. Once fully equipped, fifty MDs and seventy RNs entrained for Sussex, N.B., to await the arrival of the *Empress of Scotland* in Halifax. After a four-day sea voyage, No. 23 landed in Greenock, Scotland, and thence to a primitive military base in Yorkshire.

Number 23 and Number 24 were the last two Canadian General Hospital units to establish themselves in England prior to D-Day, 1944. I was fortunate to be attached to No. 23 which was four miles west of Watford Junction near the village of Leavesden Green. Watford Junction was the last station on the Baker-Waterloo subway line from Paddington Station, London. Our unit was located on the grounds of a mental institution. We were allowed to use a vacant three-story stone building for all our medical cases. On a lower level of land forty surgical wards were built. A covered, open concrete ramp divided these wards in two. It led down to the billets for officers and NCOs. A modern kitchen and messing halls separated the billets. These one-storied brick buildings were modern in every respect. One nursing sister and two orderlies comprised the staff of each 44-bed ward. Two semi-private rooms were set aside for the very ill. In the centre of the ramp were the operating theatres and X-ray units. Near the billets was a ward which the physiotherapist shared with the occupational therapist.

All was in readiness by D-Day, June 6th. A DeHaviland airport and factory was our neighbour. It was there that the convoys of wounded were flown in from the beachheads of Normandy. Lorries were quickly filled with the soldiers on stretchers, and in the cover of darkness, they arrived at the ramp of our unit. The stretchers were unloaded on the ramp.

Fifty MOs soon determined the severity of the injuries and the orderlies moved the soldiers to the appropriate wards. Within a week our 1200 beds were full, and long tents were hastily erected at the ends of each surgical ward for 400 additional beds. Everyone worked twelve-hour shifts, seven days a week until the Big Push in Europe subsided.

The closest buzz bomb exploded one mile from our unit. We had no warning for V-2s – we only heard the explosions. Air-raid sirens and blackouts prevailed till VE Day, May 8th, 1945.

Instant romances blossomed everywhere. Youth lived for the thrill of the moment. As a result, I became Pilot Officer Frank Anderson's wife in September 1944. I had nursed him in isolation at the "Alex" when an epidemic of scarlet fever had swept through the Manning Depot in Edmonton. Once married, no nursing sister could volunteer for service outside the British Isles so I was content to explore England and Wales when on leave.

My ward, No. 27, was full of amputees, shrapnel wounds, burn cases and a few belly wounds. Thank God for penicillin! It and morphine were prescribed the most frequently. No problem of drug addiction was evident. Guinness Stout – a bottle a day – was used to stimulate appetites, and it did the trick!

The orderlies were wonderful assistants. As soon as a patient was considered "convalescing," he was garbed in "blues," and then was expected to help with serving and distributing food trays and feeding patients. I cannot remember a cleaning staff. Each ward became a family and maintained their home. The soldiers were so thankful to be alive and headed for repatriation that they cooperated in every way. Some developed friendships with the British families in the nearby, rural communities, so occasionally AWOLs occurred. Many of our woolen bed blankets – a lovely blue colour – became coats for the deprived local lassies. Canadian food supplies found their way into the English homes, courtesy of the patients.

In April of 1945, I 'specialed' a Canadian military police sergeant from London. He was having severe convulsions, and the MO diagnosed spinal meningitis. A maximum dose of penicillin was given while orderlies restrained the sergeant. As soon as the convulsions subsided, an intravenous was started. We were in an isolated area of the darkened ward. Now the patient and myself were totally alone; it was after midnight. I sat at his bedside with my fingers constantly on the pulse of his unrestrained arm. The pulse beat slower and slower. His survival depended on that massive dose of penicillin. I had no orders but to watch him constantly. Suddenly, a small, dark-haired man wearing a clerical collar appeared. He was a chaplain. He asked that he might pray for the sergeant. I thought to myself, *"You are much too late to help this soldier."* However, I felt compelled to add my prayers to those of the chaplain's. I was unaware of how many seconds or minutes passed by. Suddenly, my fingers felt rapid pulse beats, too rapid for normal, but the heart had not given up. I shared the good news with the chaplain and he quietly disappeared into the night. That pulse beat never failed again while the sergeant remained with us for three weeks of recuperating. I assured him he was my miracle man, for whatever reason, we will never know.

This incident I relate to show the camaraderie which often occurred on our wards. 'Twas the summer of 1944 – I arrived on duty at 0700 hours and discovered a new patient sitting up in bed, totally unrecognizable for his head was swathed in bandages. It was obvious he had lost part of two arms and his two hands. All fellow patients took an immediate interest in him. They learned he had been a victim of a grenade blast in a tank. Those who were able became his hands. A small, dark, slight man on crutches became his best friend. He had had a leg off at the hip. Off to the bathroom the two would go – a most unlikely pair – the little fellow was able to assist with trousers, bodily parts and wiping. Mission accomplished! Gradually, that face emerged from the bandages – two bright, blue eyes and a reddish beard cropping out of the red burned skin, and a wide smile which captured all our hearts.

One very foggy winter night, I was biking the four miles from Watford railway station. I had been visiting my husband in Shrewsbury. It was 0400 hours. Cat-eye reflectors along the road were my only guide. I became aware of odd sounds. Clip-clop-clip-clop. I passed by a shadow on my right from whence the sound came. The shadow was a patient on crutches. One leg had a full-length plaster cast. I stopped the bike, helped him mount the seat of my bicycle, then I proceeded to pedal him the remaining distance to the staff's secret entrance into the hospital grounds. I urged him to tell no one of our experience or I would be reprimanded. I hoped that he would have no recollection of that secret entrance, for then I would really be in serious trouble.

Off-duty hours were never boring. The countryside was always beautiful even in winter. Most of us had bought second-hand bikes on arrival, so off we would go during the bright summer evenings and explore the country roads and villages. We learned the route well to Watford Junction – night or day. A half-hour subway ride took us into the centre of London. We enjoyed the best of two worlds!

My husband and I were on leave in Llangollen, Wales, when V-Day occurred. We shared in the victory celebrations at the home of the village doctor. On return to our respective units we discovered our world had been turned around and we were no longer "essential" commodities. All new orders had been cancelled, and repatriation was the name of the game.

I joined a POW ship, the *Volendam* which carried 1200 POWs back to Canada. Some of these men published their experiences through books, plays and films.

Civilian nursing had little appeal after the fast exciting pace of wartime nursing. I was ready to establish a home and raise a family. Frank chose to return to Medicine Hat and aid his father in operating the family insurance business.

I learned to be a civilian again and became very involved in community activities. Soon, I was the proud mother of two sons and one daughter. Rearing children was a challenge I loved. I also became very active in teaching Sunday School and mid-week groups. The nurse's training I had received at the Royal Alex plus my post-graduate experiences equipped me well for my roles of wife, mother, homemaker and volunteer. I maintained a keen interest in the world of medicine by being an active volunteer in our hospital auxiliary association.

Once my children left home, I furthered my education in the humanities and art by attending our community college. I have been blessed with a happy marriage, and we are the proud grandparents of five talented grandchildren.

Fifty years ago, the Royal Alexandra Hospital under R.A.F. Anderson's administration led the way in medical and nursing care in Alberta. I was very privileged to be one of the trainees. May the "Alex" long continue to give leadership in medical care and research in North America.

Patricia Hedley (Nee Porter), 1st marriage, Hall

Military History:

Service: RCAMC

Rank: Lt. Home sister

Served: 18 February 1944 to 31 August 1945

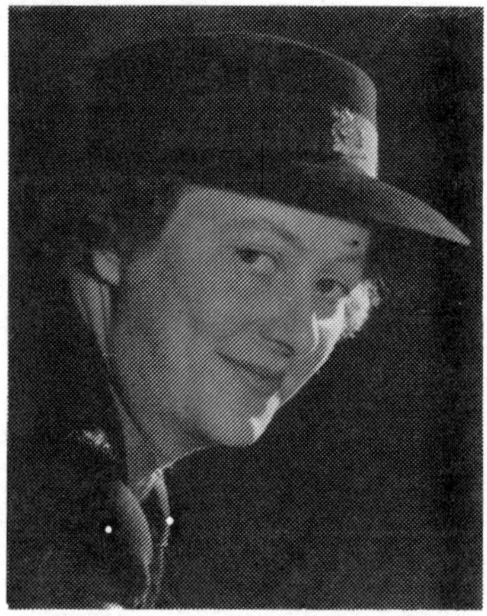

2/Lt. Home Sister Patricia (Porter) Hall

I was non-medical; I served with RCAMC as home sister from 18 Fbruary 1944 to 31 August 1945 with the rank of lieutenant.

After my first husband Lieutenant F.C. Hall was killed on active service in Sicily, I was wondering what to do, when a nursing sister suggested I apply for the position of home sister. I did this and was accepted, then proceeded to Nanaimo, B. C. for basic training. The matron was E. Rossiter. I was transferred to Terrace, B.C., then to Fredericton, N.B. From there I was sent overseas in January 1945. I was stationed at Watford (No. 23 Canadian General Hospital) and at No. 1 Neurological and Plastic Surgery Hospital at Basingstoke. I returned to Canada on the *Ile de France* and was discharged in Vancouver at No. 11 MD.

The role of the home sister was indeed a varied one, and when I came on the scene, not too important. I found there wasn't very much to do. I seemed to count a lot of blankets and sheets. I produced, or helped produce, many wedding receptions held in the mess for nursing sisters. I also did a bit of scrounging for liquor supplies and shopped for extra messing comforts – this was overseas.

In Canada there was more to do with actual housekeeping and menu planning, although the kitchen staff did not much help in this regard beyond a few recipes and suggestions. In fact, one rather amusing thing occurred shortly after I arrived in Fredericton when I went into the kitchen and said to the sergeant cook, *"I really don't know what we should have for dinner tonight."* This was Saturday – and the cook replied, *"But Sister, the beans are already in the oven!"* That was my introduction to the Maritime staple of baked beans on Saturday!

However, the home sisters who went overseas to England

and the Continent with the first units did a most important job. I have heard they did wonders setting up the various nursing sisters' messes and scoured the countryside for extra messing treats. Alice Baynes, who I believe is now in Glengarry Hospital in Victoria, is one who was often mentioned to me for the wonderful work she did, and I'm sure there are many others.

So, I think it would add to the interest of your book to interview or otherwise contact some of these persons, as I am sure they would have many interesting stories to tell. The home sisters at Taplow (Cliveden) served many a cup of tea to prominent and famous people who visited that particular showplace!

Kathleen (Walker) McCabe

Graduated from: Montreal General Hospital School of Nursing.
Year: 1943

Military History:

Service: RCAMC

Rank: Lieut. N/S

Served: 22 January 1944 to
5 July 1946

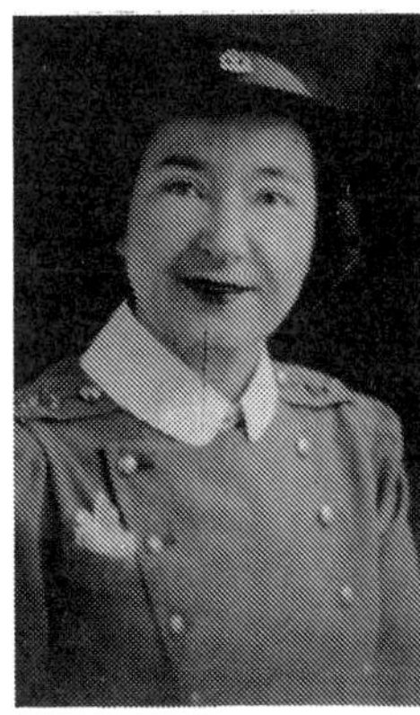

Lt. N/S Kathleen (Walker) McCabe

I became a nursing sister in the RCAMC to serve my country – Canada

The highlight of my military experience was in caring for the wounded soldiers who came to our hospital. They were brought to our hospital in England in convoys of Red Cross transport ready to be looked after by our doctors and nurses. They were brought from Italy, Germany and France.

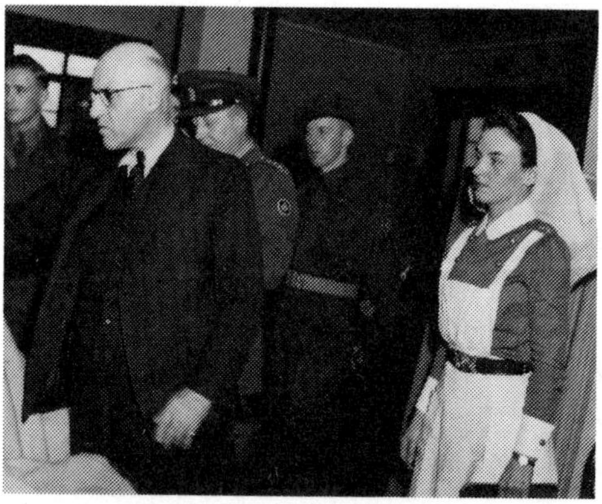

No. 23 Canadian General Hospital, Leavesden, England 15 October 1944 Pictured at a Canadian General Hospital in England are: Hon J.L. Ralston, Canada's Minister of National Defence, Col. A. A. James, OC of the Hospital and Lt N/S Banford Canadian Forces photo

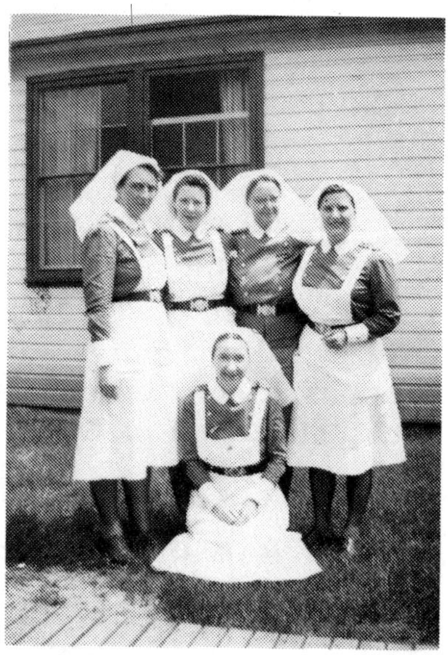

Camp Borden 1944: Nursing sisters McLean, Haggerty, Matron Percy, Hilton, K. Walker sitting

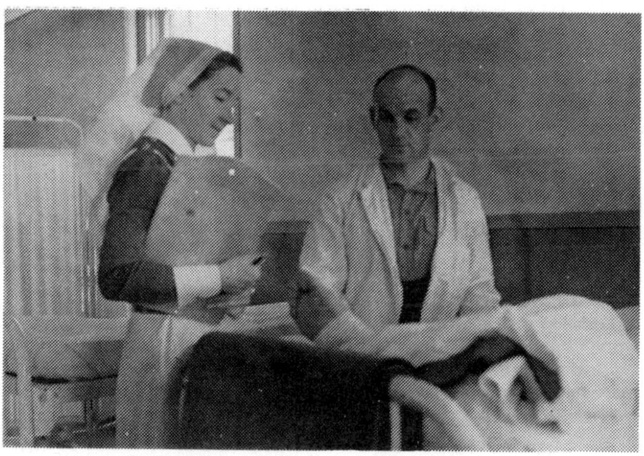

Camp Borden 1944: One of the men to be orderlies, Kathleen Walker teaching

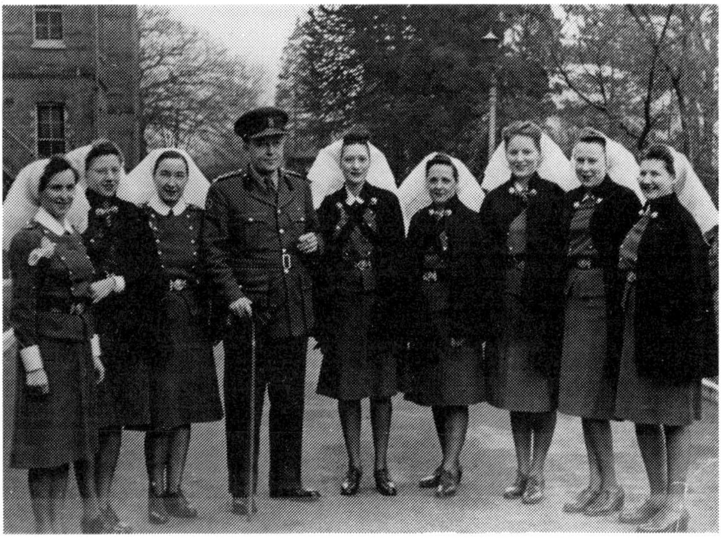

No. 23 CGH, 1944 London, England.
Left to right: Nursing sisters Bridget Reddy, Newfoundland; E.A. Kertin, Montreal; K. (Walker) McCabe; Col. James our Commanding Officer; Nursing Sisters Watt; Cooper; Bea Black, Montreal; Eleanor Wilson, Toronto; Marjorie Ward, Toronto Canadian Forces photo. Photograph by A. Louis Jarche

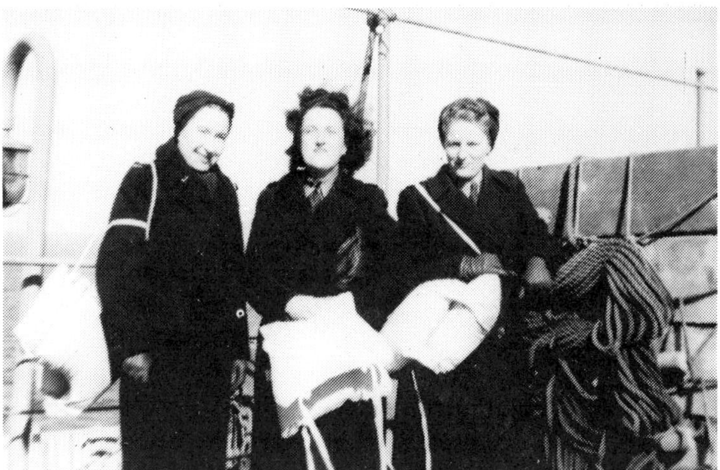

Coming home - February 1946 - on board Queen Elizabeth, *Kathleen Walker on left*

NO. 24 CANADIAN GENERAL HOSPITAL

Margaret (Kinnin) Cowie
Dorothy (Morrison) Donaldson
Irene (Knight) Logan
Eleanor (Smith) Marvin
Margaret (Neal)Taylor
Joan (Packford)Thomas
Kay (Swan)Wyatt

No. 24 Canadian General Hospital mobilized at Listowell, Ontario, in March 1944. On 1 July they were at sea and landed at Gourock, Scotland. The unit was located at Horley, Surrey, by the end of July with Major E.E. Rossiter as principal matron and Ruth E.Littlejohn as A/matron. No. 24 became a permanent installation in England and served as a base for casualties evacuated from the Continent.

By 5 February 1946 most nursing sisters were struck off strength, and by the end of February the unit was turned over to the British Queen Alexandra's Military Hospital.

Margaret Ellen (Kinnin) Cowie

Graduated from: Hotel Dieu Hospital School of Nursing, Windsor, Ontario. Year: 1943

Military History:

Service: RCAMC

Rank: Lt. N/S

Served: 11 February 1944 to 11 April 1946.

My mother was a nurse in the British Army in World War I and he was very keen on military life, it was natural for me to join the Army.

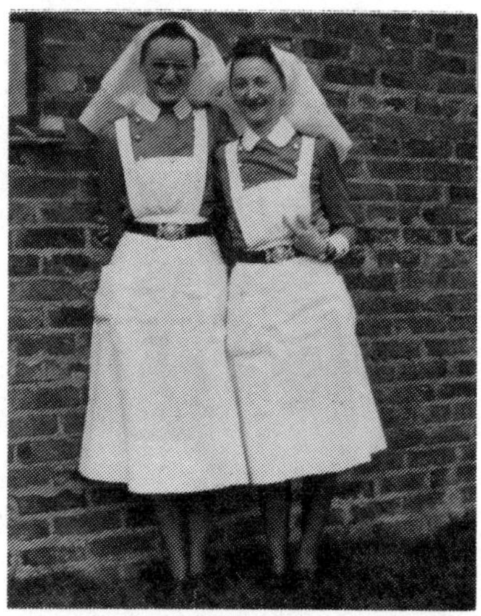

M.E. Kinnin and M.E. Broadfoot, summer of 1944 at Suffield, Surrey, England

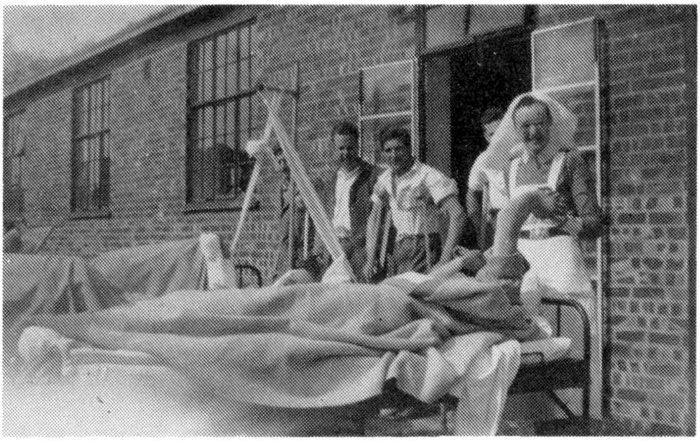

N/S M.E. Kinnin and patients,
Ward 4, No. 24 CGH 1944, England

Dorothy F. (Morrison) Donaldson

Graduated from: Hospital for Sick Children School of Nursing, Toronto. Year: 1940

Military History:

Service: RCAMC and RCAF

Rank: Lt. N/S and F/O N/S

Served: RCAMC 1943 to 1946 and RCAF 1950 to 1952

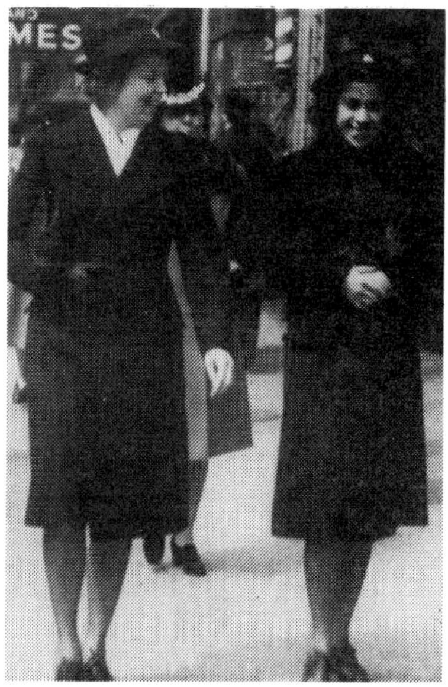

L-R: Grace (Lawrence) Mathieson and Dorothy (Morrison) Donaldson, No. 24 CGH

It is difficult to say why I chose the Service; it seemed the thing to do at that time. Looking back, the highlight seems to be the many wonderful friends I met. Many I still keep in touch with and consider close friends. I remember the many nights the V-1s and V-2s came over the hospital, No. 24 CGH, Horley, Surrey. At first they caused great concern, later, as we did not have any direct hits, they were just 'accepted' and we did not stay awake listening for them. I also recall some hilarious moments on route marches on the Moors at Scotch Corners, Yorkshire!

Irene (Knight) Logan

Graduated from: Royal Jubilee Hospital School of Nursing, New Westminster, B.C. Year: 1942

Military History:

Service: RCAMC

Rank: Lt. N/S

Served: January 1944 to February 1946

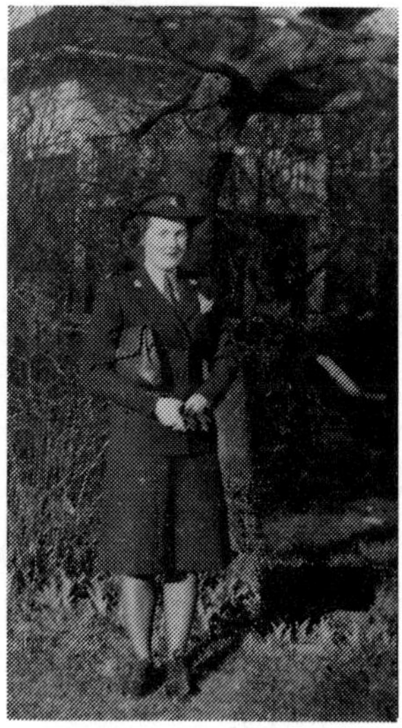

N/S Irene (Knight) Logan, No. 24 CGH

The Army provided an opportunity to do a different type of nursing; also, there was loyalty to my country. My friends were joining up; that influenced me to do the same.

I was stationed at Horley, England, at No. 24 Canadian General Hospital. I returned to Canada in July 1945 with 50 other Army nurses to go to the Far East. Supposedly, we would train in Kentucky for three months, be home for Christmas and leave via San Francisco for the Philippines. I ended up in Chilliwack. The atom bomb was dropped in August 1945.

Eleanor (Smith) Marvin

Graduated from: Prince Edward County School of Nursing, Picton, Ontario. Year: 1940

Military History:

Service: RCAMC

Rank: Lt. N/S

Served: January 1944 to June 1946

I chose military service because at the time it was the thing to do and many of my friends and relatives were in the service.

I began my military service at Kingston Military Hospital in January of 1944. I moved to Rideau Military Hospital in April

1944 and went overseas with No. 24 Canadian General Hospital in June 1944. We were truly blessed to have Edna Rossiter from Nanaimo, B.C., as matron. We were the last 1200-bed hospital to go overseas and arrived at Horley in Surrey at the time casualties were arriving following D-Day invasion – a busy time for many months. I was in the holding unit at Bramshott on VE Day enroute to No. 10 General in Turnhout, Belgium. From there I went on to No. 2 CCS at Apeldoorn, Holland, a few months later before returning to No. 22 General at Bramshott, England, for another several months, then home to Canada at the end of May 1946.I was not in the Service a long time, but was very proud that I was there.

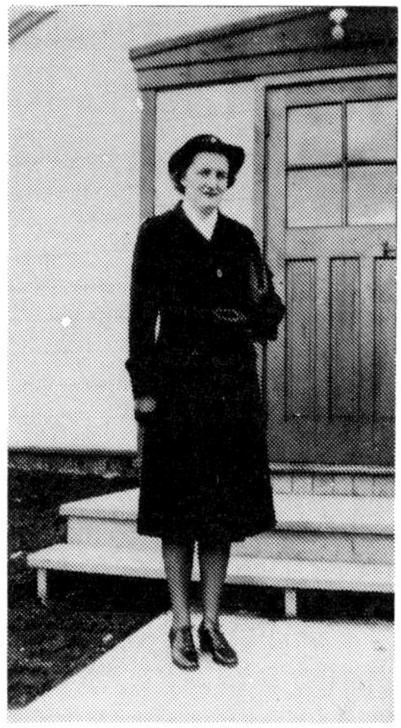

Lt. N/S Eleanor (Marvin) Smith, Kingston Military Hospital 1944

Margaret E. (Neal) Taylor

Graduated from: Saskatoon City Hospital School of Nursing.
Year: 1938

Military History:

Service: RCAMC

Rank: Lieutenant N/S

Served: 1944 to 29 April 1946.

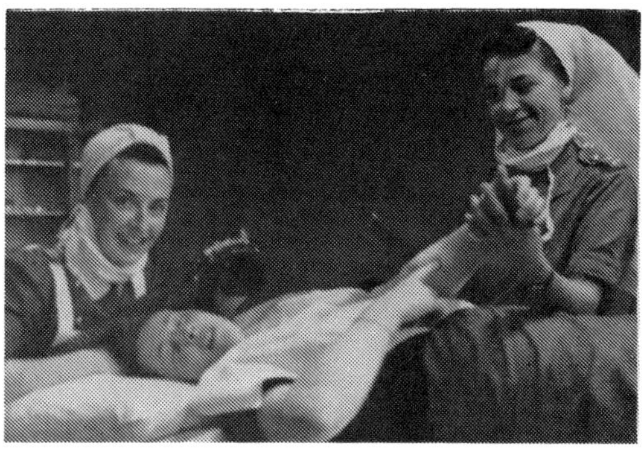

No. 24 CGH operating room, Horley, England. L-R: Peggy (Neal) Taylor, Irene Knight and Dorothy (Morrison) Donaldson

During WW II all my friends were going overseas and I wanted to be with them. My duty assignment was with No. 24 Canadian General Hospital at Horley in England.

I learned to bike during blackout in Horley. I watched V-I and V-2s go over Horley Hospital hoping none would fall.

We were lucky ones.

I watched double amputees go home alive!

Joan O. (Packford) Thomas

Graduated from: Royal Alexandra Hospital School of Nursing, Edmonton, Alberta. Year: 1940

Military History:

Service: RCAMC

Rank: Lt. N/S

Service: From 1943 to December 1945

My mother was a nursing sister (QAIMNS) in WW I; that influenced me to choose a similar career. There were many highlights in my career with the RCAMC and it all seems so long ago.

After D-Day I was with No. 24 CGH in Horley in the south of England. Large convoys of wounded would arrive at any hour of day or night – we all were on duty.

These men were flown to Gatwick (then a small airfield) and from there by ambulance to the surrounding military hospitals. There were quite a few Canadians in that area. One of the worst things was finding a patient from home, whom you knew, and so often it was fatal, and one ended up writing to the family.

From there, I went to Belgium (No. 10 CGH). This hospital was in Turnhout, a former Army barracks, walled and large. Here among our wounded were a lot of German POWs. They seemed so young. They were all housed in a separate wing. They seemed so much younger than our own boys.

Social life was inhibited here, though occasionally we got into Antwerp. During time off we investigated the town, though we couldn't go off the roads as all areas hadn't been cleared of mines.

I remember getting a ward made up for casualties – going in when the convoy arrived and finding the ward stripped – all bedding gone. Guess someone came over the wall!

Next, on to a Casualty Clearing Station in Apeldoorn. This was established in part of a mental hospital; some of the former patients were still housed in an adjoining building. The Germans had occupied this hospital before us. In the basement was a large store of lovely books about Holland, well illustrated, printed in German. We were each given one. They had also collected a large store of various kinds of liquor which they had had to leave behind. This was gradually used in the mess. They had also left behind a lot of plaster (for plaster casts). We did not wish to use this on our patients, though it was probably as good as ours. However, after the war many of the staff had obtained souvenirs, ornaments, etc., so we encased the breakable ones in plaster and they were able to ship them home safely. I was in Holland until November 1945.

The Dutch people were so kind and friendly; much more so than the Belgians. We were able to go a bit farther afield (Amsterdam, etc.,) and were welcomed even in the smallest villages.

Looking back, though, we saw such a lot of unnecessary tragedy on all sides. It was quite a learning experience for young (as we were then) nurses, and it has stood us in good stead all our lives. Most nursing sisters are very involved with community work, volunteering, etc.

Kathleen E. (Swan) Wyatt

Graduated from: Misericordia Hospital School of Nursing, Edmonton. Year: 1942

Military History:

Service: RCAMC

Rank: Lieut. N/S

Served: January 1944 to September 1945

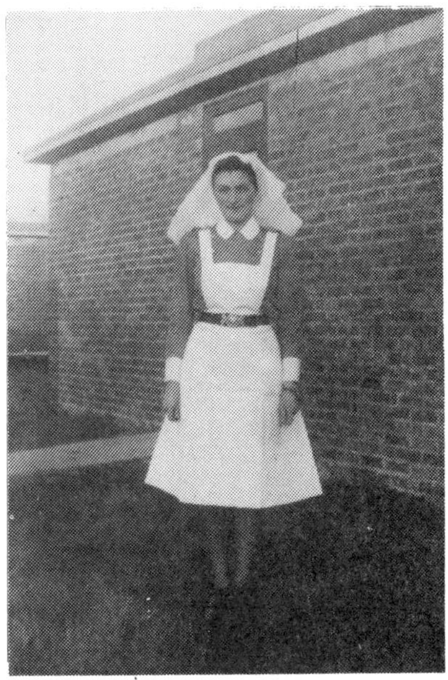

Lt. N/S Kathleen (Swan) Wyatt

When I graduated, my father was with RCE, my brother with the Loyal Edmonton Regt., and my sister with No. 15 Canadian General Hospital. So it was natural to enlist. I then had to wait to be called. In the interim I worked for the USED in Whitehorse, Yukon, on the Alcan Highway. I learned that I would not be called up while I worked for the U.S. Army so quit the end of 1943. I spent the first four months in the Army at a Lethbridge POW camp and went overseas with No. 24 General as a Second Lieutenant. We took over from No. 21 Canadian General Hospital at Horley in Surrey midst the worst of the V-1 and V-2 bombardment. It was an eye-opener and we wondered, at first, how England had stood the "real" blitz. But we got used to it very quickly as we were too busy to worry about it.

I was married in England and we went on our honeymoon in St. Ives on VE Day and as we had an extra 48 hours' leave. We spent VE I and II in London which was an extraordinary experience. My husband was with the Calgary Highlanders.

NO. 25 CANADIAN GENERAL HOSPITAL

Evelyn Blanche (MacRae) McLeod

No. 25 Canadian General Hospital mobilized at Botwood, Newfoundland, 6 January 1941 with Captain M.T. Kobrinsky, RCAMC, as CO. By 17 August three nursing sisters transferred to No. 25 General from St.John's Military Hospital – No. 26 Canadian General Hospital.

Duty at No. 25 General was considered an overseas assignment. The unit disbanded 31 July 1945.

Evelyn Blanche (MacRae) MacLeod

Graduated from: Prince Edward Island Hospital School of Nursing. Year: 1938

Military History:

Service: RCAMC

Rank: Lieutenant N/S

Served: No. 25 CGH and No. 26 CGH, 14 March 1941 to 3 January 1943

I chose the RCAMC first of all for the opportunity to serve my country, and for the opportunity to travel and have employment, which at that time was not always available.

The highlights of my military career were my assignments at the following locations:

Halifax, Cogswell Street Military Hospital, April 1941 - August 1941 - November 1941-August 1942

No. 26 Botwood Military Hospital, August 1941-November 1941

Chorley Park Military and Toronto Convalescent, August 1942 - January 1943

Retirement in 1943 ended my military career.

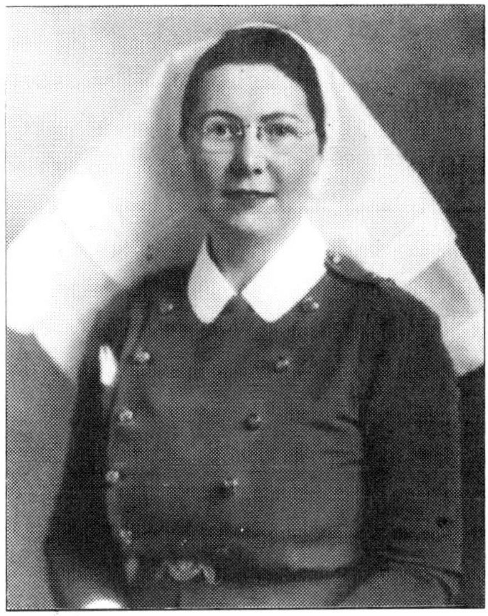

Lt. N/S Evelyn Blanche (MacRae) MacLeod, No. 25 St. John's Military Hospital, Newfoundland

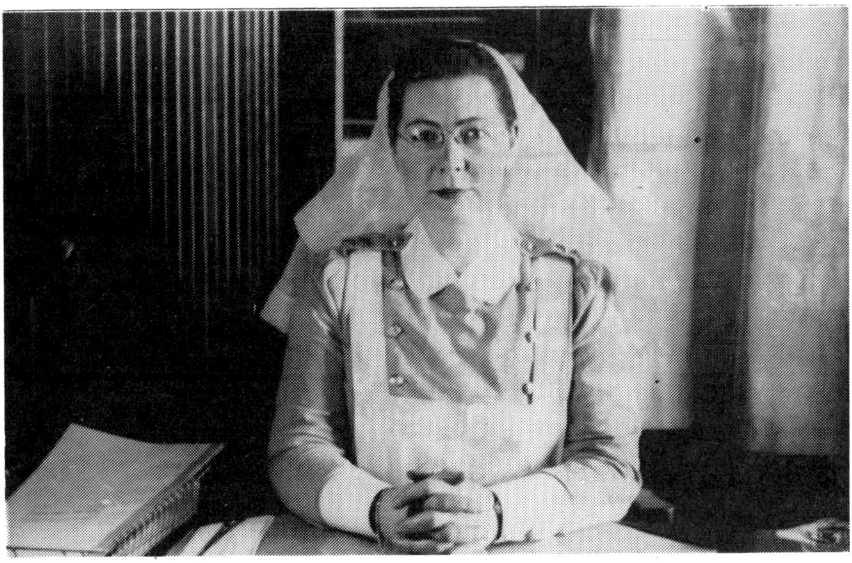

Lt. N/S Evelyn Blanche (MacRae) MacLeod, No. 26 Botwood Military Hospital, Newfoundland

NO. 26 CANADIAN GENERAL HOSPITAL

Evelyn Blanche (MacRae) McLeod

No. 26 Military Hospital, St.John's, Newfoundland, alternately known as St. John's Military Hospital and Lester Field Military Hospital, was in existence from November 1940 to July 1944 when it was disbanded. All nursing sisters were moved to Canada. Duty at No. 26 General was considered an overseas assignment.

NO. 27 MILITARY HOSPITAL

No. 27 Military Hospital, formerly known as Lewisporte Military Hospital, was in existence from 15 August 1944 to 31 December 1944 at Lewisporte, Newfoundland.

On 30 December 1944 the hospital officially closed down at Lewisporte and moved to Botwood, Newfoundland.

NO. 28 CANADIAN GENERAL HOSPITAL

No. 28 Canadian General Hospital was in existence for a brief time in Italy. On 4 February 1945, No. 1 Canadian Field Hospital was disbanded, and by the same authority a 200-bed No. 28 Canadian General Hospital was formed at the same location – a Benedictine convent at Mercogliano.

Nursing Sister E. Purdy was the acting matron for a dozen nursing sisters and one dietitian. Nursing Sister Bellis was in charge of the operating room.

By mid-April admissions ceased and patients were evacuated to a hospital ship in Naples.

The whole unit, including officers and nursing sisters, sat down to dinner 19 April 1945. This was their farewell to Italy and many months of good service by all. It was the last unit function, this being the last day No. 28 General existed as a unit.

Chapter 8

SOUTH AFRICAN MILITARY NURSING SERVICE

Alexandra Bury
Elizabeth Clement
Isabel (Morrison) Fraser
Eleanor (Edey) Hoon
Ellen Jean (Wheeler) Keays
Bodil Krag
Nancy Viola Lee
Ruth MacLennan
Emily Mayhew
Marion Cecelia (O'Neill) McColl
Doris (Bischlager) Moir
Jean (MacKay) Robinson
Helen (MacPherson) Rodin
Germaine (Quilchini) Schonek
Florence (Merlin) Shearer
Jean Snelgrove
Anne (Guthrie) Thomas
Margaret (Henderson) Watson
France (Dopson) Wilkie
Marian Williams

CANADIAN NURSES IN SOUTH AFRICA

By Alexandra Bury

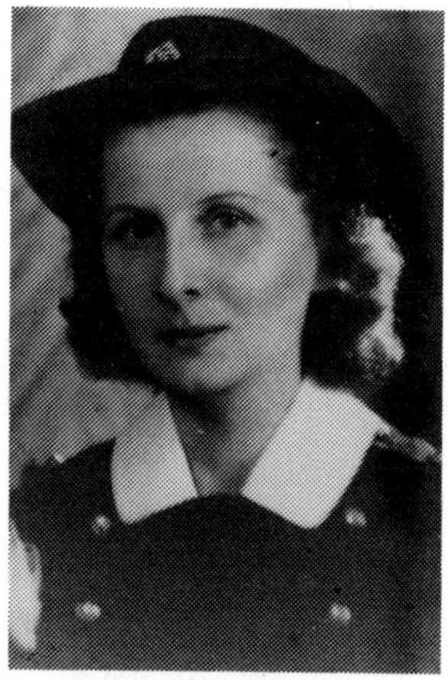

N/S Alexandra Bury, Johannesburg, South Africa 1942

When World War II broke out between England and Germany in 1939, Canada and South Africa were members of the British Empire and Commonwealth. Within a short while both countries declared war on Germany as well. In September of 1939, the prime minister of South Africa, Jan Christian Smuts, was consulted by Winston Churchill and other Allied leaders, and his main role was to mobilize his country's resources to prevent Germany and Italy from conquering North Africa.*

British troops were sent to the Middle East to protect the North African approaches to the Suez Canal. South African troops and others from Commonwealth Nations fought alongside the British 8th Army. Many casualties were caused by intense fighting, but could not be evacuated to Britain because of enemy attacks on ships in the Mediterranean and so were transported to South Africa. Although military hospitals were set up throughout the Union, the influx of sick and wounded created a shortage of qualified nurses to care for them.

During the summer of 1941, the Canadian government received an urgent request from the Union of South Africa for three hundred registered nurses. When the news of this was released across Canada, our nurses responded immediately and enlisted through the Royal Canadian Army Medical Corps. With the rank of Lieutenant N/S they wore the Canadian Nursing Sisters' uniform with pride and were attached to the SAMNSs.

In December of 1941, the first group of nurses arrived in Capetown, where a warm letter of welcome greeted them. After a short stay and most pleasant hospitality in Capetown, the nurses boarded the train for Durban, where they were soon assigned to various military hospitals in South Africa. The second group of nurses sailed for Capetown December 31, 1941. In the spring of 1942, the third and largest contingent went to England, where the nurses were divided into smaller groups for sailing to South

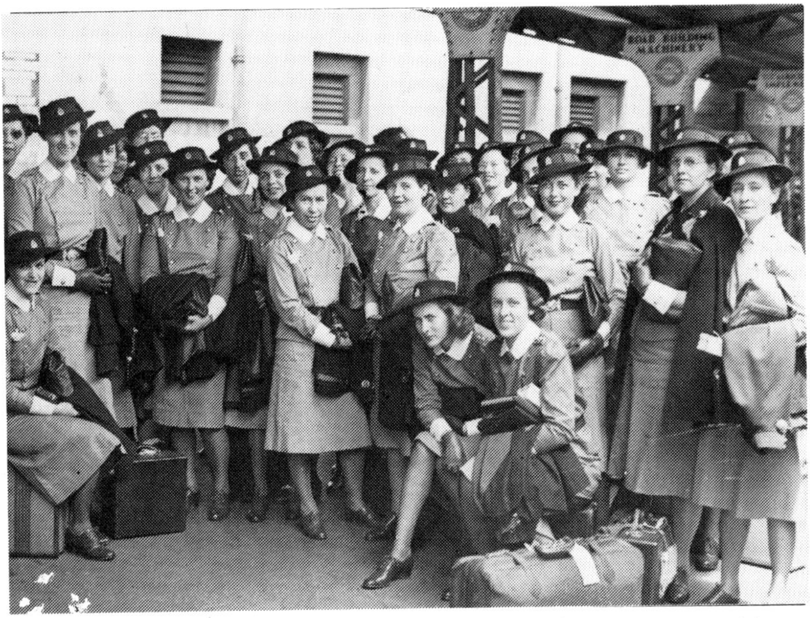

Eighty-two Canadian nurses in attractive uniforms, at present in Capetown, are the first batch to arrive in response to the Union Government's appeal to Canada for nurses. A further 220 will arrive in the future to serve in military hospitals in the Union.
The following are members of the first group who sailed on board the SS Kawsar from New York 15 November 1941 and landed in Cape Town 26 December 1941. The above picture was taken as the group disembarked from the train at Durban.
Muriel Ahier, Margaret Allan, Julia Andrews, M. Eleanor Ball, Jean Barned, Ann Brewer, Dorothy Brown, Jaqueline Brown, Alexandra Bury, Ethel Butler, Margaret Carpenter, Charlotte Cook, Annie Cullen, Marguerite Cusson, Margaret Dobson, Louise Eager, Mary Edmondson, Katherine Feisel, Gladys Fitzgerald, Helen Fountain, Marjorie Germaine, Margaret Goldsmith, Grace Govenlock, Annie Green, Zoe Harman, Julie Harwood, Dorothy Hayes, Florence Ingraham, Kathleen King, Marie La Croix, Isabel Lamplough, Mabel Lang, I. Elizabeth Langstaff, Barbara LaPierre, Edith Lewis, Elizabeth Lovegrove, May MacDonald, Nora MacNeil, Dorothy MacWade, Christine MacDonald, Marian McAfee, Laura McCluskey, Jean McIntosh, Nita McLardy, Ella McMillan, Agnes Maloney, Nona Mannix, Emily Mayhew, Ellen Meagher, Florence Merlin, Alice Monteith, Margaret Muir, Maureen O'Brian, Mildred O'Leary, Freyja Olafson, Marion O'Neill, Marjorie Parker, Violet Parker, Alma Patterson, Helen Peer, Germaine Quilchini, Bernice Rusenel, Emily Schmidt, Elsie May Smith, Orma Smith, Madeleine Steinhoff, Anne Stockwell, Edna Sullivan, Mavis Thompson, Fern Townsend, Margaret Verey, Edythe Ward, Margaret Waugh, Margaret Wastle, Ina Wetmore, Ida White, Olga Wicks, Gladys Wilkin, Mildred Wright.
Loaned by Marie (LaCroix) Smith

Africa on several different ships.

Although some Canadian nurses returned to Canada after one year's service, the majority stayed on with the SAMNS, and many were moved north to the Suez Canal and Tripoli areas. Later, a group was sent to Italy to care for the wounded of the South African Division.

The war ended and the Canadian nurses received a most welcome appreciative letter from Mr. Jan Smuts: "Now that your period of service in the forces of the Union of South Africa has drawn to a close, I wish to express to you the gratitude and thanks of all South Africans for so generously coming to our assistance in the days when we were faced with a big task.

"By your contribution you have enabled us to provide hospital accommodation for many thousands of Empire and Allied troops, in addition to our own.

"I hope that the same spirit of service and sacrifice that you have exhibited in the cause of freedom, and in cementing the bonds between countries, will enable you to contribute to the rebuilding of the shattered world.

"Your stay in our country and with our Forces in the field will remain an abiding and treasured memory. Thank you for it.

"With all good wishes for your future."

General Headquarters,

Pretoria, J.C. Smuts

Date 5/9/46 Minister of Defence

To: Mr. Smuts and the South African people:

We thank you for your very kind letters and for the opportunity to be of service to your country. It was indeed a privilege to nurse the brave young servicemen who fought so courageously for our freedom.

Alles van die beste

300 Canadian N/S

* The New Encyclopaedia Britannica, Volume 10, 15th Edition, 1994. Chicago. Page 905.

Elizabeth Louise Clement

Graduated from: Royal Columbian Hospital School of Nursing, New Westminster, B.C. Year: 1930

Military History:

Service: RCAMC and SAMNS

Rank: Captain

Served: April 23, 1942 to Aug. 13, 1946

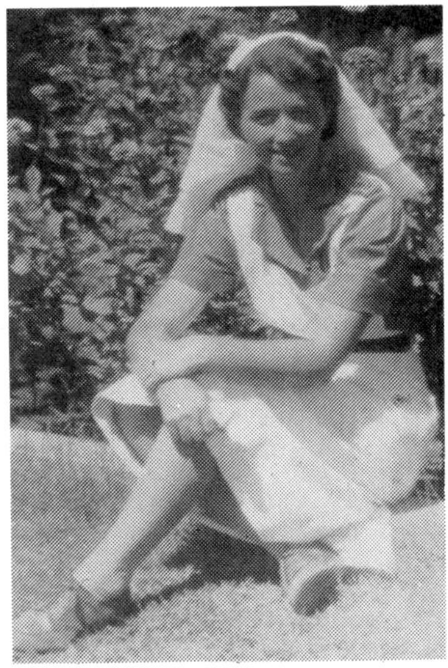

N/S Elizabeth Clement on the grounds of the Kenya Club, part of our garrison at Helmich, Egypt 1945 The Kenya club was a place to have afternoon tea.

There was little hope in 1941 of getting into the Canadian Army as a nurse. So when it was advertised that the Army needed 300 nurses for South Africa, I hurried to apply.

In late July 1941 the Union of South Africa asked the Canadian Government to recruit three hundred graduate nurses to staff several new hospitals in that country. This was agreed to and the information broadcast over the radio and published in the newspapers.

The nurses would be attached to the SAMNS, referred to henceforth as the SAMNS and would come under SAMNS rules and discipline and pay scales. The contract was to be in effect for one year with a chance to extend the service for the duration and six months after the nurses had been in South Africa for a while. All nurses would enter the service as staff nurses and some would be promoted to nursing sisters before leaving. Others would have a chance for promotion during their service. Uniform to be worn would be Canadian, i.e., the uniform of a nursing sister. Each nurse would have $150.00 given to her to purchase her uniforms.

What they forgot to mention was that in South Africa the SAMNS had to pay for their board, lodging and laundry; something that was provided for in the Canadian Army. No one thought to question this point. This reduced our take-home pay considerably.

At that time it was almost impossible to get into the

Canadian Army, so many nurses who wanted to serve applied and were quickly accepted. In British Columbia recruiting was done by Colonel Gordon Kenning at Work Point Barracks, Esquimalt.

Unknown to us, and probably unknown to anyone in Canada, the SAMNS was not considered a part of the Union Defence Force. Nurses did not receive commissions, although they wore military uniforms, badges, were governed by military rules, and were required to salute senior officers and return the salutes of others when wearing walking out uniform. This strange situation probably stemmed from the fact that in South Africa women were, at that time, still considered to be chattel. This situation was further borne out when the time for demobilization came; women received very small gratuities. The South African sisters always said that women and natives got the same amount. The gratuity paid after four and one-third years' service was fifty pounds, an equivalent of $150.00 at that time, compared to over $1,100.00 given to Canadians for the same service.

Due to the disparity between the treatment of Canadians in the SAMNS and those in the RCAMC, the Government of Canada passed an Order in Council on November 15, 1945. It gave those in the SAMNS the same benefits as these in the RCAMC.

We were advanced the sum of $150.00 to purchase uniforms; however, the bare minimum, according to the list supplied to us, cost approximately $300.00, not to mention the white panama hat and white shoes and dunnage bag that we were told to buy when we were in Montreal.

It was obvious that no one in the RCAMC knew much about the South African climate, for we were sent off to sunny South Africa with light-weight great coats – really just summer coats. Many of us were stationed in Johannesburg at an elevation of over 5000 feet where winter is really cold and the wind blows across the open veld, and then blows some more. Needless to say, our coats were inadequate. Those in our group were accepted October 1, 1941. We were supposed to sail from New York on the MV *Selandia* early in January. From Christmas week until April 1942 we received telegrams and letters every two weeks saying – you are leaving – you are not leaving – your ship has been confiscated by the American government. Now you will be leaving, sorry General Smuts has insisted that you go in convoy. Finally, on April 23, 1942, St. Georges Day, we left Victoria at 2:00 P.M. by boat for Vancouver. In Vancouver we were joined by several other sisters. Again, in Montreal, some B.C. girls joined us as they had been visiting across Canada.

The group from British Columbia consisted of nursing sisters Lillian McMillan, Gwendolyn Stevenson, Bodil Krag, Kirsten Krag, Thelma Baker, Nancy Lee, Audrey Ann Hopkins, Gladys Berndt, Agnes Griffiths, Doris Bischlager, Betty Putnam, Marian Williams, Elizabeth Clement, Marian Dobbie, Edith Coles, and Margaret Robbin.

In all, there were one hundred thirty of us who left from Halifax in convoy. We had no idea where we were going until we asked some of the civilian passengers on MV *Andes* on which we sailed. All we knew was that the tickets for the *Selandia* out of New York had been collected with our passports which had the U.K. added to them when they were returned.

In Montreal, Miss Mary Mercer was placed in charge of the draft. She had been in the RCAMC at Camp Borden. On the second day in Montreal we were told that our trunks had been moved from the Windsor Station to the Bon Aventure Station. We were told to take our dunnage bags and repack so that we had sufficient clothing for both warm and cold weather. We were to take enough to last at least two weeks as we would not have access to our trunks during the voyage. When we boarded the ship we were told to report to a certain area at 4:00 P.M. to identify our luggage, and our trunks were delivered to our state rooms.

We travelled in convoy, and the *Aquitania* with her distinctive four funnels was our constant companion throughout the eight days it took to reach Iceland. There the convoy left us and we travelled at top speed through the Irish Sea with two Corvettes as escort to Liverpool. We had only two scares, one at 4:00 A.M. when the escort came on a German submarine which surfaced. The gunfire awoke us but it was the depth charges that we really felt and heard. The second was in the Clyde when there was a sub directly in front of us submerged with probably only fifteen feet of water under her. Our ship turned to port and the escort swept in depth charging as they came. We never learned what transpired.

From Liverpool we travelled by a cold, cold troop train to No. 15 Canadian General Hospital at Bramshott. No meals were served on the train and we had breakfast about 5:00 A.M. Lunch consisted of two hard ships buns with a thin slice of meat, and an apple and orange. We couldn't eat because track workers looked at them so longingly when we opened our lunches around 10:00 A.M. while the train was standing still in the marshalling yard of Liverpool. We had to open the window and give them to the men for their children.

We spent about three weeks in England. During this time we were allowed ten days' leave and an advance on our salary of ten pounds. Miss Agnes Neil, Matron-in-Chief, had made arrangements for us to lodge in reasonably priced clubs and hotels in London. Some sisters went to Scotland and other parts of England. The South African Government entertained us at SA House and took us on a bus tour of London. The British Overseas League took us on a bus tour with other service men and women, to Windsor and Hampton Court. British Columbia House gave us theatre tickets. In all events we were treated very well. Our only problem was the respirator and tin hat with which we had been issued. They were so heavy to carry about all the time that our shoulders were very tired after we had walked around London all day.

Toward the end of May we were alerted to be ready to leave on short notice, and gradually, each day, one or more groups of around thirty nurses disappeared from the mess. When it was our turn we left from Maplehurst Station. While waiting for the train to come, our trunks and bags were all on the platform, all stencilled N6 and just our names, no rank or unit. There was a strange looking man peering at them, and it was whispered among us to be careful what we said as he might be a spy!

We stayed overnight in London at an ATS barrack. It had recently been bombed and in many of the rooms the walls had been broken and had been cemented up, and outside the ground was deep in broken glass and other rubble.

The next morning we proceeded to Euston Station where we boarded a troop train. We had no idea where we were going. We thought that when we got to Redding, which is a divisional point, we would be able to tell whether or not we turned north or whatever. The station names were all removed and it was impossible to tell. Finally we came to a port and left the train at the quayside. There was quite a stir when we came aboard the SS *Staffordshire*; no one knew that there were going to be any women on board, not even the OC Troops. Officers enjoying cabins to themselves had to move out; bathrooms had to be relabelled; everyone stared at us but very few deigned to speak to us. We had not been introduced! The port was Avon Mouth, and although the OC Troops did not know we were coming, some of the Naval officers did. A waitress in the village asked one of the South Wales Borderer officers if he was going on the ship with all the women, and this was the day before we arrived.

The South Wales Borderers, the Welsh Regiment, and a Major Paterson were some of the first to make our acquaintance, and gradually we were accepted. The convoy collected in the Firth just below Glasgow, and after sitting there for two days we were off zig-zagging across the Atlantic until we were nearly back to America. We even passed through the Gulf Stream just off the Caribbean. We didn't know it at the time, but I found out where I had been on my way home after the war. After two weeks of sailing we entered the harbour of Freetown, Sierra Leone. Here we sat in our ships for one week while the convoy watered and oiled. No one was allowed ashore; however, the naval contingent decided that the Army OC Troops really couldn't tell them, the Senior Service, what to do, so they went away. They returned with fresh, very green looking bananas. They turned out to be ripe – the kind that don't turn yellow.

When we sailed we were accompanied by two battleships, the *Rodney* and the *Nelson*, which were at Freetown when we arrived. All the naval ships preceded us out of the harbour and through the mine field line ahead. When they got outside, they depth-charged the whole area as they swept westward, then they had gun practice. It was a terrific sight. Then we followed them out through the mine field and the convoy formed up, the battleships always in the middle.

The day before we reached Cape Town the battleships left us and I have never seen a more beautiful sight. It was a lovely, sunny day. The water was that deep blue that is only seen in the southern Atlantic. The convoy parted and the two battleships, with all flags flying and the sailors in their tropical whites standing on every turret and every gun sailed down the lines of ships, turned at the southern end and sailed back again, their flags saying *"Safe Journey and God Bless."* It had been a happy journey, marred only by the sudden death of an elderly naval officer who was on his way to Aden. He had been unwell and only that day had been allowed up on deck by the doctor. That evening it was the nursing sisters' turn to entertain. We were putting on a melodramatic mime, called the "Light House Keeper's Daughter," when the sister representing Poop Deck Paddy the Light House Keeper who was the first character on stage, looked into the audience and saw this officer in the midst of a heart attack. It put a damper on our farce, but the show went on without a hitch.

On arrival in Cape Town July 1st, 1942 we lived on the ship for a couple of days until train transportation could be arranged to Johannesburg. There our group was assigned to Baragwanath Military Hospital. This hospital was occupied but had not been officially opened. It was partly medical and surgical and partly a TB hospital, and held 1000 beds. The administration block was on level ground at the top of a hill and the hospital fanned out from three ramps down the hill. Each ward was a separate entity with lawn between it and the next ward. Wards 1 to 8 were surgical wards and were situated off an enclosed corridor that led to the OR theatres and X-Ray department. The other corridors or ramps were open but did have a roof. Each ward consisted of a large ward for 24 patients and two side rooms for ill patients, a doctor's room, treatment room, nurses' office, kitchen, sluice room, and bath rooms for patients. Each ward had a stoop the full length of the main ward. At first there was no grass between the wards and the dust blown up by the wind was quite a problem to the wards. As soon as spring arrived in September the ground was cultivated and grass sown which improved the situation in the wards.

Patients came to us from the Middle East and from India arriving in Durban by Hospital Ship. They arrived at our hospital by train and were loaded off at a small station nearby as we were five miles south of Johannesburg and right out in the country.

This hospital was financed by money from Britain, built by South African labour and four-fifths of the professional nursing staff was Canadian. General Smuts remarked that, due to these facts, it was a unique hospital.

The people of Johannesburg were very concerned with the welfare of the patients and each ward was adopted by some business or group of people. They visited the boys, saw that they had note paper, books, smokes, candy and fruit. At Christmas every patient got a gift. In one ward that I worked in they collected enough film, and it was in short supply, to take every boy's picture either alone or in a group, and had enough developed so that they could send them home to their families. Besides this, they provided a turkey so that there would be two turkeys for dinner instead of one, and a great big beautiful Christmas cake.

One Christmas a group gave sufficient money so that all the female patients and the nursing staff could all be taken to town to see the Pantomine which is an annual event at Christmas time.

Gradually, after the first year, Baragwanath was changed from a medical and surgical hospital to a totally tuberculosis hospital. This change provided some benefits for the staff. The beautiful swimming bath built by a swimming club in Johannesburg was now entirely a staff pool, the tennis courts, too, reverted to staff entertainment. However, lawn bowling was a sport that the patients could indulge in.

A lovely little red brick chapel was built close to the wards. The nursing staff provided the blue carpet for the middle aisle and the blue cushion kneelers. This chapel was used by all denominations. If you were not Anglican or Roman Catholic you were classed as non-conformist.

Miss Gladys Sharpe was the first senior matron, but she left to go on the hospital ship for a trip before she left for Canada at the end of her year's contract. She was followed by Miss Henrietta Fick, an Afrikaans matron. There was always a senior matron and a junior matron. When she was transferred, we had a Miss E. Stoney, and she was our lass from Lancashire. She was loved by all. She developed cancer of the throat and died at Robert's Height Hospital in 1947. She had been awarded the Royal Red Cross in 1944 and the Florence Nightingale Medal in 1947 while she was a patient in hospital.

Our staff consisted of approximately eighty Canadian sisters, twenty South African sisters and probably about two hundred nurses who were trained in service and had been recruited from every profession and business. They had left their jobs to help care for their wounded and ill servicemen. There were about three male orderlies in the whole hospital. There were Women's Auxilliary Services, sergeants' mess and officers' mess; the cleaning and dish washing was done by civilian natives at one time and then by native soldiers.

Our living quarters were long, brick bungalows with six separate rooms that opened out onto a stoop. There was no plaster lining and the floors were covered with a reddish-brown, very poor linoleum. The beds were folding camp cots with very thin mattresses, and the army blankets would have been more suitable for covering a horse than a person. Later on, we got spring-filled mattresses and white blankets. There was no heating of any kind in our rooms unless you could find an electric heater in town. During the first winter this was impossible. The Ablution block was shared by four bungalows and there was no heat in there either, so baths were taken very quickly. When you were on night duty you moved over to the night hut and slept there, which was a good thing as it was very quiet there.

Our mess had a large dining room and a lounge, and between our mess and the WAS (Women's Auxiliary Service) mess there was a small canteen run by one of the nurses. The money from this canteen supplemented our rations in the form of catsup, pickles, ice cream and extra milk. The mess was supervised by a home sister.

Prior to the official opening of our hospital by Field Marshall Jan Christian Smuts, the Canadian sisters were introduced to the Afrikaans' language in the form of the national anthem "Die Stem," which is always sung in Afrikaans. As we comprised the largest groups, and as the staff were supposed to sing the national anthem, it was necessary for us to learn it. We had it written out in phonetics, and we practised every evening. Then came the big day and we were all lined up in front of the Administration Block; the band struck up "Die Stem." We opened our mouths to sing, but the band played too fast and we never sang a word.

The days, months, and a year passed; some Canadians went home at the end of their first year. Some of us decided to stay and signed on for the duration and six months. All those remaining signed what was known as the Blue Oath which stated that we were willing to serve anywhere the SA Defence Force went. Some South Africans refused to go outside their own country. Those who signed the Blue Oath wore orange flashes on their epaulettes.

After Miss Sharpe returned to Canada we had no one of our own to turn to. We were having difficulty getting new uniforms and it took about six months for a parcel to come from Canada. The Canadian Army was wearing summer uniforms with open necks and short sleeves to work in, and here were we in a subtropical country still wearing starched collars and cuffs. One of the sisters was on vacation in Cape Town so she went to see the trade commissioner and told him of our troubles. It was not long until material and the pattern for the summer uniforms were available, and all we had to do was order them and they were made for us. The matron-in-chief tried to find out who had gone over her head, but no one ever told. Of course, probably only a few of us knew.

In September or October of 1944, in an attempt to improve the trained staffs' pay, it was decreed that all trained nurses would have the rank of captain. Now, quite a number of new sisters were recruited around this time and they all came into the service wearing three pips. This infuriated the staff nurses who had given two or three years' service, as they felt any promotion should be a reward for the time and effort that they had put into their work. So we refused to put up another pip. This went on for about two weeks, although the order was on the mess notice board. Then one evening the matron and sisters were invited to the sergeants' mess for a party. (There was no snobbishness in the Union Defense Force. I have seen parties in the sisters' mess when there was everything from a private to a general present). When different ranks were invited to a party, either the officers or the other ranks were invited by written invitation; the others were invited by word of mouth. On this particular evening, I felt that we could not embarrass the matron by appearing improperly dressed. At this time I was the senior sister in the mess. I went around to all those who were going to the party and suggested that we had made our protest and that now we should give in and put up our third pip. Everyone agreed and we all walked over to matron's cottage and proceeded to the mess with her. No one ever said, *"You didn't obey orders."*

From time to time drafts of staff left our hospital for Egypt or Italy. In February 1945 I was lucky enough to be sent in charge of a draft from our hospital to Egypt. We travelled to Durban where we were joined by two smaller drafts. After some delays we were on our way in the MV *Selandia*, the same ship I was supposed to sail on from New York in the spring of 1942. She was a small ship and I would rather go from Durban to Suez in her than across the Atlantic. There were no stewards on board and we had to do all the odd jobs like sweeping out our cabins, cleaning bathtubs. The other ranks swept the corridors, companion ways and the lounges. There were some civilian wives of high ranking officers on board and they took a very dim view of the whole affair. For four hours we degaussed the ship to prevent magnetic mines being attracted to our hull. This consisted of travelling up and down and around two buoys just off Durban bathing beach. The Indian Ocean here is very shallow and the surf comes tumbling in and anyone who was going to be sea sick was, long before we left the beach. When we had passed the Island of Madagascar the sea calmed out and everyone enjoyed the rest of the trip. Even though it was wartime, the usual fun took place when we crossed the line. It was an uneventful but happy trip.

No. 5 South African General Hospital was situated in the Helmieh Garrison. There was space for another tented hospital, but the 64th British Hospital was next door and we admitted troops (other than South Africans) on alternate days with the British Hospital. Our hospital was mostly tented, although the orthopaedic, surgical and acute medical wards were in buildings. Most of the tent wards were what was known as EP. IP. tents, i.e., European Personnel and Indian Personnel. These tents were double and could be arranged to take advantage of any cool breeze by closing one door and opening another on the side where the breeze is. They also had ventilators in the roof. The floors and walls were cement and the tent was pitched on top of the cement wall giving it great height, and so, improved ventilation. The other tents were marquees pitched on cement floors level with the ground.

Each ward had an ablution block and a kitchen. There was hot water only in the ablution block and this had to be carried to the kitchen to wash dishes or to the ward to bathe bed patients. Our South African native soldiers who looked after our kitchens were not slow to exploit the fact that the Egyptian men who were around the camp were very, very poor. Our boys dried out all tea leaves and coffee grounds that had been used. They kept them all in tin cans and then bartered them for work. The Egyptian men carried all the water from the ablution block to the kitchens, being paid in crusts, used tea leaves or coffee grounds.

In our service rooms or duty rooms we didn't have any electric or gas sterilizers. We used fish boilers with methylated spirit for fuel. It was a long time since any proper wicks had been available so two-inch gauze bandages were inserted where a wick should have been and they worked perfectly. All water for tea was heated on a primus stove.

When on night duty one usually had several wards to oversee; there would be a nurse on each ward and the sister travelled between giving medication and checking very ill patients. On one occasion I had three wards in buildings. First came an orthopaedic ward. It was at the bottom of a small hill and had a mud wall about three feet high surrounding it to keep the sand from drifting in. There was room between this wall and the building to walk. The young nurse on that ward was very nervous and was quite sure someone was skulking around in the space between the walls. I had to take her and a torch and creep through this space to convince her that there was no one there. My second ward was a surgical ward in a building at the top of the small hill. It was a very old wooden building and white scorpions used to drop out of a hole in the ceiling on to the chart desk. The third ward was just over the hill about fifty yards. It consisted of two buildings with an EP IP tent in between for a duty room for the staff. There was a hole in the cement floor right under the sister's chair. Every night it would be full of the most enormous earwigs; our cure for this was to move the chair pour meths (methylated spirits) into the hole and light it.

One night I was down in the first ward when suddenly many shots were fired. There were terrible screams and sirens sounded. Looking out you could see tracer bullets flying. All this sound and fury came from the direction of Ward 3. I ran as fast as I could over the desert to the ward on top of the hill, but everyone there was quite all right . On I went, quite sure that I would find the nurse at No. 3 stabbed, shot or worse. When I got there she and the ward MO were sitting playing crib. He had been working on files and they were having a little relaxation before he turned in. The whole thing started when the guards found a WOG (Western Oriental Gentleman) breaking into the fumigation building to steal blankets.

Sisters acted in cooperation with the laboratory. On a medical ward, whenever a patient was admitted with a high fever the sister immediately started taking blood slides for malaria and sent them at once to the lab. It was not wise to leave a blood slide on a desk or table for even a few minutes as the flies would eat all the blood in no time. As soon as a positive slide was obtained the sister immediately instituted the treatment laid down for that type of malaria and the MO was notified as soon as possible.

In the native medical wards we had many strange tropical diseases. Kala-azar, elephantiasis, bilharzia, guinea worms, tape worms by the score, typhus and leprosy, just to name a few.

VE Day was celebrated in fine style with very little work done during the day and a huge dance at Hyde Park Corner (a club-type place in our garrison). Later, about three of the sisters and three doctors danced the Palaise Glide all the way to the officers' mess – about half a mile. The South African officers' mess had been a stable in the First World War but had been done over during the Second World War as there was no need for a horse stable. We entertained the British general, Medical Services Middle East, that night. He wanted to fry eggs for all of us but the kitchen was locked. Our colonel said, *"Let him break down the door, we don't have a General to break down our kitchen door every day."* So the door was broken down. He tried to light the primus stove and nearly lit the mess, so he decided to make Bombay oysters for us. Every glass had a raw egg broken into it, then a dash of Worcestershire Sauce, and then it was "down the hatch." Lucky if you didn't break the yolk. There was no getting away – he stood over everyone till they drank their oyster.

VJ Day was less exciting, but of course everyone got extra days off in lieu of the actual day. Vacations were nearly always spent in Palestine. You went there by train and returned by train; but travelling around in between was usually done by hitching a ride.

Christmas was a special time in both the Union and in Egypt. We always decorated the wards with streamers and Christmas trees if available. The traditional colours for Christmas in South Africa are pale blue, peach and pink. They thought the soldiers very strange when they wanted green and red to trim their wards. We always had a big mess dinner before Christmas Day with turkey, plum pudding and the lot even though it was boiling hot and the middle of summer. Of course, in Egypt it was winter. On Christmas Eve we always sang carols in every ward, and up patients would join the carolers as we moved along. It was always very dark so we carried storm lanterns on the long window poles and wore South African nurse's capes turned inside out so that the scarlet showed over our white aprons.

In September 1945 the hospital was due to close, but as the repatriation of the soldiers was not as fast as had been expected the colonel asked us to stay on. We didn't get away until the middle of February. On our return to the Union we were met at Durban by the matron-in-chief. She gave us all, regardless of whether or not we had been given leave in Egypt, one month ex north leave and one month leave as long as it didn't override our leave cycle. As my leave cycle started on April 23 (the day I had started from Victoria), I lost about four days' leave. However, I had been given two weeks' leave while in Egypt, so we were extremely well treated.

The esteem in which the nurses and sisters were held by others is born out in the following poem:

CHRISTMAS 1945
No. 5 South African General Hospital Helmieh, Egypt
Published in the paper *Hospital Gen.* by J.G.

WOMEN IN WHITE

To all the praise for men and women who,
Served and fought in khaki and two shades of blue.
Add this in testimony for those who served in white,
Long after battle, in their own grim pain allaying fight.
These few, the host,
Who warred with foes in water, sand and blood,
Who cleansed the wounds, or scraped away the mud,
Or washed away the filth and pus to bring to light of day
A semblance, torn and shattered of the former human clay.
They carried on the trivial round, the common load,
They stood with cup in hand, or jar or flask
To moisten parched lips, or ease the pain wracked
Temple of the Holy Ghost.
They kept their records, they made their routine rounds,
Alert and highly sensitive to the varied suffering sounds,
They kept their nightly vigils, they toiled through torrid days,
To help their suffering comrades, thro' many healing ways,
They earned the gratitude of those for whom they cared,
Theirs is the honour in the knowledge that they shared
With their brothers in the battle to set mankind free,
Their Glory is plainly written for everyone to see.
"As much as ye did it unto these ye did it unto Me."

In January we started to close down and pack away all the hospital equipment. We also had to clean out our bungalows. As there had been nursing staff in these rooms for over five years, it is easy to imagine the amount of accumulated junk there was in cupboards. However, the garbage trucks never got very much. As fast as any piece of clothing, old shoes, old suitcases, etc., etc., was thrown out, there was a flutter of a white robe and some Egyptian gentleman grabbed it. Finally, in mid-February, we left and travelled by train to Tewfick, a military port near Suez. We were embarked by tender to our ship as we were not allowed to go into the city and to the quayside as there was a plague there. After a voyage of fifteen days we were back in the Union.

Following my long leave I was posted to Wynburg which is just a suburb of Cape Town. Several other Canadians arrived; however, they were in transit and didn't have to work. I had been posted there and had to work, although we were all waiting for a ship to take us home. I worked in the Theatre and really enjoyed it. We left for home on the *Cape Town Castle* July 15, 1946, and arrived home in Vancouver on August 13, 1946.

I had two memorable short leaves for VE Days and VJ Days; one spent in a British leave camp outside Alexandria at Agmi, included trips to the battle field at El Alemain and a day at Sin Bish beach.

The second was a trip to Luxor and Karnak with a side trip to the Valley of the Kings.

Isabel (Morrison) Fraser

Graduated from: Victoria General Hospital School of Nursing, Halifax, Nova Scotia. Year: 1940

Military History:

Served: SAMNS and RCAMC

Rank: Lt. N/S

Served: March 1942 to May 1946

I decided to join the Army (RCAMC) as many of my classmates had the same idea! Three of us joined the SAMNS from Halifax, along with 300 other nurses from Halifax to Victoria, B.C. (The other two nurses were Jean Desmore and Dorothy Wiswall). We left Canada March 1942. Two of us left South Africa after one year and returned to Canada and joined the RCAMC in Halifax. I served in England with No. 23 CGH. Later I was assigned to Germany and remained there until 1946 when I sailed for home.

My husband and I were married in September 1946 and lived in Sydney, Nova Scotia, where Kenneth practised medicine for nearly forty years. He passed away in 1989, and now that I am widowed I travel to see grandchildren in Edmonton and Ottawa.

Eleanor E. (Edey) Hoon

Graduated from: Ottawa Civic Hospital School of Nursing.
Year: 1936

Military History:

Service: South Africa Military Nursing Service

Rank: Nursing Sister

Served: July 1942 to Sept. 1945

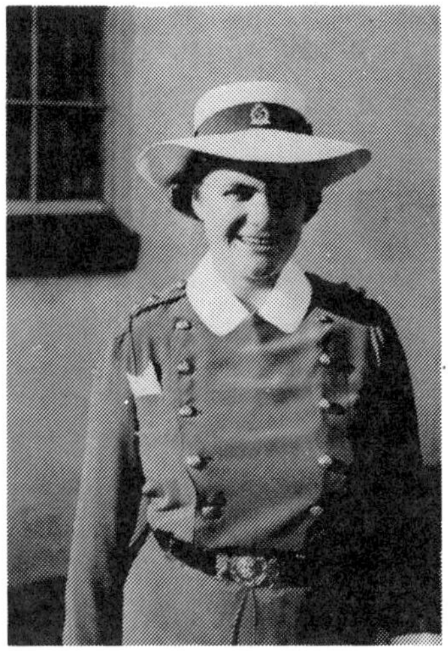

N/S Eleanor (Edey) Hoon

The opportunity was there – newspaper article wanting nurses in South Africa and I wanted to be in the Army. I chose to accept the SAMNS

It was a pleasure meeting British soldiers (patients). The comradeship with other nurses continues to this day.

I was born and grew up in Ottawa, Ontario. Following high school graduation in June 1933, I entered the Ottawa Civic Hospital Training School of Nursing in September 1933.

After graduating in 1936 I did some general, then private duty. Came the war and in 1941 I enlisted to go to South Africa. Two groups had already left and arrived in South Africa. Finally, after being collected right across Canada by train, we boarded the *Andes* for England. We were divided into five groups – each on a different ship, and proceeded to Durban. The largest group continued to Baragwanath Hospital outside Johannesburg. From here some returned to Canada after one year of service while others stayed on. After one and a half years there, I was transferred to Wynberg Hospital near Capetown. That's where I met Len, a sailor in the South African Navy. We were married in 1944, came to Abbotsford, B.C., where we have lived happily ever since.

Ellen Jean (Wheeler) Keays

Graduated from: St. Boniface Hospital School of Nursing, St. Boniface, Manitoba. Year: 1941

Military History:

Service: SAMNS

Rank: Captain

Served: December 1941 to December 1944

The Army provided an opportunity to serve my country as well as travel.

I was posted to Durban Sydenham Military Hospital for approximately five months. I was on a chest ward (medical). Because of the humidity I requested a transfer to an inland hospital. Edna (Pool) Jackson and I were then sent to Piet Retief, Transvaal. It was a small 120-bed hospital in three buildings. Two buildings for whites and one for natives. It was a general hospital – but wonderful experience, all in all. It was a different and challenging experience.

When the South Africa 106 Hospital was closed down we were transferred back to Quassasin, 70 miles from Cairo. I was back on medical wards taking care of patients with communicable disease, skin disease and some post-surgery depending on staffing.

We lived in tents while in North Africa and had excellent military accommodation while in South Africa.

I loved the country of South Africa. I sincerely hope the whites and natives can come to a peaceful solution.

Bodil S. Krag

Graduated from: Royal Columbian Hospital School of Nursing, New Westminster, B.C. Year: 1935

Military History:

Service: SAMNS

Rank: Lieutenant N/S

Served: April 1943 to Nov. 45, 3 years 7 months

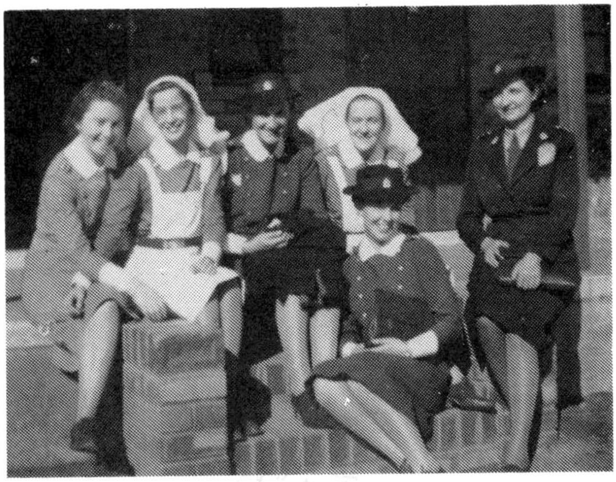

Nursing sisters Elizabeth Clement, Bo Krag, Nancy Lee, Kay Krag, Marian Williams, Agnes Griffiths

Canada was at war, I was a nurse and nurses were being called for so it was natural for me to join the Army. I had been in England when war was declared.

We were advised to return to Canada and join our own units. There were many tourists in England and war didn't strike for about a year. I joined Civil Nursing Reserve, but returned to Canada and joined SAMNS for Africa. South Africa wanted nurses in the military hospitals. After over a year there, I went to Egypt for the duration. It was wonderful experience; we worked under canvas on the desert sands of Egypt.

I returned to work in Shaughnessy Military Hospital, still receiving the military casualties from U.K. and Continent before their embarkation home. I spent two leaves seeing the Holy Land and Jerusalem.

Nancy Viola Lee

Graduated from: Vancouver General Hospital School of Nursing. Year: 1932

Military History:

Service: SAMNS

Rank: Lt. to Captain

Served: April 1942 to September 1945

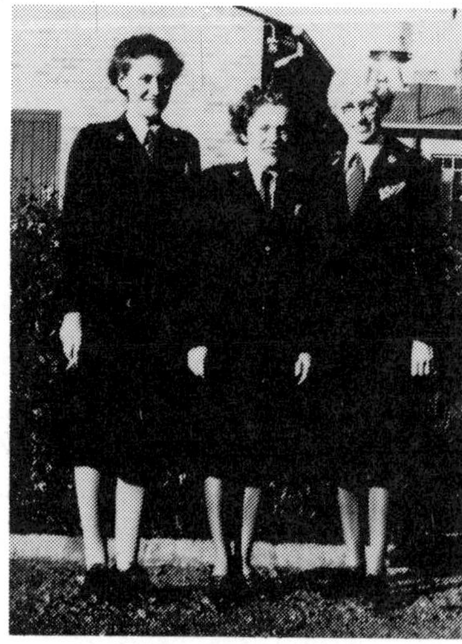

Capt. Nancy Viola Lee, D. Wiswall, A.Henderson at Teupe

I think many of us were anxious to "do our bit" when the 2nd World War broke out, I know I was. It was a tense time.

When we opened 108 SA Mobile in Florence, Italy, we were closer to the front (12 miles) more than we had ever hoped to come. We admitted a wardfull by the end of the day. It was practically empty by 10:00 A.M. the next day as long as air evacuation was possible. This happened daily. Florence was a wonderful city to be in, if and when we had a day off.

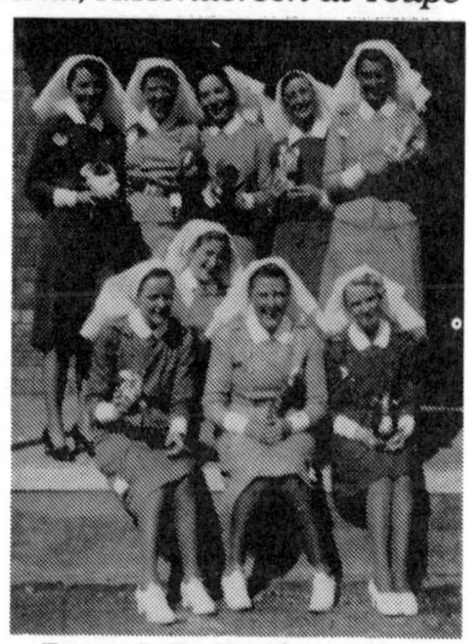

Rear: L-R: E. Clement, L. McMillan, G. Stephenson, Bodil Krag, N. Lee. Front L-R: K.Krag, E. Coles, D. Bischlager, M.Dobie

On VE Day, I was in a very small hospital in Montegnana nursing several German POWs who were too ill to be evacuated. My orderly at night was a German POW who, in civilian life, worked for Mercks in Frankfurt. He spoke no English; I spoke no Italian. It was surprising how we managed to communicate and both agreed in our thanks that the war was finally over. He was terrified that he would be sent to Russia and I wonder what became of him.

My 13 months in Italy are full of memories; I was fortunate to be sent there. My time in the South African Military Nursing Service was an unforgettable experience.

Ruth C. MacLennan

Graduated from: Toronto General Hospital School of Nursing.
Year: 1940

Military History:

Service: SAMNS and RCAMC

Rank: Lt. and Captain

Served: 1940 to 1944

In Canada I was stationed at military camps in Toronto, Chorley Park, Camp Borden, Hamilton, and on the *Lady Nelson* hospital ship, Halifax, N.S.

I had my picture taken in South Africa with General Smuts when he opened our large military hospital at Baragwanath, Johannesburg.

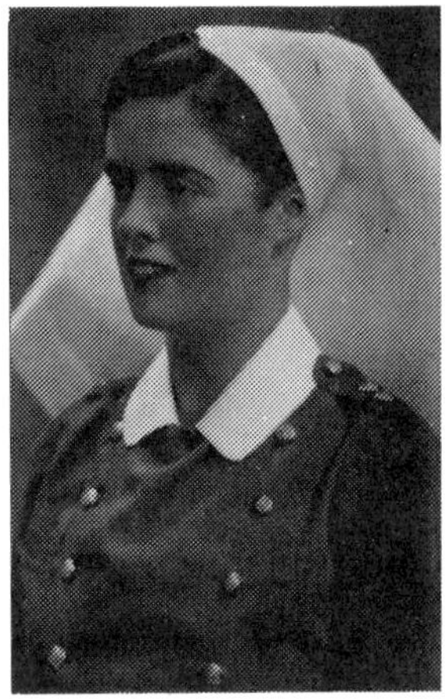

Captain Ruth C. MacLennan

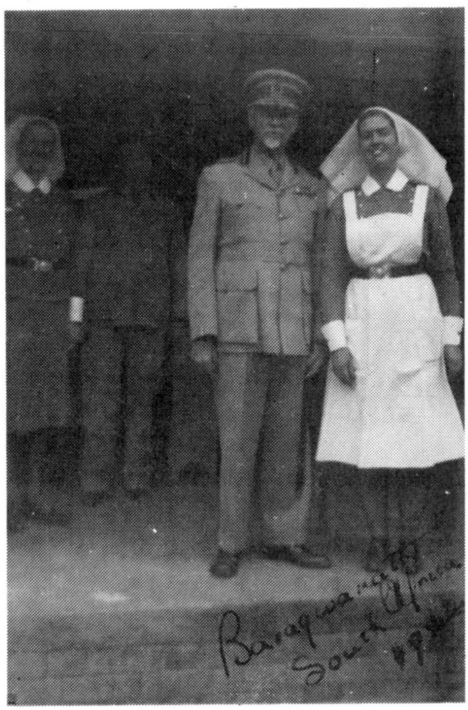

The opening of the military hospital at Johannesburg, South Africa General Smuts, N/S Ruth MacLennan, Baragwanath, South Africa

Emily Elizabeth Mayhew

Graduated from: Royal Alexandra Hospital School of Nursing, Edmonton, Alberta. Year: 1940

Military History:

Service: SAMNS and RCAMC

Rank: Lt. N/S

Served: December 1940 to November 1944 in SAMNS then in the RCAMC until the end of the war on the *Lady Nelson* Hospital ship.

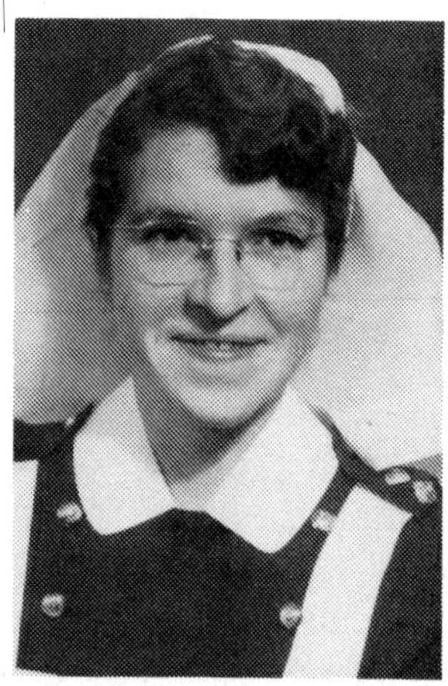

Lt. N/S Emily Mayhew

I knew a war was coming soon. I wanted to be a nursing sister so I resigned from teaching at the Indian Residential School, Edmonton, and went in training at the RAH. I graduated in September 1940 and went over with the first group of Canadian nurses to South Africa. In January of the following year I was in charge of a surgical ward in a tent in South Africa.

When I was on night duty, a storm was threatening but all the windows and doors were open. One of my patients I was worried about had finally gone to sleep when I heard a loud strange sound in the ward. At first I had difficulty locating it, until I came to his bed. I waited – all was quiet, he slept on. As soon as I left, the sound came again. So this time I shook him to find out if he was all right. Then I discovered a dog was snoring under his bed; it had come in for shelter.

Another time we were very anxious about an RAF pilot in a side ward. That morning I was afraid we were going to lose him, and forgetting, went into the big ward looking very sober. Immediately the men called out *"Where is our sunshine"?* They always called me Sunshine, so I had to turn and joke with them.

Many of the incidents are tinged with humour, as we were not only treating the body, but the mind as well. I am happy to say when I was transferred to another hospital the RAF pilot was able to take my arm and walk to the gate with me.

It is most difficult to give highlights, especially of nursing in

South Africa, as there were many on and off duty.

On the hospital ship in the Canadian Army I not only nursed, but I entertained the patients by playing the violin in the ship's orchestra and giving vocal solos.

We were docked, empty in Halifax, ready to go back to England. The two padres were good friends. One was a Baptist, the other a Roman Catholic. I had never seen the little priest smile.

There were only curtains to our sleeping quarters. One night I woke to feel some heavy body running over me. I put out my hand and felt a rat's head with its whiskers and nose between my thumb and first finger. The rat was as startled as I was and squeaked and leapt for the porthole, fell back on me, and this time got up my pyjama sleeve. I leapt to the floor. The rat again scrambled to get out, and this time disappeared through the port hole. I ran for the first man I could find. He was the priest, I imagine, going over his prayers. I dragged him into the room telling him to make sure the rat had gone. He pulled all the trunks out from under the bunks and looked in every corner until I was satisfied, but I saw his lips going up at the corners in suppressed mirth. The next day the whole ship had heard about it and the little priest smiled at me every time he saw me although I was not of his flock!

In all my travels I have circled the globe. I have nursed in a mission hospital as a relief nurse in Northern Zambia, which was an unforgettable experience, but my retirement is the busiest and happiest period of my life.

Marion Cecilia (O'Neill) McColl

Graduated from: St. Joseph's Hospital School of Nursing
St. John, New Brunswick. Year: 1934

Military History:

Service: SAMNS

Rank: Lt. N/S

Served: 1941 to February 1943.

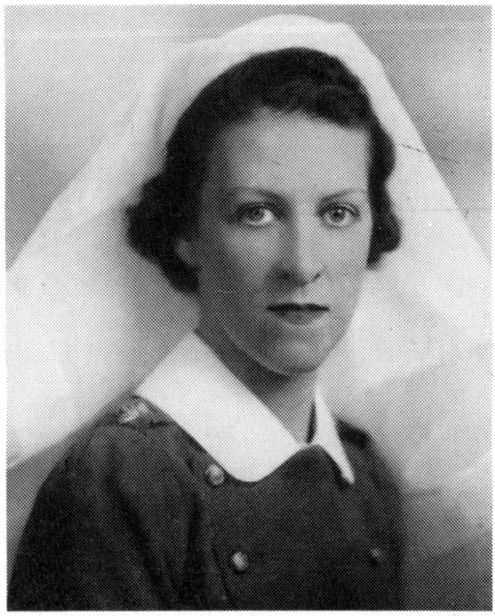

N/S Marion Cecelia (O'Neill) McColl

The Army provided a chance for adventure as well as war service.

I was in first group of 100 Canadian nurses recruited for South African service. We left from New York on the Egyptian ship, the SS *Kawsar*, bound for Capetown via Trinidad and Recife.

I was stationed in a British Hospital, Oribi Hospital, Pietermaritzburg, Natal.

Doris G. (Bischlager) Moir

Graduated from: St. Joseph's Hospital School of Nursing, Victoria, B.C. Year: 1937

Military History:

Service: SAMNS

Rank: Captain

Served: April 1942 to March 1945

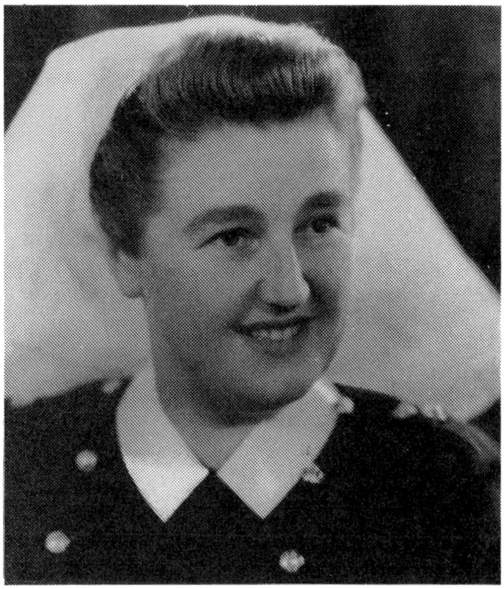

N/S Doris (Bischlager) Moir

There was a request from South Africa for nurses. My father served in both wars as a chaplain and my brother was killed while serving in the RCAF; that was enough to convince me to join the Army. I wanted to be a part of the war effort.

I spent one year in Baragwanath Military Hospital, Johannesburg. That was followed by six weeks at Transit Hospital, Clearwater, Durban.

My next assignment was six months at new European Military Hospital, Cairo, Egypt. After Egypt I spent one year with the South African Military Hospital at Bari, Italy.

I married in August 1944 to a British artillery captain in Bari; we met on the boat going to South Africa.

Jean E. (MacKay) Robinson

Graduated from: Saskatoon City Hospital School of Nursing.
Year: 1937

Military History:

Service: SAMNS

Rank: Lt. N/S and Captain N/S

Served: April 1942 to October 1945

My military experience was not too amusing, but unusual and stimulating. Excerpts from my five-year diary assist me in my recollections. On 19 April 1943 I left Francistown, Bechuanaland Protectorate, where I had been on leave in Maun, a guest of Mr. & Mrs. Bruce Rutherford. He was assistant district commissioner of the British protectorate between South Africa and Southern Rhodesia. At 12:30 A.M. I was in Bulowayo for seven hours. I helped officiate at a birth on the train (Cape to Cairo train) at 8:20 P.M. between Bulowayo and Livingston, Northern Rhodesia. Capt. Davidson of the British Army Medical Corps officiated. He was returning from leave in the Cape Province to his unit in Kenya. On 20 April 1943 we arrived at Victoria Falls at 6:45 A.M. Capt. Davidson accompanied our mother and new baby to the hospital in Livingstone and then returned to the Falls where he had planned to stay a few days.

The Belgian couple with a child and a female relative were returning to the Congo from a leave in Capetown when she went into labour. The patient was most cooperative; the birth was normal, so we were lucky. The dining car steward supplied a large bowl of hot water, a bottle of Dettol, a piece of string and a pair of scissors. I was grateful for a supply of Kleenex I had in my luggage. It had arrived from Canada just before my leave. I cleaned off the baby boy and wrapped him in a towel for there was no layette. The train officials supplied a fresh bedroll for the mother so she was freshened up.

I visited her in the hospital before my three-day visit to Victoria Falls was over and received such a warm welcome. They had named the baby Daniel. He could be a grandfather by now!

Helen (MacPherson) Rodin

Graduate of: St. Paul's Hospital School of Nursing, Vancouver. Year: 1939

Military History:

Service: SAMNS

Rank: Nursing Sister in Canadian nurses uniform on British rates of pay and rations.

Served: December 1941 to October 1945

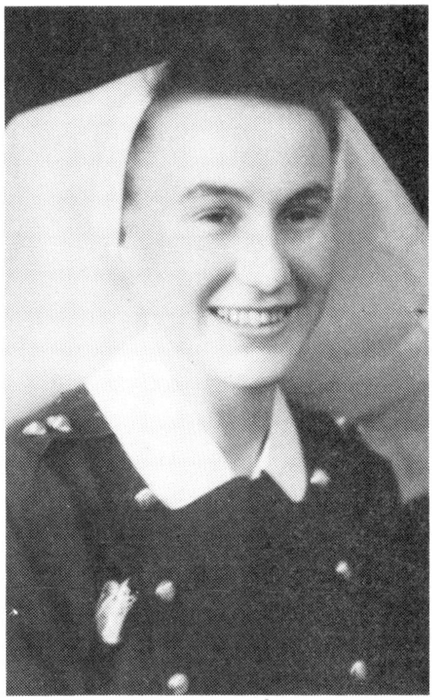

Lieutenant N/S Bee (Helen) (MacPherson) Rodin.

I was anxious to nurse in war conditions. I was too young for the Canadian military but eligible for South Africa so in December 1941 I joined the South Africa Military Nursing Service.

My first duty assignments were at the South African hospital at Roberts Heights and at Ladysmith. I next was stationed at No. 106 South African Hospital at Quassin and Tripoli, furthest out in the desert, then at No. 5 at Helmiah. From there, I was assigned to No. 108 in Italy, starting in Florence then Orvietto, Bologna and Milan.

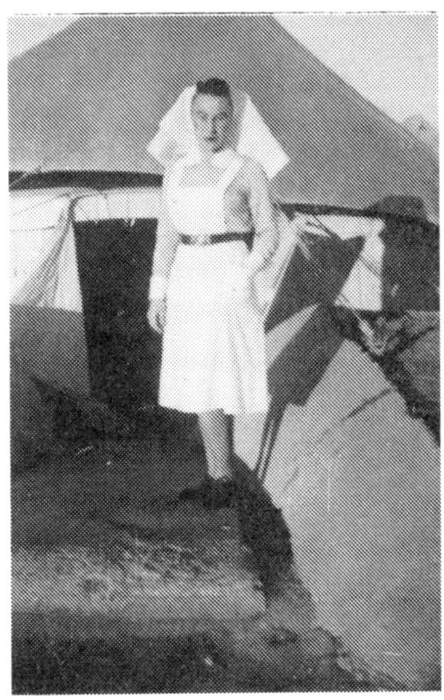

N/S Bee MacPherson, tented ward at Quassiv.

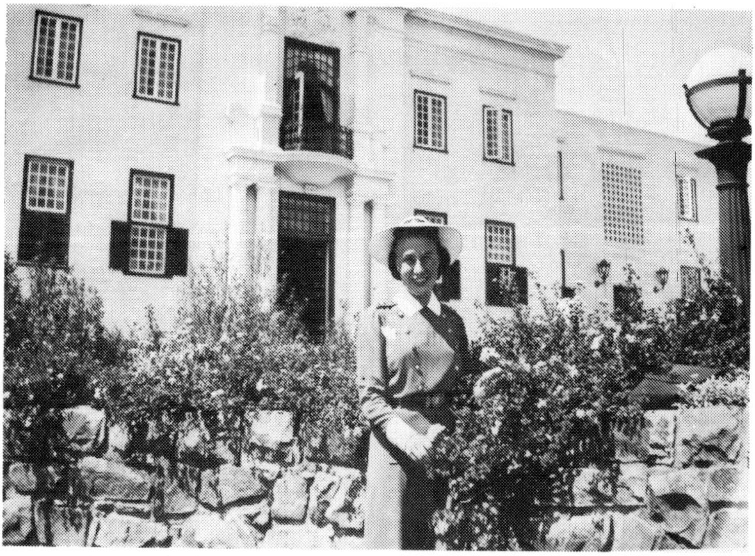

Bee MacPherson visiting General Smuts Pretoria home.

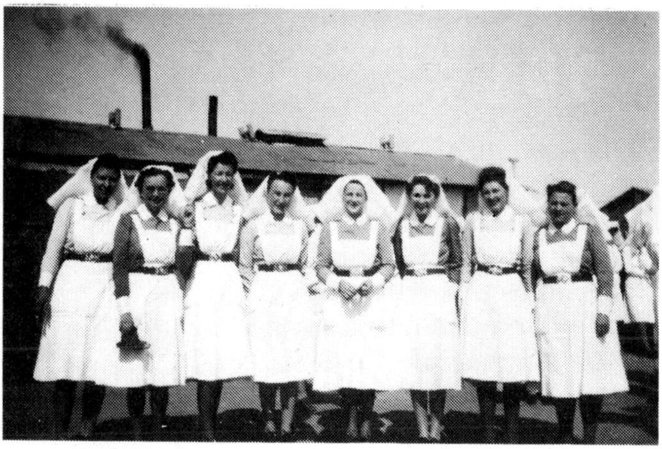

The Canadian sisters back at No. 106 just before breaking up: L-R: Cal Lewis; Muriel Ahier; Margaret Wastle Birnie; Gar Bradshaw; Mildred Wright; Phil Hurrex; Ida White. Jean Wheeler took the picture.

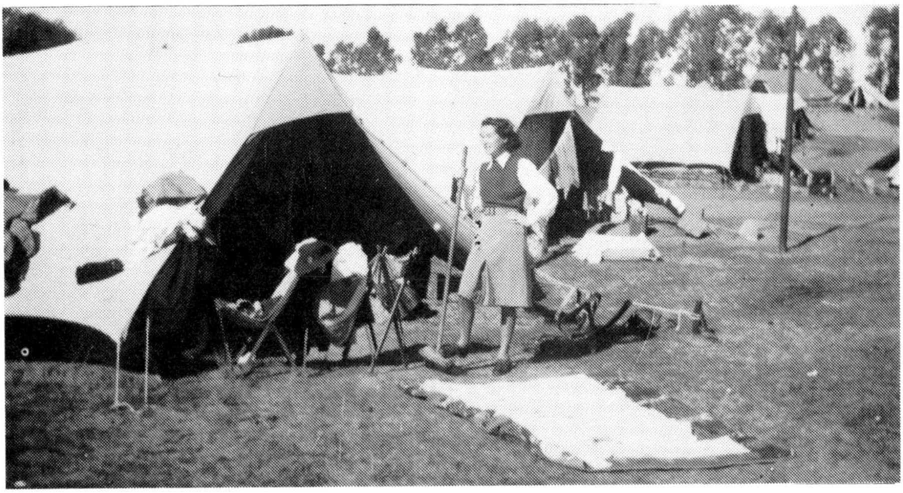

Our tents in Tripoli, N/S Bee MacPherson

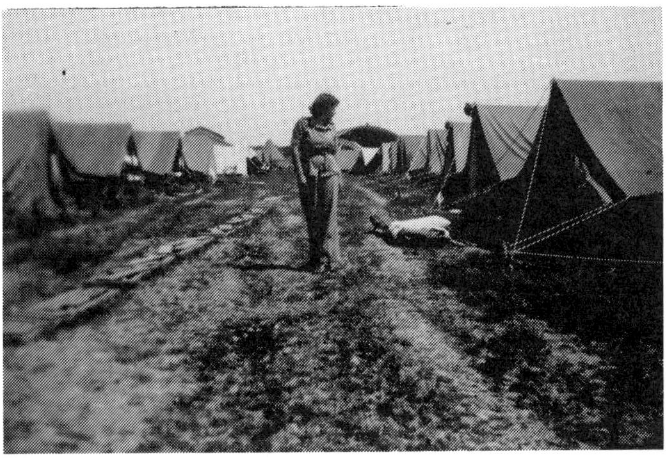

*Mud in Bologna; our tents. The hospital itself looked as though the circus had come to town.
Big tent tops - though a little more orderly arrangement.*

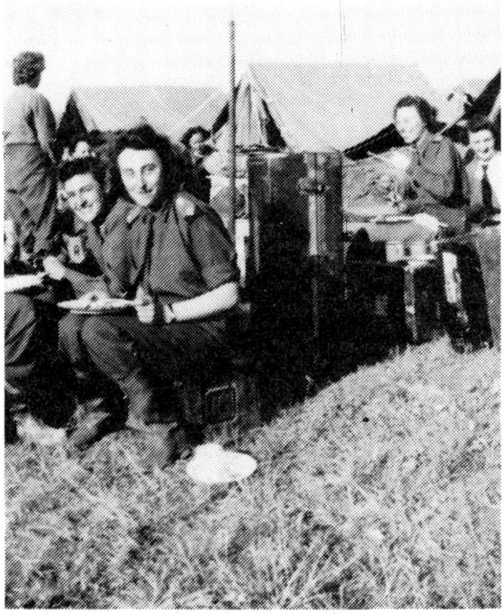

On the move again. Breakfast.

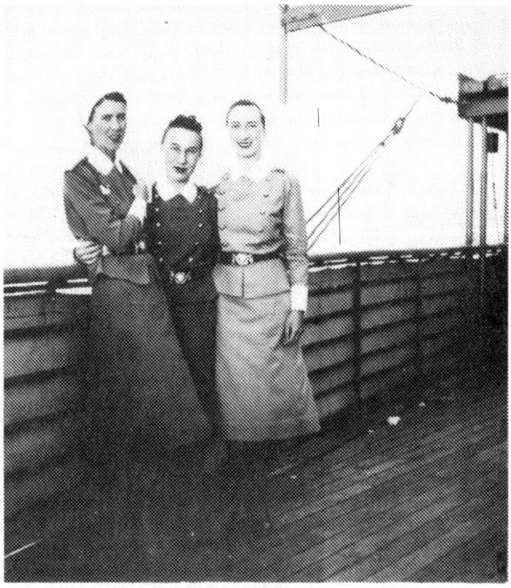

On board the "El Nil" : Frances Dopson Wilkie; Bee MacPherson Rodin; Nancy Islip Stent.

Germaine Strong (Quilichini) Schoneck

Graduated from: General Hospital School of Nursing, Edmonton, Alberta. Year: 1932

Military History:

Service: SAMNS

Rank: Lt. N/S

Served: November 1941 to July 1943

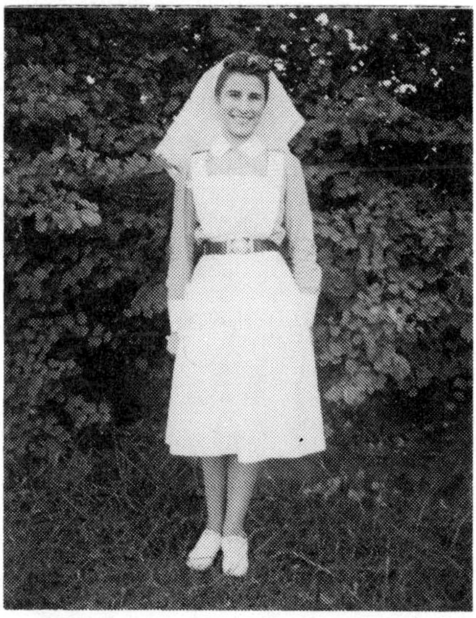

Germaine (Quilchini) Strong Schonek Barberton Military Hospital in an outlying area of the Transvaal, 1942 Our work uniform. Coming off duty

When there was a call for nurses to serve overseas I wanted to do my duty and nurse the wounded, but I was terrified at crossing the ocean because I could not swim! I thought about it for a few months and decided that if I was supposed to drown, it would be God's will and I would drown here anyway – in the river or lake.

So early in 1940 I made up my mind to put my name down for service anywhere in the world, and in 1941 I volunteered to go to South Africa. From then on I never worried about drowning, even when we were being chased by German subs.

I arrived in Capetown on Boxing Day, 26 December 1941 with the first group of Canadian nursing sisters. Soon afterwards we went to Durban where we were given postings to various military hospitals. With a group of friends, I went to the Roberts Heights Military Hospital in Pretoria.

Early in January 1942 we were assigned to various wards. I happened to look in a ward we were passing and a voice called, *"Come in!"* – which I did. This was my first contact with a war casualty – a flying officer in the South African Air Force, Fighter Squadron. He was in a body cast which concealed his many fractures and the bandages on his head covered his entire face with the missing teeth, except for the blue eyes which looked at me intently. Nice eyes. His name was Peter Strong and he insisted that I promised to come and see him again. As I went out, I remembered that once someone had said, *"If you like a man's eyes, you will marry him."* Well, I thought to myself, *"Not that wreck!"*

A few days later I was posted to the Barberton Military Hospital in an outlying area of the Transvaal. There we nursed a great many patients suffering from acute malaria, causing frequent attacks of chills and very high fever, with many times severe complications such as anemia, etc. But I remember that during one month, out of a thousand very sick patients, we lost only one. Barberton was also the camp hospital where all the casualties from Abyssinia (Ethiopia) and the Middle East were brought on their way to different military hospitals in the Union of South Africa.

Then, before long, I was so unlucky as to get cerebral malaria. Although I was very ill, I recovered to return to nursing in a month's time. After this, I was posted back to Roberts Heights Hospital and assigned to a surgical ward where all the patients were war casualties; young men with a variety of wounds. We were very short staffed; short of doctors as well. We had the responsibility of doing major dressings and performing duties such as taking out stitches, ordering quinine or other medications as indicated. We were extremely busy working long hours – more than twelve. By the end of the day I was exhausted – too tired to eat! I recall one patient who was so badly injured that he had been told by his doctor he had only one month or so to live. In spite of that, we did not give up on him and gave him as intensive care as possible. He recovered and sent me a dozen roses later when he went home.

Some of the other patients who come to mind: one critically wounded soldier who suffered a complication, pneumonia, for which nothing much could be done. Feeling that something should be tried when I came on duty on the night shift, I asked the sister who was on days if the doctor would mind me trying mustard plasters on the patient. She told me that the doctor did not expect this man to recover and would not object to this treatment. So I applied mustard plasters to his chest, back and feet which were ice-cold. By morning the patient seemed to be better as his circulation had improved. The day sisters and I continued this treatment and then, little by little, he got better. His wife, who remained in the room with him, later thanked me very sincerely, as she believed that the mustard plasters and the special care saved her husband's life.

Another one of my patients: a handsome young man, was very depressed, his injuries not being that serious but he was no doubt suffering from shock too. For days I worked on him every chance I got to make him smile into a mirror or even into space whether he felt like it or not. It took a while, but in time he began to feel better about himself and life. After he was discharged, I received some beautiful handkerchiefs (I still have one) from him and a note saying that he was happily married and never forgot what I told him – to remember to smile.

It gave me a good feeling knowing that I was of some help to those fine soldiers who fought for our freedom.

While nursing at Roberts Heights, I also discovered that my first-day acquaintance, Peter Strong, was still in an adjoining ward and he could see me as I walked by his room. (Some time later he told me that he had written to his parents in England to tell them that he had met the girl he was going to marry.) In 1940 he had been posted as a fighter pilot in the Middle East and while fighting in Abyssinia, crashed with such force that he had to be dug out from underground.

One day, while still wearing his cast but bandages off (he was handsome), Peter asked me if I would escort him to a hospital concert. Although I was very tired, I did. He could not sit down, so we just stood by the door. Another day he asked me to go to The Fountains, a restaurant in a lovely park, for lunch with him and we arranged to go the next day, July 1st, 1942. He was still on crutches with his leg in a cast. To my surprise he asked me to marry him. I was so stunned I couldn't answer him – and he said, *"I knew you would!"* The next day Peter brought me a beautiful diamond engagement ring which I accepted. We were married later that month and after our wedding in Durban, I continued on staff until July 1943.

During his two-year hospitalization, Peter developed osteomyelitis in his leg and arm. He could never again bend his right knee. As soon as he recovered, with his right leg in a caliper, he went right back to flying and then became an instructor until the end of the war.

After the war, my husband pioneered the air route over the Drakensburg Mountains and the first airmail Service to Basutoland (now Lesotho). He was known by the natives and people in South Africa as, "The White Bird Man." Peter and I enjoyed life in South Africa where our four children were born. After twelve and a half years there, we decided to bring our family to Canada and settled in Edmonton, Alberta. I did not earn any special medal for my service with the SAMNS, but I was greatly rewarded – I brought home a hero!

Florence (Merlin) Shearer

Graduated from: Halifax Infirmary School of Nursing. Year: 1940

Military History:

Service: SAMNS

Rank: Lt. N/S

Served: 1941 to 30 December 1942

It was difficult to get into the Canadian Army so when I heard of the requests for duty in the SAMNS, I responded. Our group had nurses from every province in Canada.

The only fear we had was that the sister ship of the SS *Kawsar* had been sunk in the Atlantic.

However, we arrived in one piece in spite of the Cape Rollers!

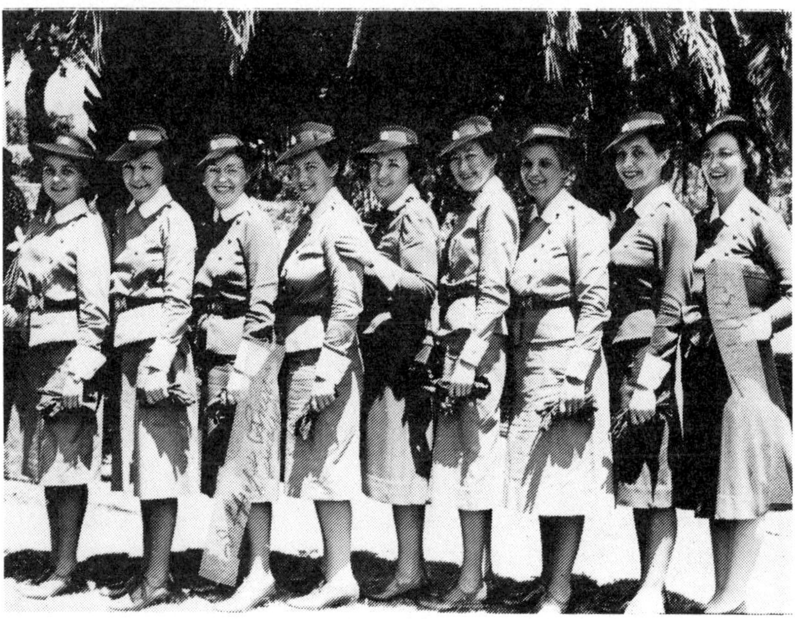

Canadian nurses on loan to South African Army, the group represents nine provinces of Canada and was taken at Mayor James luncheon for us in Capetown on arrival. L-R: Marguerite Cusson - Nanaimo, BC; A. Green - Prince Edward Island; D.I. Hayes - Quebec; Ethel Butler- Nova Scotia; Elizabeth Lovegrave-Ontario; Margaret Goldsmith - NB; Margaret Waugh - Manitoba; Kathleen Fiesel - Saskatchewan; Jean McIntosh - Alberta

M. Jean Snelgrove

Graduated from: Prince Edward County Hospital School of Nursing, Picton, Ontario. Year: 1940

Military History:

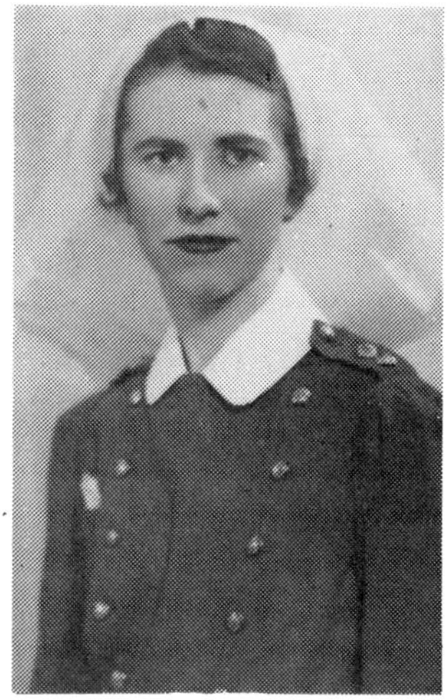

N/S Jean Snelgrove

Service: SAMNS and Royal Canadian Army Corps

Rank: Lt. N/S

Served: April 1942 to February 1944: SAMNS
February 1944 to May 1946: RCAMC

One of the highlights of my military career included a three-week stint in the service of the British Navy. Lt. N/S Alice Coneybeare (nee Robertson, now deceased) and I had applied for permission to return to Canada after one and a half year's service in South Africa. We were given the opportunity to return home via England on a British hospital ship, caring for two VAD English nurses who had become ill in South Africa.

On arrival in England we were met by a Canadian Army vehicle and taken to the Canadian Red Cross nursing sisters' club in London. We were somewhat financially embarrassed at this point as we were unable to collect our pay when leaving the ship. Consequently, we began to make the rounds of the war offices. First we went to the South African office where we were told they were no longer responsible for us. Next to the Canadian headquarters where we tried to enlist on the RCAMC but were told we must return to Canada first and re-enlist at home. We were feeling rather bereft at this point but pressed on to the offices of the British Admiralty where the personnel were absolutely splendid. We were given a sympathetic ear and partial payment for our services on the hospital ship. The balance came after we arrived home.

Even though this terminated the Navy's responsibility for us, they arranged our return to Canada and we sailed two weeks later on a little passenger ship, the SS *Bayano*. We were never really sure just which country was actually responsible for us. We were two Canadian nurses in Canadian uniform of the RCAMC. We had left home to serve with the SAMNS, left South Africa with the British Navy and home from England on a small passenger ship where we were the only two military personnel on board!

All in all, a most memorable experience and certainly unique compared with my other wartime nursing sisters. I wouldn't have missed it for the world!

Anne (Guthrie) Thomas

Graduated from: University of Alberta Faculty of Nursing, Edmonton. Year: 1932

Military History:

Service: SAMNS

Rank: N/S - Captain

Served: 1941 to 1946

No one thing influenced me to join the Service, but as a trained nurse, I had a strong desire to "join up."

I was on a visit to South Africa when war was declared. There was no shipping to get me home, so I joined the SAMNS.

My first posting was with a CCS (Casualty Clearing Station) to Kenya, where our duties were mostly nursing patients with tropical diseases. It was no great hardship to be there in the Highlands of Kenya; beautiful country, beautiful climate. It was peaceful there, in spite of war to the north.

From Kenya I went to what was then Italian Somaliland, to Mogadishu. The country had just been taken over from the Italians by Allied Forces. Food was scarce – the population was hungry and so were we until we began getting fresh food shipments from Nairobi.

After several months we went back to Kenya for a short time before being loaded onto a hospital ship to go to Egypt. We had quite a large hospital on the Canal zone – wards in Nissen huts and we lived in tents.

After the Germans were defeated in N. Africa and the armies were moving to Italy, we were moved to Tripoli in readiness to take casualties from Italy. And take casualties we did. After several months we went back to Egypt. At this time I had completed four years in N. Africa so I was sent south. I worked in the Voortrekkerhoogte (ex Roberts Heights) Military Hospital outside of Pretoria for a few months until I was released from the SAMNS.

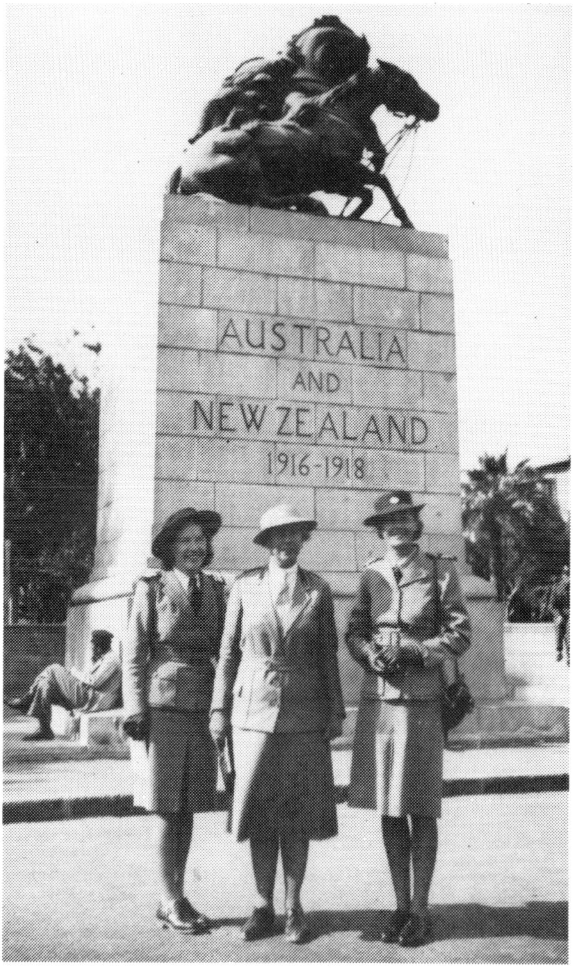

L-R: Captain Anne (Guthrie) Thomas at Port Said, the matron of the British Hospital I was seconded to at the time, and one of the South African nursing sisters

Margaret (Henderson) Watson

Graduate from: Fisher Memorial Hospital School of Nursing, Woodstock, New Brunswick. Year: 1941

Military History:

Service: SAMNS.

Rank: Lieutenant N/S

Served: December 1943 to May 1946

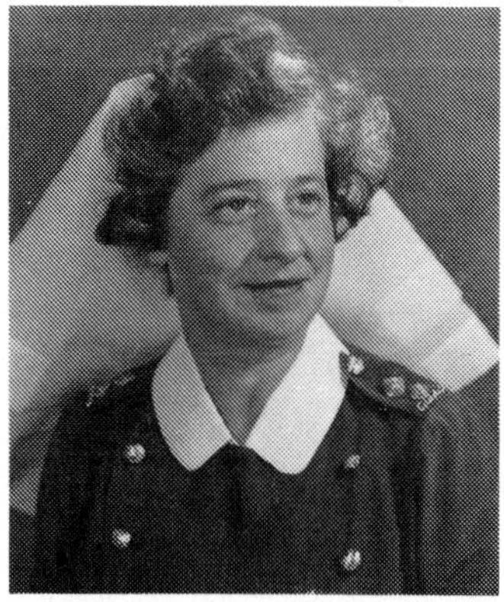

N/S Margaret Henderson

The world was at war. Everyone was going into the service, so I wanted to go too! I chose the SAMNS.

I truly enjoyed the city of Johannesburg, South Africa, the beautiful countryside and flowers and beautiful friends.

I met my husband, Major G. Robert Watson, of Ottawa, at a dance in Halifax when we returned to Canada. Bob was in charge of all war brides arriving in Canada. He had to see that they arrived at their destinations safely.

My time in the service was lots of fun; I have wonderful memories.

Frances E. (Dopson) Wilkie

Graduated from: St. Joseph's Hospital School of Nursing, Victoria, B.C. Year: 1934

Military History:

Service: SAMNS and RCAMC

Rank: 1st Lt., promoted to Captain in South Africa

The War – the excitement, being where the action was, being in the service – all of this was important to me. I would not have missed it.

My first military experience was with the SAMNS. I recall

with great pleasure the tea in New York that American nurses gave for Canadians. We had never been together before. When we took our greatcoats off, none of the 80 nursing sisters had their names on their uniforms (yet)!

When I returned from South Africa I joined the RCAMC and went overseas with No. 22 Canadian General Hospital. One of the highlights for me was sitting out on a moonlight night, watching the buzz bombs go over.

Helen Marian Williams

Graduated from: St. Paul's Hospital School of Nursing, Vancouver, B.C. Year: 1936

Military History:

Service: SAMNS

Rank: Lt. N/S

Served: 21 April 1942 to 4 November 1945

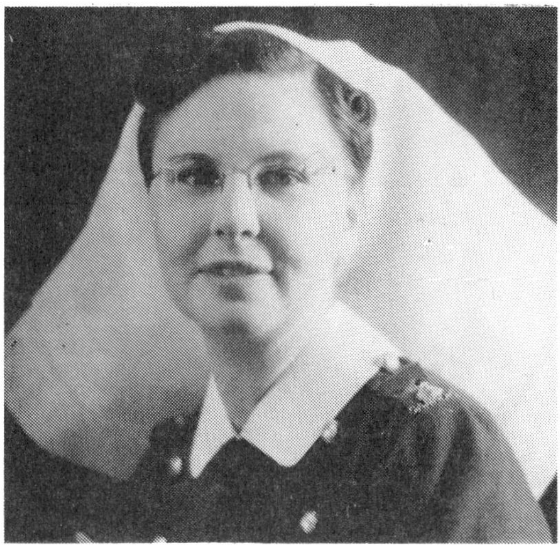

N/S Marian Williams

In wartime there was a need for nurses. I recall hearing on the radio that South Africa requested 300 Canadian nurses.

That, plus the fact that I had relatives in that country, influenced me to join SAMNS in 1942.

I was assigned to Roberts Heights Military Hospital in Pretoria for my first year in South Africa. The following two years were at Springfield Military Hospital in Durban. Our patients were members of the Army, Navy and Air Force including men training under the Air Commonwealth Training Plan and from war zones in North Africa and later Italy.

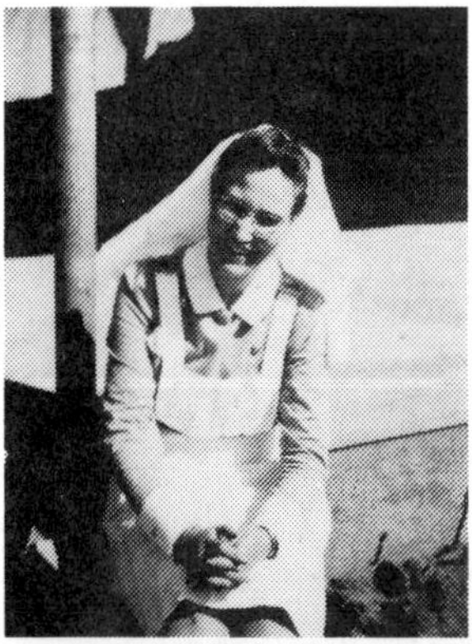

Lt. N/S Jean (McIntosh) Elleker, Petermaritzberg, South Africa Oribi Military Hospital

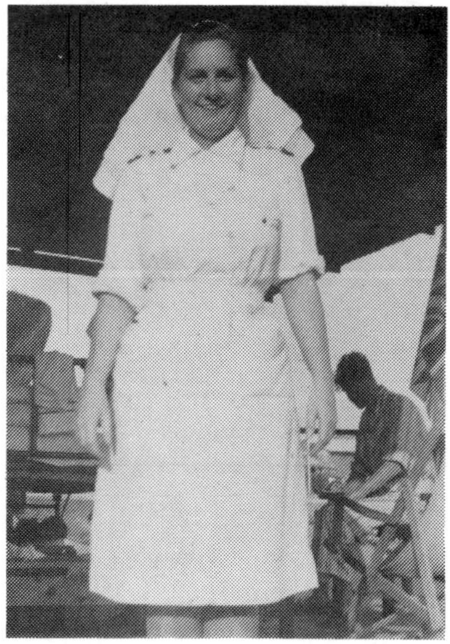

South African nursing sister

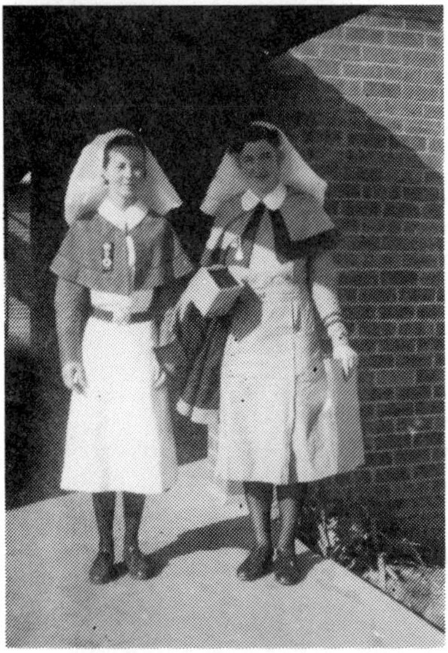

Nursing sisters Tiny Croger, British Navy, McDonald, British Army. Canadian nurses worked with British Army and Navy at Petermaritzberg, South Africa

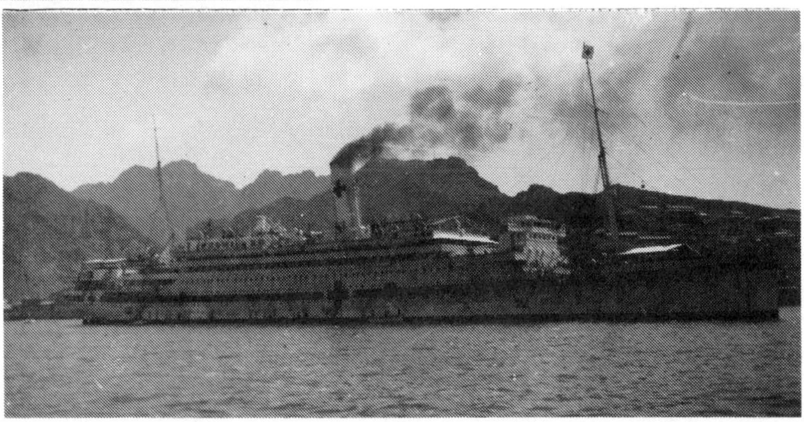

British Hospital Ship Atlantis; brought wounded from Lybia through Durban 1941 to 1945, from Durban the wounded came by train to Petermaritzberg, South Africa

Chapter 9

COLLECTION OF PHOTOGRAPHS

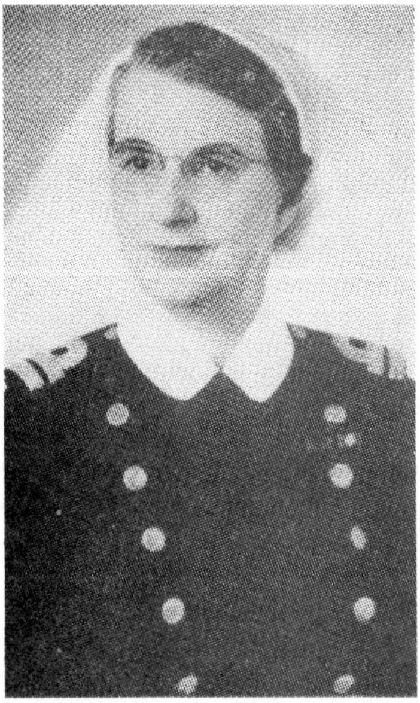

Mrs. Evelyn Stibbard, Matron in two Naval hospitals

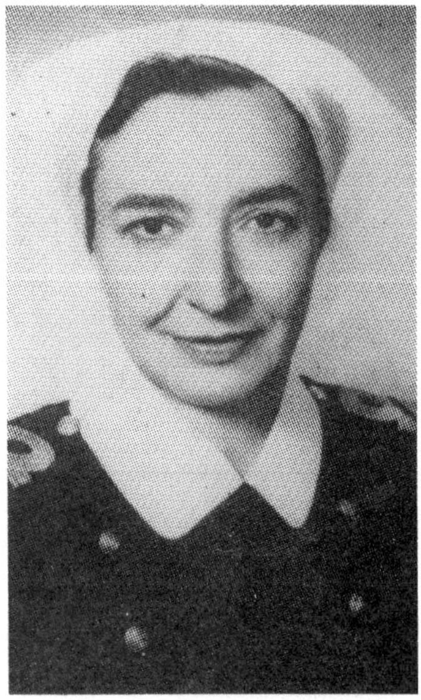

Mrs. R.D. Millar (Ellen Cameron) Matron in Naval hospitals

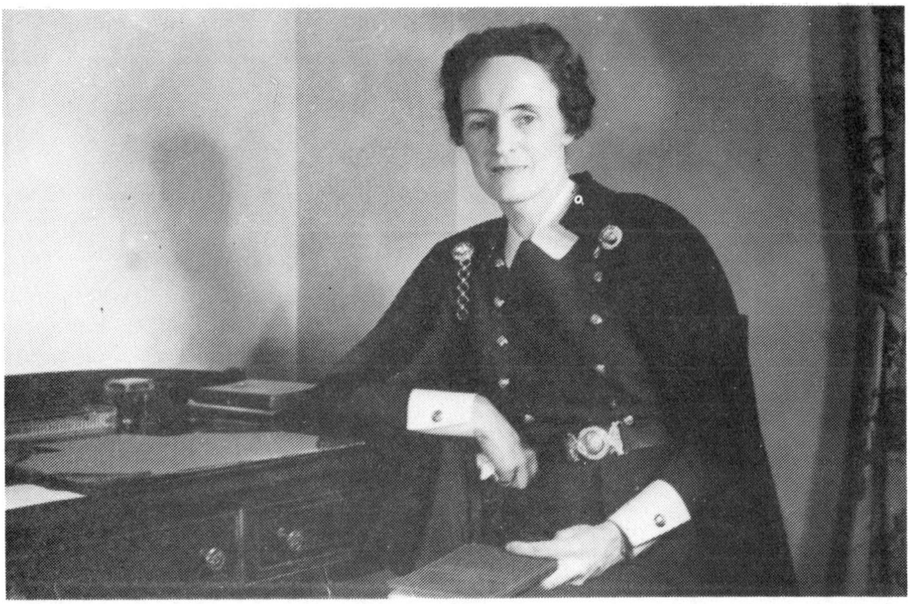

N/S Christine MacDonald, a graduate of Saskatoon General Hospital, matron in charge of the first contingent of nursing sisters to join the South African Military Nursing Service

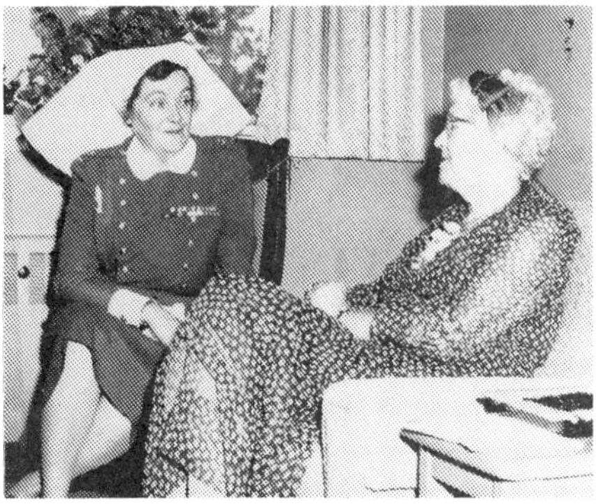

L: Major Margaret Dodderidge
R: Emma Pence, retired Matron-in-Chief, RCAMC

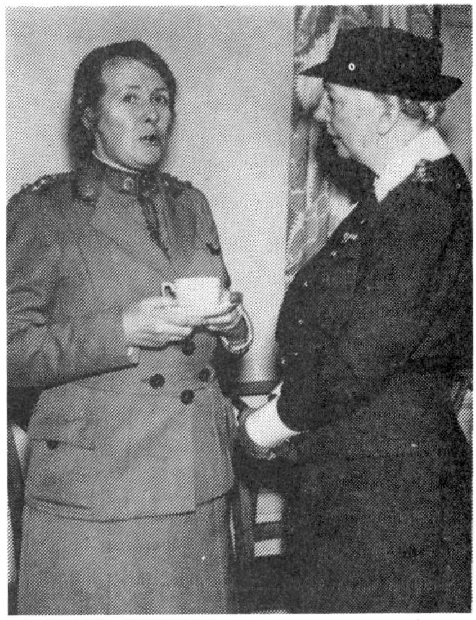

Right: Miss Elizabeth Smellie, Matron-in-Chief RCAMC with Dame Katharine Henrietta Jones, Matron-in-Chief of QAIMNS (now QARNC) at a reception in London given by Miss Agnes Neill 1943
Canadian Forces photo PMR75-224

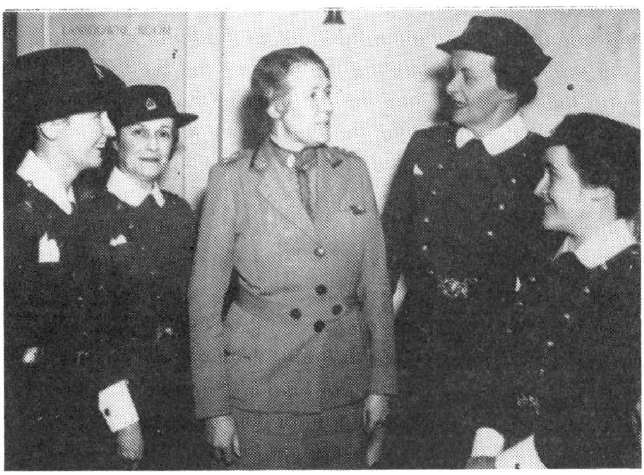

L-R: Principal Matron D.M. Riches of No. 8 CGH, attached to CMHQ of London; Principal Matron M.R. Shaffner of No. 15 CGH; Katharine Henrietta Jones, Matron-in-Chief of QAIMNS (now QARNC); Principal Matron A. Neill, CMHQ; Principal Matron Mary Minor (Mills) No. 16 CGH at a reception given in London by Miss Neill, 1943
Canadian Forces photo PMR 75-223

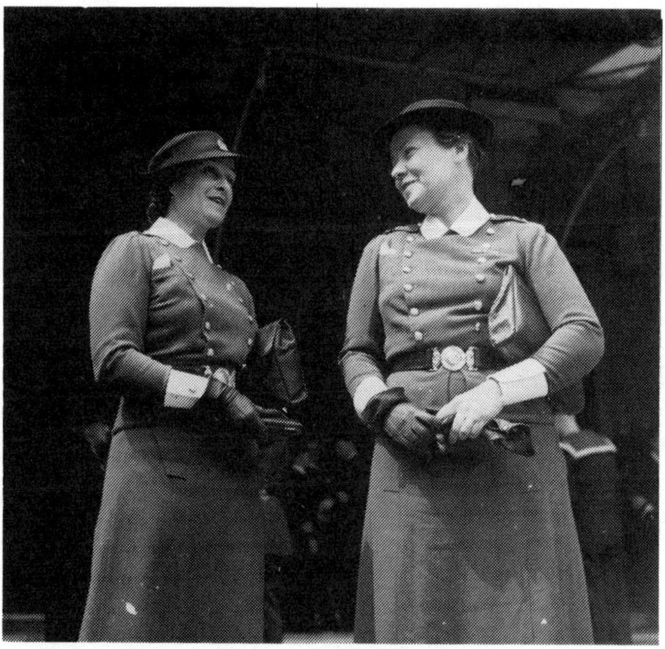

Majors M.R. Shaffner (left) and A.J. Macleod, Principal Matrons, RCAMC, after RRC investiture at Buckingham Palace, London, England, 1944. Canadian Forces photo, the National Archives of Canada 20526

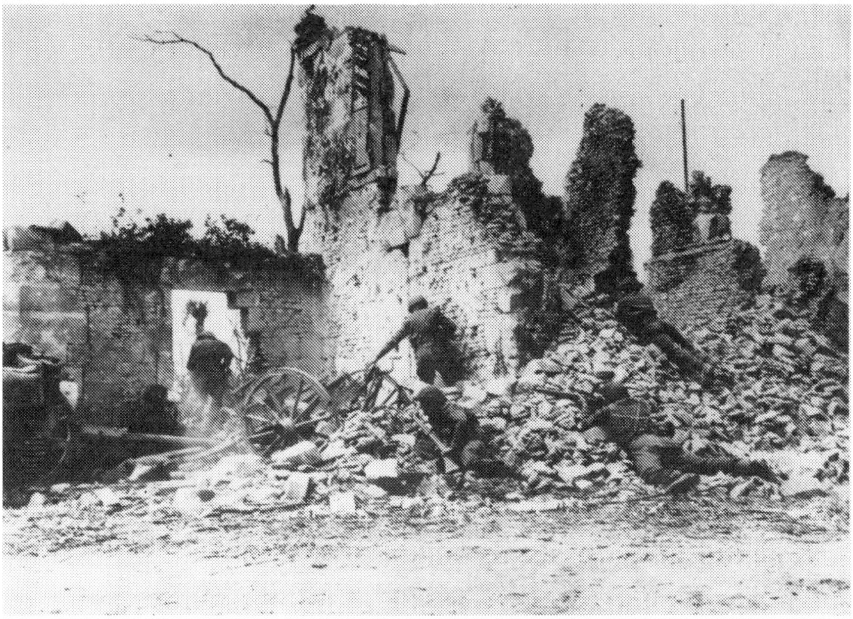

BATTLE FOR CAEN.
Photo shows: Looking for snipers in Le Bijude.
337150: British Newspaper Pool Photograph No. 337150. L.N. II

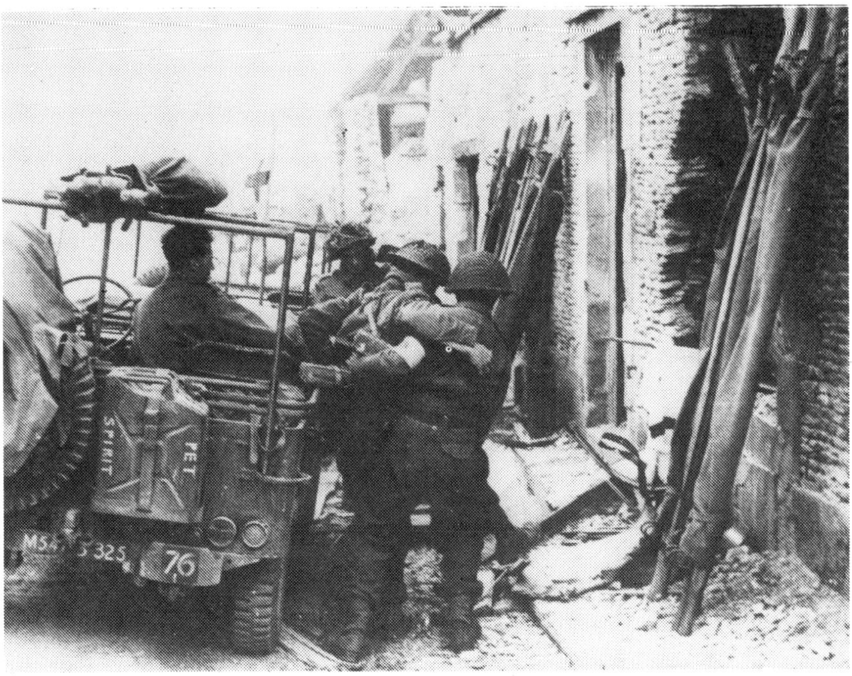

THE CAPTURE OF CAEN, July 9, 1944.
B 6740 XP: BRITISH OFFICIAL PHOTOGRAPH NO B 6740(XP)
War office Photograph-Crown Copyright Reserved.

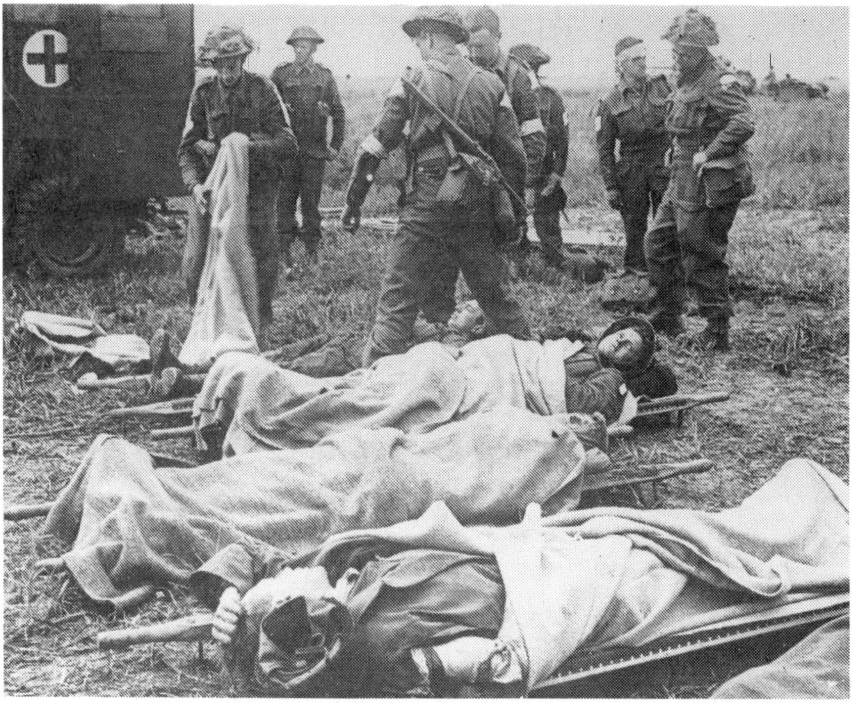

NORMANDY: THE BRITISH ADVANCE EAST OF TILLY (Issued June 1944) B 6005 (WPL) BRITISH OFFICIAL PHOTOGRAPH NO. B. 6005(WPL) Crown Copyright reserved.

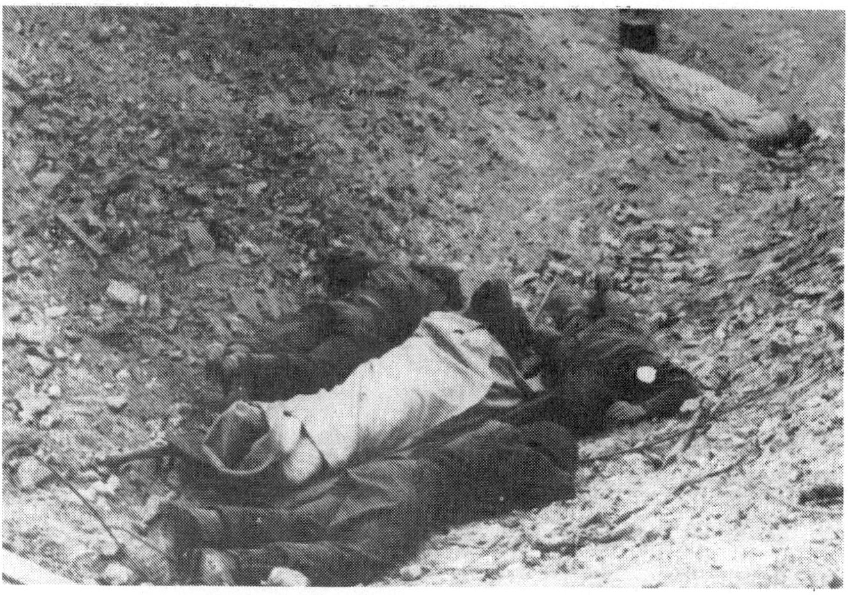

NORMANDY: SWIFT TREATMENT AND EVACUATION OF WOUNDED. B 6825: British Official Photograph No. 6825 (XF) War Office Photograph - Crown Copyright Reserved

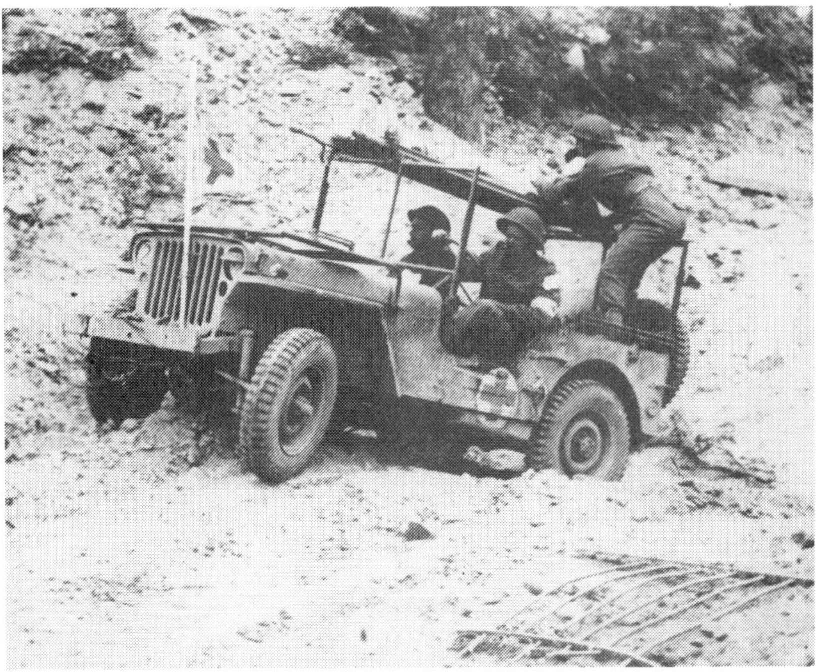

NORMANDY: SWIFT TREATMENT AND EVACUATION OF WOUNDED issued August 1944. B 6827: BRITISH OFFICIAL PHOTOGRAPH NO. B 6827. (XP - C) War Office Photograph Crown Copyright Reserved.

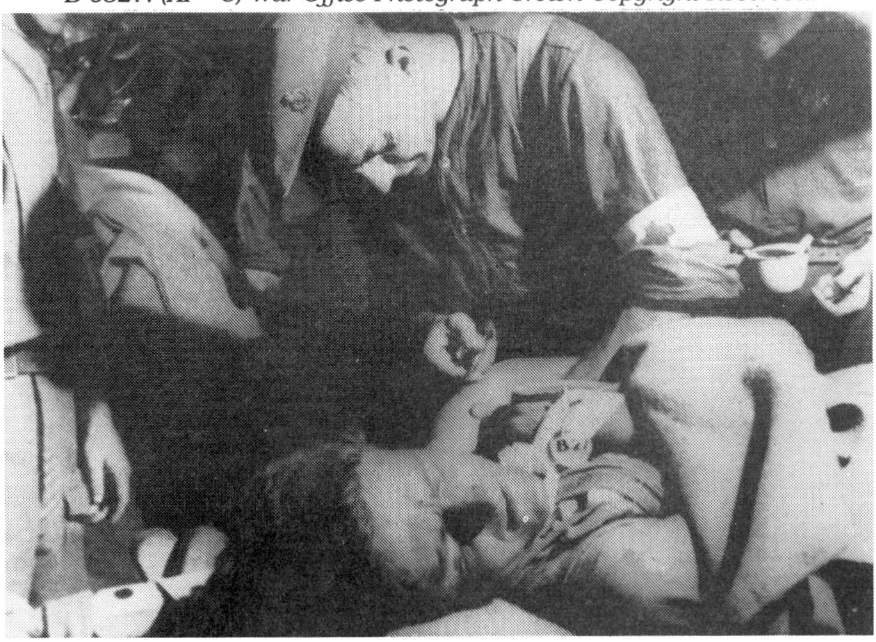

B 6843 XP: War Office Photograph Crown Copyright Reserved. NORMANDY: SWIFT TREATMENT AND EVACUATION OF WOUNDED. B 6843 XP: War Office Photograph Crown Copyright Reserved.

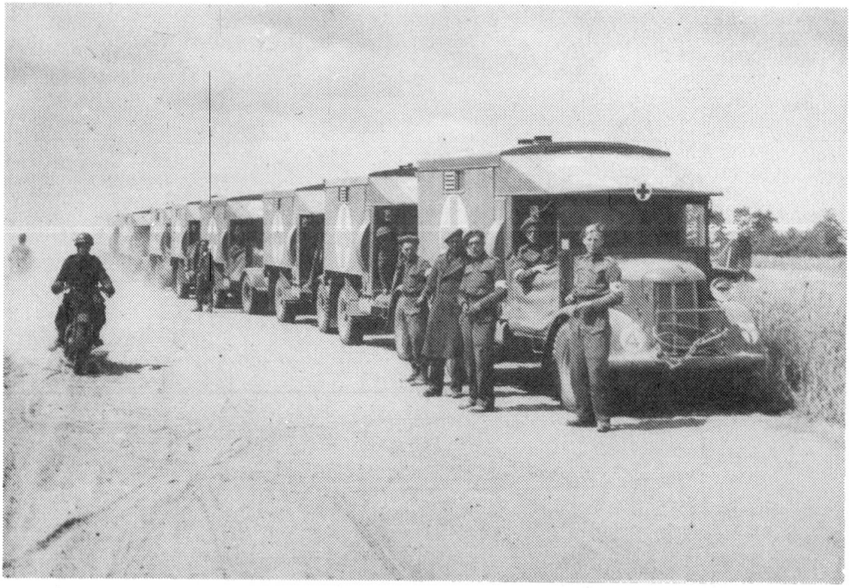

LIBERATION OF EUROPE: AIR AMBULANCES FLY WOUNDED FROM FRANCE TO ENGLAND. CL 170 WA: BRITISH OFFICIAL PHOTO.CL 170 WA. CROWN COPYRIGHT RESERVED. 18644.ER. CL 170 WA.

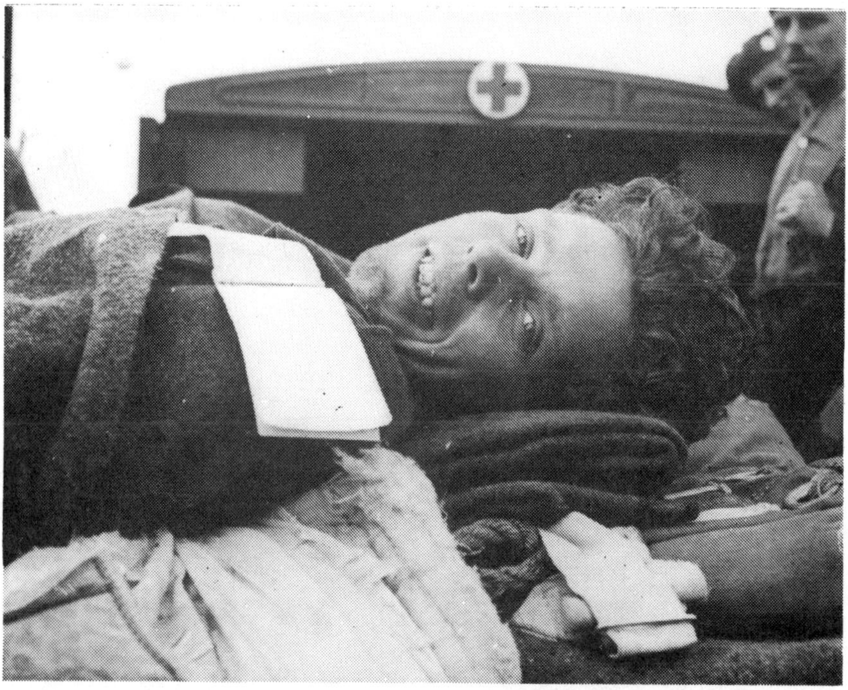

Issued July 1944. LIBERATION OF EUROPE: WHEN THE WOUNDED ARRIVE BACK HOME. BH 23818 XC: BRITISH OFFICIAL PHOTOGRAPH NO BH 23818 XC. War Offfice Photo-crown copyright reserved.

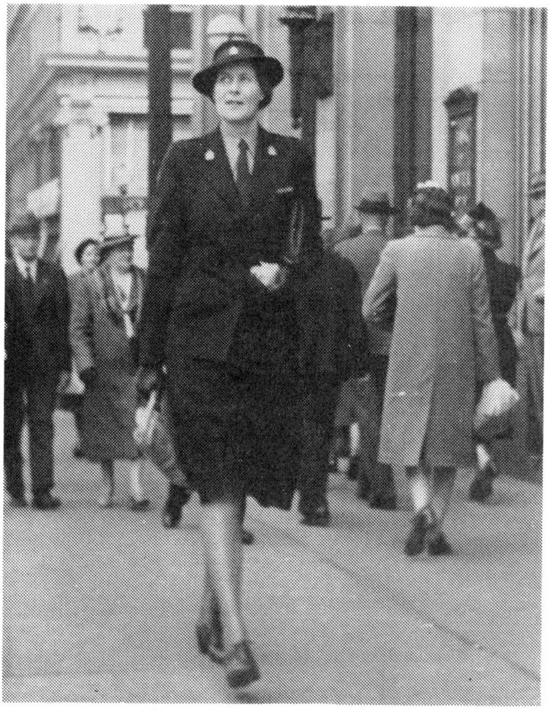

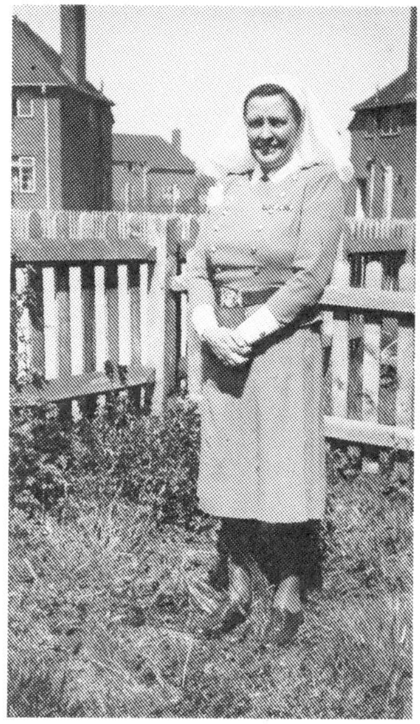

Matron Mima McLaren, 1944, No. 8CGH

*Matron Edna Rossiter served overseas as matron of Nos. 24 and 12 Canadian General Hospitals. Post war she was appointed as nursing consultant for the western region and later became director of nursing at Shaughnessy Hospital, Vancouver. Her earlier work in organizing military hospitals in British Columbia when she was Principal Matron Pacific Command brought her the award of the Royal Red Cross in January 1944.**

**Canada's Nursing Sister's, G.W.L. Nicholson, p 211*

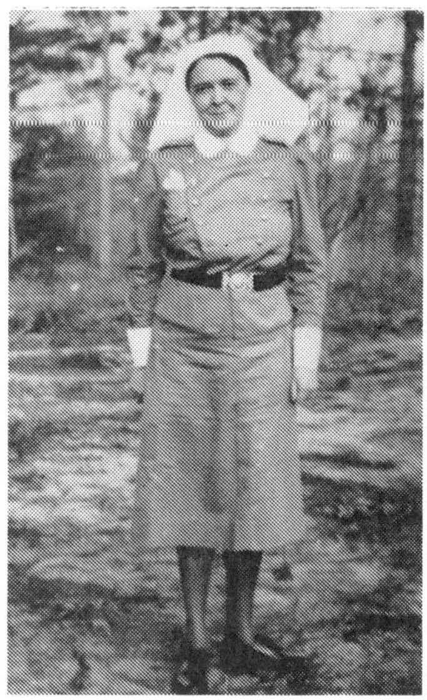

N/S Dorothy Percy Camp Borden Military Hospital 1941

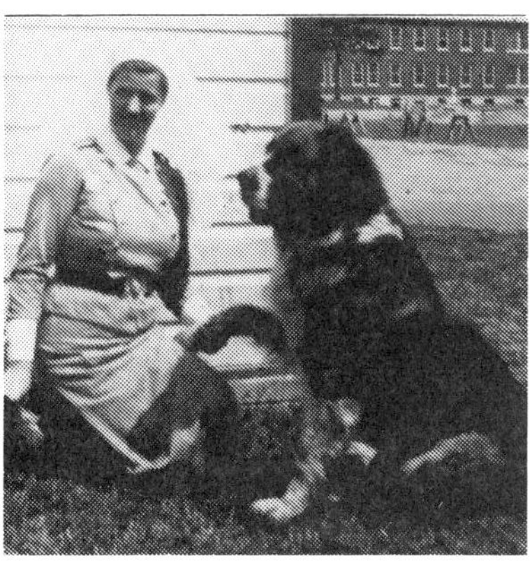

Camp Borden Military Hospital 1941
N/S Gladys Sharpe and Duke
Canadian Forces photo PMR228

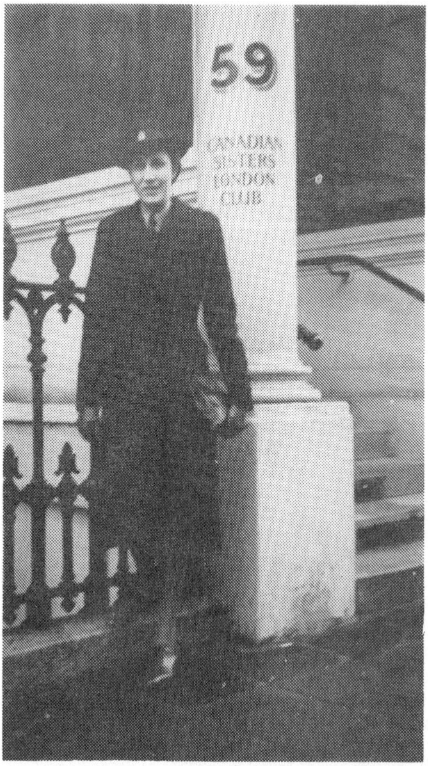

N/S Club, London 1943,
Lt.N/S Helen Bright

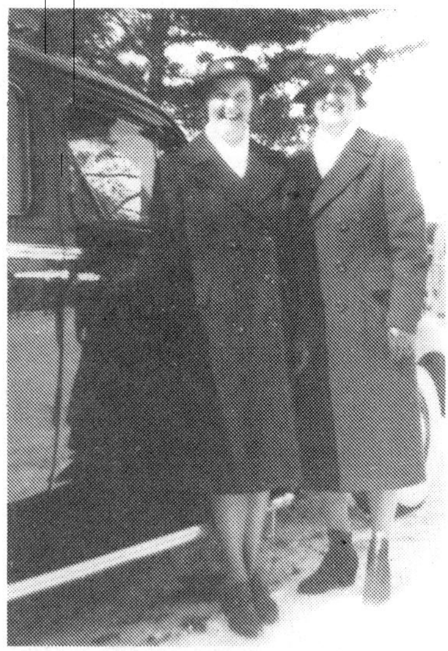

Camp Borden Military Hospital
1941 L: Gladys Sharpe
R: Blanche Herman
Canadian Forces photo
PMR75-226

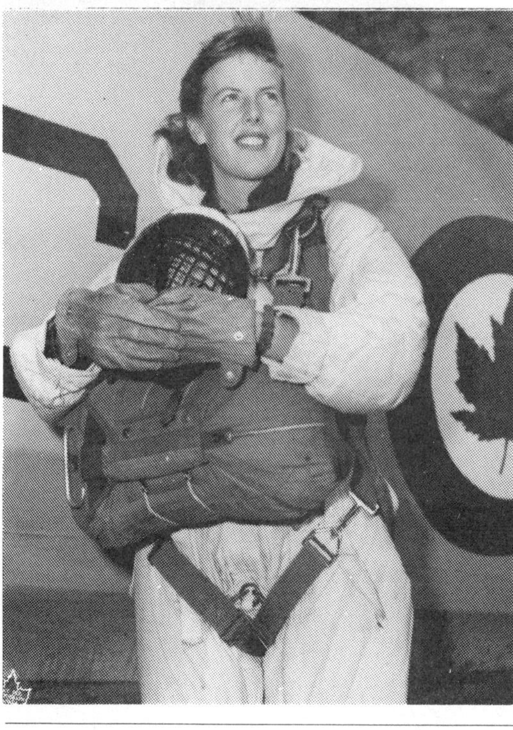

P/O Marion MacDonald,
RCAF rescue team
Canadian Forces photo
PL-52586

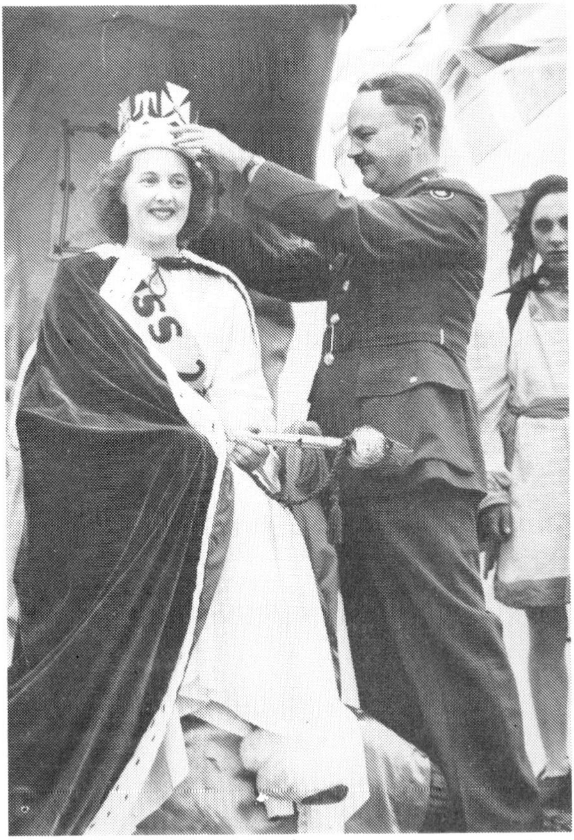

Lt. N/S I.G. Knight being crowned Queen of No. 24 CGH on their birthday Canadian Forces photo 55202

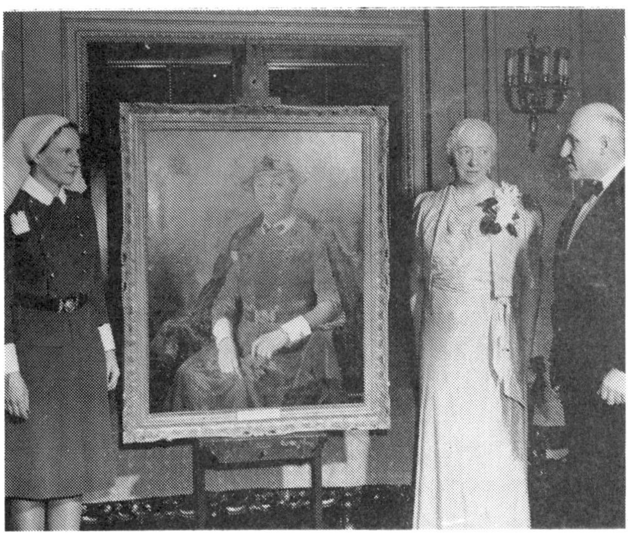

Unveiling of portrait of Colonel Elizabeth Smellie, Ottawa, ARTIST: Ford L-R: Colonel D.I. (MacRae) Warner; Colonel Elizabeth Smellie, RCAMC, retired; Col. J.L. Ralston, Minister of National Defence, retired. Canadian Forces photo. Edna Rossiter donated this photo to Sheila (Rankin) Zerr, History of Nursing member,BC.

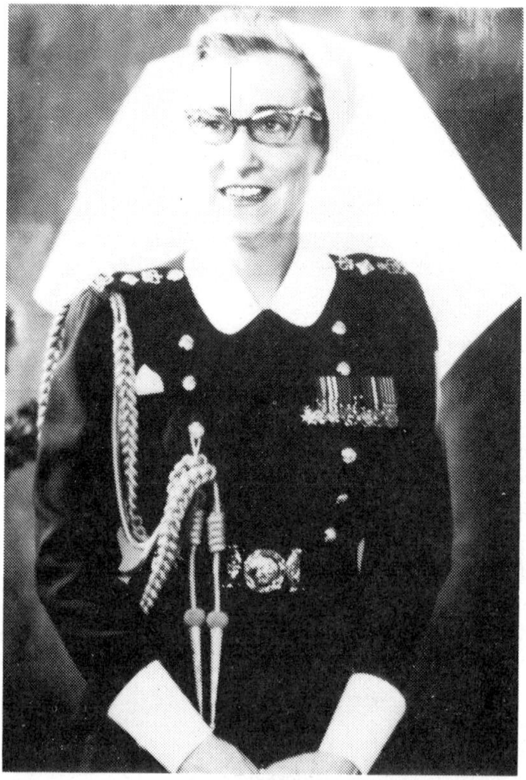

Lt.Colonel H.J.T. Sloan, Ottawa 1969 Matron-in-Chief CFMS 1964-1968

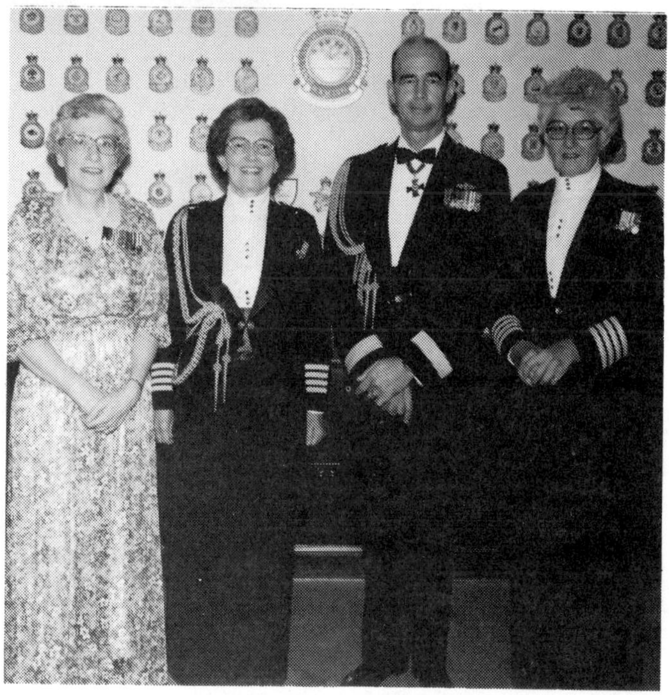

18 July 1980 Ottawa L - R: Lt.Colonel H. Sloan, retired; Colonel Helen Ott, Director Nursing Service; Surgeon General W. Leach; Colonel Jessie Lawson Director Nursing Service, retired. Canadian Forces photo

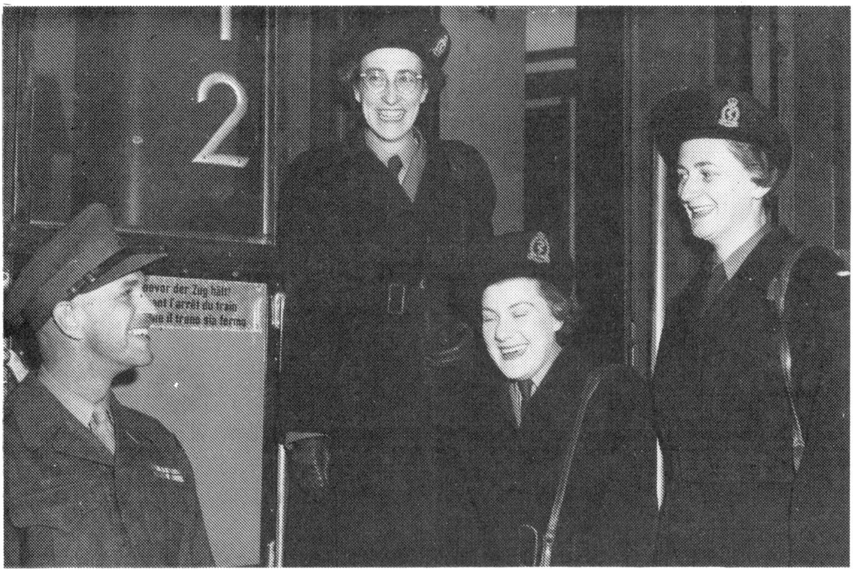

Arrival of first Canadians to join the British Military Hospital at Iserlohn as part of NATO. L - R: LTC J. Barr, CO, Capt. Matron Hallie Sloan, Lt. N/S Rita Roy and Lt. N/S Susanne Pelessier
Canadian Forces photo EF 3758

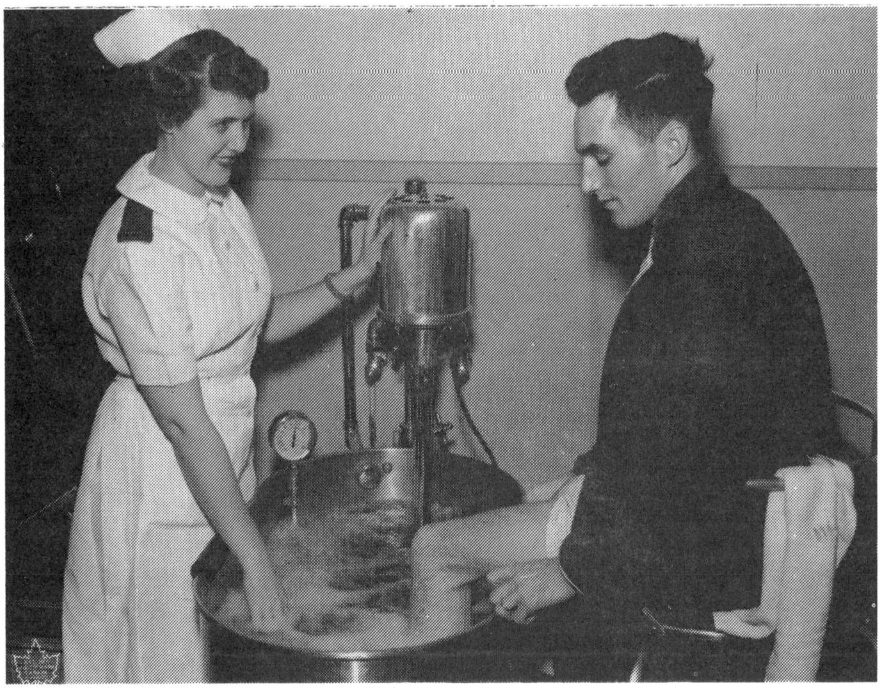

Flying Officer Dorothy Finch, of Toronto, a physiotherapy specialist supervises "Whirlpool Bath" being given to Sapper Harold Jones, of Newmarket, Ont. at Rockcliffe Hospital. Canadian Forces photo.

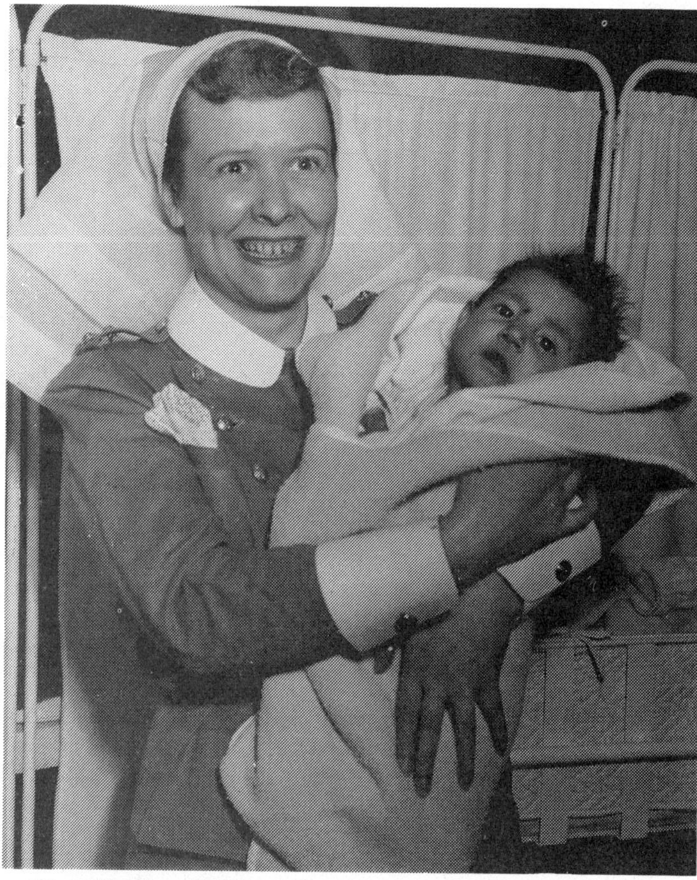

Lt. N/S Muriel (Clift) Hein with patient. Churchill Military Hospital. Canadian Forces photo PC-1606

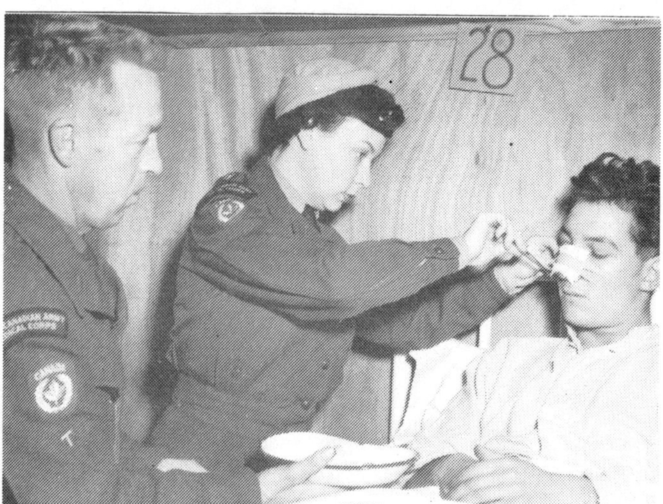

Changing a dressing in Korea 11 November 1953 N/S Marie Dunkerley Canadian Forces photo SF 8652

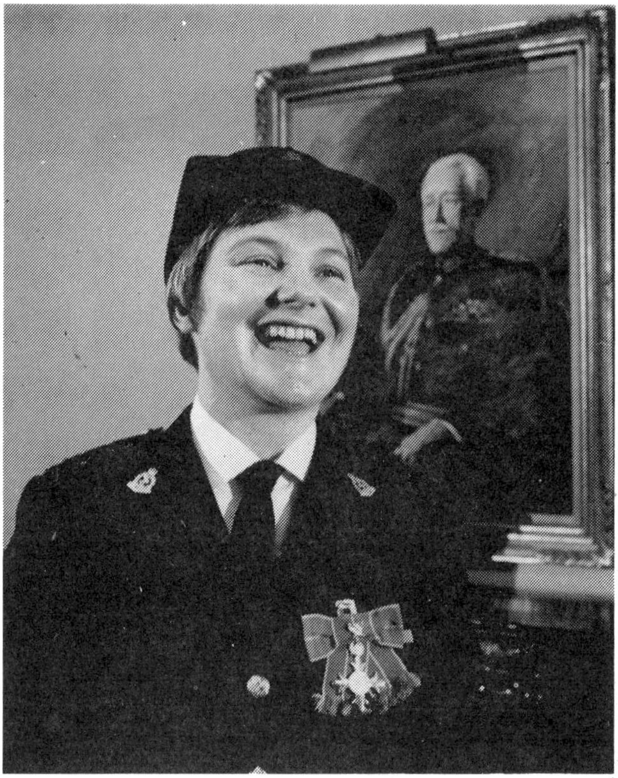

Captain Joan Cashin, MBE
Captain Joan Cashin having just been made a member of the Order of the British Empire for her heroic efforts at the scene of a crashed Czechoslovak aircraft at Gander Newfoundland in September 1967. N/S Cashin who was serving with No. 226 Aircraft Control and Warning Squadron, tended the injured at the scene and was credited with saving several lives.
Canadian Forces photograph PL- 53267 1967

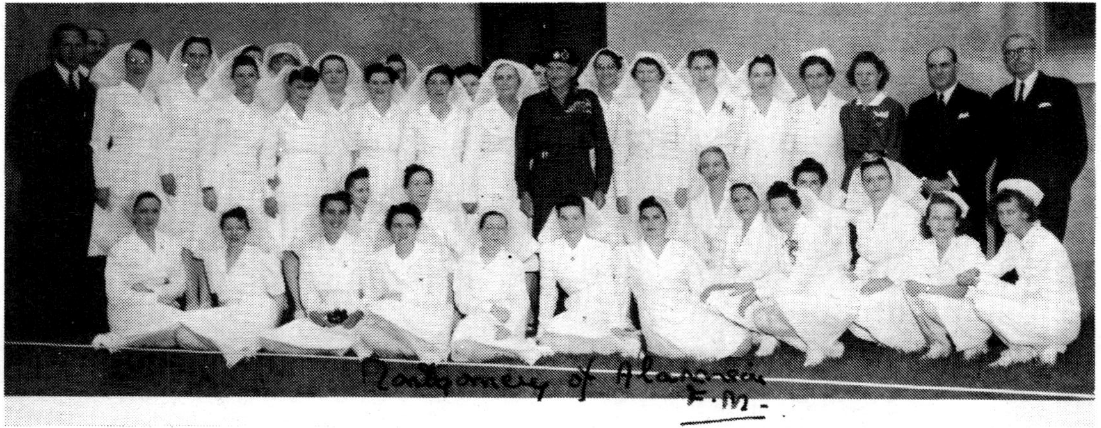

Field Marshall Montgomery visits Camp Hill Hospital, Halifax.
Miss S.C. MacIsaac, RRC, Matron, Camp Hill Hospital, 1946, on Field Marshall Montgomery's right
N/S L. Fitzgerald WWI, 7th from left in back row
Canadian Forces photo

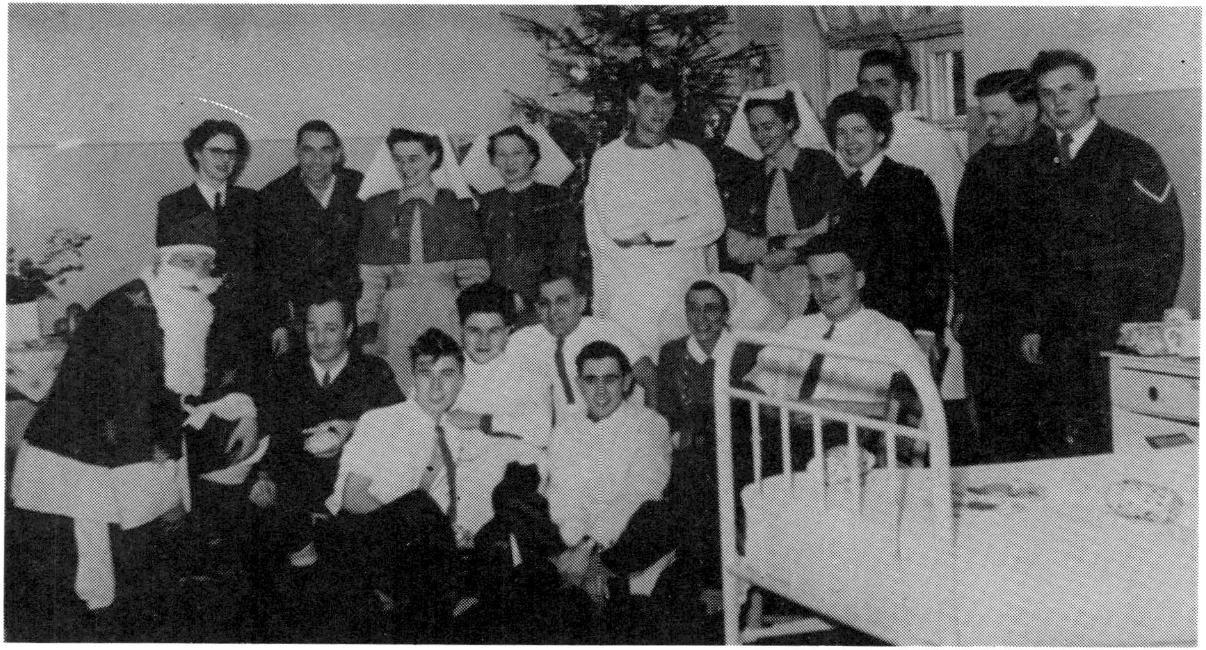

Christmas 1954 at British Military Hospital, Iserlohn, Germany. Lt. Nannette Isard in Queen Alexandra's Royal Army Nursing Corps uniform, first on right, Head Nurse, Surgical Ward; Major Edna Longridge, Centre, Deputy Matron, 2nd in charge; Capt. Hallie Sloan, Canadian Matron, seated, first nursing sister on right; with Santa Claus, patients, orderlies and others making the "rounds" Christmas Day. BMH was an SS barracks (German) during World War II. Very little was done to make it hospital like. It was cold, drab and very difficult to clean. NOTE: the bed mattress was three "biscuits" filled with straw. A large patient was difficult to nurse as the three parts separated. So the Canadian nursing sisters tied the sheet at top and bottom making a "fitted" sheet. This was 1954. The British Quartermaster was unhappy because the strain caused the sheets to tear and wear out. I will never forget working this Christmas Day. The wards were cold and uninviting, although efforts to improve the situation were made by the various head nurses. Loaned by Nina Rumen.

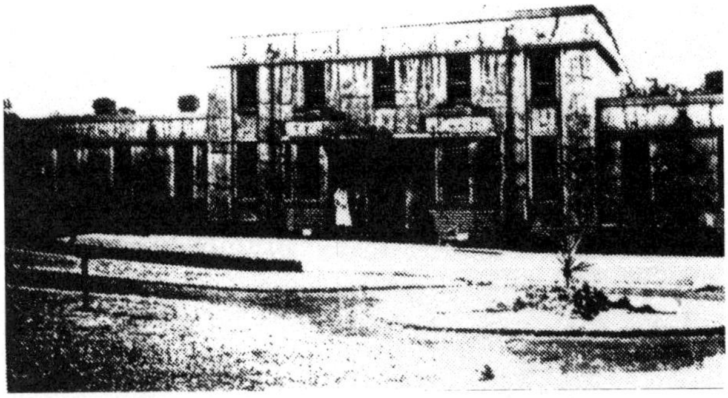

RCN Hospital, HMCS Niobe, Scotland
Loaned by Joan (Story) Giles

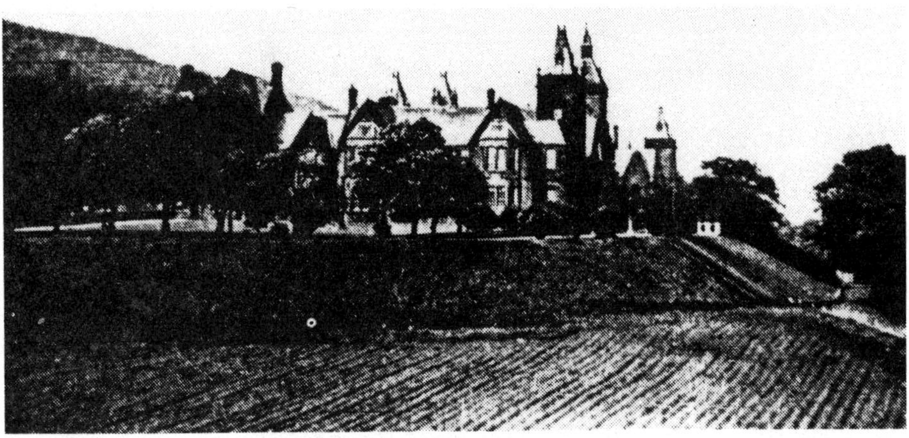

RCNH, HMCS Niobe, Scotland
Loaned by Joan (Story) Giles

Chapter 10

DIEPPE POEM

Irene Stephenson Mercier, No. 10 CGH has submitted this poem since her 1994 return to Dieppe

Dieppe Then and Now

by Irene Stephenson Mercier

The guns have long since been silenced,
The memory of battle has dimmed
The beach looks serene and inviting
Which once with gunfire was rimmed

The waves are lapping the shoreline
Which once encountered the dead
Where others lay mortally wounded,
And the waters ran rivers of red

The beach is still rocky and bouldered
Where tanks became mired and lost
The sea wall lies grey in the sunshine
Which was reached at such terrible cost

Ask why their commanders had sent them
To a battle they never could win.
Even the enemy wondered
Why our forces still kept coming in

Their fate was sealed in that moment
For they would see loved ones no more
And one choice they were given
To die on the water or shore

The seabirds are flying above me
They fly without fear overhead
The white clouds look soft and appealing
Like blankets to comfort the dead

The breezes blow softly and gently
My cheek is caressed by their breath
With no hint of the awful carnage
Of bloodshed, destruction and death

I feel that they know I am listening
To the sounds of that long ago day
And am seeing the boats overloaded
As they toss in the waves of the bay

I hear the noise of the battle
As it rages by night and by day
While before me the scene is quite peaceful
With laughter of children at play

History may always record it
As a battle that had to be
A prelude to others that were to come
Before the world could be free

They did not seek fame nor glory
They died so that we could be free
May the valour of men on that fateful day
Never fade from our mem—o—ry.

Chapter 11

SERVING WITH THE ROYAL CANADIAN ARMY MEDICAL CORPS IN CANADA AND NATO

Noreen Cambon
Jean (Wallace) Campbell
Louise Chausse
Mildred Cohoon
Betty (Chinn) Dewick
Luella Downing
Patricia (Ferris) Gill
Mary Hemphill
Jessie C. Larmon
Edith (Landells) Lees
Mary (Patton) Luco
Thelma (Horton) McLean
Edith (Kidd) O'Donoghue
Claire (Bourret) Phillips
Rita Mary (Hart) Santell
Helen Saunders
Lille (Tattrie) Sheehan
Muriel Joyce Sinclair

Noreen Cambon

Graduated from: Vancouver General Hospital School of Nursing, Vancouver, B.C.

Military History:

Service: RCAMC/CFMS

Rank: Major

Served: 1950 to 1968

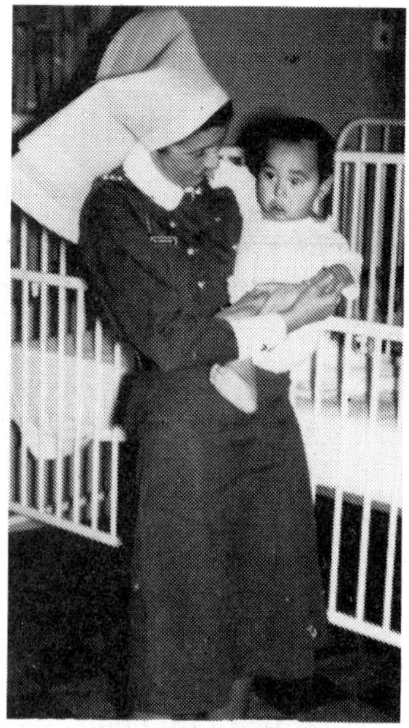

Churchill Military Hospital. Lt. N/S Noreen Cambon with patient

Having spent four wartime years in the RCAF (Women's Division) and then taking nursing at Vancouver General Hospital and immediately joining the RCAMC, one has to believe service life was my cup of tea.

I could tell many tales but shall pick an interesting incident from my posting to Fort Churchill, Manitoba, and to the British Military Hospital, Germany.

Fort Churchill was a very interesting posting. To be truthful, we nursed mostly Indians and Eskimos as the troops seemed very healthy.

There I met Farley Mowat in a bar downtown. I also visited a hermit (well educated but now a loner.) He did not seem to mind my occasional visit. One of the incidents I still remember with chills was being spotted by a polar bear. These beautiful beasts who travel very quickly are not friendly to people. Some of our buildings were connected by tunnels. We travelled through these tunnels but there were open patches between. Fortunately, I had a head start on my friend and reached the door safely. Polar bears are beautiful beasts but not for petting! I am thankful I did not become a polar bear snack.

BMH Iserlohn, Germany, was an interesting place to spend two years because we worked long hours but then had very generous time off to see Europe. We lived in what used to be quarters for Nazi troops. The quarters were nice but we were padlocked in at night and told it was to keep out the Polish guards. Being "free" Canadians, we all resented this and used to say what if there were a fire and we could not find a key?

My brother and sister-in-law were in London at the time taking their specialities, ENT and ophthalmology. One time I went to visit them and they took me to visit a doctor and his wife in a beautiful home. The doctor asked me what I thought of BMH Iserlohn. Naturally, I was very vocal about being padlocked in at night. On the train back to London Ken, my brother said, *"By the way, Noreen, you were talking to the head of the British Medical Service – a Brigadier General."* Two days later I arrived back at my base in Germany. I found the padlock had been removed! I always kept silent till now.

H. A. Jean (Wallace) Campbell

Graduated from: Regina General Hospital School of Nursing.
Year: 1942

Military History:

Service: RCAMC

Rank: Lt. N/S

Served: 2 April 1945 to 28 April 1946

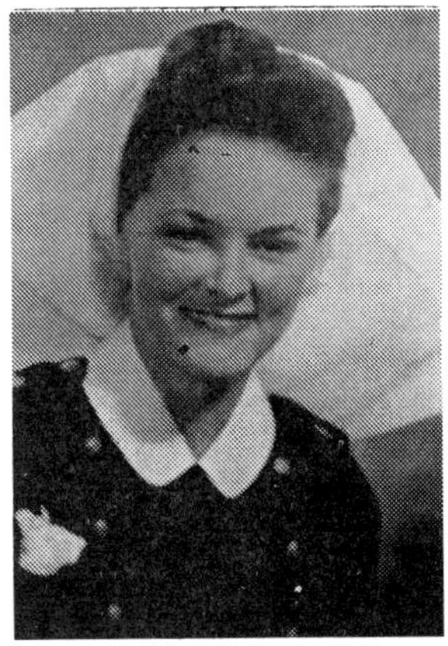

Lt. N/S Jean (Wallace) Campbell, Dundurn, Saskatchewan, 1945

I hoped to obtain a varied nursing experience and perhaps to travel when I joined the Army.

My entire service was at Dundurn Military Hospital, Saskatchewan. I cared for many interesting patients. I met my future husband there, Capt. A.M. Campbell.

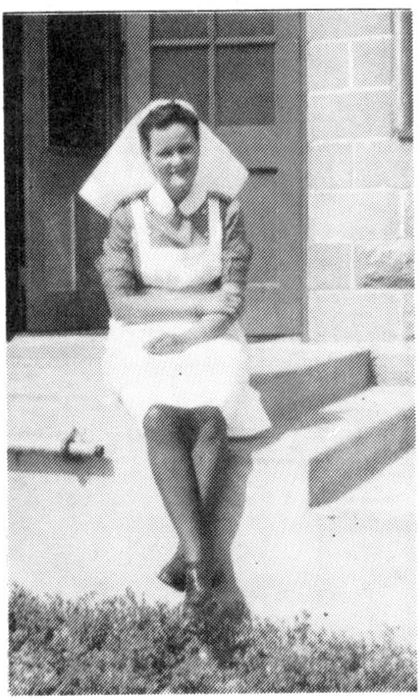

Lt. N/S Jean Wallace, Dundurn Military Hospital, Saskatchewan, 1945

Louise C. Chausse

Graduated from: Edmonton General Hospital School of Nursing. Year: 1935

Military History:

Service: RCAMC

Rank Lt. N/S

Served: November 1943 to November 1946

I took my basic training at Nanaimo Military Hospital then I was sent to Pacific Command Headquarters (old Hotel Vancouver) to be in charge of sick bay for CWAC personnel. I also met incoming female troops and arranged accommodation for them in Vancouver.

I had duty aboard troop trains, usually from Vancouver to Winnipeg and I met troops coming from overseas and returning to Vancouver. I also met troop trains from the U.S. with Canadian soldiers returning from Hong Kong.

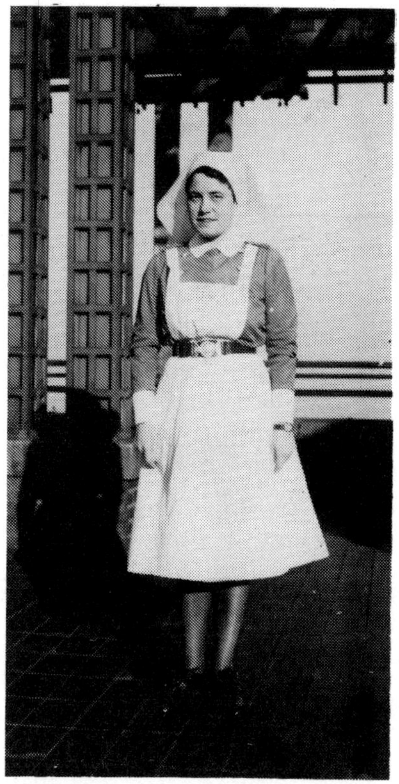

Lt. N/S Louise Chausse at old Vancouver Barracks

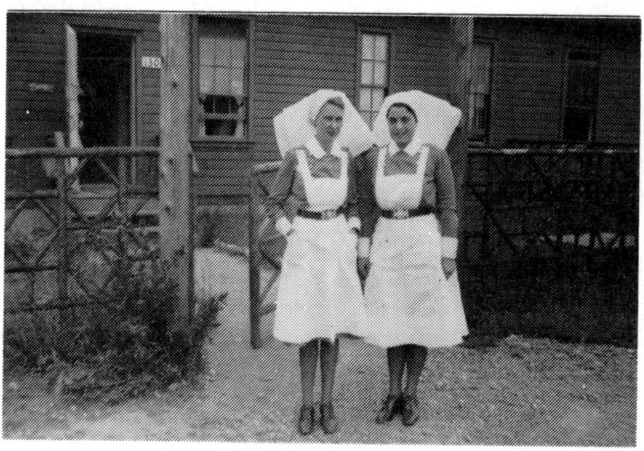

Nanaimo Military Hospital
L - R: Nursing Sisters Winnie Blackburn; Louise Chausse

CN HOSPITAL TRAIN

Hospital on Wheels

This exhibition of a full-sized reproduction of a military hospital car is presented by the T. Eaton Company Limited, in cooperation with the Canadian National Railways, to acquaint the public with the methods used to bring wounded servicemen home to Canada with the maximum of comfort. The photographs on display show how wounded troops are cared for on board the *Lady Nelson*, Canada's senior hospital ship, former flagship of the Canadian National (West Indies) fleet.

An exact duplicate in all its details, the model was made to the specifications of the Canadian National's approved design. The interior layout was planned by CNR medical and mechanical experts in association with officers of the Royal Canadian Army Medical Corps (which staffs the cars in service) and the design was adopted by the government as standard for Canadian "hospitals on wheels."

To date, the Canadian National have built ten hospital cars and an auxiliary unit in their car shops. The first car was delivered in July 1940. Eight of the eleven have air-conditioning

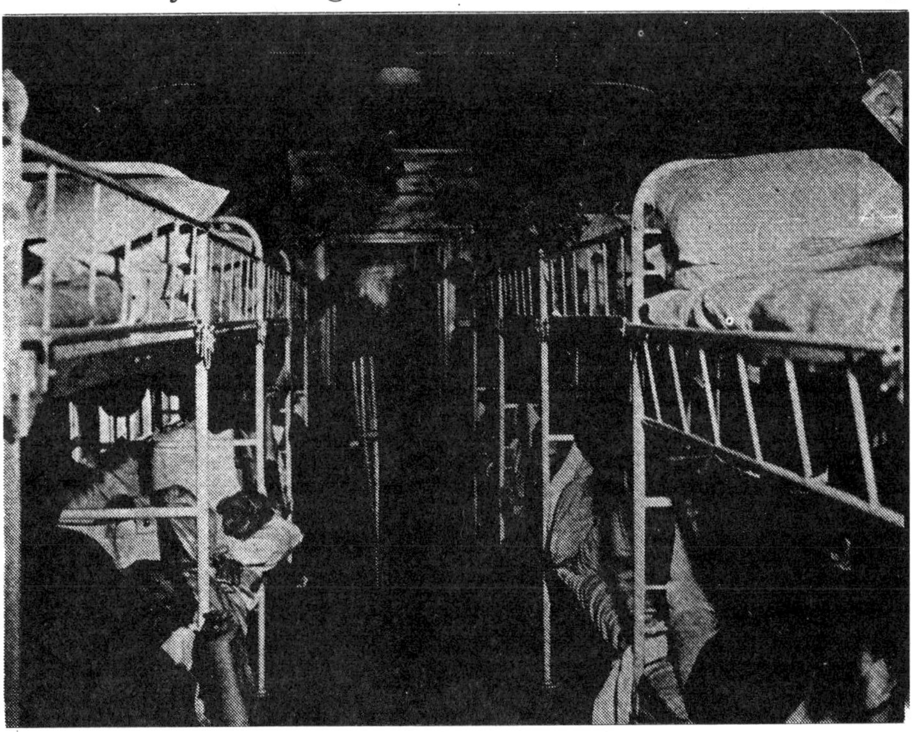

Hospital on wheels

equipment and all were converted from all-steel parlor and sleeping cars. They are 75 feet long by 10 feet high. There are 28 beds in each car. They interlock in continuous construction, with one post serving two beds, which makes for greater length and rigidity. For the protection of the patients, the upper beds are equipped with drop side safety guards. Each bed has its individual lamp with swivel reflector shade, ash tray and call-bell button. Special tea trays and glass holders are provided.

In the utility room or dispensary are two gas plates and one electric, for the preparation of light diets. Cupboard space is provided, a refrigerator compartment, two sliding kitchen work boards, a cracked-ice container, and a new type of sink designed and located to lessen fatigue.

The interior colour scheme is sea green for the walls, a white ceiling and mottled rust marboleum for the floor covering. Standard Canadian National passenger car green is used for the exterior, with black roof, and the lettering is in gold.

Canadian men wounded on active service overseas are assured of the most efficient and sympathetic care on their journey home. *

* Photograph and caption courtesy of Alberta Association of Registered Nurses Archives, Edmonton, Alberta.

Mildred Cohoon

Graduated from: St. Paul's Hospital School of Nursing, Vancouver, B.C. Year: 1927

Military History:

Service: RCAMC

Rank: Lt. N/S

Served: 1943 to 1946

I chose to join the army out of patriotism. My duty assignments were all in Canada:

Military Hospital, Terrace, B.C., Military Hospital, Harrison Hot Springs., Military Hospital, Camp Wainwright, Alberta.

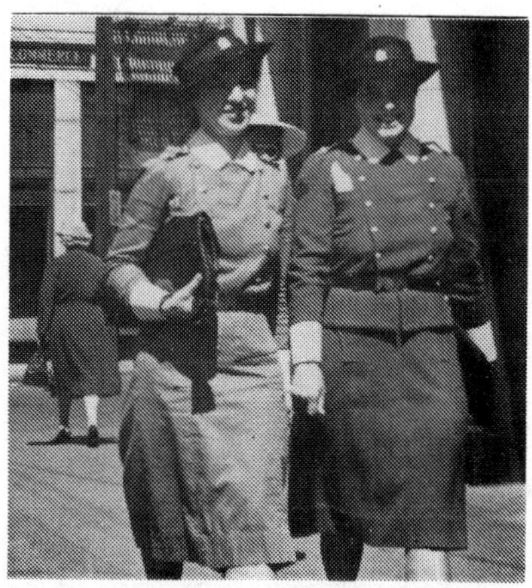

L - R: Nursing sisters Mildred Cohoon; Louise Chausse

Luella M. Downing

Graduated from: Regina General Hospital School of Nursing.

Military History:

Service: RCAMC

Rank: Lt. N/S

Served: 1942 to 1945

I was working in the operating room at the Shaughnessy Hospital in Vancouver in 1941 when I decided to become a nursing sister. I was not permitted to leave the military hospital then (Shaughnessy) but my father became ill in Saskatchewan so I had to go home and resigned from the Hospital.

After six months at home, I applied to the Army and was accepted. After basic military training at Camp Borden, I served the Army in Kingston and was then sent to Nova Scotia to organize and operate an operating room at Acadia.

I was put on draft for overseas but taken off the night before I was to leave and sent to Edmonton, Alberta, to work in the operating room. I had special operating room training with Dr. Penfield at the Neurological Institute in Montreal and was needed in the University Hospital in Edmonton for OR work as many soldiers were returning with head injuries.

I was there until September 1, 1945 when hostilities ceased and the war was over!

Betty C. (Chinn) Dewick

Graduated from: Royal Alexandra Hospital School of Nursing, Edmonton. Year: 1940

Other: Diploma in Public Health Nursing, University of Alberta (1943)
M.D., C.M. Queens University, Kingston, Ontario (1954)

Military History:

Service: RCAMC

Served: 1 November 1944 to 3 June 1946

My father was quarter-master sergeant for local militia unit (pre-war), 19th Alberta Dragoons and was QMS at Prince of Wales Armouries, early in WW II.

When I was in training at the Royal Alexandra Hospital, my father was stationed at Prince of Wales Armouries across the street. When we saw bonfires we knew they were burning clothing that was infested with lice.

Post war when I got my MD through Department of Veterans Affairs, it was quite a struggle. I worked with the travelling clinic for TB control, then when it got too hard to lift the heavy equipment, I went into radiology.

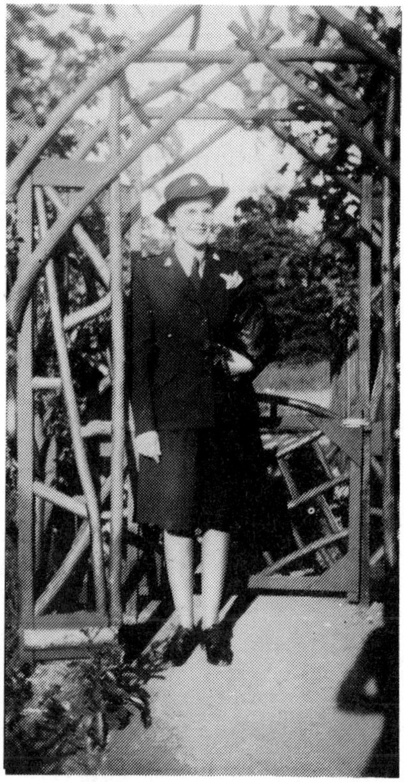

Lt. N/S Betty (Chinn) Dewick

Patricia (Ferris) Gill

Graduated from; Ross Memorial Hospital School of Nursing, Lindsay, Ontario. Year: 1949

Military History:

Branch of service: RCAMC

Rank: Lt. N/S

Served: Fall 1952 to Winter 1954

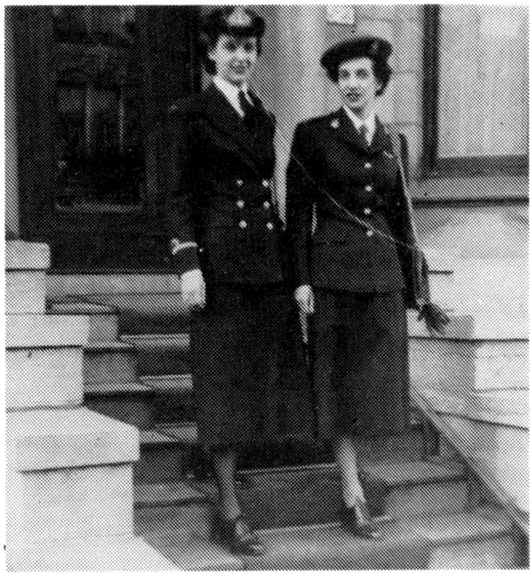

Montreal 1952. L-R: Gwyneth (Ferris) Molloy, my sister – a Sub-Lieut. WRCNS (Reserve); Patricia (Ferris) Gill

Having spent three of the war years in the WRCNS, I realized the joys of service life. I made a decision to continue that service in the medical field.

Following a post-graduate course in obstetrics nursing at the Margaret Hague Maternity Hospital in Jersey City, N.J., and a short hospital working experience, I joined the RCAMC. in 1952. When dependant care was initiated at some of the camps, I was posted to the military hospital at Camp Shilo, Manitoba, to set up the obstetrical unit there. The QM was constantly amazed at the weird-seeming supplies being requisitioned from him.

By the time the unit was in full swing, I was leaving to be married. When we left on our honeymoon there were lots of jokes such as: "Ha-Ha, you'll be a patient here in nine months." Guess what – I was! The amazing bit was that the MO on duty when I was in labour was fairly newly posted and hadn't delivered a baby in fifteen or more years. She sat beside me reading a manual and saying, *"Pat, I'm so glad you're a nurse – you can tell me exactly what's happening."* Now, she was a neighbour and had even removed sutures from our cat after its surgery so I had considered her a friend. However, that night I could have killed her! Anyway, all went well and I was later overwhelmed with visits from staff members from kitchen, garden, maintenance and administration as well as medical. It was great – a fun and happy time.

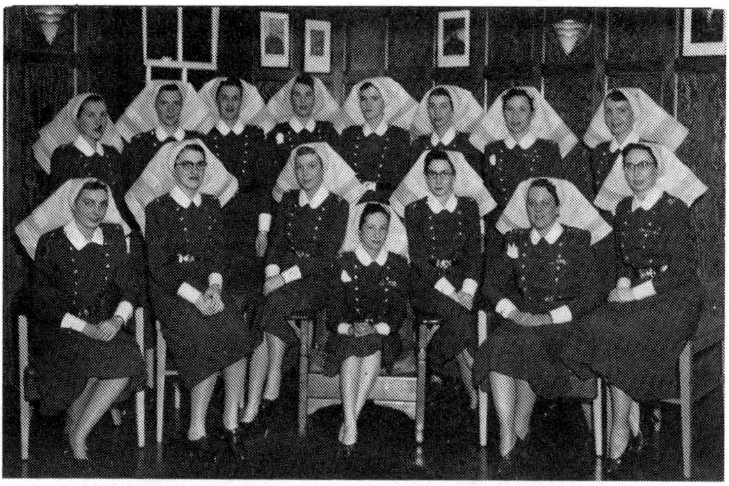

Nursing Sisters course at Camp Borden, 1952
L-R: starting at rear: Vivian Treacy, Hazel Kydes, Yonty Ontychuk, Fran Cowley, Mary Sranford, S. Loeser, Betty Smith, Zolande LeBlanc, Marie McKinney, Patricia (Ferris) Gill, Agathe Cloutier, Matron-in-Chief Major Andrews, Leopoldine Asselin, V. Kenney, M.E. Scoyer.

Mary S. Hemphill

Graduated from: Toronto General Hospital School of Nursing. Year: 1940

Military History:

Service: RCAMC

Rank: Lt. N/S

Served: April 1942 to September 1943

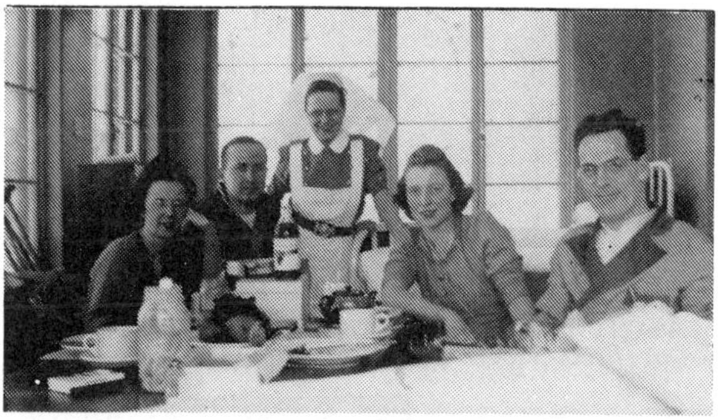

N/S Mary Hemphill; Capt. McKinnon; N/S Laura Larkin; N/S Arlene Winterton, physiotherapist who was in the accident with me.

I wished to make a contribution in the war effort. However, my active duty was extremely short – I was involved in an accident at Camp Borden in May 1942. The result was a compound, comminuted fracture of tibia and fibula (left leg) – was discharged in 1943 from Christie St. Hospital on small pension.

Jessie C. Larmon

Graduated from: Archway Hospital School of Nursing, London, England. Year: 1941

Other: Midwifery 1942/43

Military History:

Service: QAIMNS and RCAMC

Rank: Lt. N/S

Served: 21 February 1944 to 26 November 1946 and 13 years (R)

I was born in Winnipeg and went to England as a teenager. I took my nurses training at Archway Hospital in London then took one year of midwifery in Manchester.

I joined QAIMNS in February of 1944 and was posted to 110th British General Hospital at Bayeux, Normandy, in July, 1944. From there, I moved with my unit to Bruges, Belgium, in November and remained there until May 1945.

My next assignment was India in July 1945. I served at Chindwara for a year. After leave in England, I was posted to Mestre-Venice for five months until my release from QAIMNS 26 November 1946.

I next served with the RCAMC (Reserve) in the 17th Medical Company, Winnipeg, for 13 years.

Edith (Landells) Lees

Graduated from: St. Joseph's General Hospital School of Nursing, Vegreville, Alberta. Year: 1944

Military History:

Service: RCAMC and RCN

Rank: Lt. N/S and Sub. Lt. N/S

Served: April 1945 to May 1946, RCAMC
1946 to 1947, Merchant Marine
1948 to 1951, RCN

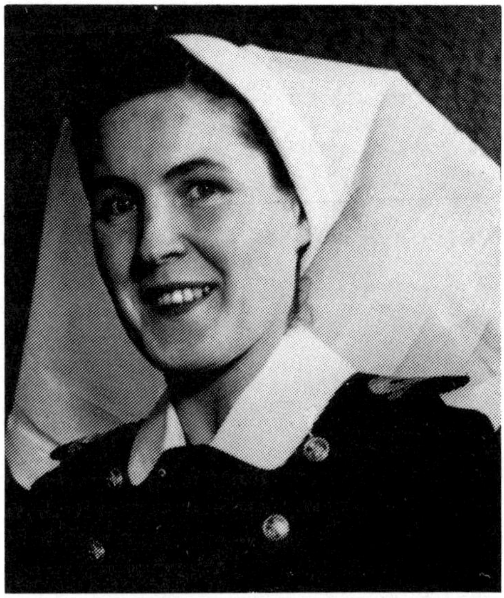

N/S Edith Landells

My aunt, Margaret Jane Landells, was stationed overseas in England and in Salonica, Greece, during World War One. She was a very positive influence in our lives, I only wish I had recorded more of her Army experiences. My brother Jack was another great influence in my life. He chose a Naval career and we spent many anxious months when he became a prisoner of war in Germany. There never was a need to make a decision, I always knew I would go into the Army.

My Army career was brief, VE Day was announced shortly after I was in the service. As countries in Europe were liberated, my brother was released, and one happy day he came to Dundurn, Saskatchewan, where I was stationed to tell me of his experiences as prisoner of war in Germany.

Again, there was no choice, the Army didn't need nurses, there weren't going to be anymore wars and I was discharged from the Army at Regina, Saskatchewan, in 1946.

I was fortunate to sign on with an Australian cargo ship, the SS *Rabaul*, for a year. They were transporting war brides from Canada to Australia and from Australia to Canada and the U.S. and required a medical person aboard. There was, as yet, no commercial traffic in the Pacific and passengers travelled by cargo ship.

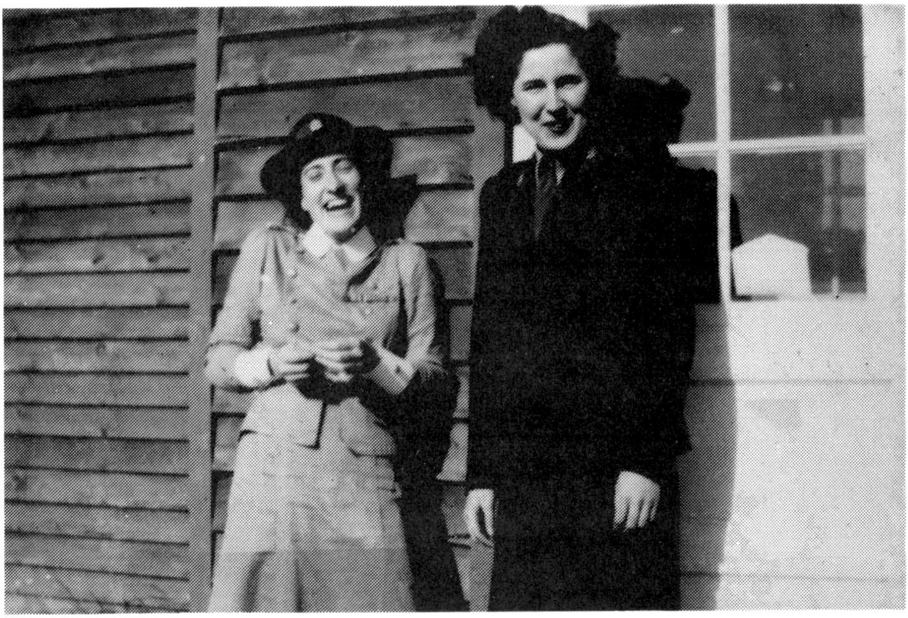

Dundurn Military Hospital, Saskatchewan 1945
L - R: Lt. N/S Hallie Sloan; Lt. N/S Edith Landells

When I heard the Navy was accepting nurses I applied and became a member of the RCN. My Navy experience was limited to RCNH *Stadacona* and *Cornwallis* in Nova Scotia. There was no opportunity for overseas duty when the Korean War came along and by this time I realized the career advantages were with further education in nursing, and therefore, worked to that end.

After retiring, I wanted to utilize my education for some definitive achievement and chose to author this book. So I end as I began, working with Canadian military people; a perfect ending for this phase of my retirement.

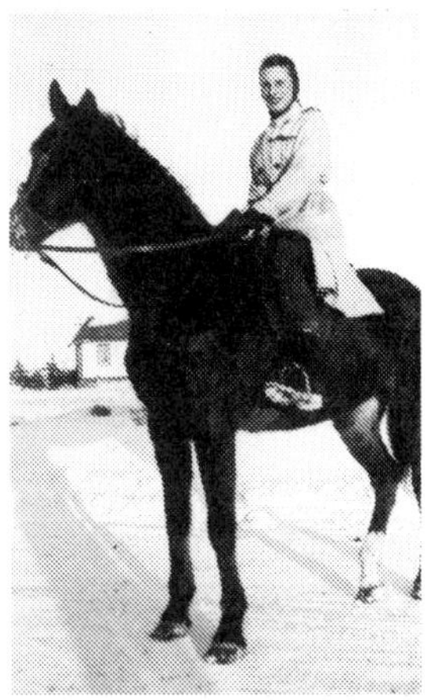

VAD Henriette Trudeau and horse, Dundurn 1945

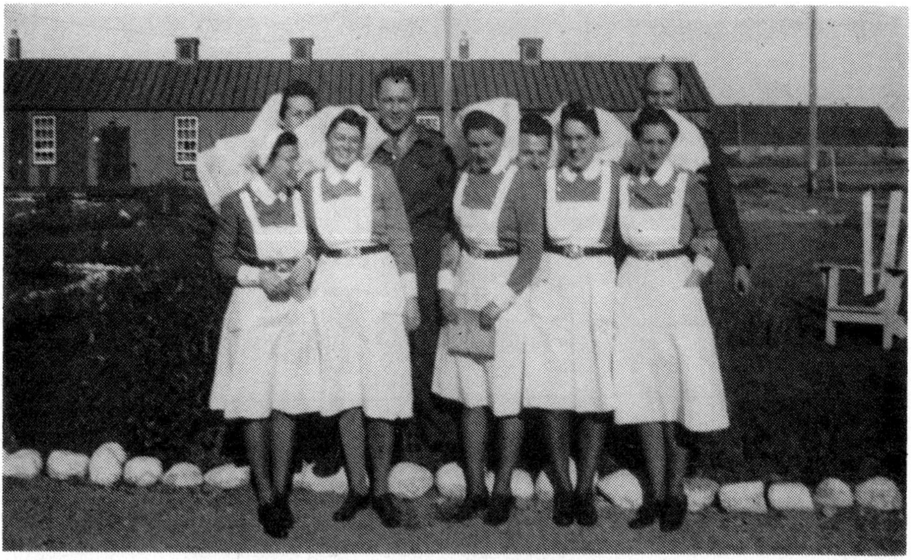

Military Hospital, Camp Dundurn, Sask. 1945
Front Row, L - R: Nursing Sisters Hallie Sloan, Marty Loken, Edith Landells, Madeleine Shockey, Helen Roth,
Back Row: N/S Ruth Frache, Dr. (name unknown), Major Marinker, Lt. Col. Bell.

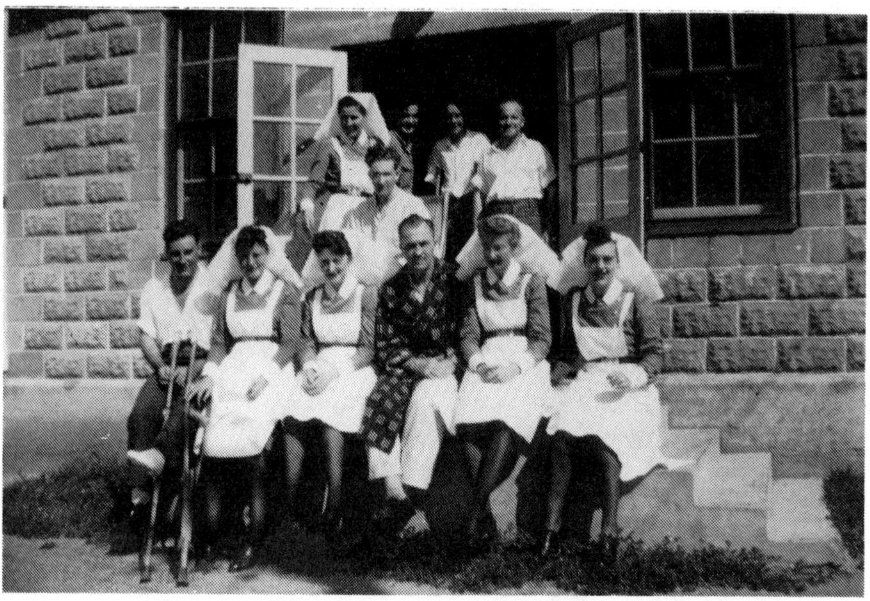

Military Hospital, Camp Dundurn, Saskatchewan 1945
Front row L-R: Nursing Sisters Betty Ramage, Catherine Cush, Victoria Batter, Madeleine Shockey.
Back Row: N/S Edith Landells and patients.

Mary Gertrude (Patton) Luco

Graduated from: Edmonton General Hospital School of Nursing. Year: 1939

Military History:

Service: RCAMC

Rank: Lt. N/S

Served: 1943 to 1945

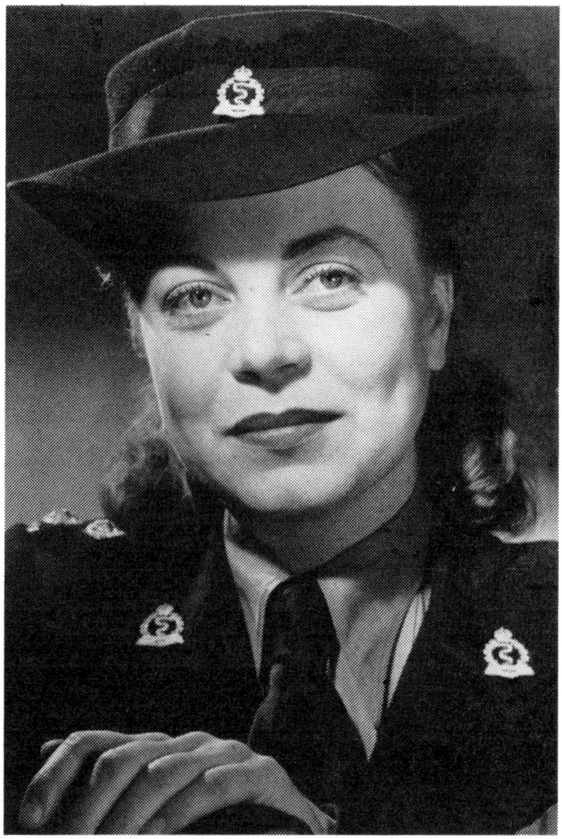

Lt. N/S Mary (Patton) Luco

After my graduation in 1939, at the age of 21, I applied immediately to the Royal Canadian Army Medical Corps; it was the right thing to do. Of course, patriotism and new adventure were important considerations. The call came four years later.

The Army provided first class transportation across Canada by train. There were weekend passes to Montreal and Toronto. We enjoyed the camaraderie of our peers and watched the return to health of the returning soldiers at Rideau Military Hospital.

I have maintained a lifelong friendship with Enyd (Skipper) Forrest, now in Winnipeg.

There are great memories.

Thelma C. (Horton) McLean

Graduated from: Saint John General Hospital School of Nursing, N.B. Year: 1935

Military History:

Service: RCAMC

Rank: Lt. N/S in charge

Served: April 1941 to March 1943

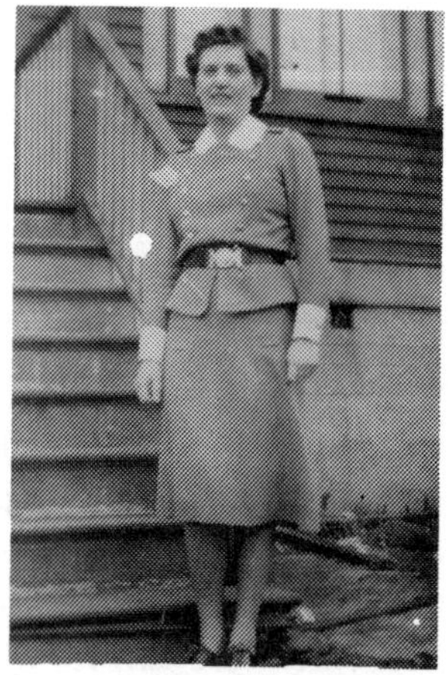

Lt. N/S Thelma (Horton) McLean

My purpose in joining the service was to serve Canada. All of my military service was in Canada: Howe Lake Military Hospital (Saint John, N.B.); Fredericton, N.B. Military Hospital – Sussex, N.B. Military Hospital; St. James Military Hospital (Saint John, N.B.).

Edith (Kidd) O'Donoghue

Graduated from: St. Paul's Hospital School of Nursing, Vancouver, B.C. Year: 1944

Military History:

Service: RCAMC

Rank: 1st Lieutenant

Served: February 1945 to May 1946

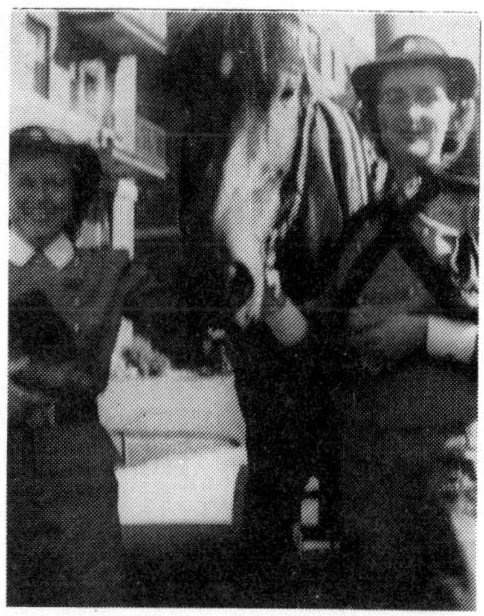

L-R: Nursing sisters Edith (Kidd) O'Donoghue, Gloria Wilson. me - a horse - my roommate Gloria Wilson

War time influenced me to choose military service. I was unable to get a visa to work for United Airlines in the U.S.A. I went with a friend who had an appointment at RCAMC.

My military experience – that is what it was – an experience – another world.

Claire (Bourret) Phillips

Graduated from: St. Paul's Hospital School of Nursing, Saskatoon, Sask. Year: 1940

Military History:

Service: Canadian Army (active)

Rank: Lt. N/S

Served: May 1945 to August 1946

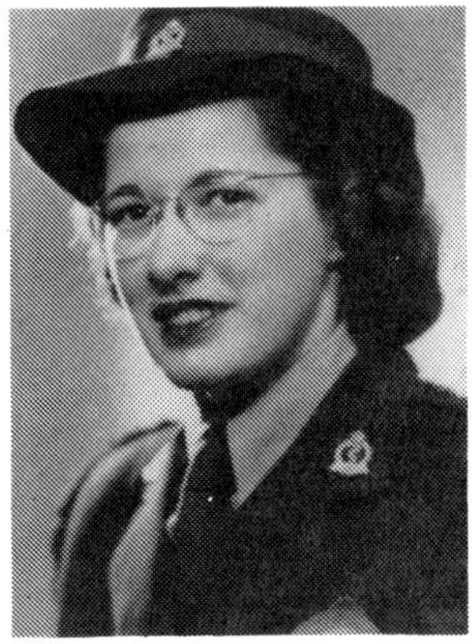

Lt. N/S Claire (Bourret) Phillips

I wanted to serve in the military.

The highlight of my military experience was caring for the Hong Kong veterans on their return to Canada.

Rita Mary (Hart) Santell

Graduated from: Brockville School of Nursing, Ontario. Year: 1936

Military History:

Service: RCAMC

Rank: Lt. N/S

Served: 1942 to 1947

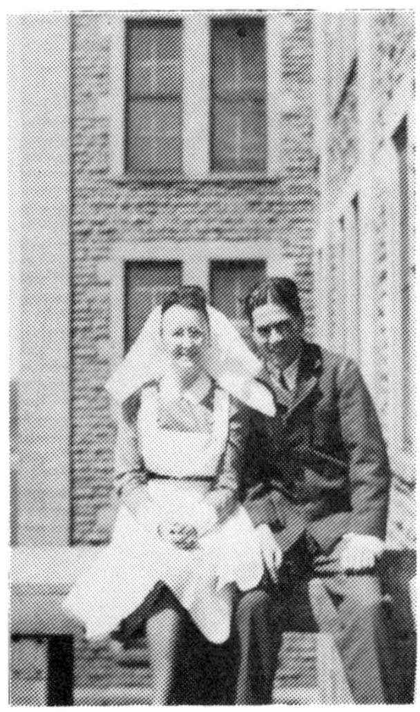

Rita (Hart) Santell, Kingston Military Hospital with one of my patients, 1942

I was nursing in Toronto at Mt. Sinai, 1942, when I decided to join the RCMAC. I was sent to Kingston Military for about a year. I was then transferred to Rideau Military Hospital in Ottawa, Canada, in order to be closer to my father. My father was very ill at home in Cobden, Ontario, about 80 miles away. I spent most of my weekends in Cobden until my father died in 1943.

In early 1944, I was transferred to

the Embarkation unit in Halifax. This was the hospital train unit. I could not go overseas with my unit, No. 2 Canadian General Hospital, because of eye trouble.

We met the ship as our wounded boys returned home and transferred them to their destination in Canada. Each of us was in charge of one hospital car. Our pharmacy was at the end of the car where our dressing trays, drugs and supplies were kept.

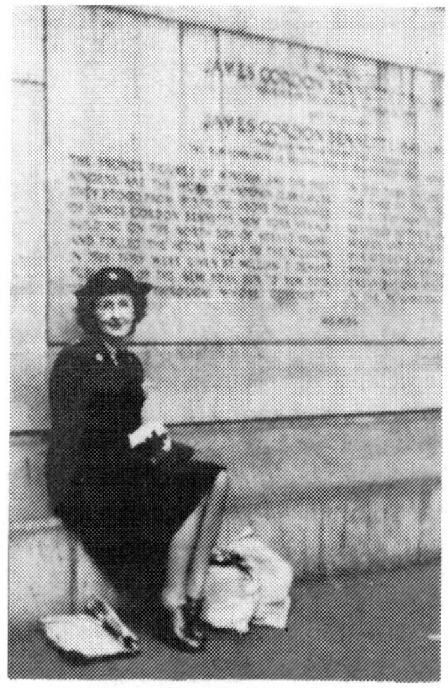

Rita (Hart) Santell. embarkation unit, Halifax 1944

Sometimes our car, or mine rather, would go to Vancouver or Winnipeg. We even went to New York to pick up the wounded a couple of times.

I found it interesting, naturally; one had to learn to balance a tray, or a basin filled with water going through the Rockies. I had a few spills, but on the whole, became very good at it.

We had our boys that needed dressings, or any special care on the bottom bunks, the ones who were able to help themselves were placed on the top bunks. They even taught me to play cribbage on the trains.

I travelled back and forth on the hospital trains from 1944 to 1946. From 1946 until 1947 we travelled across the Atlantic on the hospital ship *Letitia* bringing back the war brides – 22 crossings. This was quite an experience in itself.

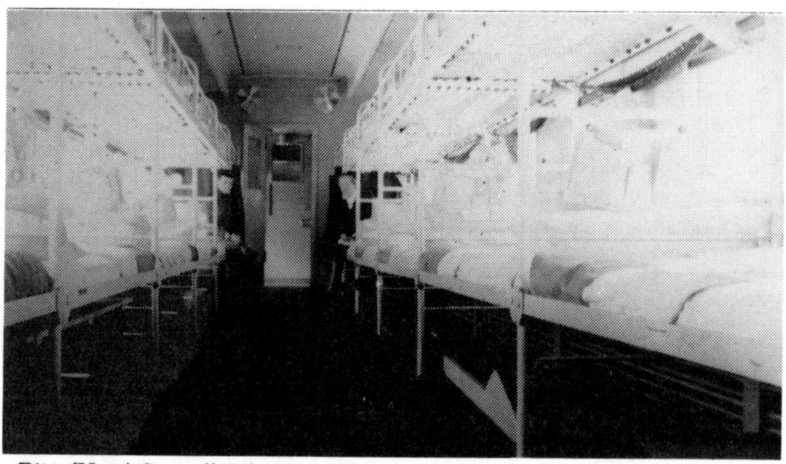

Rita (Hart) Santell - this is what our hospital train cars looked like.

Helen A. Saunders

Graduated from: Vancouver General Hospital School of Nursing. Year: 1939
Basic RN and B.A. and B.A. Sc. (Nursing), University of British Columbia, 1940

Military History:

Service: RCAMC

Rank: Lt. N/S

Served: June 1944 to September 1945

I only joined to do my part in the war effort. I did not choose military nursing as a career.

I was never posted outside of British Columbia and have no real "highlights" to report on my personal experience in the Army. I served 17 months in the RCAMC during World War II and joined up for the obvious reason – to use my nursing ability to help my country at that time.

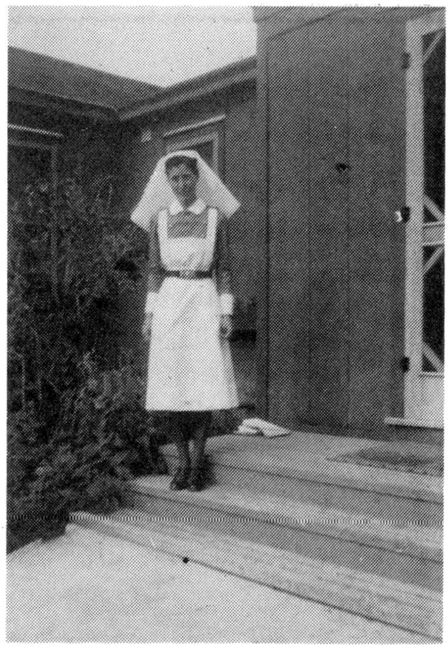

Lt. N/S Helen Saunders

Lille Elizabeth (Tattrie) Sheehan

Graduated from: St. Paul's Hospital School of Nursing, Vancouver, B.C. Year: 1939

Military History:

Service: RCAMC

Rank: Lt. N/S

Served: April 9, 1945 to May 14, 1946

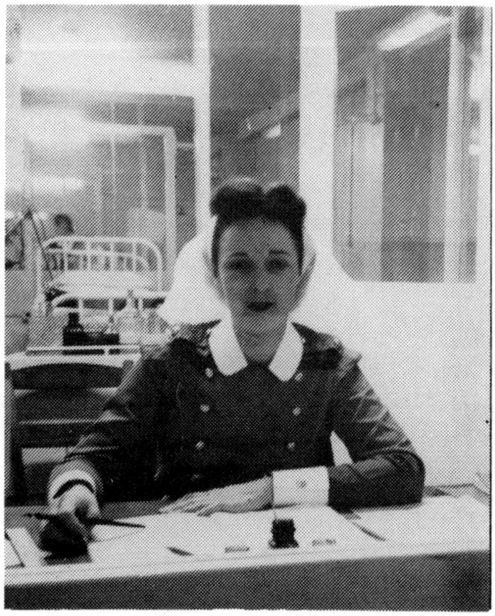

N/S Lille Elizabeth (Tattrie) Sheehan

When I joined the Army I wanted to contribute to the war effort. I was posted directly to Montreal Military Hospital on Queen Mary Road in April 1945 from Vancouver, B.C., where I enlisted

After a qualifying course at Camp Borden, I was promoted to Lieutenant N/S from 2nd Lieutenant and continued to work at Montreal Military Hospital until the war ended.

My military experience was limited as I was in the Army such a short time. I felt that being there to nurse and encourage the many military casualties that arrived from overseas mostly was my contribution to my country, Canada.

I enjoyed my work there and met many fine soldiers and military personnel.

I had hoped to go on a hospital ship but was told that the nurses who had been overseas had first chance to do so. Needless to say, I was very disappointed.

An interesting, rather humorous side occurred when Hilda

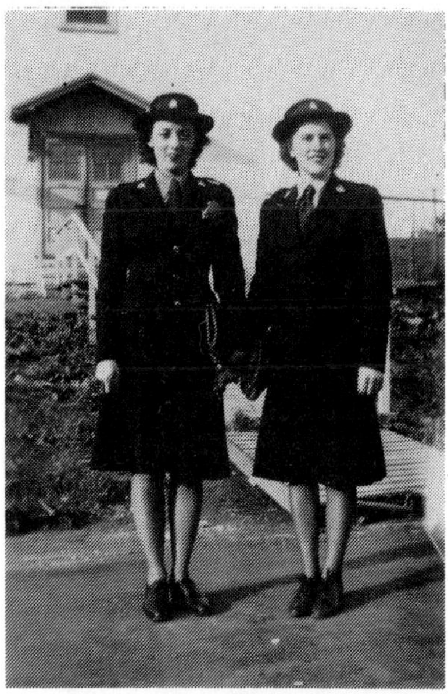

L - R: two Vancouverites Lille (Tattrie) Sheehan and Hilda (Vaughn) Doupe

Vaughan (Doupe) and I were sent across Canada, one via CPR and the other via CNR. We were sent to Farnham, Quebec, (on strength) which was a POW hospital 40 miles from Montreal. It's needless to say that there were no women there and we were sent back to Montreal post-haste. Included among the patients was one very famous POW whose name I can't recall – sorry. I was able to see them as they filed in to dinner.

You will, no doubt, have many interesting experiences described to you from nurses who served overseas as I have heard from them at the various functions I have attended as a member of the Nursing Sisters Association.

Muriel Joyce Sinclair

Graduated from: St. Thomas' Hospital School of Nursing, London, England. Year: 1954

Other: Sick Children's Hospital, Edinburgh, Scotland, RSCN

Military History:

Service: RCAMC (Reserve)

Rank: Captain

Served: 1957 to 1972

My experience was that of a part-time Reserve Militia nursing officer; I was the training officer for No. 18 (now No. 17) Medical Company in Winnipeg. I qualified at Kingston, Ontario, as a major, but as there was no establishment at that time, 1971 or 1972, for a female major, I did not get promoted!

Chapter 12

SERVING IN KOREA

Dorothy Doyle
Olga (Hannas) Dube
Elizabeth (Pense) Neil

KOREA

At the outbreak of the Korean War, the RCAF had 13 qualified flight nurses, a number of whom were attached to the U.S. Air Force for duty in flying casualties from Japan to San Fransisco. In mid-1951 the first large-scale hospital airlift carrying Canadian casualties to Tacoma, Washington, took place. From there, the casualties were transferred in a converted RCAF Dakota air ambulance to Edmonton and other DVA centres. One flight nurse and flight medical assistant cared for the patients enroute.

During the Korean War, RCAMC nursing sisters served in hospitals in Kure, Japan, and in Seoul, Korea. In the spring of 1953, nursing sisters were employed with a Canadian Field Dressing Station at Touchong, 20 miles north of Seoul, where a total of 112 surgical and medical cases could be accommodated.*

THE WAR IN KOREA 1950-1953

On June 25th 1950 North Korean forces crossed the boundary between North and South Korea and advanced on the South Korean capital, Seoul. American Forces were ordered into action. At the same time the United States requested the United Nations to legitimize its intervention. Canada, among those member states of the U.N. endorsed the American action.**

* Courtesy *Carillon*, August 1987. Public Affairs Division, Veterans Affairs Canada, Minister of Supply and Services Canada, 1987.

** *Canada's Soldiers, 3rd Edition* by George F.G. Stanley, Macmillan of Canada/Toronto. pp.399-406

Dorothy E. Doyle

Graduated from: St. Francis Xavier University, Antigonish N.S. Year: 1939
B.Sc. Dietetics. Internship, Victoria General Hospital, Halifax, N.S.

Military History:

Service: RCAMC

Rank: Captain (Diet)

Served: December 4, 1950 to December 25, 1964

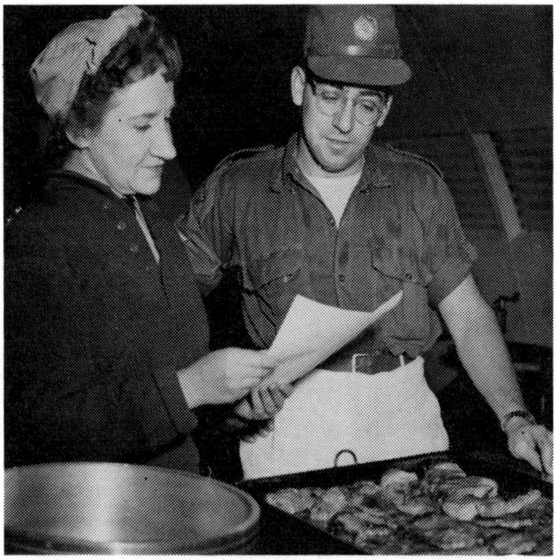

Nursing sister Dorothy Doyle at 25 Field Dressing Station, Korea 11 November 1953
Canadian Forces photo SE8658

I was encouraged by an Army dietitian and a good friend to join the Service.

I joined the Army in Montreal and served at Montreal Military Hospital; from there I was assigned to Calgary Military with a summer at Wainwright (a horrible experience). Then to Calgary again. Then back to Montreal spring of 1953, and on to Korea with 25 Replacement Group at 25 Canadian. Field Dressing Station.

Korea was an interesting posting – a wonderful group of people, both professional and non-professional. Everyone pitched in with ideas for improvements; from these we ended up with a fairly good kitchen and storeroom. Refrigeration was limited so great care in handling foods, etc., was necessary (perishables).

A steam table was put together – very unique, using oil drums and M-37 burners to heat the water to heat the steam table holding food pots. Next, a portable one was put together; oil drum, a wheel, or I should say tire from a helicopter, a top to hold containers, water heated with an M-37 burner. Therapeutic diets were organized, a cook was assigned and a special refrigerator was acquired.

The U.S. Army was most generous with supplies to me; cleaning equipment, M-37 burners and even ice cream. The supply people were most helpful; they never were empty handed when they dropped in.

As I've looked back over the years, it was quite a challenge, and, as I repeat, the staff was always willing to help and bring forth their ideas.

Some of the Korean kitchen workers were quite good, particularly if we kept an eye on them. One particular lad was a cleaner and he thought I was just wonderful. He always wanted to do the right thing, and to make sure he had completed his various tasks he would ask me to inspect so he would know he was doing his work well. He had heard I was going on R & R (they knew everything) and wanted to ask me if I would buy him something in Japan. He tried very had to explain to me what he wanted, I couldn't figure it out. Finally, he sat down in the mess hall at a table, made a little square with his hands on the table, then put his hands to his ear, bent his head as if sleeping and made a noise like an alarm clock; that is what he wanted. I was able to act this out for years and had everyone laughing, a real funny incident. Now, I have forgotten my acting routine.

We had great fun with the house girls; they never moved quickly and we would say hubba, hubba (meaning hurry, hurry), they would take hours to brush our shoes with great giggles. We all had many laughs, some incidents that I would never want to see in print.

Korea was a wonderful experience and my being so fortunate to join the 40-year pilgrimage to Korea, October 1993, was most exciting. A great group; very well organized and we all enjoyed the social activities too. It was busy and tiring; however, for me a wonderful opportunity.

After Korea, I spent 1954-59 at Toronto Military Hospital in Sunnybrook Hospital. I worked on the military wing and also DVA wards. It was most interesting and I really enjoyed my years there.

From 1959 to 1964 I was at RCASC School of cookery. It took me a year to get used to living in camp. I should say I got used to it, but really never cared for teaching.

Olga Yvonne (Hannas) Dube

Submitted by her sister, Dorothy Hannas Loveniuk

Graduated from: Misericordia Hospital School of Nursing,Edmonton, Alberta. Year: 1950

Military History:

Service: RCAMC

Rank: Lt. N/S

Served: Korea

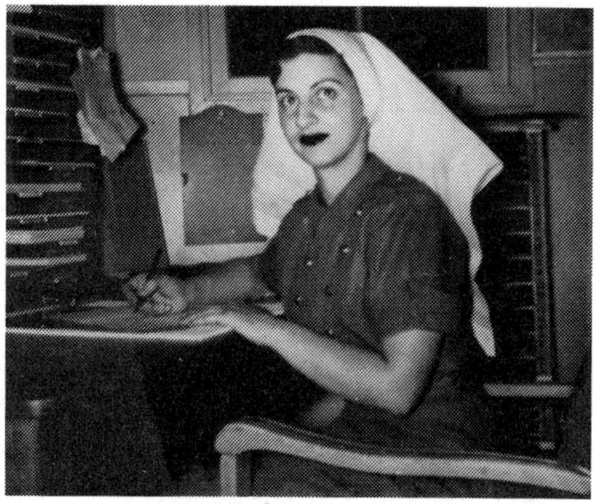

Lt. N/S Olga Hannas Dube

I remember how excited Olga was when she was accepted into the Army. Olga was a superb nurse; she received many awards upon graduating. She was the class valedictorian.

While stationed in Korea, Olga made friends with a talented seamstress. She decided she wanted her wedding dress made by this friend. The dress was ordered in good time, but with the postal service or whatever, the dress had not arrived. Olga made up her mind to wear her formal dress attire for the wedding ceremony. We all felt badly that the dress had not arrived on time, and everyone expected to see her walk down the aisle in her uniform. But when the wedding song began to play and she walked into the chapel on the arm of her brother, she was in the most gorgeous wedding gown we had ever seen. It was made of a beautiful white satin, with hand-sewn pearls in orchid design. The story is that the dress arrived two hours

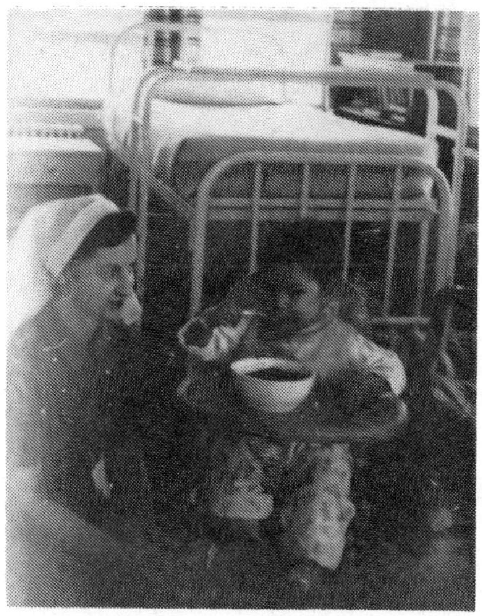

Lt. N/S Olga Hannas Dube and patient in Korea

before the wedding ceremony and she kept it a secret from all.

Olga and Ray Dube were married in Vancouver at Cherry Hill, in a tiny chapel on the beautiful grounds of Army quarters. There were four children. They had a very happy marriage, but unfortunately a very short one. Olga was diagnosed with breast cancer and died two and a half years later. It was a very difficult time for the whole family. We still miss her warmth, generosity and love.

Elizabeth (Pense) Neil

Graduated from: Hamilton General Hospital School of Nursing, Hamilton, Ontario. Year: 1933

Military History:

Service: RCAMC – Permanent Force

Rank: Major

Served: 2 September 1939 to 2 November 1960

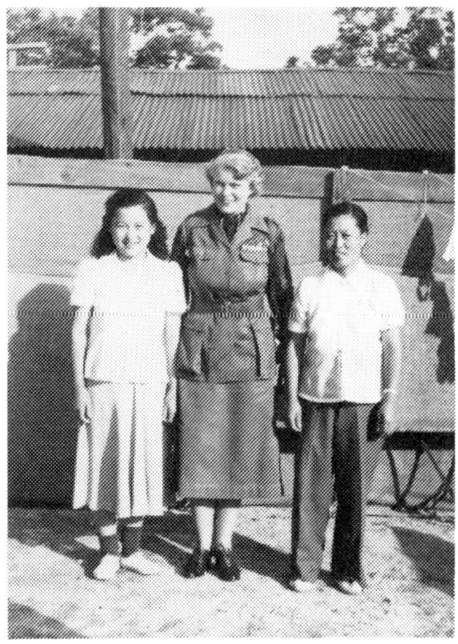

Korea, with our housegirls (maids) at Touchong

During the Korean conflict nursing sisters of the RCAMC served in Kure, Japan, and at Seoul and Touchong in Korea. In March 1951, Canada agreed to assist in staffing a 400-bed British commonwealth hospital in Kure, Japan. At that time there was no commonwealth hospital in Korea. All cases requiring more than minimal care had to be sent back to Japan. In September of 1952 the first commonwealth nurses arrived in Korea; two Canadians, two Australians and two British nursing sisters. Canadian Captain Elizabeth Pense was now matron of the newly formed British Commonwealth Communications Zone Medical Unit. She was responsible for establishing nursing services in an old school building.*

In a letter to her family dated 23 September 1952 she describes the situation: "This is to be a 100-bed hospital, though we have 112 patients at the moment. The outside of the buildings looks quite respectable, but inside it is not too good. Plaster falls from the ceilings, and they tell me that when it rains I will need an umbrella in my office.

"Our quarters have possibilities, but at present are very bare. We have a bed each, some nails on which to hang our clothes, a bucket latrine, a narrow table for the wash basins, some pails for the Korean house girls to bring up water. That is about all at present, but they are trying to get us some furniture. We are hoping to get some curtains soon. As we have no blinds, we have to undress in the dark.

"For the first few days we had to rely on sponge baths – usually cold – but now they have arranged for us to have the use of showers for half an hour each day. The showers are good, but built for tall men. One of our sisters, an Australian, has to have hers standing on a chair, in order to reach the taps!

"Looking back over this, it seems that I have nothing good to say

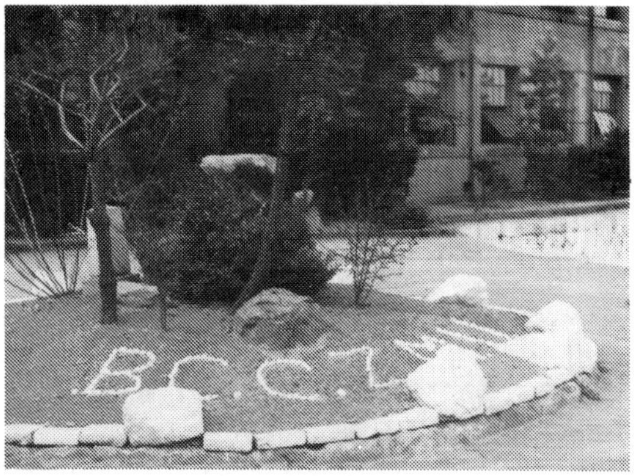

British Commonwealth Communication Zone Medical Unit

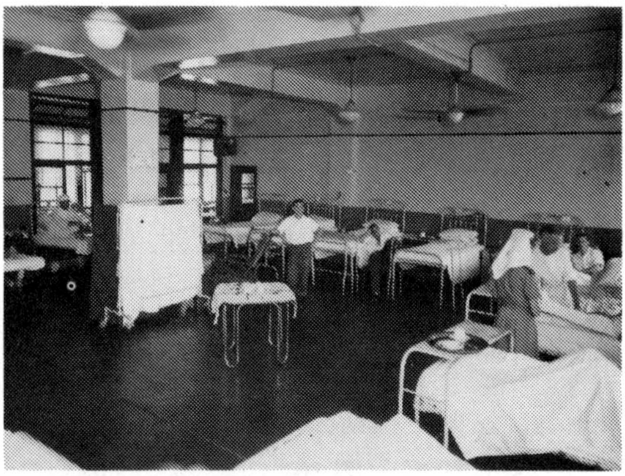

A section of a surgical ward of 20 beds (4 sections to a ward) total 80 beds, Kure, Japan. Canadian Forces photo SE4589

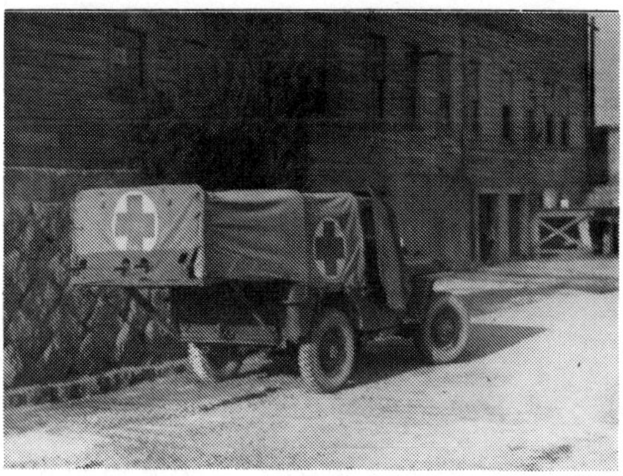

Ambulance receiving patients, Korea 1952

about the place. Actually, it is much better than I had been led to expect, and I am thrilled to be here. In Japan I had no real job to do, and was pretty bored. Here I have a very interesting one with congenial people, and a chance to put some of my ideas into place. We have a very good group of medical officers, and they have been extremely cooperative.

"The weather has been lovely since we arrived here, much like a September day at home. They tell me we should have another month of this, and then it will turn cold. When it does, we will go into battle dress."

*Nicholson, G.W.L. *Canada's Nursing Sisters*. Pp. 213-215.

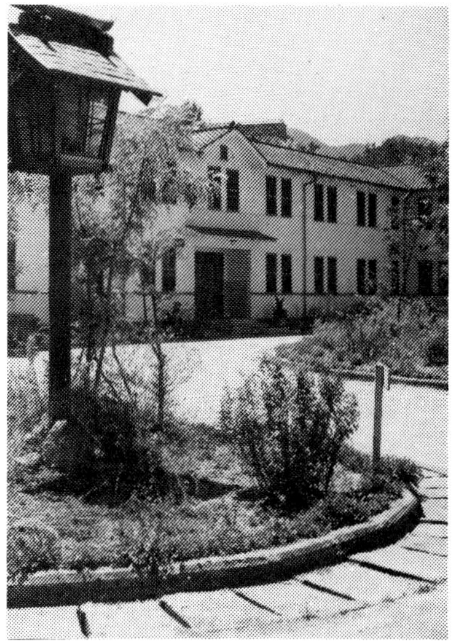

N/S quarters Commonwealth Hospital, Kure, Japan Canadian Forces photo 4603

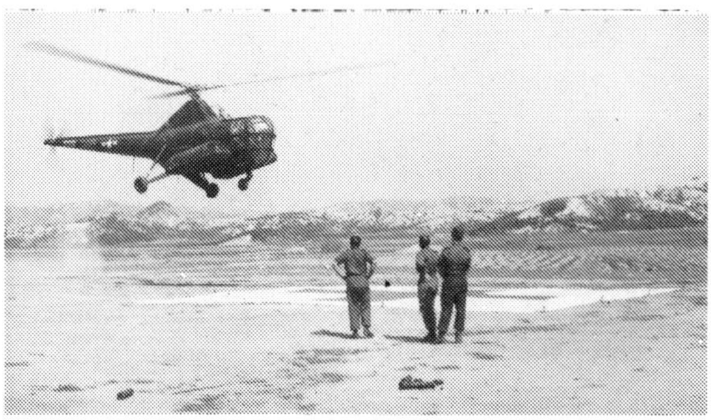

Receiving patients, Korea 1952

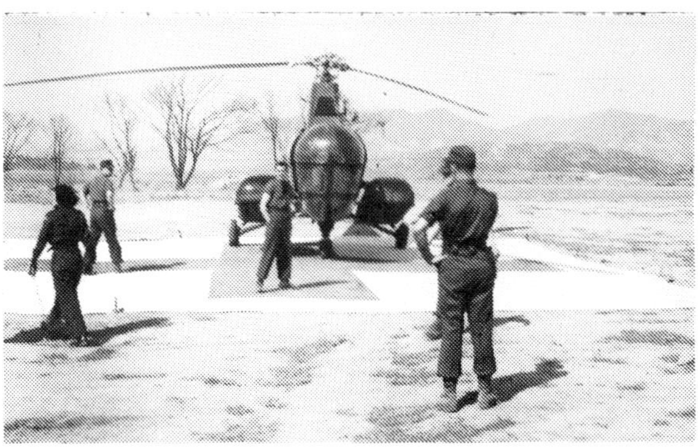

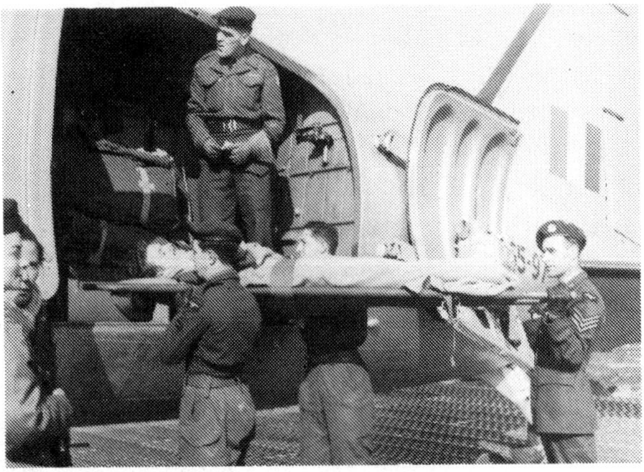

Evacuating patients

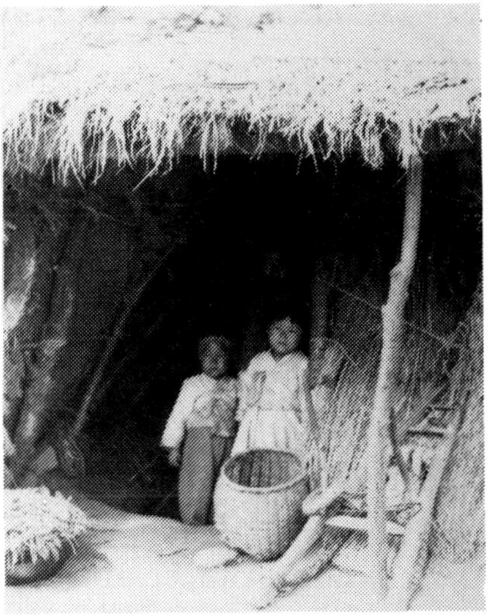

Korean children

Chapter 13

SERVING IN THE PERSIAN GULF WAR AND SOMALIA

Persian Gulf War
Somalia, Operation Deliverance

Rebecca (Gowthorpe) Patterson

Graduated from: Mack Centre for Nursing Education, Niagara College, St. Catharines, Ont. Year: 1987

Military History:

Service CFMS

Rank: Lieutenant (N) Navy

Served: January 1989 to present

Tradition, excitement, travel, ability to train in many different areas; two careers in one – officer and nurse. I have always felt great patriotism towards Canada. I truly believe this career is the best way to give something back to Canada.

The military life was very much a part of my upbringing. Though dad left the RCN in 1968 and mum had to leave the service after her marriage in 1962, the discipline that they had both learned was instilled in all of us children. Throughout my teenage years I was a member of the Navy League Wrenettes and Sea Cadet Corps in Thunder Bay Ontario. My siblings also participated and my father was a chief petty officer 2nd class with the Naval Reserve Unit. The decision was always ours as to whether we chose to remain as members. We did so with great enthusiasm. My mother remained a staunch supporter of her family and at times felt rather wistful watching us on parade.

After graduation from Mack Centre for Nursing Education in 1984 it only seemed natural that I apply to the Canadian Forces. While waiting for acceptance in the CF I worked as an ICU nurse at a local hospital.

I was accepted into the CF in January of 1989. I spent 13 weeks in Chilliwack, B.C., doing basic training with all the other new officer cadets. Infantry tactics, leadership skills, military indoctrination and intense physical training were all part of the training. I wasn't recognized as a nurse until almost a year into my military career!

My first posting has been to National Defence Medical Centre in Ottawa. I have worked in the ICU as officer in charge of the recovery room and head nurse of a 39-bed general surgery/orthopedics ward.

I have also been fortunate to be a member of 1 Canadian Field Hospital during the Persian Gulf War and of the medical team during Op Deliverance in Somalia. On 11 November 1993 I was honoured to be chosen as the nursing officer to represent all military nurses – past and present – on the National War Memorial (literally standing front and centre) in Ottawa for the Remembrance Day Services.

PERSIAN GULF

My first operational deployment was during the Persian Gulf Crisis. On 17 January 1991 war broke out in the Persian Gulf. Canada had committed 1 Canadian Field Hospital to assist the British Army 33rd Field Hospital to support the imminent ground war. In less than 24 hours, approximately 485 members comprised of nursing officers (32 including yours truly), medical officers, medical assistant and numerous support staff were ready to deploy from Canadian Forces Base Petawawa. Our group also contained one platoon of RCR infantry soldiers to provide stretcher bearing capabilities and security for the hospital

Prior to deploying, we were all given a crash course in nuclear/biological/chemical warfare since the threat of chemical warfare was great. At the end of this training, we were all able to put on and remove gas suits, gloves, boots and masks in seconds. Training also included the care and decontamination of patients and their injuries in such conditions and small arms training. All personnel were issued with a 9mm pistol for personal and patient protection.

The whole hospital finally arrived in Saudi Arabia by mid-February in 1991. The Field Hospital itself was located with the British Army, approximately 40 km from the Saudi/Kuwait/Iraqi border. Since it was winter, it rained non-stop and the camp was a quagmire. Patients were treated both medically and surgically by Canadians. This included Allied troops and a number of starving Iraqi troops. Iraqi soldiers had been told terrible things about how we would treat them (i.e., poison them, etc.); before they realized that we meant no harm they took much encouragement to let us treat or feed them.

Not all members of the Field Hospital made it up to Al Kasuma where the hospital was set up. Due to the short duration of the war and the relative high risk of transporting Field Hospital personnel by road, it was decided that a number of personnel would remain at base camp in Al Jubayl – 250 km south and wait the return of the others. There, we occupied time by providing sick parade functions for our troops, by writing letters, shopping (albeit in closely male supervised groups), in the near-by town and by visiting the huge British and American Field Hospital set ups (300-500 beds each) in town.

Our stay was brief – two months (mercifully) for all the ground troops. This was the first deployment of a Canadian Field Hospital since Korea. We returned home none the worse for wear in March of 1991.

SOMALIA

The following is an account of the experiences of Lt. (Navy) Rebecca (Gowthorpe) Patterson during Operation Deliverance with the Canadian Airborne Regiment Battle Group from 1 January to 6 June 1993 in Belet Huen, Somalia.

My second memorable deployment occurred from 30 December 1992 to 5 June 1993. I was a member of the Forward Surgical Team sent to provide medical and surgical support to the Canadian Airborne Regiment Battle Group deployed in Somalia. The mission was to help re-establish a country torn apart by war and starvation.

The medical platoon consisted of 53 personnel. One (1) surgeon, one (1) anaesthetist, two (2) general duty medical officers, three (3) nurses (two operating room trained and myself – an intensive care nurse). The remainder of the platoon was composed of medical assistants, operating room technicians, X-ray

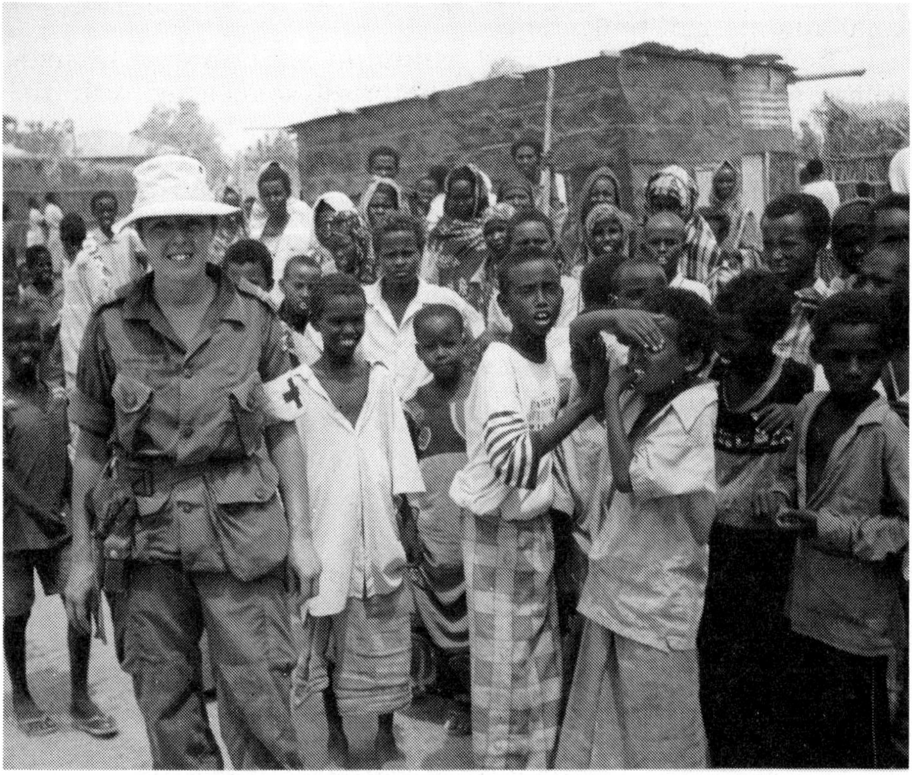

May 1993, Belet Huen, Somalia, Operation Deliverance
Canadian Airborne Regiment Battle Group
Lt. (N) Rebecca (Gowthorpe) Patterson with local Somali youth

and laboratory technicians and preventive medicine technicians.

We set up our tiny hospital just outside the town of Belet Huen which was located 250 Km north of Mogadishu and 40 Km from the Ethiopian border. There was an operating room set-up, a pre-operative/ICU area which could hold two patients, and a ward which could hold up to 10 patients. We were located in a destroyed building that we cleaned up by hand.

I was one of three nursing officers sent on the experience of a lifetime. Lt.(N) Dianne MacIntyre and Capt. Val DeJesus were deployed as part of the Forward Surgical Section (both are OR nurses) and I were sent to perform Pre-op/Post-op/ and ICU duties since I am a critical care trained nurse. I also performed officer in charge duties for the Holding Section. This proved to be the largest part of my duties. Because the two sections were co-located, both areas could be covered by one nursing officer. By the end of the deployment it was obvious that one general duty nursing officer wasn't quite enough!

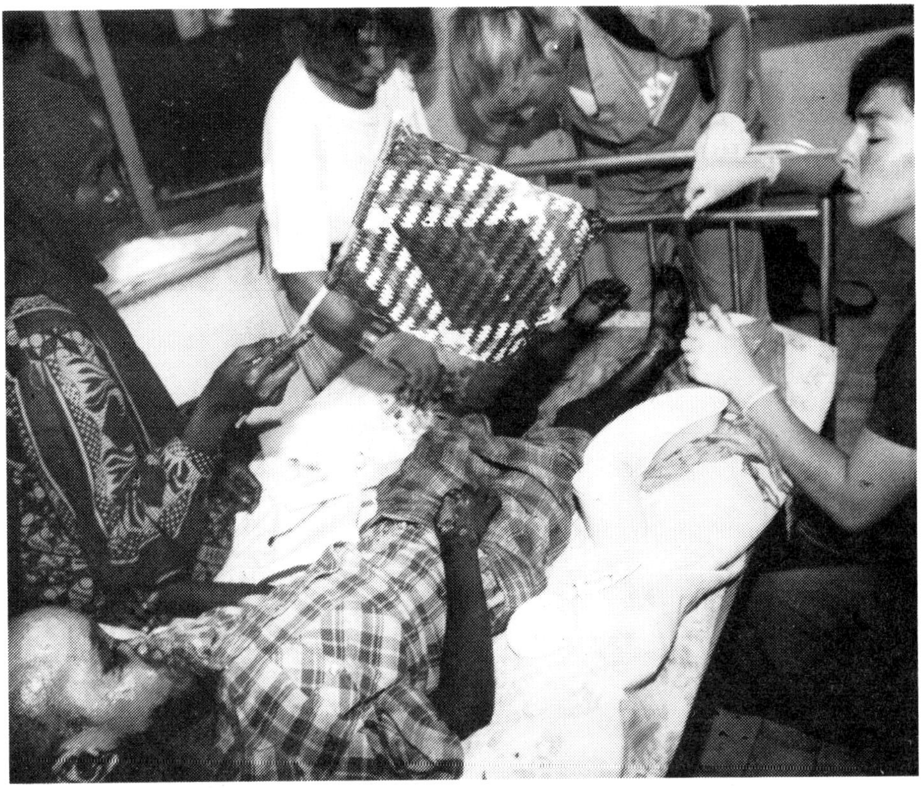

Louise Atkins & Maggie Wideau, U.S.A., and young Somali with his mother. She later became a friend of mine. Her name was Zahar and she was a veterinarian prior to the war and spoke 4 languages fluently. The boy was burnt. Rebecca Gowthorpe, far right.

Unable to work 24 hours a day, seven days a week, it became essential to involve as many people in direct nursing care as possible. Not a day went by when there wasn't something to do. This caused our deployment to fly by and provide me with some of the best and most interesting experiences of my career.

Creating a hospital out of the remains of a burnt-out laboratory building built by the West Germans prior to 1990 was a great challenge. The lab had been used to conduct animal testing for various diseases that run rampant in the Third World. It took seven days to completely clean and set up the hospital. Though the roof remained intact, animals had lived and died within the walls. Somali nomads had set fires inside to cook food, and human waste littered each room. Since the previous Western occupants had had to escape in a rush, there was also a multitude of broken glass, used needles and syringes and discarded computer disks. It took a huge amount of effort from all ranks with a severely restricted water supply to hand clean the fine ceramic tiles that covered the floors and went half way up the walls. Any wiring, pipes, toilets, etc., of any value had been taken away.

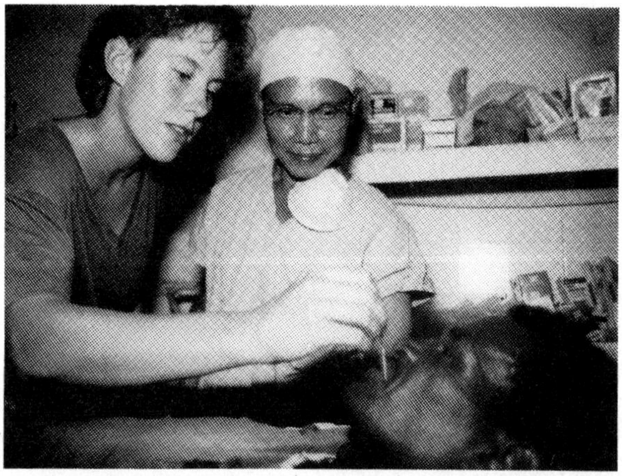

AB Joanne Robertson, a Med A with 2 FD AMB and Captain Val Dejesus, an NO from CFB Halifax, attend to a wounded Somalian
Canadian Forces photo

Thanks to connections on HMCS *Preserver* which was floating off shore near Mogadishu, we were able to have all the floors and walls spray painted white. It cleaned the place up nicely and gave a few sailors a chance to see how the Army lived!

HOLDING SECTION

Since the Surgical Section and Holding Section were co-located both areas were covered by one nursing officer who was appropriately trained. The Holding Section was comprised of fifteen medics trained predominately at the QL3-5 level (privates and corporals). The hospital had seven to nine beds depending on the need and one to four ICU beds as required. Rarely were the holding beds empty. We cared for approximately 140 patients over a five-month period ending 31 May 1993. We treated Canadians, U.S. and German servicemen, Somali nationals and relief workers from the various organizations that had established themselves in the area.

The majority of cases treated – at least 85-90% were for severe nausea, vomiting, diarrhea or non-malarial febrile illnesses required three to four days of hospitalization. Due to extremely harsh environmental conditions, hospitalization in what eventually became an air conditioned environment was essential to prevent severe dehydration and heat illness.

Other cases seen: post insect bite cellulitis; traumatic injuries requiring surgical intervention; critical incident stress reaction; relief workers with malaria.

Nursing services were performed in two different areas: caring for our troops and performing humanitarian work at the local hospital.

Caring for the troops was very similar to Canada. The biggest challenge came not from the type of care we were required to give, but the continual fight with the environment to keep the equipment and ward running. The heat and dust were major challenges.

The heat ranged between 30 degrees centigrade at night into the mid 40's during the daytime. Inside the hospital building the temperature remained a fairly constant 32-35 degrees centigrade. The installation of large air conditioning units could cool the ward to approximately 27 degrees. It became a standing joke that anyone who stayed inside for too long was "only hurting themselves" when they were required to venture outside.

Thermometer watching (located on an outside wall by the P. Med. office) was also a hobby that troops took up. I'm sure every letter home had at least one reference to the latest reading!

Heat was also responsible for the failure of rechargeable batteries and the questionable quality of some of the local anesthetics used for minor surgical procedures.

Exhaustion of Holding Section shift workers was also evident. "Days off" were not always a reality due to the multitude of other taskings for the troops as well as shift work. Heat made it very difficult to sleep in the tents that were staff quarters so after some trials it was decided that shifts would run from 0500 hours to 1700 hours and 1700 hours to 0500 hours. Since we were so close to the equator, the sun was up by 0600 hours and had set by 1800 hours. By running the shifts at those hours, everyone got some time to rest during the cool parts of the day.

Dust was ever present and always blowing around – that was the other major problem. Talc-fine dust would clog up equipment and coat everything. Every day patients would have to be dusted off and the wards swept out.

Morale became a large issue with in-patients. Extreme heat coupled with harsh living conditions and an uncomfortable illness thrown in for good measure brought on different responses. The troops considered illness a weakness and constantly asked when they could return to their units. American troops, on the other hand, didn't want to go! They were given no R(est) and R(ecreation) or phone calls and felt things were quite excellent where they were!

As previously mentioned, providing care at our hospital was not so different until we received four Somali patients.

Mohammed, Abdi, Olad and Abdi stayed with us for over a month. They required complex dressing changes and nursing care. As business was brisk elsewhere in the hospital and the fact that these patients required more complex care, the care was divided up between the three nursing officers, Sgt. Ashman and MWO Pare.

Religious and dietary restrictions proved to be a challenge. Food for all people in the camp took the form of IMPs or hard rations "boil in a bag." The Somalis ate what we did but we had to be careful about anything with pork products. Ever think how many I(ndividual) M(eal) P(ackages)s have possible pork products in them? – wieners and beans, sausage and hash browns, ham omelette.

The Med A's of Holding Section deserve a big congratulation for overcoming religious, language and cultural boundaries with these patients. Our friends were reluctant to leave in the end, and they left feeling positive about their experience with the Canadians.

At the local hospital medic OS D. Nearing provided formalized first aid training to Somali guards at the relief agencies. His presentation was utilized to train teachers at the local schools which had been reopened by Canadian troops.

Humanitarian aid (voluntary) was also done at the local hospital three days a week. We taught local nurses about asepsis, basic nursing care, and proper operating room techniques. This experience proved to be very rewarding.

My time in Somalia went very quickly. While I was there, I was fortunate enough to have a visit from my then fiance. He was in Nairobi working as a logistics officer sending relief supplies to us and Sudan.

The deployment was an exceptional experience for me and one I would be willing to partake in anytime in the future.

Information Report by Lt. (N) Rebecca (Gowthorpe) Patterson
after she returned from duty at Belet Huen in Somalia
June 1993

I became involved with providing humanitarian aid down at the local Belet Huen Hospital in January 1993. We had proposed to the International Medical Corps that we help provide teaching and support at the hospital. By the time we had left in June of 1993, we had provided over 4,000 hours of support.

Belet Huen was the only hospital in Somalia that was not looted by bandits so the hospital structure that had been built by the Italians in the early 1980s still stood. Sadly, due to lack of pay and fear for their own well being, many of the local doctors and nurses had left the hospital leaving a few determined people to provide very rudimentary care to the patients that were there and also to manage a few pharmaceutical supplies that were available.

International Medical Corps took over support of the local hospital at the end of January 1993 and were also the providers of all the medication. Again, sadly, many of the medications and drugs that were intended for patient use were looted soon after they had entered the hospital pharmacy and sold on the local market or were taken for personal use of the staff.

The hospital was broken down into a number of wards. There was a pediatric ward, a male medical ward, a male surgical ward, a female medical surgical and everything else ward, and a baby delivery unit.

The assessment of the situation by myself, Mary Louise Van Aiken, and later Maggie Wideau and Hoppy Whitman from International Medical Corps revealed that the teachings of basic nursing skills were required for the general nursing staff. It was decided that Lt. (N) McIntyre would work with the operating room staff and that I would help teach the general ward nurses about basic asepsis, drug administration and basic nursing skills.

It should be noted that most of the nurses there were not nurses at all. Many, as I had stated previously had fled when the war started. Most of the nurses who worked on the ward were trained by the Italians prior to the outbreak of the war in 1990 and had stuck around. Any other staff that were working on the floors were interested people who had come in off the street and stated an interest in nursing and were being trained accordingly, and the training was based on what the nurses who were there decided was appropriate.

Training was one of the other areas we found dramatically lacking because the Italians had run the hospital right up to 1990 using the Somalis as the regular staff; there was no form of education or upgraded education for anybody there. It was also true that when the Italians were present, the Somalis were never given any positions of authority and very often were delegated to work positions. One of the areas that we decided to tackle was basics in service education, which is something we do here in Canada. What it allows people to do is upgrade their skills through classes that are provided throughout the working day.

We also decided, after having a look around the hospital, that a major cleanup was in order. The hospital was built in the form of a hollow square with all the wards facing into a courtyard. Before our arrival, dirty needles, used dressings, bed pans and human waste were just thrown outside the wards onto the ground. To say this created a health hazard was an understatement and it was given a priority for action.

Contaminated needles carried the hazards of hepatitis (rampant in the Somali population), HIV and a variety of other illnesses. After much brainstorming, we decided to introduce sharps containers. This is a system we use in Canada to collect used needles all in one place for safe disposal. We came up with the idea of old water bottles on each ward to collect sharps. One thing we forgot was that empty water bottles were a hot commodity for the locals and our sharps containers kept disappearing. We then started cutting holes in the bottles and provided extensive explanations which were given by a Somali interpreter as to how important it was to protect themselves as well as everyone else. Sadly we were not able to convince them as to the importance. I went away for two weeks on leave, and on my return I was told through the interpreter that the pediatric ward had thrown their containers away because they didn't think I was coming back! I wondered then if it was me or the uniform they cooperated with.

A great contribution we did make was to the use of a proper wound dressing team. Highly-motivated staff quickly picked up the techniques and hopefully decreased the high post-operative infection rate that was prevalent in the hospital. We communicated the concept of bacteria spreading between different patients in the form of hand-drawn pictures of small monsters travelling on the forceps of the dressing team members from one patient to the next.

The biggest test of our teaching skills came in the form of a 14-year-old boy who had second degree burns to at least 80% of his body after playing with fuel that had ignited. He had been left to die because one small infection to the burnt area could have killed him. He became our darling. We taught the Somali staff how to debride (remove dead tissue) him over a six-week period.

It is agony to have dead tissue removed and the best pain medication we could give him was injectable Aspirin. The Somali staff considered it prestigious to work with us and willingly helped and learned while we were there, but paid no attention to the patient when we were not there.

The boy did heal eventually. He was an orphan who lived with his grandfather. The grandfather had been sergeant major in Sid Barres military police force. They were a pleasure to care for and it was obvious they were pleased to see us. The grandfather told me that if he had been younger, he would have asked me to marry him. We both laughed.

There is a very sad conclusion to the story. When the boy was better, he developed a fever, headache and vomiting. All the doctors, both western and Somali, decided there was nothing wrong with him based on shabby lab work done by the local laboratory. He was sent home and was dead with cerebral malaria within two weeks. I had given him a photo of Ottawa covered with snow (which was very hard to explain). The delight on his face of being given this gift is how I will always remember this brave young man.

The most touching thing the grandfather did was to ask me (through an interpreter of course) if I would take a picture of him in his uniform. I, of course, agreed. The next day I was at the local hospital – he turned up with a bag under his arm. When he saw me he was very excited and ran off into the courtyard. When he returned, he was wearing an obviously old uniform meticulously pressed and repaired. His shoes had seen better days but were buffed to a high gloss and also repaired perfectly. He put his forage cap on, pace stick under his arm and stood smartly at attention to have his photo taken. I had the photos developed in Kenya when I was on my next R&R and presented it to him along with a photo of his grandson when I returned. They were so excited. It is probably the only memory the grandfather now has of the boy. What was more amazing was that he had no fear of being seen in the uniform of an army controlled by a despised man!

We spent many hours teaching the staff about basic hygiene, nursing skills and care of hospitalized patients.

Of course, not all our experiences were as positive. There was a small courtyard where we set up a chalkboard and small pieces of equipment. Each Thursday, Louisa and myself would teach classes to the Somalis. There were a number of stone benches that surrounded this tiny courtyard. We came in one day to find all the courtyard smeared with oil; Louisa looked at me and said it was because they were threatened and didn't want us to teach, and this turned out to be the case. It was very difficult to get the chairs clean and none of the staff came back to the area that had been sabotaged because of this reason.

We also became very frustrated with the fuss that went on when we delivered drugs (or rather IMC did). No matter what method of control we implemented, we were unsuccessful. Valium was a hot item because the locals would use it to come down off of a chat high. It was frustrating because the people who really needed the medications couldn't get any; the only place they could get drugs was out of the local pharmacy which had received the stolen goods in the first place.

There were many humorous events that occurred when blending the two cultures. To begin with, Lt. McIntyre and myself were a great source of curiosity to the local nurses. We found that as time went by, the best nurses to work with were the ones on the male surgical ward. When we first arrived on our initial tour, they were very interested in how Diane and I were dressed. First of all, they had to assess that we really were women and they wanted to know how old we were. When they found out that we were well over the age of 25, they wanted to know if we had children. It was as if they were trying to find something in common with us. When they found that we had no children they were shocked and they tried to figure out just why we were in the military. The conclusion they came to – as much to our amusement as theirs – was that we were in the military because we were barren and that was the criteria for being allowed to join! Working with them during that time, I made some very good friends with the nurses. Most had a few rudimentary words of English which they had learned in local schools prior to the war and they were very interested in what my plans were. I was due to get married after returning from Somalia and they wanted to know when I was having babies. This was the point they felt they had in common with me, and we all did much laughing comparing our cultural differences.

The patients themselves were very happy to have Canadians helping out with their care. We were concerned initially because we were military, but very soon after arrival they got used to the concept that we wore uniforms but we were also there to provide medical care and to teach their people. We had to be careful that we did not take over control or do all of the care for the staff. This is a tendency North Americans have and it took a lot of control not to do the same in an environment where they had to learn to do it themselves. The Somalis were very pleased that we were happy as well because they were guaranteed to receive good care. It got to the point that there were some long-term patients there who, whenever we went to do our rounds early in the morning, would greet us and by the end of our tour were particularly anxious that we not leave, because they knew they would really miss us. We had a lot of offers to trade wives, T-shirts, whatever.

Another factor that had to be considered when working with the Somalis was their concept of life and death. Death is not the most significant event in the family history, possibly partly due to their religious beliefs and probably partly due to the austere conditions in which they live. Death is very much an everyday part of life. A family member dies and that family member is quietly taken away, and the family mourns. They do not possess the ability to provide sophisticated medical care and they don't expect it. An elderly man ran into the hospital compound one morning and collapsed on the ground. People stood around until he died and the family took him away. It was quite a new concept for us all to grasp.

We knew we were accepted into the local medical staff when they started to invite us into their lives. The surgical team was invited to a local wedding and all of us received gifts from the staff when we left.

There were many incidents of kindness on behalf of the CF and the Canadian people. They are as follows:

The preventive medicine tech was consulted to set up water sanitation systems for the NGOs.

Hospital beds, equipment and supplies were donated by Trenton Memorial Hospital which was flown by Canadian aircrews from Trenton via Nairobi, Kenya to Belt Huen, Somalia.

Generators were supplied and repaired by the maintenance staff from the Airborne Regiment.

Running water was supplied by the maintenance staff who helped fix the pump in the local well, and repaired the water tank that belonged to the hospital.

X-ray equipment was all broken in the hospital. The Signals Platoon attempted to fix it and spent a great deal of time doing so.

The donation of at least $250,000 worth of medical supplies to the local hospital through IMC for the Somali people was a gift from the Canadian Government.

Individual soldiers donated children's clothing which was sent from home by the families.

Medical assistants developed programs such as first-aid programs that were to be taught to all the local schools in the area.

Though things were not always perfect, I truly believe that we helped to make a difference. The Somalis said that they were very sad to see us leave. Recently, I met some of the German doctors who replaced us and they assured me that the hospital is functioning quite independently now.

Barbara (Soanes) Gowthorpe

The following narrative is included because of the mother-daughter military affiliation. Barbara Gowthorpe, Royal Navy, married a Royal Canadian Navy man and their daughter Rebecca [Gowthorpe] Patterson) is a career nurse in the Canadian Forces.

Graduated and became a State Registered Nurse and a State Certified Midwife in England.

Military History:

Service: Royal Navy

Rank: Nursing Sisters didn't carry a rank but we were treated as officers.

Served: United Kingdom and Malta

My name is Barbara, but I have always been called Bunty by my nearest and dearest, and especially my dear maternal grandfather. He was a fisherman from an east coast port in England. My mother and I were the only ones in my immediate family who were passionately addicted to the sea. This was the reason, I think, that I always wanted to be a sailor. However, in 1953 when I left high school, the idea of such a thing for a girl was as remote as the moon. Consequently, I became a state registered nurse and state certified midwife by the age of 23.

During World War I, my paternal grandfather was on a fishing boat which was fitted with a gun and became an armed trawler. They were torpedoed by a German submarine and he was killed. During World War II, two of my uncles were killed at sea. My generation didn't have anyone interested in joining the Navy except me, so I applied to the British Admiralty and was accepted as a nursing sister in the Queen Alexandra's Royal Naval Nursing Service.

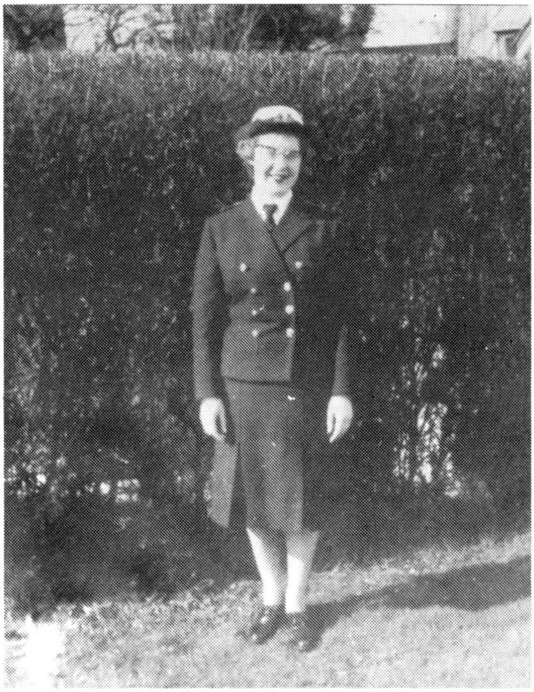

Nursing sister Barbara Soanes, Royal Navy, Norwich, England 1961. Mother of Lt (N) Rebecca (Gowthorpe) Patterson, CFMS

The nursing sisters didn't carry a service rank but we were treated like officers in every way. I started my service career in the Royal Naval Hospital, Haslar, Gosport. I learned a great deal and looked after cases of "the bends" and various tropical diseases of which I was completely ignorant before this. All was going well with my career until I had a patient in my ward who became very important to me in a non-professional way. In the 1960s we had to leave the service upon marriage, and when my posting came up to go to Malta, I knew that I would not be able to spend two years on the Island. The matron-in chief told me that I would have to accept the change.

The Royal Navy was taking over the David Bruce Military Hospital from the Army and I was one of the first to go there, mainly to work in the midwifery ward. We looked after service wives, including those of the Maltese Regiment. I was startled and rather appalled to have a couple of patients in my first week there who were delivering babies that they knew were already dead in utero. One lady was enduring her 17th pregnancy, and had only four living children. She sadly informed me that it was "Gods Will." The Maltese girls were beautiful, but their lives were so hard that by the time they were 30 they looked a great deal older.

The Island of Malta is very hilly and we used buses a great deal to travel around. On the bus, the driver does not sit directly behind the driving wheel, but behind and to one side of it. They consider that God is really driving. As the bus leaves, everyone on board crosses themselves! When you come to a steep hill, everyone gets out and walks behind the bus, to the top, including all the old ladies with their mountains of shopping.

I had to give three months' notice of my impending marriage, so my stay on Malta was only a few months. I returned to England and married my submariner stoker who was training in British Submarines. He had six more years to complete in the Royal Canadian Navy, so I became a happy Canadian and produced two daughters and a son. I never dreamed that my second daughter would become a nurse, and subsequently, an officer in the Canadian Armed Forces (N). She obviously takes after her mother and father! Perhaps one day she will do what I always wanted and get the chance to serve on a ship.

Chapter 14

CANADIAN FORCES MEDICAL SERVICES

The following address was given to the Nursing Sisters Association at their biennial meeting in Edmonton, 10 June, 1994 by Col. Marielle Gagné, Chief Nursing Officer Canadian Forces

THE CANADIAN FORCES MEDICAL SERVICES

At the end of WW II, the Royal Canadian Navy, the Canadian Army and the Royal Canadian Air Force had their own separate medical services. Some cooperation existed between these services; but essentially, they each were autonomous. Military hospitals and clinics were spread across the country and medical care was provided to military personnel, their families and to veterans.

In the mid-fifties, a review of the organization and provision of medical services was carried out; as a result, the three medical services were unified to reduce the unnecessary duplication of medical facilities between services, to standardize professional and technical training as well as personnel administration, and to achieve an economy of resources. This unification took effect on 15 January 1959 with the formation of the Canadian Forces Medical Services (CFMS) under the direction of one Surgeon General. The CFMS did not include medical personnel from the Reserve Forces; these personnel remained under the control of their respective service.

This reorganization which included the establishment of several regional medical headquarters both in Canada and abroad (Atlantic, Québec, Ontario, the Prairies and the Pacific as well as Germany) was fully implemented by 1963. Regional surgeons were responsible for the provision of medical support to service members and their dependants within their respective region and acted as medical advisors to senior regional operational commanders. Medical training was standardized; rank structures and promotion policies were adjusted to give equal opportunity for promotion to all members of the Canadian Forces Medical Services. Training for both officers and non-commissioned members (NCMs) was concentrated at the medical school in Borden and medical personnel became eligible to serve with either service regardless of their respective uniform.

Further changes occurred in 1967 with the unification of the three Services. Functional commands were then established and the role of regional commanders enhanced; they were given more control of medical resources within their regions.

In the early 70s, upon the adoption of the national health policy, the provision of medical care to dependants was gradually transferred to the provinces except for those units where care was not available elsewhere. Veterans' care was also gradually transferred to the provinces. Today, NDMC is the only military hospital which provides medical care to veterans albeit the veterans' ward will be relocated to the Perly Hospital once its construction is completed (about 1996).

In the late 80s, the Canadian Forces hospitals were grouped under one headquarters called the Canadian Forces Hospitals and Medical Supply System (CFHMSS); this HQ is responsible for the provision of fourth line (hospital level care) health care to military personnel. This formation will be renamed Canadian Forces Medical Group (CFMG) this fall.

Current Medical Facilities. The following is a list of medical facilities:

a. Canadian Forces Hospitals (50 beds and over, institution providing fourth line care): NDMC, Halifax, Valcartier.

b. Canadian Forces Base Hospitals (5-50 bed institutions providing primary care): Esquimalt, Comox, Chilliwack, Calgary, Edmonton, Winnipeg, Borden, Trenton, Petawawa, St. Jean (Qc), Gagetown, Greenwood.

c. Canadian Forces Base Clinics (an out-patient clinic with no beds): North Bay, Shearwater, Goose Bay, Toronto, St. Hubert (Qc), Geilenkirchen (Germany).

The CF has three field ambulances which are responsible to collect and transport casualties in time of conflict. These field ambulances are staffed by medical officers, medical assistants, administrators, etc. They are currently being deployed in the former Yugoslavia, on a rotation basis; and for the purpose of this mission, their establishment is augmented with a surgical team. This team consists of one surgeon, one anaesthetist, one intensive care nurse, two operating room nurses and two operating room technicians.

Primary care for operational units such as regiments, battalions, squadrons, etc., is provided through a Unit Medical Station (UMS). These UMS are established for medical officers and medical assistants, or medical assistants alone depending on the size of the unit being supported; in the case of smaller operational units, medical care may be provided by the closest medical unit. Aeromedical evacuations are carried out by personnel employed at air command units. Medical care aboard ships is provided by medical assistants with the three larger ships or supply ships also being established for a medical officer.

CFMS STRENGTH

The strength of the Canadian Forces is now less than 75,000 with about 18,000 officers and 62,000 non commissioned members (NCMs); female personnel represent about 11.2% of the total strength. The Reserves included about 34,500 members. The CFMS strength is 2,728. This includes 1,043 officers and 1,685 non-commissioned members. Of the officers, 348 are medical officers, 370 nursing officers, 143 are health care administrators and the remaining 185 include pharmacists, physiotherapists, social workers, and medical associate officers (radiology, laboratory, biosciences, preventive medicine). Among the NCMs, 1,375 are medical assistants, 310 are either operating room technicians, laboratory technicians, X-ray technicians, preventive medicine technicians or aeromedical technicians.

HISTORICAL PERSPECTIVE NURSING OCCUPATION

Nurses have been affiliated with the military since the North-West rebellion in 1885. Since then, they were deployed during the Boer War, WW I, WW II and the Korean War. Between the Korean War and 1990, nursing officers worked in peacetime conditions, and often times operational requirements were forgotten. Then came 1990 and the Gulf War.

During this conflict, nursing officers were deployed in Saudi Arabia with the Canadian Field Hospital, aboard HMCS *Protecteur* and USN *Mercy* and as members of critical stress teams. A total of 35 nursing officers served with 1 Canadian Field Hospital, six served aboard the USN *Mercy* and four on HMCS *Protecteur*. Nursing officers have since been deployed in support of UN missions to Somalia and to the former Yugoslavia for a period of six months, as members of the surgical team attached to the Field Ambulance. One team was deployed to Somalia, while a fifth team has just left this past May for the former Yugoslavia.

By the way, I would like to say that we are no longer called nursing sisters. Times have changed and there are now several male nursing officers within the occupation; in fact, they represent 14% of our total strength. Since the early 70s we have been called nursing officers as opposed to nursing sisters; also, we no longer wear the veil or the cap and we identify ourselves by rank and name as opposed to "sisters."

UNIFORMS

In 1967, upon unification, all service members wore a common "green" uniform. In the mid 80s, the CF went back to the three colour uniforms. Although members now affiliate with one environment, i.e., Air Force, the Army and the Navy, it does not affect the employment of medical personnel. An Army nursing officer can be employed with the Air Force, and Navy nursing officer with Army, and so on.

NURSING OFFICER RANK STRUCTURE

With the recent closure of units including Canadian Forces Europe, the strength of the nursing occupation has decreased. The current manning level of the occupation is 370 the following structure: Colonel: 1, LCol: 2 , Maj: 25, Capt/Lt: 342. Over one-third of the nurses are married with the majority being married to service members. Career managers do their utmost to post married members to the same unit or base, but a "husband and wife" team cannot be employed in the same chain of command (in other words, one cannot be a supervisor to the other). Female personnel can have children and remain in the Forces as long as they are willing to meet all service requirements (including operational deployments).

ENROLMENT

Nurses can join the Armed Forces as a Direct Entry Officer after completing nursing training or under the Regular Officer Training Plan at which time they could be sponsored for the duration of their studies. The latter programme results in a period of obligatory service. There is also a possibility for a non-commissioned member to become a nursing officer under the University Training Plan for Men.

The initial period of service is nine years. On completion of this period, nursing officers are eligible for an intermediate engagement which will bring them to 20 years of service. At that time, they become eligible for an indeterminate engagement, i.e., until age 55. Nursing officers can be employed in hospitals, clinics or at the Canadian Forces Medical School, and they can also be employed as staff officer (mostly out-of occupation).

TRAINING

Upon joining the Forces all officers must go to the Basic Officer Training School for a period of 10 weeks. This training is completely integrated and nursing officers is only one of the occupations represented. They learn the basic rudiments of the military including leadership skills, rules and regulations, military skills, field exercises, etc..

The next course is the Basic Nursing Officer Course. This course introduces students to the Medical Services, and places some emphasis on the clinical skills which they will need while employed in a hospital or clinic and during contingency deployments. In the course of their career, nursing officers can train in the following specialties: intensive care, operating room nursing, psychiatric nursing, community health nursing and obstetrics (a basic course required prior to a posting to an isolated area).

OPERATIONAL TRAINING

Operational training includes a three-week basic field course, aeromedical evacuation, cardiac life/trauma support. Several staff/nursing administration courses are also offered to nursing officers to prepare them for positions of an administrative nature. These courses are either given within the military or through civilian institutions. Additionally, they have the opportunity to be sponsored for Baccalaureate of Nursing or Master of Nursing studies.

Chapter 15

SERVING WITH THE ROYAL CANADIAN NAVY

Dorothy (Price) Airey
Nora (Wilks) Britton
Monica (Laturnus) Drew
Joan (Story) Giles
Marjorie (Cowan) Horton
Doris G. (Heels) Jackson
Ann (Mossman) Kaump
Rosine (Gammon) Long
Clara (Watson) Meade
Helen Ott
Marian (Duncan) Pangman
Jean (Glanville) Smyth
K. Elizabeth (Gardner) Smythies
Lilla Wright

During World War One hospital care for the Navy was provided by the RCAMC. By 27 July 1917 a medical facility opened at Admiralty House on Gottingen Street, Halifax, Nova Scotia, with accommodation for 50 patients. There was a surgeon, three medical officers, two registered nurses and ten sick berth attandants.

It was officially named Royal Canadian Naval Hospital on 26 October 1917. (1)

Not so well known was the existence of a Naval hospital ship on the West Coast during World War One.

SS *Prince George* was chartered as a Royal Canadian Fleet Auxiliary vessel and fitted out as a hospital ship complete with operating room on the upper deck and staffed with a medical officer, six registered nurses and two sick berth stewards engaged locally. Only the nurses didn't have reserve training. (4)

Because there was evidence of German naval activity on the West Coast, SS *Prince George* left Esquimalt to join the *Rainbow* which was protecting two Royal Navy sloops. They met north of San Francisco without encountering enemy ships, so they returned to Esquimalt. Because of possible enemy action near Prince Rupert, the *Prince George* continued on to that area, again without encountering the enemy. After 47 days of service, the *Prince George* was returned to her owner 23 September 1917. (4)

ROYAL CANADIAN NAVY, WORLD WAR TWO

As in World War One, there were no Naval hospitals by the outset of World War Two. The medical care for RCN personnel was provided by RCAMC medical officers. Members of the sick berth branch provided most of the nursing care. Facilities ashore were sick bays, one in Halifax, and one in Esquimalt. Local military and civilian hospitals provided additional care. (2)

The RCN expanded rapidly in World War Two. Separate hospitals and nursing sisters were needed to care for the sick and wounded. The RCN nursing branch was established in late 1941. Temporary Naval hospitals were constructed at Halifax and Esquimalt. Permanent hospitals were added later. As Naval bases opened, hospitals were built or acquired at Cornwallis, Sydney and Shelburne in Nova Scotia, St. Hyacinthe in Quebec, St.John's in Newfoundland and Greenoch in Scotland. There were three special units at Montreal and St. Agathe in Quebec, and at Kingston, Ontario. (1)

On 29 December 1941 nursing sisters Olive Olga Wilson, Mary B. Brydon and Joan M.D. Russell were retired from the RCAMC for the purpose of joining the Naval nursing service. From the original three nurses recruited in December of 1941, 343 were recruited by the end of the War. Marjorie Gordon Russell became the first woman to fill the position of matron-in -chief of the Royal Canadian Navy Nursing Service with the Royal Canadian Naval Hospital at Halifax as her headquarters. (3)

When the medical branch was restructured effective 1 August 1951 it consisted of four sections; medical officer (surgeon); medical administrative officer (MAd); nursing officer (MN); and medical technical officer (MT).

The distinguishing colors were maroon, although surgeons continued to use scarlet. (4)

References:
1. *Three Centuries of Canadian Nursing*, John Murray Gibbon and Mary S.Mathewson. The Macmillan Company of Canada Limited 1947. pp.458-60
2. Martime Command Museum, Admiralty House, CFB Halifax, N.S.
3. Department of National Defence, Ottawa, Canada. 28 August, 1941. Quote No. 54-27-93-3
4. *Operation Sick Bay: The Story of the Sick Berth & Medical Assistant Branch of the Royal Canadian Navy*, Lieut.Commander (MAd) S.T. Richards, RCN (Ret'd), Cantaur Publishing, West Vancouver, BC. pp. 23-25; 45; 51-53; 167; 205

Dorothy I. (Price) Airey

Graduated from: Victoria Hospital School of Nursing, London, Ontario. Year: 1936

Military History:

Service: RCN

Rank: Sub-Lieut. Nursing Sister

Served: February 1942 to May 1944

My first husband, Capt. F.W. Wiggins, Permanent Force, was killed overseas in 1941 and I felt I must go into the Service to help.

My posting in Esquimalt at HMCS *Naden* was particularly interesting and the leadership of Matron Olive (Wilson) Roblin was truly a pleasure. Our friendship is ongoing and she has moved to Stratford, Ontario, and joined our Nursing Sisters Unit in London, Ontario.

Nora (Wilks) Britton

Graduated from: Toronto General Hospital School of Nursing. Year: 1940

Military History:

Service: RCN

Rank: Sub-Lieut. N/S

Served: November 1942 to June 1945.

I was nursing in Bermuda at the time of Pearl Harbour and decided I would join whichever service would take me. Soon after returning to Canada from Bermuda, I was called by the Royal Canadian Navy. After serving a short time in Halifax, I joined the first nursing sisters already stationed on HMCS *Niobe* in Scotland. We took a circuitous route through rural U.S.A. arriving in New York only to find our ship, the *Queen Elizabeth*, had already departed. We were taken out by tugboat to meet the great *QE* and climbed over the side. Seventeen excited Canadian nurses were given a royal welcome.

Monica (Laturnus) Drew

Graduated from: St. Joseph's Hospital School of Nursing, Victoria. Year: 1941

Military History:

Service: RCN

Rank: Sub-Lieut. N/S

Served: December 1, 1944 to May 17, 1946

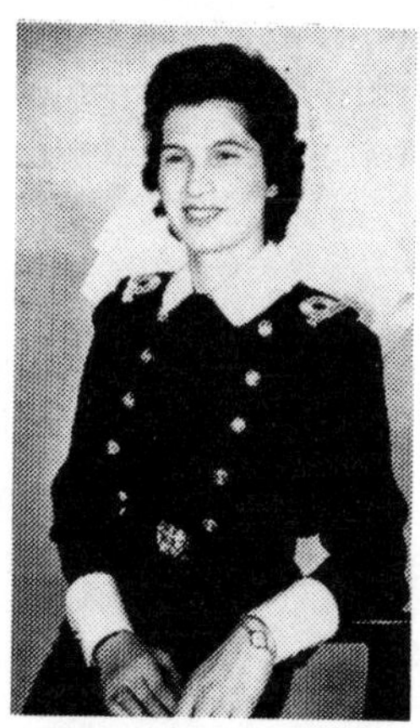

Sub-Lieut. Monica (Laturnus) Drew

When I chose a military career I wanted to help, I wanted to be a part of the war effort. Also, two of my brothers were killed, one in the Army and the other in the Air Force.

My military experience consisted of general duty nursing at HMCS *Naden*, Esquimalt, B.C.

Joan (Story) Giles

Graduated from: Halifax Infirmary School of Nursing, Nova Scotia. Year: 1940

Military History:

Service: RCN

Rank: N/S, Sub-Lieut. RCN (T)

Served: February 9, 1942 to July 12, 1946

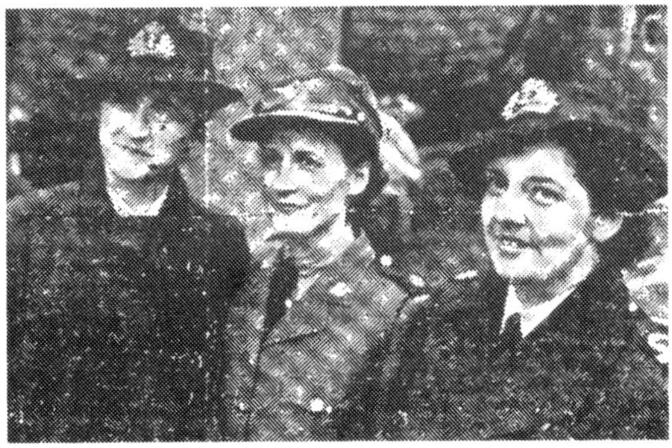

Major Alice Sorby, CWAC and nursing sisters S. Beck and J. Story arrive in England

I think one of the reasons I chose a military career was the fact that my father had been in the First World War and a prisoner; and also, having come in contact in my hospital with the Merchant seaman who had been sunk off the coast of Nova Scotia.

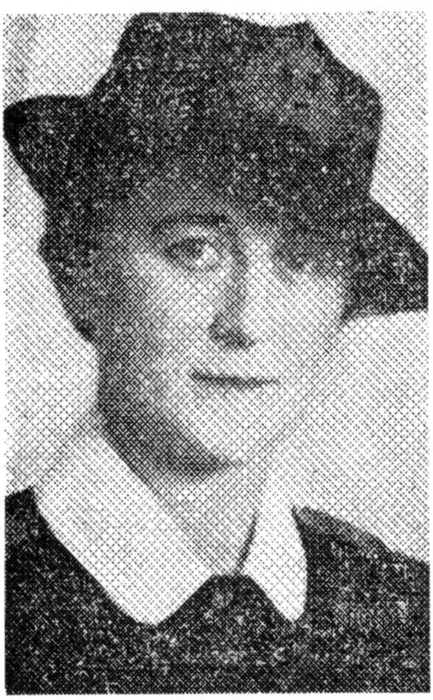

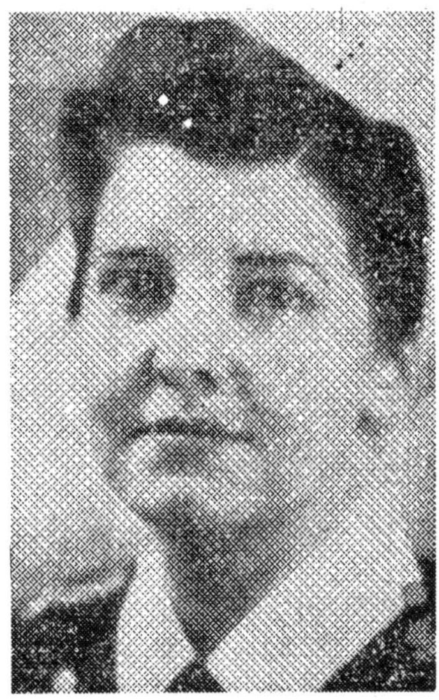

Two Halifax women are the first in a group of six Royal Canadian Naval nursing sisters to arrive overseas. Nursing sister Shirley Beck, left above, of Middle Musquodoboit, was accepted as a navy nurse in December 1941. Nursing sister Joan Story, right above, Halifax, was accepted in the Naval nursing service in February 1942.

ROCKHEAD HOSPITAL

After being in the Navy a month I was put on night duty in old Ward A to hear in the night report. There was a very sick young patient from St. Pierre and Miquelon, a boy seaman in the Free French Navy. He was diagnosed as having a suspect pneumonia. He did not speak any English, and for some reason, neither understood what was said, nor could make himself understood. When I neared the bed, there was a very offensive odour. It immediately reminded me of some of my last days in training when I was one of the nurses assigned to nurse a Merchant Navy man with typhoid fever.

I knew it was urgent to isolate him immediately, and as the one private room on the ward was occupied, I cleared the MO's office of desk, etc., and we moved the bed in. I tried my schoolgirl French on him. He understood me and I found out the pain was in his abdomen, not the chest. Next A.M. he was transferred to RCN Rockhead Hospital for Infectious Diseases.

I don't know whether or not it was because of this that I found myself six weeks later on the way to take up duty on that ward. Imagine my surprise when the first room I went into, I saw my boy seaman and was greeted in English. I neglected to say I had given him my French grammar before he left. When he was finally discharged a few weeks later, he made quite a speech to all.

I must say the hospital was quite an education. It was very old, uneven floors, no running water, no cupboards in the rooms. Isolation techniques were very primitive and to get the SBAs to remember to maintain technique was a job in itself. Each room had a small table outside the door with a basin of water, a scrub brush and green soap, a coat rack and gown. The staff all had masks and the female staff dispensed with their veils for OR caps.

We were kept very busy as all personnel from the Army, Navy and Air Force were sent there. It seemed all those recruited from the farms and small communities across the country, not being exposed to childhood diseases, fell like flies. The beds gave way to bunks, and at one time there were 120 cases of mumps as well as everything else in abundance! It is nice to be able to say that there were no cases of cross infection at that time. In mid-July of 1942 I was posted overseas.

In the spring of 1944 I was again posted to Rockhead and found many changes – a matron and a big increase in staff. The upper floor was a psychiatric ward and had its own staff. By this time, there were Wrens as well as the male sick berth attendants. There were many funny moments at Rockhead too. I will never forget coming on duty at midnight and needing to ask the duty MO for an order. I knocked on the door, was told to come in, and found him sitting on the radiator playing a flute. At one time, another sister was asked to play the Ouija board with him.

It is customary in the Navy for officers at Christmas to serve the meal at lunch time, which the MOs and nursing sisters did before we had our own meal. When it came our turn, we had just finished when some SBAs came with a large box and presented it to me. It was one box inside another, and when we finally got to the final box, found it contained a baby bottle of rum! This poem appeared in the bottle:

'Twas the night before Christmas
and all through Rock-head
Not a creature was stirring
They're probably all dead;
But not Sister Story
'Cause she's in her glory - -
Drinkin rum from a bottle instead.
She must drink in one gulp,
Or be kissed to a pulp - -
By the Tiffies who said she was scared.

In late 1945 after peace was declared, the personnel, of course, started returning home; the matron left Rockhead and I was appointed acting matron and stayed there to close the ward and move it to a ward in the old original RCN hospital until I left in May 1946 when I received my discharge.

MEMORIES OF HMCS *NIOBE*

Having been bombed out at Plymouth in 1941, the base had been moved to Scotland and now occupied the lands of the former Smithston Asylum and Poor Farm. (I always wondered where they put all the former inmates.) The entrance to the grounds was over a bridge above the rail track, and many a member of the personnel had a severe shock in the very dark night-time hours. Not realizing that the track dipped down quite sharply, it looked as if the train was coming right at you.

The base consisted of a huge, ancient-looking building and a modern 100-bed hospital. There was a farm attached, including pigs and the Fever Hospital, which was independent of the base. The hospital was about 500 yards from the main building.

The four nursing sisters from the East Coast were informed mid-July they would be going overseas, and were sent to the office of the officer responsible for the movement of personnel overseas. We asked if there were any particular items we should take with us. He said we would be able to have trunk, duffel bag and suitcase. The things suggested struck us as funny – an evening dress, pants on board ship, bedspread, travel rug, as much toilet paper as we could get in and Moirs Chocolate Mounds – they were about a half-inch across and filled with vanilla cream!

We went aboard the Cunard ship SS *Cameronia*; a very old vessel. We proceeded to sit and wait for the girls from the West Coast, N/S. L.E. Wright and N/S F. Hodson and the rest of the complement – Army, Navy and Air Force. There was also Major Alice Sorby, the first CWAC officer to go over.

There were two bands aboard, so we did not lack entertainment – an Air Force band and an Army band.

We sailed on August 6th in a convoy of 42 ships made up of escort ships and the first of the U.S. troops going overseas, and our ship, the *Cameronia*, which every morning at daylight would be lagging well behind. Apparently, the captain did not like convoys. This went on for two or three days until there was a signal from the leader of the escort vessel (I think by this time we had changed to RN escort); he proceeded to ride herd on us by having a large Naval vessel on each side of us. We were then told to be quiet or the Germans would hear us.

The convoy split and the majority went to Iceland; we proceeded to the Clyde, where we parted company with our escort. When we saw the first signs of bombing, everyone moved from port to starboard; the ship tipped so we were ordered to boat stations until we reached Glasgow. We were met by an officer and driver, and after a hair-raising drive on the left hand side of the road, arrived at Greenock on August 18th, 1942.

On arriving at the quarterdeck we were piped aboard by the Bos'n, and this occurred every time we returned from the hospital. Our quarters were just above the quarterdeck, and completely separate from other rooms. There was not a sentry posted but the door was under the eye of the sentry on duty below. We met the captain and our fellow officers at dinner in the officers dining room. Afterwards, except for formal occasions, we had our own mess.

An amusing incident was the fact the captain insisted we go to the greenhouse to see the passion flower in bloom; we had not even unpacked!

Next A.M. we were introduced to the hospital staff and patients. The PMO was Surg. Commander R. Ruttan and the Surgeon, Lt. J. Frost. We were all presented with huge keys which had to be carried at all times in the hospital, as every door, when shut, would automatically lock. The keys were about five inches long and resulted in many holey apron pockets! The doors were soundproof and had only a small round window at eye level. I was locked in the pharmacy.

Nursing Sister Wright's description does not need me to repeat or to add to her improvisations. We received a very seriously injured Army private (he had walked in front of a Bren gun) and the surgeon called for a gastric suction, so an MO asked me to help find it in the pharmacy, the SBA in charge not being on duty. There was not one, so he proceeded to find bits and pieces to make one; all was complete except for a small balloon for the end of a tube. I suggested the thumb of a rubber glove – not big enough. He decided to use a condom, and it worked. I don't know who was blushing most, both being on the quiet side.

N/S Beck was matron in charge and N/S Tilling was in charge of the OR. Two of us worked shifts 8-4 and 4-12; the night hours were covered by an SBA and the duty medical officer who was quartered in the hospital.

The weather was very depressing and from the time we landed until mid-November we hardly saw the sun. It was always, "Scotch Mist." Our favourite walk off duty was climbing up behind the base to the Cut; a walk stretching for miles around the town water supply and miles of heather. I remember not being able to resist pulling a huge clump and putting it on the hearth in front of the blocked fireplace in the bedroom, and the huge black slug which greeted us in the morning – it was about four inches long, ugh!

So many funny things occurred, it is hard to know what to include. Christmas was fun, despite being so far from home.

It started when we got the holly and found it had no berries, so I got some straws and tied short pieces on it. I found the straws in the shop where we used to buy books; and then we decided to make ornaments. The holly looked very realistic and some of the wardroom guests wanted to know where we got it, as none of it had berries that year.

I remember our own entertainment when we decided to ask one of the SBAs if he could get us some wine, so Beryl said to get three bottles. When he brought them, he said he had a bottle of brandy for the nursing sisters from the SBAs. She put it all together in the wardrobe. Then, when she got the three bottles to give to the wine steward to mix, she just grabbed three bottles. We invited our guests for wine and the Christmas cake we had from home. The event was a great success. Everyone said the wine was excellent! After dinner we were invited to the wardroom, and those not invited wanted to know what we had served; I guess the guests had felt no pain! Poor Beryl, when she realized what had happened.

Another incident worth mentioning, I think, was the ENSA concert. The ship's company was assembled with the officers and the nursing sisters in the front row. The concert was good, and the fact there were ladies was greeted with glee. Most of us soon realized our "ladies" were male but two of the sisters didn't tumble. Their faces were a riot at the end of the concert.

Then there was the evening dress – a housecoat we got in a fancy dress shop in Glasgow, despite not having coupons. It was beautiful.

Speaking of Christmas, we were informed that it was customary for all officers to go to the CPO and POs mess on Christmas Day. Being the only two not on duty at the time, we had to attend. That horrible beer with the pieces in it. Not being a beer drinker, I could not face it and was told it was insulting if I did not drink it all. I managed a few mouthfuls and someone took pity on me and transferred it to their glass.

I must mention, the base was getting larger and larger each day and we were very busy and very relieved when in March five more sisters arrived, N/Sisters White, Patterson, Henderson, Wilks and Palmquist. With the increased staff it was much easier; several purchased bicycles and many trips and picnics were held when off duty.

In September, five of the "old originals" and one who came in the spring were transferred back to Canada. We sailed on the *Queen Mary* on September 29, the day before my birthday. It was quite eventful, transferring from the tender to the *Mary* at

Greenock. Not easy with choppy water. We expected a rapid trip home but the subs were waiting for us just outside the Clyde and we zigzagged all over the Atlantic. We were as far south as the Sargasso Sea and saw flying fish. This time we were not the only females aboard; there were 26 war brides going to the States, and then there were the German POWs quartered in the swimming pool!

We landed in New York and were taken to the Barbizon Plaza Hotel where they were expecting six male sub-lieutenants! We had to pay our own hotel bills, and after two days were taken to the station and supplied with tickets for the train. All was well until we hit Boston and found we had to change stations to proceed to Halifax. By this time five of us were broke and it was not until we were well into New Brunswick that Lilla Wright found she had a small cheque in her purse. We arrived in Halifax in the middle of the night and found my father at the station to meet me. He had the means of finding out when we were arriving, (RCMP. Supt. J.C. Story) after my call from New York as soon as I landed.

A few days later the separations began, but by room-mate, Lillian Wright and I are still best friends.

Marjorie (Cowan) Horton

Graduated from: Regina General Hospital School of Nursing. Year: 1934

Military History:

Service: RCN

Rank: Lieut. Nursing Sister and Matron

Served: 24 February 1942 to 2 November 1945

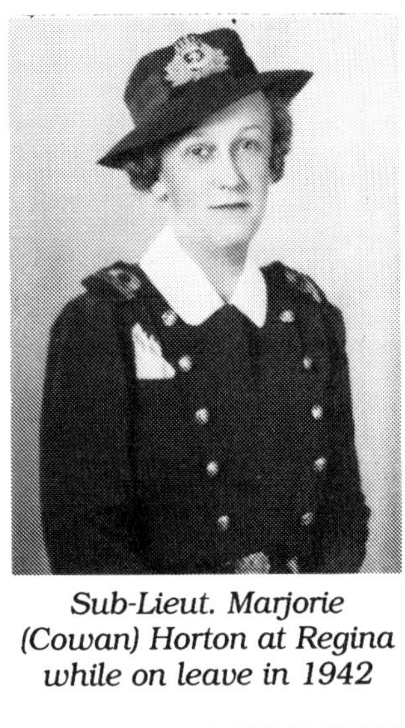

Sub-Lieut. Marjorie (Cowan) Horton at Regina while on leave in 1942

When we first became nursing sisters, we (at that time) did not return a salute; we were told to acknowledge a salute with "a smile or a nod, but never a wink." In due course, we had a class to teach us the correct Naval salute.

To go back to 1942 – seven of us

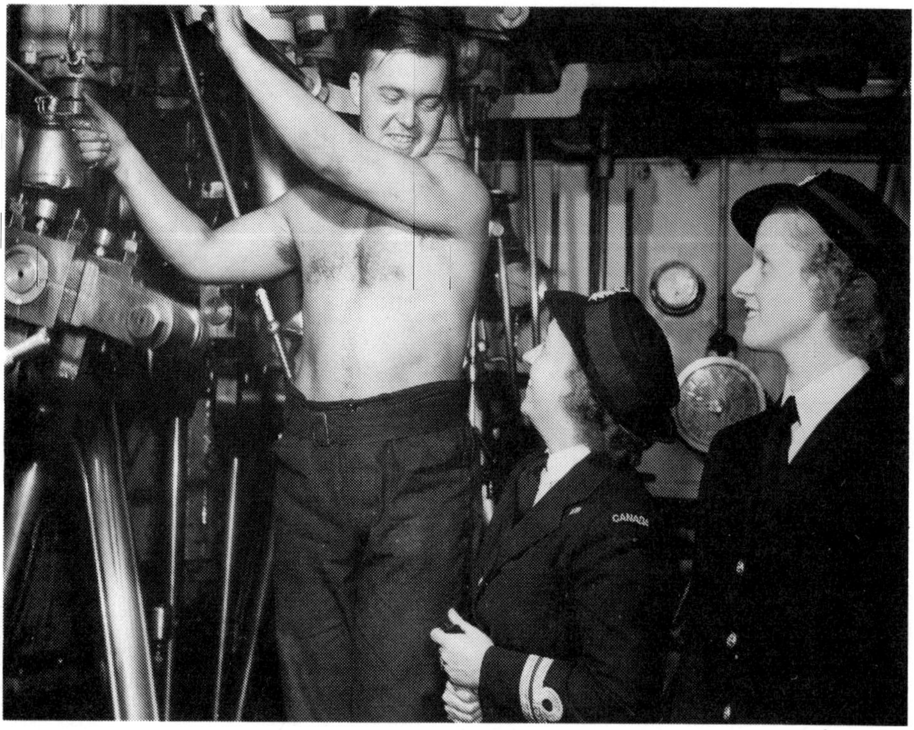

NAVY NURSES
Final step in a course outlined for Naval Nursing Sisters to make them more familiar with the history, routine and operations of the Royal Canadian Navy is a trip at sea in a minesweeper. Hottest place aboard ship is the engine room, but the nurses included it in their tour of inspection. ERA Don Smith, RCNVR, Winnipeg, explains the workings of the ship's engines to Matron Marjorie Cowan, Regina and N/S Audrey Hunter, Montreal. Canadian Forces photo S2060-4. Photographer R. Keegan, RCNVR Sept. 16th 1944.

arrived in St. John's; we used a part of the St. John's General Hospital's nurses residence until our own building was ready. We had a busy summer with many casualties. In October, Matron Evelyn Stibbard told Agnes Wilkie and I to decide which one would go out on leave. We tossed a coin – Agnes won and went with dietitian Margaret Brooke to visit friends and family in Winnipeg.

I have a letter Agnes mailed to me 10 October 1942 from Montreal enroute back to St. John's, which I received 13 October 1942 at RCNH St. John's. She told of their train trip back to Montreal and described a fancy breakfast they had enroute to Montreal. They were to catch the passenger car-ferry (the *Caribou*) at North Sydney ferry terminal the evening of October 13th.

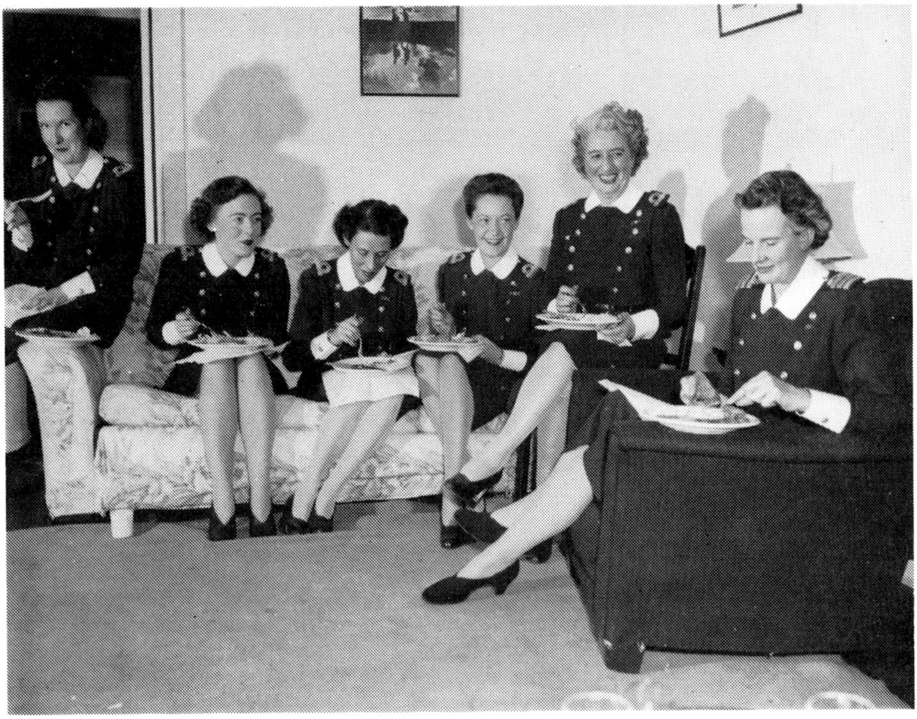

A picture taken of some of the nurses, during a visit by Marjorie Russell to St. John's, NFLD. From left to right: Eleanor Waines; Pat Rand; name unknown; Hope Thompson; Perry Harper; and Marjorie Russell.

On pages 76 and 103 of the *Night of the Caribou* by Douglas How, which tells about the ship being torpedoed that night, the two nursing sisters are frequently mentioned. It is also noted that Agnes became the first Canadian nursing sister to die due to enemy action in World War Two.

At the time of the 50th year since it happened, Madeleine (Connolly) O'Dea sent a copy of the St. John's newspaper with the write-up as well as a picture of the staff at that time. Maddy and I keep in touch with Christmas letters. She lives in St. John's.

In August 1944, five of us went on a mine sweeper to clear the channels for the ship bringing Winston Churchill to Quebec City for a conference with Roosevelt and MacKenzie King to discuss the Allied invasions of Italy and France. We did not know until we were at sea that it was a special trip because of Churchill. We saw the ship in distance and that was as close as we came to seeing Mr. Churchill!

During the day, a corvette came into view returning to

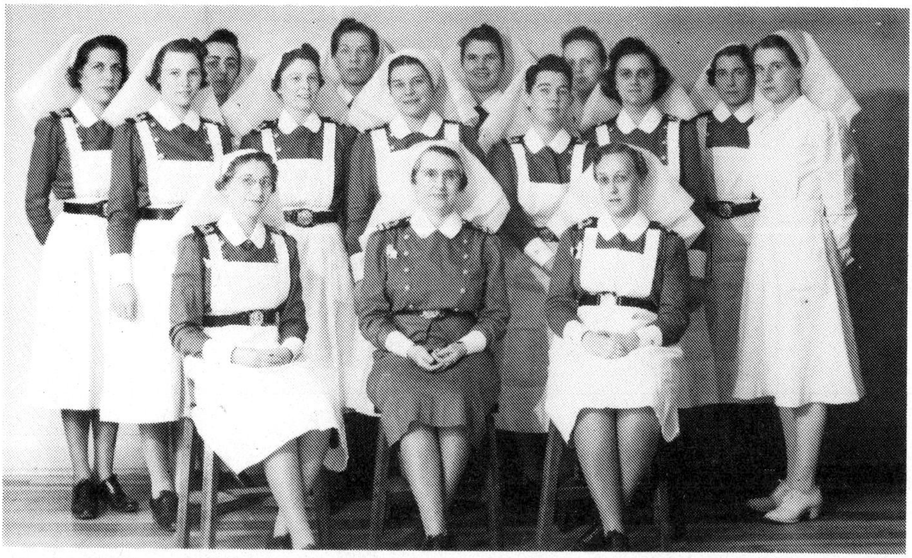

Back row from left: Edna Belden Rosier; Dorothy Halpenny; Jessie Muir Dodds; Margaret MacLean; Madeline Connolly O'Dea.
Middle row from left: Margaret Greene Oke; Gladys Carley; Margaret Waterman; Betty Summers; Dorothy Sanderson.
Front row from left: Agnes Wilkie; Mrs. Evelyn Stibbard; Marjory Cowan Horton.
Canadian Forces photo NF 497

Canada. I recognized the ship's number, and the captain was a friend. An officer on the minesweeper asked if I would like to send a message. I said, *"Yes. Welcome back to Canada."* The officer came back with the reply, *"The matron is invited aboard."* I asked how? Was I to swim ? No, they'd rig up a bos'n (boatswain) chair to take me to the other ship. I replied, *"Thank you very much, but not today."*

A few weeks after our trip on the minesweeper, my friend, the captain, presented me with a lamp made from a four-inch shell. The chap (sailor) who lost the winning pool from their expected time of arrival in Halifax made it for me. The engraving on the lamp merely states the date, ship name and: "The Matron was afraid to get her feet wet." How true.

When visiting Ottawa some years ago, my husband and I went to the parliament buildings. We stopped to see the book called, I believe, the *Book of Memory* which lists all those who lost their lives while defending their country. The caretaker of the book opened it up for Morly and I to see Agnes' name. A page is turned every day as I recall.

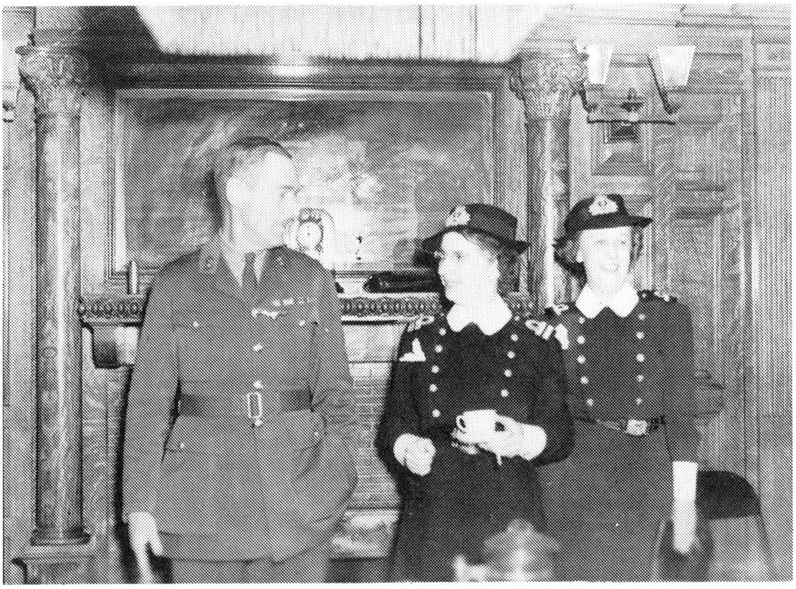

L-R: Army Colonel; Mrs Evelyn Stibbard; Marjorie Cowan Horton.
photo taken at Army mess, St. John's, NFLD.

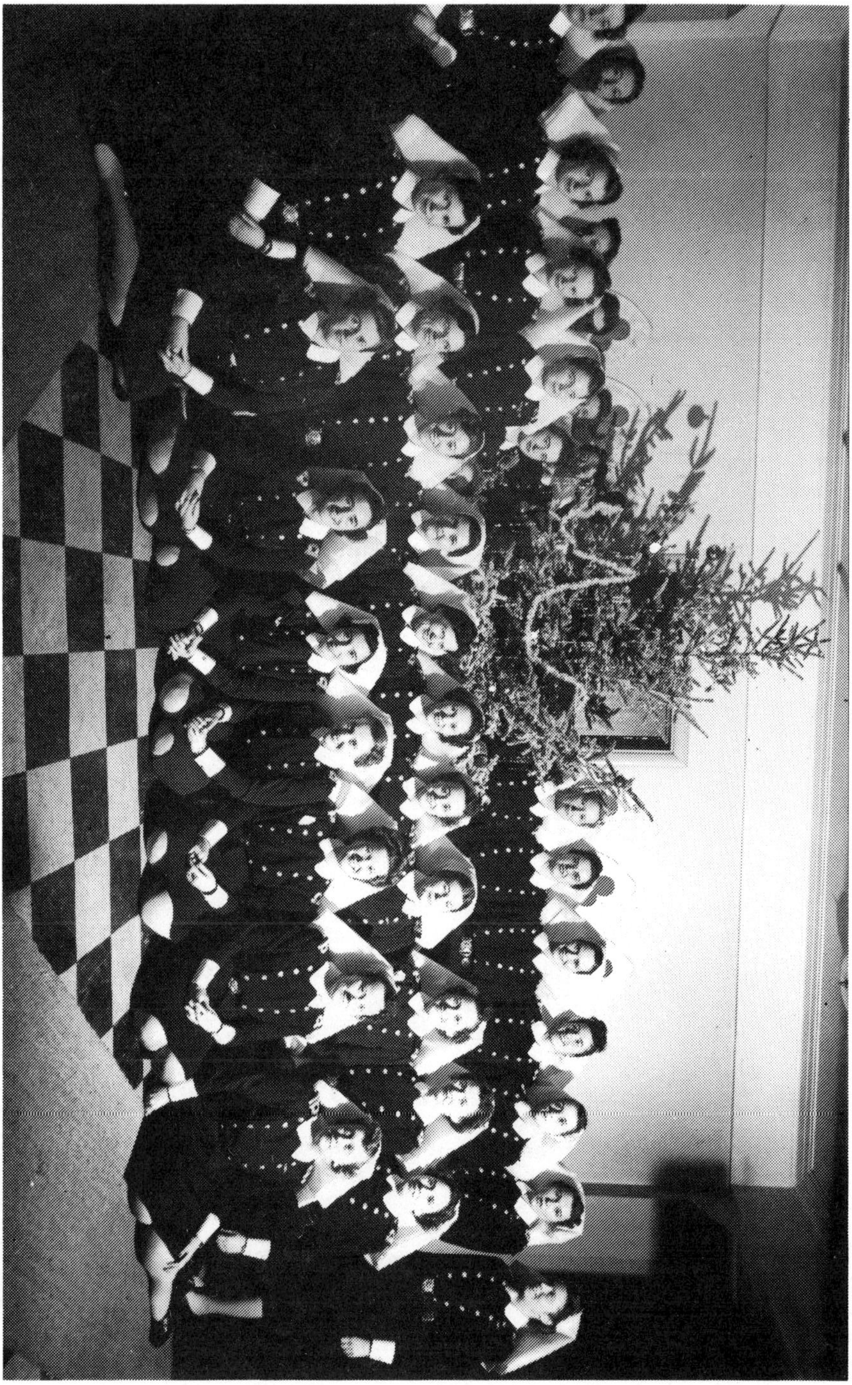

HMCS Stadacona, Royal Canadian Naval Hospital, Halifax, after Christmas carols on the wards December 1944.

Doris G. (Heels) Jackson

Graduate from: St. Andrews Hospital School of Nursing, Midland, Ontario. Year: 1942

Military History:

Service: RCN

Rank: Sub-Lieut. N/S

Served: 1944 to November 1947

It was wartime and I wanted to be associated with any of the Services. I signed up for all three – the Navy answered first. I loved it!

One the highlights of my military experience was being attached to RCN Hospital at HMCS *Stadacona* on VE Day and being downtown to witness the devastation of the riots. The Navy personnel were then confined to barracks for a short period.

I was at HMCS *Stadacona* helping to set up wards where we expected the survivors of a torpedoing just off Halifax, namely the Bangor mine sweeper vessel HMCS *Esquimalt*, which was sunk on April 16, 1945 with the loss of 44 lives. The 26 survivors were treated for the effects of their long immersion.

I was in Halifax when the troop ship, *Ile de France*, returned from overseas carrying nearly 10,000 servicemen.

It was a very exciting time in my life as I recall!

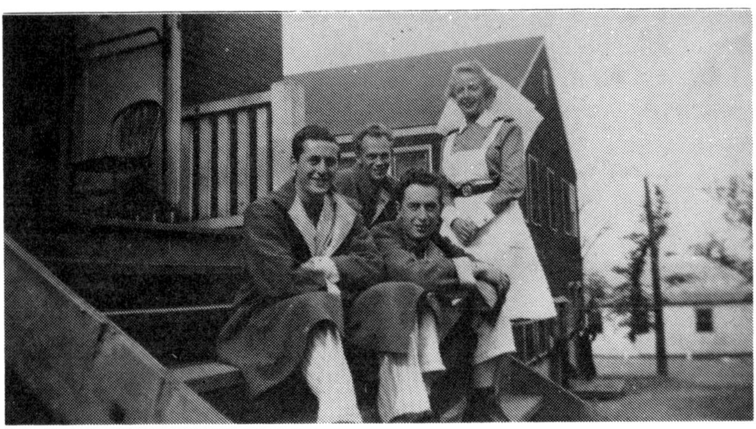

Sub-Lieut. Doris (Heels) Jackson and patients in one of the annexes at Royal Canadian Naval Hospital, HMCS Stadacona, *Halifax, NS, 1944*

Anne (Mossman) Kaump

Graduated from: Royal Jubilee Hospital School of Nursing, Victoria, B.C. Year: 1942

Military History:

Service: RCN

Rank: Sub-Lieut. N/S

Served: 16 October 1944 to 23 March 1946

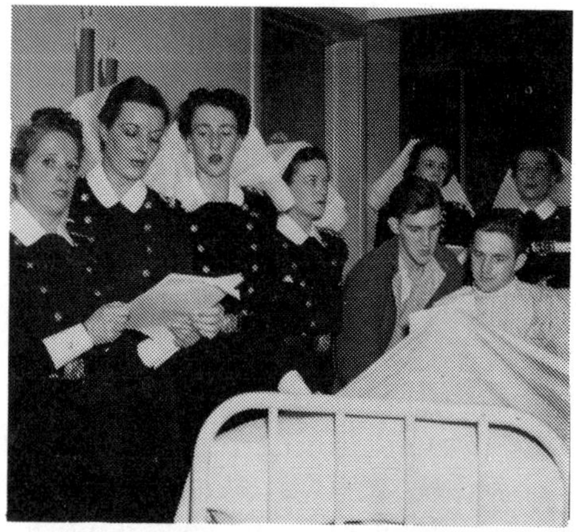

Carol singing Christmas eve 1945, RCNH, HMCS Cornwallis
L-R: Isobel Sloane, Anne Mossman, Daphne Hemmel, Rae Fellowes, name unknown, Marian Haig, two patients.

I didn't want to stay home and worry. I would rather be trying to help in some way so I chose to join the Navy as a nursing sister.

We had two weeks basic training in Halifax – you should have seen Navy nurses trying to march as one "right wheel," etc., (one always went left). I spent a year at HMCS *Cornwallis*. There were teenage boys learning gunnery and navigation in a hurry before being sent out in "Escort Corvettes" to convoys that dipped and rolled at the same time.

After the war I was sent to *Ste. Hyathcine*, Quebec, to what had been a Naval signal school. It was now an empty base except for the RCN Hospital turned over to DVA for returning Hong Kong POWs, mostly French-speaking ones who all had T.B. It was staffed by Navy doctors and nurses until enough civilians could take over.

Rosina Marion (Gammon) Long

Graduated from: St. Joseph's Hospital School of Nursing, Toronto, Ontario. Year: 1939

Military History:

Service: RCN

Rank: Sub-Lieut. N/S

Served: January 1, 1943 to September 17, 1945

Canada was at war. Joining the Service seemed the right thing to do.

I was the operating room supervisor and assistant matron at the Naval hospital, HMCS *Naden*. I met many wonderful people and made many friends. We still keep in touch!

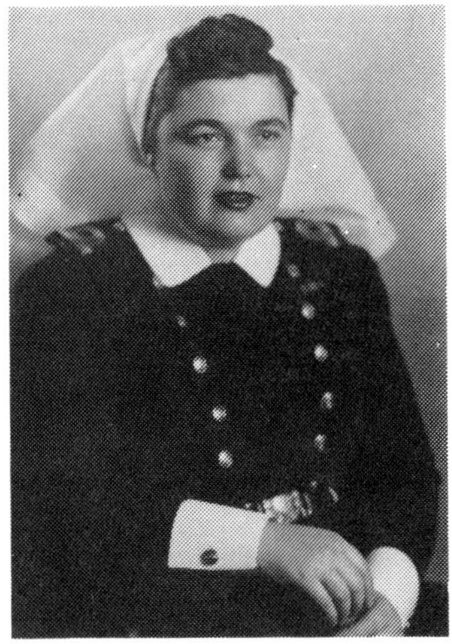

Sub-Lieut. Rosina (Gammon) Long

Clara (Watson) Meade

Graduated from: Victoria Hospital School of Nursing, London, Ontario. Year: 1940

Military History:

Service: RCNVR

Rank: Sub-Lieut. N/S

Served: October 20, 1944 to February 28, 1948

The Navy gave me an opportunity for a new experience. I wanted to join the Army but my father passed away in November 1940, so I stayed home for a while. I finally joined the Navy and was stationed at HMCS *Stadacona* for my entire military life.

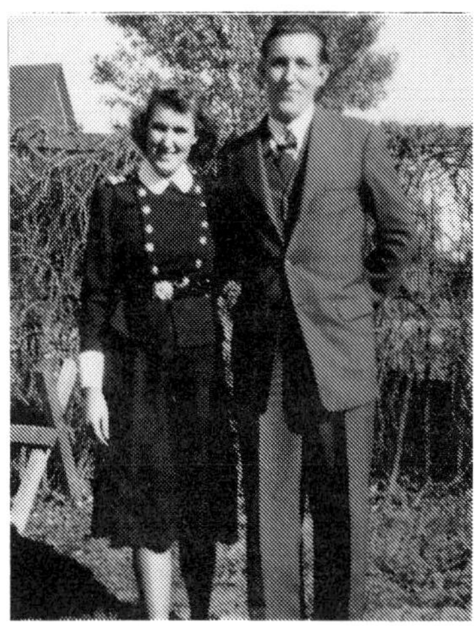

Clara (Watson) Meade and her brother, Alvin Watson, October, 1944, London, Ontario

I was working at a small hospital on the Basin that had communicable diseases and psychiatric patients. I had my patients outside playing volleyball one night about 6 P.M. when a bomb was dropped on board a ship in the harbour. We were all thrown to the ground by the blast. My boys kept calm – to my surprise. Windows were broken in the hospital and we were ordered to evacuate the rest of the hospital. We finally transported to Halifax by 8:30 P.M.

Helen F. Ott

Graduated from: Toronto Western Hospital School of Nursing. Year: 1948

Other: Clinical Supervision, University of Toronto; Nursing Service Administration; University of Western Ontario: Military Nursing courses-Canadian Forces Medical Service, and U.S. Army Nurse Corps.

Military History:

Service: RCN & CFMS

Rank: Captain (N) on retirement, (Colonel)

Served: March 15, 1954 to April 4, 1984.

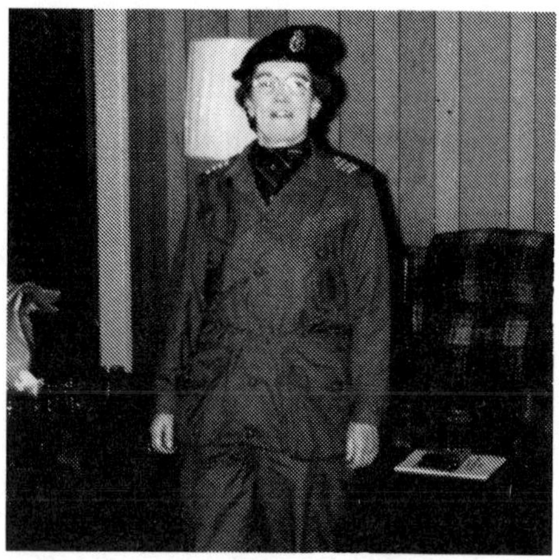

Col.Helen Ott wearing combat gear on a visit to the Basic Officers Course, Chilliwack, BC, 1983

I chose a military career because I wanted something different.

There is little of interest in my career for anyone but myself and my contemporaries: the ups and downs of peace-time nursing, integration of medical services, changes in military nursing education, officer professional development, broadening the scope of duties of Nursing Officers.

Capt. Helen Frieda Ott

Joined RCN at HMCS *Star*, Hamilton, Ontario 15 March, 1954 as A/S Lt (MN)

Appointments and Promotions

15 Mar 54: RCNH *Stadacona*

Sep 54: S. Lt(MN) General Duty Reg. N. (Medical nursing)

Mar 56: Lt (MN) Clinical Instructor

Jul 58-Dec 60: Medical Branch School, HMCS *Naden*, Instructor of Medical Assistants

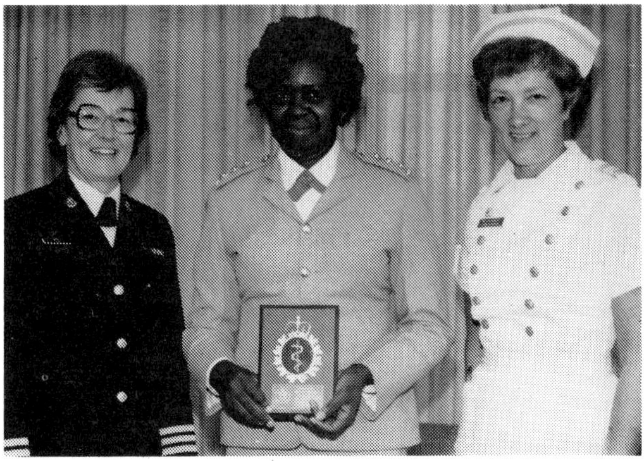

NDMC, 1977
L - R: Lt.Col. Helen Ott; Capt.Marion Comfort Anyagi, Ghana, Africa, attached to NDMC for training and experience; Major Marie Craig Canadian Forces photo

Dec 60-Aug 64: Canadian Forces Medical Training Centre, Camp Borden. Instructor of Medical Assistants and Nursing Officers

Sep 64-May 65: University of Western Ont. London, Ont. (HMCS *Prevost*)

Nursing Administration Certificate

May 65-Dec 66: C.F. Hospital, HMCS *Naden*

Asst. Matron, Clinical Instr.

Dec 66-Mar 69: Base Medical Centre, CFB Petawawa

Matron (Senior Nursing Officer)

Mar 69: Promoted LCdr-Seniority 1/69

Mar 69-Jul 70: Regional Matron, Central Command (Oakville)

Jul 70: to CFB Trenton, same appt.

Sep 70: Mobile Command Hq, St. Hubert as regional Senior Nursing Officer

Jul 73-May 76: CF Medical Services School, CFB Borden

O-I-C. Medical Assistant Training

Promoted to Commander, Seniority January 76

May 76-May 79: National Defence Medical Centre as Director of Nursing

Promoted to Captain, Seniority January 1979

May 79-Apr 84: Director of Nursing Services CFMS NDHQ

1968: Uniforms changed to tri-service green

1985: Uniforms reverted to different uniforms for each service

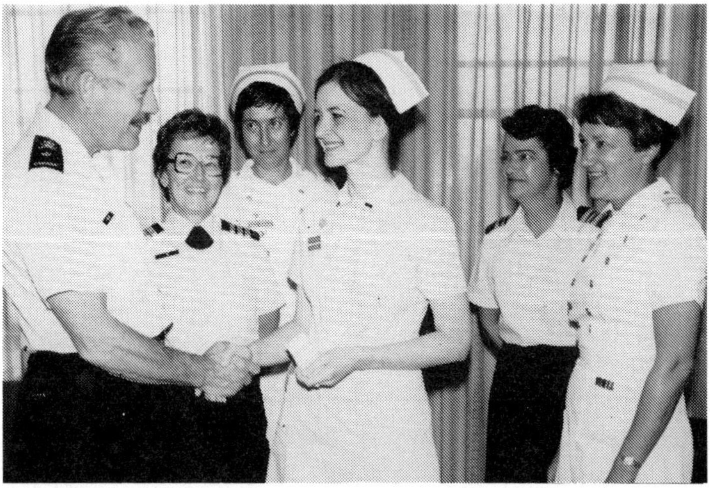

L - R: Brigadier General Frank Cullen, Dryden, Ont., Commandant, National Defence Medical Centre, Directorate General of Medical Services. Lt.Col. Helen Ott, Port Colburne, Ont., Director of Nursing Services, Major Huguette Theriault, St. Antoine, Que. Marielle Gagne, Rimouski, Que. receiving her Majority, 1977. Major Colleen Howard, St.John, N.B., Major Marie Craig, Ste. Anne des Monts, Que. Canadian Forces photo

Decorations/Awards

Canadian Forces Decoration with 1 rosette. 15 Mar 54-4 Apr 84
*Commander in the Order of St John 1990
125 Anniversary medal (for work with Friends of the Canadian War Museum) 1992
*Serving Sister 1963
Officer Sister 1982
Commander Sister 1990

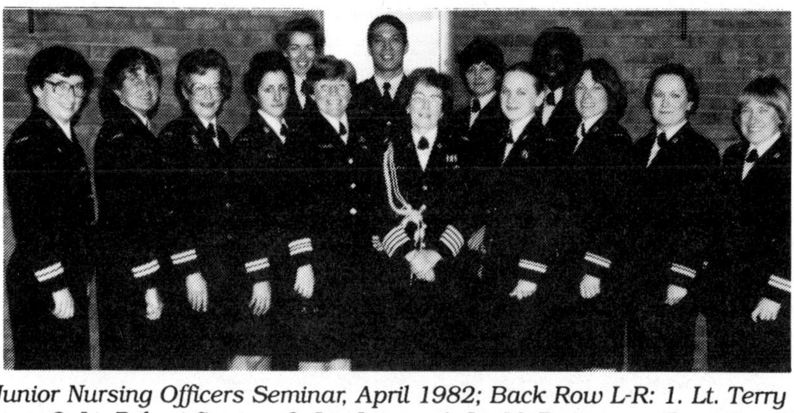

Junior Nursing Officers Seminar, April 1982; Back Row L-R: 1. Lt. Terry Ettinger; 2. Lt. Robert Santos; 3. Lt. Jutras; 4. Lt. M. Rousseau; Front Row L-R: I. Capt.Gwen Sear; 2. Lt. Julia Czerniski; 3. Capt. Carol Trites; 4. Capt. M. Desjardins-Messier; 5. Maj. D. McClelland; 6. Col. Helen Ott; 7. Lt. Furlong; 8. Lt. Gagnon; 9. Lt. Fraser; 10. Capt. M. Turnbull

Marian C. (Duncan) Pangman

Graduated from: St. Boniface Hospital School of Nursing, St. Boniface, Manitoba. Year: 1940

Military History:

Service: RCN

Rank: Sub-Lieut. N/S

Served: August 1944 to December 1945

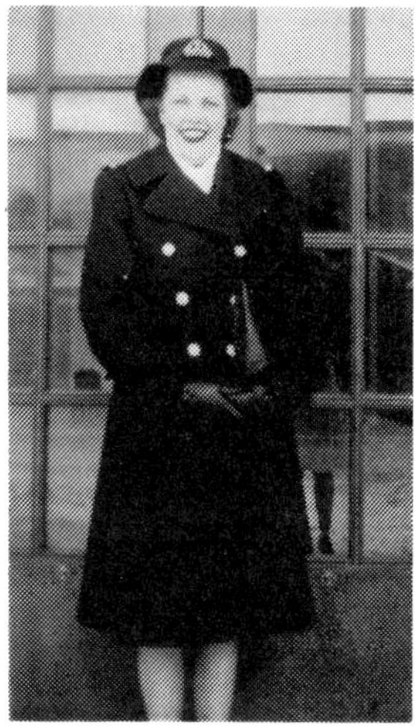

Sub-Lieut. Marian (Duncan) Pangman

Two things influenced me to choose the service. First, patriotism: I had a brother in Royal Canadian Air Force. Also, I was looking for adventure. I was stationed first at HMCS *Stadacona*, Halifax , Nova Scotia. My next duty assignment was at HMCS *Protector*, Sydney, Nova Scotia.

I worked in the operating room. One job I had was to do gastric analysis in the morning on young sailors who had just crossed the Atlantic. I really felt for them – the stress they were under. The North Atlantic was a rough trip; many of these very young men had symptoms of ulcers.

Jean Elaine (Glanville) Smyth

Written by her daughter, Dreena (Smyth) Taggart

Graduated from: Royal Columbian Hospital School of Nursing, New Westminster, B.C. Year: 1940

Military History:

Service: RCN

Rank: Sub-Lieut. N/S

Served: October 1941 to December 1943

Mom was very patriotic and wanted to do something for her country. She was most proud of her uniform and having been given the chance to wear it. I would have to say the highlights for mom were; having the chance to meet so many wonderful people in the service; having the chance to help so many people who were ill; having the chance to possibly learn so much more and to travel abroad, helping others.

Her military time was at HMCS *Naden*, Esquimalt, Victoria B.C. 1940 - 1941 General duty nursing, Port Alberni General Hospital. 1941 - 1943 Nursing Sister, Royal Canadian Navy, Victoria. 1943/45 Private Duty Nursing, Victoria. 1950/52 General duty, Victoria General Hospital (was St. Joseph's Hospital), Medical Nursing, and Isolation. 1952/60 Clinical Instructor, Victoria General Hospital, Medical and Geriatric Nursing. 1960/77 Coordinator/Head Instructor, Practical Nursing Program, Camosun College, Victoria.

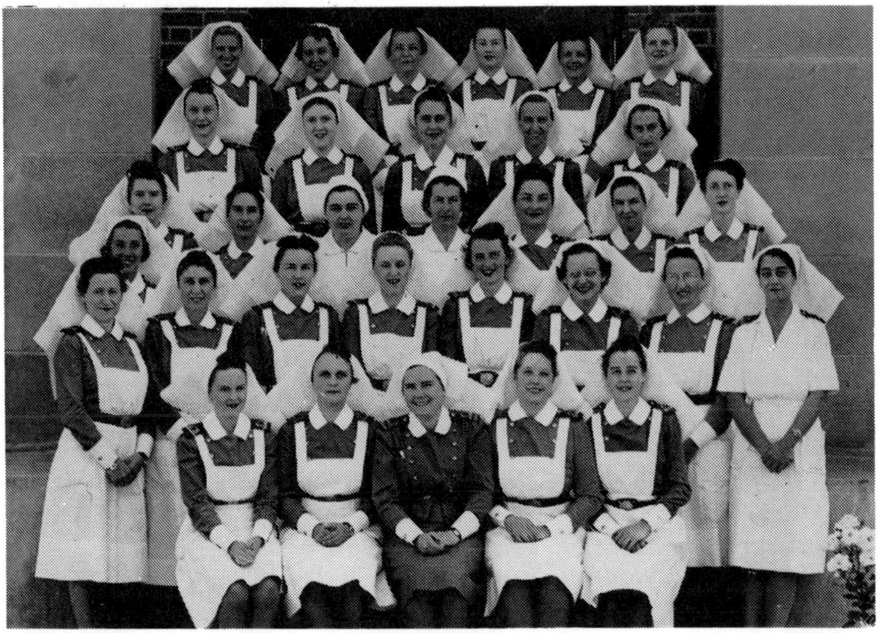

ROYAL CANADIAN NAVY NURSING SISTERS - HMCS Naden, Esquimalt, BC 1943. STARTING TOP ROW LEFT TO RIGHT EACH ROW: Lorna Harris; Doretta Reid; Vivian Knight; Jean Milne; Francis McDonald; Jean Glanville; Doris Carlson; Dorothy Doyle; Connie Bates; Jean Harris; Mary Pogson; Betty O'Neill; Violet Cantwell; Rose Gammon; Joan Russell; Ethelwyn Mackie; Barbara Player; Daphne Hemmel; Gwen Newton (alone) Elenor McPhail; Nora Cornwall; Helen Mutrie; Helen McPherson; Peggy McLeod; Norah Cooke; Grace White; Doris Hember; Mabeth Kerslake; Dorothy Wiggins; Matron Olive Wilson; Belle Sloan; Joan Sparrow. loaned by Mrs. D. Taggart, daughter of Sub-Lieut. N/S Jean Glanville Smyth

Katherine Elizabeth (Gardner) Smythies

Graduated from: Montreal General Hospital School of Nursing, Montreal. Year: 1941

Military History:

Service: RCN

Rank: Sub-Lieut. N/S

Served: 1st February 1945 to December 1948

I had a classmate in the Navy, that influenced me to choose the Royal Canadian Navy.

Lilla E. Wright

Graduated from: Royal Victoria Hospital School of Nursing, Victoria, B.C. Year: 1940

Military History:

Service: RCN

Rank: Sub-Lieut. (Lieut. in Reserve Navy in 50's)

Served: April 24, 1942 to November 26, 1945

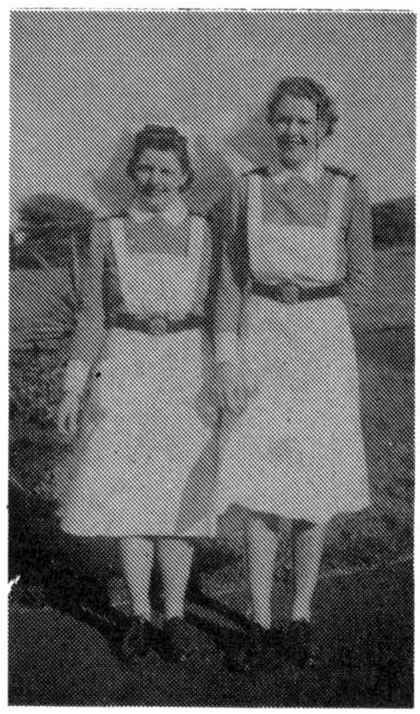

HMCS NIOBE 1942 - 1943.
L - R: Sub. Lieut. Nursing Sisters Joan Story and Lilla Wright.

Private duty nursing in Victoria was sometimes embarrassing (particularly home cases) when there was a war going on. I wanted to serve my country.

On April 24, 1942 I was the 12th nursing sister to join HMCS *Naden*, Esquimalt, B.C. Three months later, Faith Hodgson and I were the two West Coast nursing sisters appointed to HMCS *Niobe*, Scotland, joining Beryl Rutherford, Shirley Beck, Hazel Tilling and Joan Story in Halifax, after our train trip across Canada.

Joan (Story) Giles has written about the convoy of 42 ships.

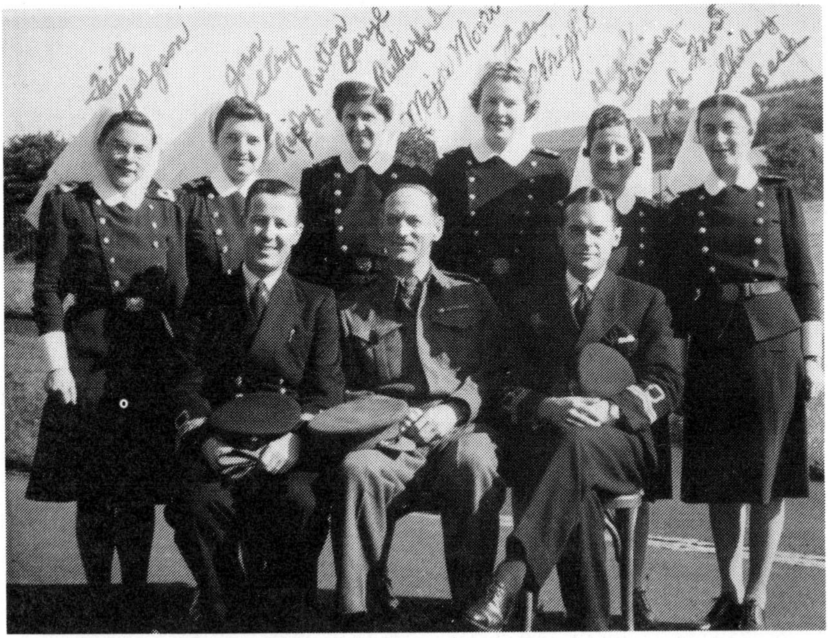

HMCS Niobe, 1942. L -R: Front Row: Surgeon Lt. Cmdr Ruttan, Victoria, B.C.; Major Moore, dentist; Surgeon Lt. Frost, Vancouver; Back Row: Faith Hodson, Alberni, B.C.; Joan Story, Halifax; Sister-in Charge Beryl Rutherford, Montreal; Lilla Wright, Tryon, PEI; Hazel Tilling; Shirley Beck, Halifax.

There was much excitement about the arrival of six nursing sisters at *Niobe*. Two sailors were dispatched to meet us at Liverpool where it was anticipated we would dock. They reportedly had a great time there while we disembarked at Glasgow, and then they dead-headed back!

(Joan Story writes of our arrival and introduction to our quarters for the next thirteen months).

As our hundred-bed hospital was built for mentally confused patients; all doors had locks. We had beds in the surgical ward, but there was not one with a Gatch frame. When it was necessary to elevate a patient's head or leg, we used a chair-back under the mattress. Two wards had double-decker bunks, and I have stood on a chair to sponge a patient in an upper, and knelt on a pillow on the floor to treat someone in a lower. One learned to improvise.

The U.S. Navy had a base, *Roseneath*, across the Clyde River but with only pharmacists' mates to give primary care in a Quonset hut. We used to have some of their personnel requiring bedside nursing. We were envious of the fruit brought by their visitors from *Roseneath*. In a market once, I recall Joan paying $4 - $5 for 1 lb. of grapes, and $1.50 for one peach.

The Americans were generous with their hospitality, inviting us for dinner and entertainment. On one occasion, we saw Bob Hope and Frances Langford, and on another occasion, Bebe Daniels.

At Christmas we had a tree in our surgical ward, and it was amazing how creative our patients and sick berth attendants were in decorating it. Pipe cleaners with cotton batting and coloured plastic drinking straws were fashioned into interesting shapes. A few drapery cords and tassels were used as garlands.

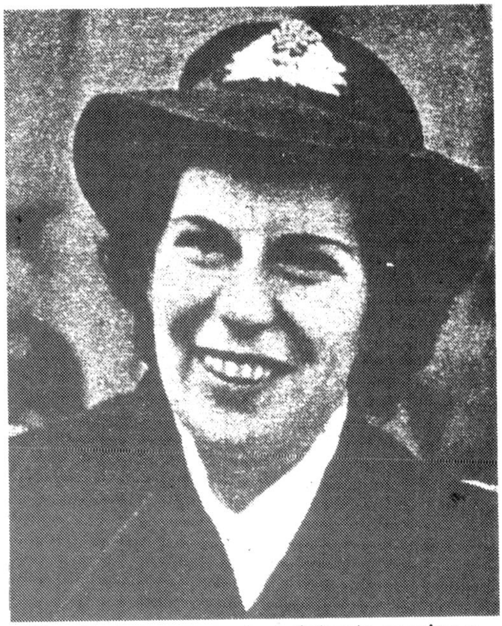

The first navy nursing sister to receive a decoration in this war from the king is RCN Sub-Lieut. Edna Belden, Toronto, seen here at Buckingham Palace after receiving the Associate Royal Red Cross Medal. It was for devotion to duty during the fire in the Knights of Columbus hostel, St. John's, Nfld., in December, 1942.

Gourock's industrial plants had been bombed before our arrival, but we did not experience any air raids during our thirteen-month stay. Blackouts, however, were observed.

In Scotland during the summer it was light enough to play tennis until 11:00 P.M., but the days were depressingly short in the winter. When walking to the hospital for our 8:00 A.M. shift, we used our torches, directed at the ground, and when we returned at 4 - 4:30 P.M., the stewards were closing the blackout curtains.

Food was rather an obsession with us. We were supposed to have one egg a week, but this was not always possible. I recall crossing the Clyde River to Dunoon and cycling 15 miles to Loch Eck, where they served a boiled egg with afternoon tea! Powdered eggs could be prepared quite agreeably in small quantities, but when baked in large pans for a long time, they were stiff and unappetizing. In our nursing sisters' small dining room there was a gas radiant, and in the winter we used to stick a fork in our coarse, dark bread and make our own toast in front of it. Much has been written about sausages in Britain during wartime, and our bangers were no exception. Our rations were adequate to maintain our health, and we didn't really suffer, but we did appreciate our parcels from home.

Others may write of *Niobe*, but Joan (Story) Giles and I are the only living members of the original six nursing sisters who all stayed together for six months of our thirteen-month stay. Joan and I worked the same 8 - 4 and 4 - midnight shifts; shared a cabin, and are still friends after 51 years!

During the next two years I served in HMCS *Stadacona*, Halifax, and HMCS *Protector*, Sidney, N.S. "Rockhead" was part of my Halifax experience, and although Joan Story said there was no cross infection, I developed scabies! (I used to pull up the blankets during night rounds.) Snow used to drift around the windows; winter nights were grim.

At the time of the Ammunition Dump Explosion in '45, I had recently finished reading Hugh McLellan's book, *Barometer Rising*, about the 1917 explosion. In the recent one, our RCN Hospital and nursing sisters' residences were the only buildings, north of North Street, not evacuated. That night my colleagues and I took shelter under dining tables, in our uniforms! In the end, there were no casualties, but we relived the stories of 1917 that night. I thought of the people of Halifax who lived under such threats of destruction during two World Wars.

Post-war, I used my DVA Rehabilitation Grant to obtain a diploma in public health nursing from McGill University, Montreal. During five years in Calgary (eight in Alberta) I joined the Reserve Navy in HMCS *Tecumseh*, spending two weeks each summer where it all began, at HMCS *Naden*, Esquimalt. Returning permanently to the West Coast, I did public health nursing in Victoria and Esquimalt for twenty years, before retiring in 1978.

In Victoria, we have an active unit of the Nursing Sister Association of Canada. In 1992, we hosted over 300 nursing sisters at the National Biennial meeting. We thought it might be the last, as our membership ages – however, another Biennial is scheduled for Edmonton in June 1994.

As our world becomes more unstable, it is hoped that Canada will continue to prepare personnel, including nursing officers, as they are now called, to meet the need.

We pass the torch to a new generation.

Chapter 16

SERVING WITH THE ROYAL CANADIAN AIR FORCE

Anne-Marie Bélanger
Dorothy (Mulholland) Bourke
Agnes (Olson) Clerf
Marion (Patterson) Ferguson
Anne Harman
Kathleen (Willis) Holl
Marjorie Jackson
Ruth Laberee
Grace (Woodman) MacEachern
Enid (Faulkner) Matheson
Mary (Ross) Middlemas
Audrey (Adams) Nettleton
Ruth (McTavish) Pearce
Shirley Robinson
Mary (Murray) Rogers
Rena V. (Mayson) Roskilly
Maureen Seymour
Signe (Johnson) White
Isabel Ziegler

Personnel of the RCAMC provided the medical care for RCAF personnel at the beginning of the Second World War and Army nursing sisters were posted to RCAF stations. As the Air Force expanded and the British Commonwealth Air Training Plan was organized, the need for a separate medical organization became apparent.

The medical branch of the RCAF was established by order-in-council in September 1940 and on 28 November the RCAF

Nursing Service was authorized. The position of principal matron was not filled until April, 1943, when Flight-Lieutenant (N/S) J.E.C. Porteous assumed the appointment. The first 12 nursing sisters in the RCAF transferred from the RCAMC. In all, 481 nursing sisters joined the RCAF during the war, 68 of them serving overseas.

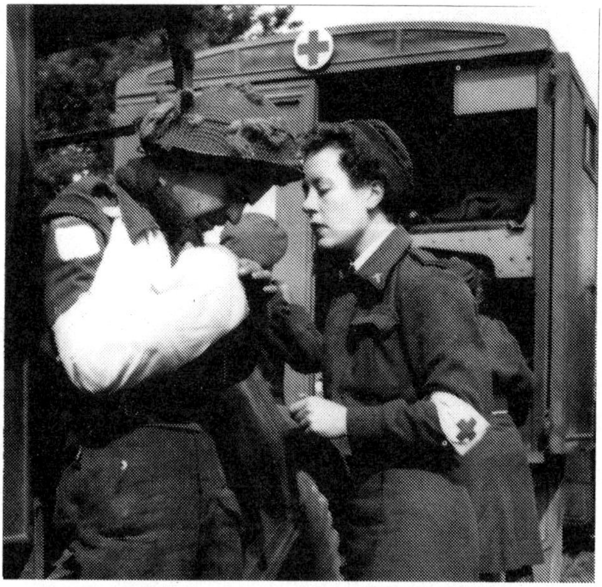

Pte. F. Madora with sister M.F. Giles at RCAF airport in France, 16 June 1944. National Archives of Canada, Ottawa PA 131427, photographer Ken Bell

Col. Smellie helped organize the new nursing service and acted as their matron-in-chief until 1943 when Matron (later Principal Matron) Porteous took over the responsibility.

During the Korean Conflict 1950 to 1953, RCAF nurses assisted with the evacuation of casualties. RCAMC nursing officers served with the British Commonwealth General Hospital in Japan and with two small units in Korea.

When Canadian Forces were posted to Europe as part of NATO forces, RCAMC and RCAF nurses were sent with them.

Not so well known is the fact that two Air Force nursing sisters landed in Normandy with an (RCAF) Mobile Field Hospital 13 days after D-Day, F/O Dabina Wyn Pitkethly of Ottawa and F/O Dorothy Mulholland of Georgetown, Ontario, the only medical unit in which RCAF nursing sisters served in Continental Europe. They were the first Canadian service women to cross the channel after D-Day.

The Mobile Field Hospital was similar to a casualty clearing station. This 100-bed unit was under canvas and gave early treatment to the sick and wounded before sending them on to a base hospital or returning them to duty.*

* Canada's Nursing Sisters. G.W.L. Nicholson, Hakkert & Company, 1975. pp. 189-195.

Anne-Marie Bélanger.

Submitted by her sister Marie Thérèse Bélanger.

Graduate of: St. Sacrement Hospital School of Nursing and Laval University, Quebec City.
Year: 1953

Military History:

Service: RCAF

Rank: Colonel

Served: Permanent Force

Colonel Anne-Marie Bélanger, OMM, CD, Canadian Forces

Colonel Bélanger was born in St. Redempteur, Province of Quebec on 26 July 1931. She resided in that province until she joined the Royal Canadian Air Force in 1954. She completed her secondary education at l'ecole normale de Levis in 1949. She graduated as a nurse from St. Sacrement Hospital School of Nursing and Laval University, Quebec City, in 1953. Following graduation, she remained on staff at St. Sacrement hospital as head nurse of the Department of Obstetrics from June 1953 until May 1954.

Colonel Bélanger enrolled in the Royal Canadian Air Force as a pilot officer in June 1954. On completion of Basic Officer Training in November of that year, she was posted to RCAF Station Rockcliffe Hospital. There she was employed in general duty nursing and as a head nurse of

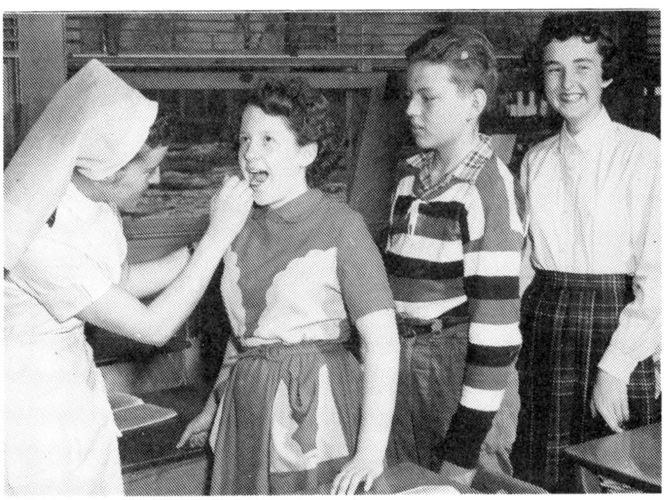

N/S Anne Marie Bélanger, RCAF school nurse and dependants. Canadian Forces photo PL 101748

the Out-Patients Department. She was promoted to the rank of flying officer in March 1955. In February 1958, she was granted a permanent commission. Subsequently, she was posted to 4 (F) Wing RCAF Station Baden-Soellingen, Germany where she served for three years as head nurse in the various departments of the base hospital.

On her return to Canada in February 1961, she was appointed senior nurse officer at the base infirmary, RCAF Station Centralia, Ontario. She was promoted to the rank of flight lieutenant in March 1961.

Colonel Bélanger attended Ottawa University in 1962-1963 and obtained a diploma in nursing education. She was then employed as a clinical instructor at the base hospital, RCAF Station Cold Lake, Alberta, from July 1963 until February 1966.

She spent the following three years at the National Defence Medical Centre, Ottawa, Ontario. There she held successively the positions of clinical instructor, head nurse medical ward, head nurse surgical ward, surgical supervisor and in-service education coordinator.

In April 1969, she was posted to the Canadian Forces Medical Service School, CFB Borden, Ontario, and appointed officer in charge of the Basic Nursing Officer Course. She was promoted to the rank of major in March 1970.

Colonel Bélanger returned to Ottawa University in September 1970 and in May 1971 was awarded a Bachelor of Science in Nursing, majoring in nursing education and public health. Following graduation, she served a second tour at the Canadian Forces Medical Service School as officer commanding, Medical Assistants Training Company.

Colonel Bélanger attended Canadian Forces Staff College, Toronto in 1973 - 1974 and afterwards was appointed Director of Nursing, Hôpital des Forces Canadiennes, Valcartier, PQ.

In May 1976, she was promoted to the rank of lieutenant-colonel and posted to National Defence Headquarters, Ottawa, where she held the appointment of Personnel Careers Officers-Nursing.

She was promoted to her present rank, colonel, in September 1978. Upon graduation from National Defence College, Kingston, in July 1979, she returned to National Defence Headquarters as director of women personnel.

Colonel Bélanger was awarded the Canadian Forces Decoration in 1968, the Order of Military Merit in 1973, the

Order of St. John of Jerusalem and the Silver Jubilee Medal in 1978. On 1 April 1980 Colonel Bélanger was appointed Honorary Aide-de Camp to the Governor General. She was a member of the Order of Nurses of Quebec, of La Société Historique du Québec and of the Canadian Research Institute for the Advancement of Women. She was also an honourary member of the Association of Military Surgeons of the United States.

Dorothy I. (Mulholland) Bourke

Submitted by her son, D.M. Bourke.

Graduated from: Wellesley Hospital School of Nursing, Toronto. Year: 1936

Military History:

Service: RCAF

Rank: Flight Officer N/S to Principal Matron/Squadron Leader

Served: World War II

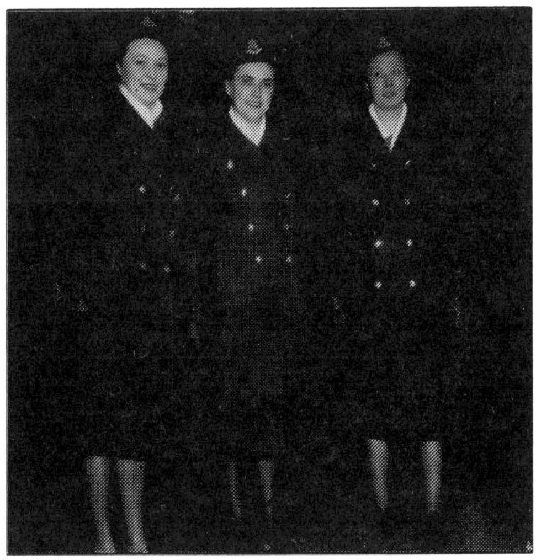

L-R: P/Matron M.T. Montgomery ARRC-Gravenhurst. N/S D.I. Mulholland RRC Georgetown. N/S D.C. Lindsay. At the Palace after Molly Mullholland (in the centre) got her ARRC

My mother graduated from Wellesley in 1936, joined the RCAF and was stationed in London during the war. At the time of VE Day she was principal matron of the RCAF nurses overseas. Mother's wedding cake was made by the RCAF nurses at East Grinstead, which was the burn unit where she was stationed at one time. Mother passed away on 20 April 1994 in Kingston, Ontario. I am donating her decorations to the RCAF Museum, Trenton, where she was stationed before going overseas.

She had hundreds of wartime photos, which unfortunately were destroyed in a fire in 1978.

I have many letters sent home to her mother during the war. I have not yet had time to give them the attention they deserve.

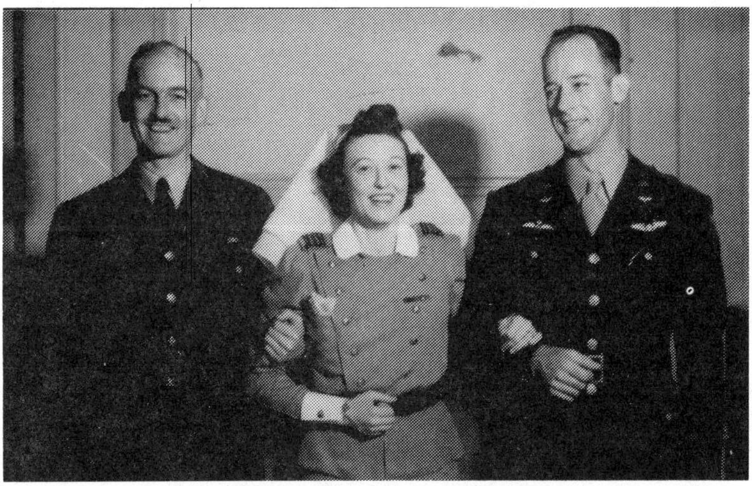

Dorothy Mulholland married in uniform.
L: Dr. C. Noble - Chief RCAF overseas. R: Capt. D.W. Bourke USAAF. Dr. Noble gave my mother away. Reception was at Air Marshall Johnson's Suites, RCAF Officers mess, London.

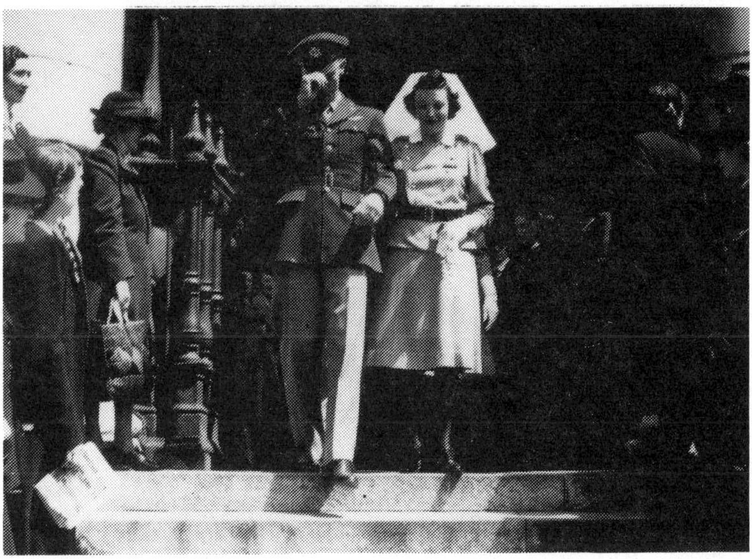

My parents. Married 07 July 1945 St. Martin in the Fields, London.

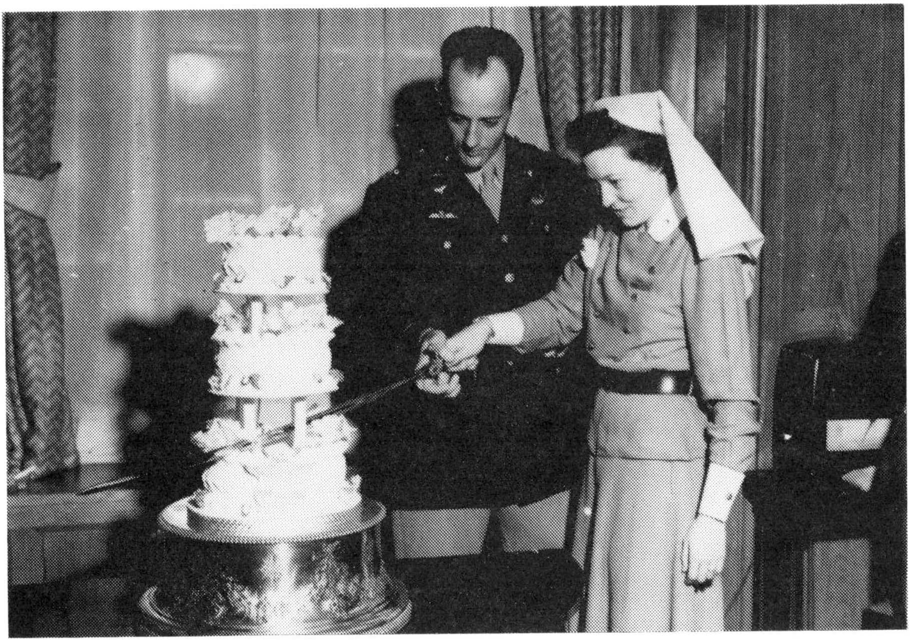

RCAF hospital personnel at East Grinstead made the cake, it was cut with a German dress sword presented by the hospital unit at Hanover, Germany. Then to the Wellington club for dinner given her by her Director of Medical Services, G/C Noble, Master of Ceremonies
Loaned by her son D. M. Bourke

*The following article is from a 18 June 1944 newspaper, name unknown. **

FIRST NURSES IN FRANCE TRAVEL IN TENT CARAVAN

By Mollie McGee
(From yesterday's late editions.)

London, June 18. – The first two Canadian women on official duty in France were Flight Officers Molly Mulholland, Georgetown, and "Pit" Pitkethly, Ottawa. Both are nursing sisters with an RCAF mobile hospital. This tent caravan hospital travels on wheels, can be set up in a few hours, accommodates up to a hundred patients – which can be extended to 200 – and is usually attached to an airfield.

The commanding officer is Wing Cmdr. "Mickey" Growse, London, Ontario, who with the chief surgeon Sqdn. Ldr. Chick Church, has been working in France with part of the unit since D-Day. The remainder of the unit rolled down to the embarkation port under the leadership of Sqdn. Ldr. Chauncey Patee, Montreal doctor, and went aboard like any other Army or Air Force unit. Every one, including the girls was in dusty blue battledress, ready to go to work on the other side with the advance party.

TRAVELLED IN JEEP.

The nurses were sitting in a jeep they were driving themselves when they reached the embarkation point. They told me they had slept in their clothes in one of their ambulances on two nights while journeying down, and had spent the other two nights in transient camps especially set up for the use of embarkation parties.

As they are the first women to use these camps, which are in temporary huts and tents, they found some difficulties. They said they locked themselves in the officers' shower room in a Nissen hut the night before until they had time to wash their dusty hair and have a thorough clean-up.

Thoroughly enjoying the experience, the nurses said they intended wearing their battledress slacks all the time except in the operating room, for which white gowns are provided.

TORONTO MATRON ASSISTS

Accustomed to battle conditions, they have been living and working in tent hospitals at several airfields in the last few months.

They said they had been much helped by RCAF Matron (Monty) Montgomery, Wellesley Hospital, Toronto. It was she who suggested that flying boots be procured for the girls. The rest of the staff followed suit. Each girl has with her a bed roll, sleeping bag, 60 pounds of personal belongings, including underwear, as well as folding baths, buckets and wash basins. They saw to it that officers' mess equipment included a flat iron that could be heated anywhere, although the hospital has its own power plant.

Said FO. Pitkethley: "We don't expect to have to carry much as long as the jeep works, but we are prepared, as we have route-marched seven miles frequently in practice in full equipment." FO. Mulholland said she was "Thrilled to pieces," enjoying every minute. She said she could not wait to get there.

Both girls are attractive brunets. They are not tall, which they say is handy, as the patients are on stretchers or safari beds just off the ground.

The sea was smooth as they sailed into the twilight and it was difficult to distinguish the girls in blue from the men in blue. "We are just part of the air force, like the boys," they said.

* A thorough attempt was made to determine the name of the newspaper without any success.

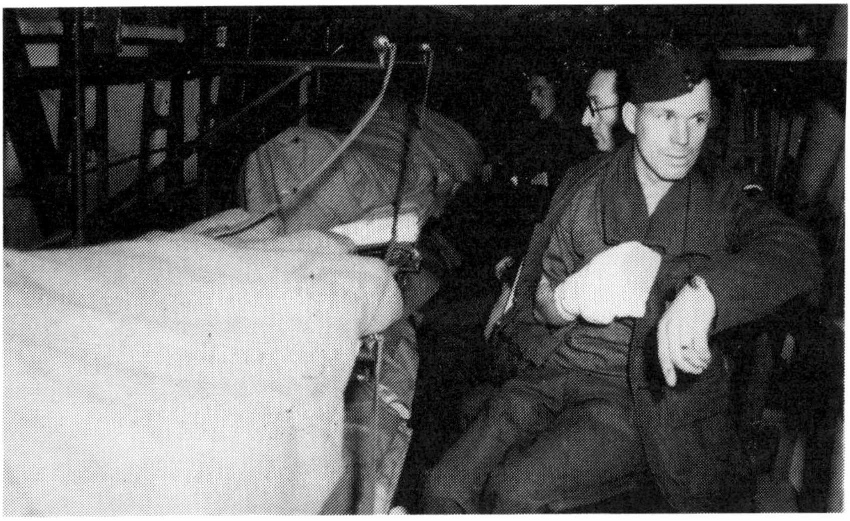

Inside view Air Ambulance, Air evacuation No. 52 MFH France

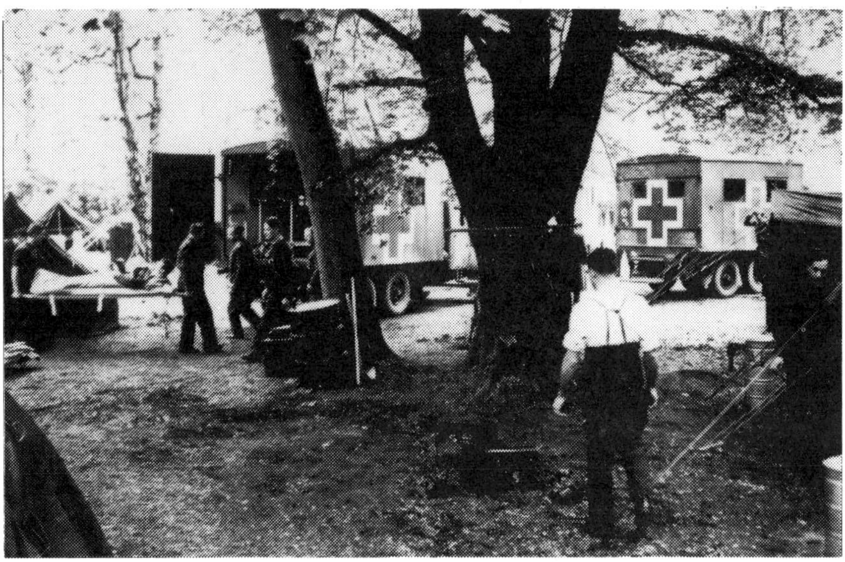

Evacuation No. 52 MFH (all Canadian) France

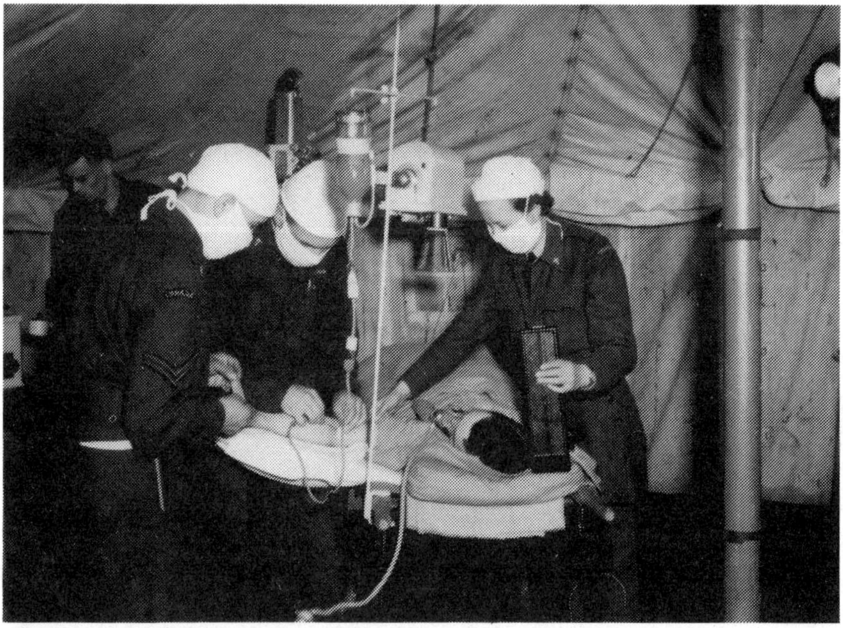

Surgery set up. N/S Pat Kelly on right. Unit under canvas. Living and sleeping in slit trench in France. The sisters loved it.

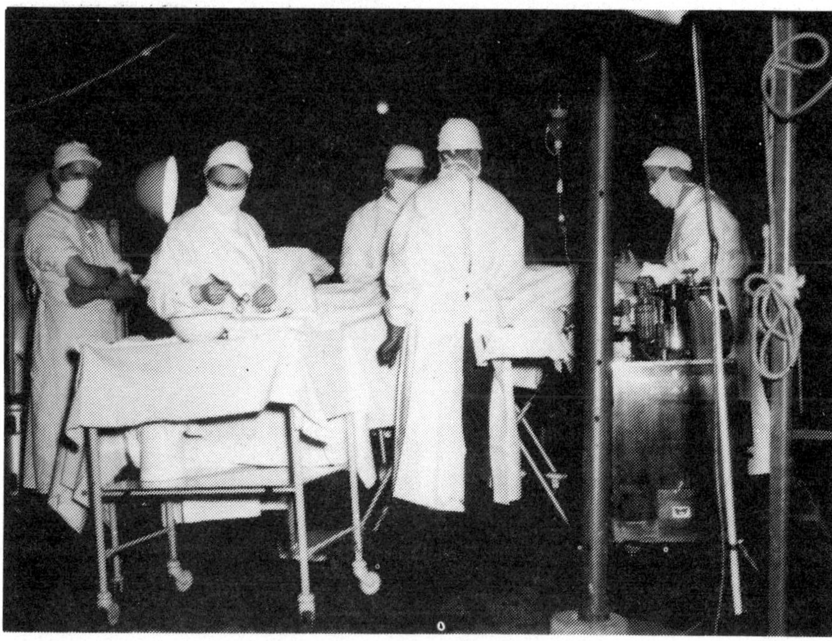

Surgery set up No. 52 MFH France

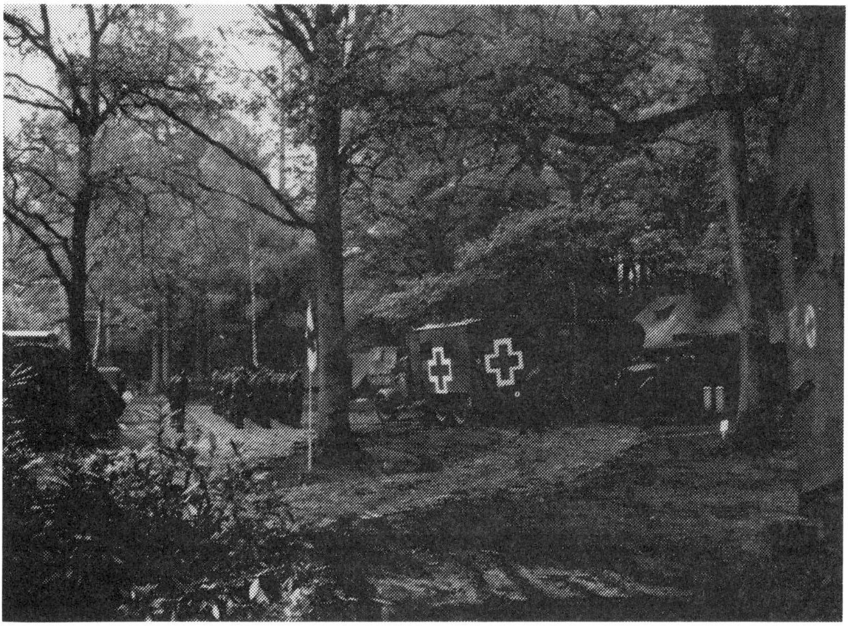

No. 52 Mobile Field Hospital, France

Agnes (Olson) Clerf

Graduated from: Royal Alexandra Hospital School of Nursing, Edmonton. Year: 1940

Military History:

Service: RCAF

Rank: Flying Officer

Served: 22 February 1943 to 5 November 1945.

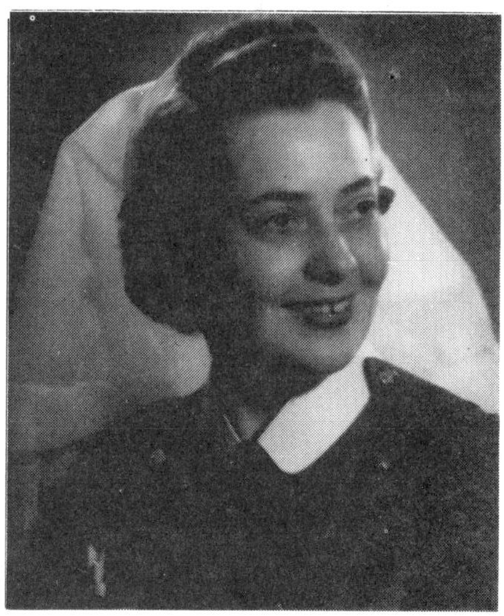

F/O Agnes Clerf

I wanted to serve my country. My friends were going into the Service. I disliked the matron who was in charge of our hospital. All this influenced me to join the RCAF as a nursing sister.

I began my career in the RCAF with a suddenness that

would take your breath away. I left Kimberley and was taken on strength as a civilian nurse at No. 3 Manning Depot in Edmonton, February 22, 1943.

I obtained my commission and was sworn in at Calgary June 20, 1943. We did general duty nursing; also helped with inoculation parade. I enjoyed my time in Edmonton where I met many people including Australians, New Zealanders and British Airmen.

On August 30, 1943, I proceeded on temporary duty to No. 2 Composite Training School (KTS) in Toronto. It was like going back to school but not really learning anything. However, we went on tours including Niagara Falls, museums and art galleries.

In early 1944 another nursing sister (Ida Craig) and I were transferred to No. 4 Repair Depot in Scoudouc, New Brunswick, to open the hospital there. It was an exciting time and I have only good memories of the time spent there. We had only one doctor and I assisted with the first baby born on the base. The doctor (I think his name was Lorrie) was married to a socialite and they lived on a huge estate in Shediac, New Brunswick.

I was young and naive but I figured I wouldn't have the chance again so I took off by myself to see New York. The Forces got reduced rates for shows, etc. I went to the Metropolitan Opera, Radio City Music Hall (1st showing of National Velvet), "Father Knows Best," and shopped at Saks Fifth Avenue. I have wonderful memories of this visit to New York.

Back on base we met many of the Airmen returning from Africa. One of them took me to a dance in Greenwood, Nova Scotia, in a small Canadian plane. We didn't wear slacks so I had to put a parachute over my skirt.

In the fall of 1944 I was transferred to Gander, Newfoundland. After being in a small hospital with two nurses it was quite a shock to be in a much larger hospital with surgery, etc. Besides the airmen, we looked after civilians who came by boat, dog sled or walked. There was no town, only a little store and very few roads. I made one trip up the coast by small plane to bring a pregnant woman to hospital.

Many famous people and entertainers came to Gander because of the American Base. We were invited to the American base for social affairs. In fact, we were about to have a barbecue the day that President Roosevelt died.

On my return to the Mainland I had an interesting posting

to Halifax. While there, I accompanied a hospital train which was loaded from the hospital ship in the harbour. We accompanied them as far as Montreal and I kept wondering how did I ever get picked.

Well, the war was grinding to a halt and I was posted from Gander to Dartmouth, Nova Scotia, where I was released from active service on November 5, 1945.

I returned to Kimberley, worked for a time, married and in 1961 went on staff and worked for 10 years until my retirement.

For all this I was awarded the Canadian Volunteer Service Medal and Clasp.

Marion (Patterson) Ferguson

Written by her daughter, Mrs. Jessica Barnett.

Graduated from: St. Boniface Hospital School of Nursing, St. Boniface, Manitoba. Year: 1932

Other: Post Graduate, 1933, Mental Health Centre Brandon, Manitoba

Military History:

Service: RCAF

Rank: F/O (N/S)

Served: 21 April 1941 to 6 November 1945

Marion was among the first 19 nurses to enlist as a nursing sister in the RCAF. She was first assigned to Carberry No. 33 Service Flying Training School where she and two other nurses set up a hospital at the RAF training base near Carberry, Manitoba.

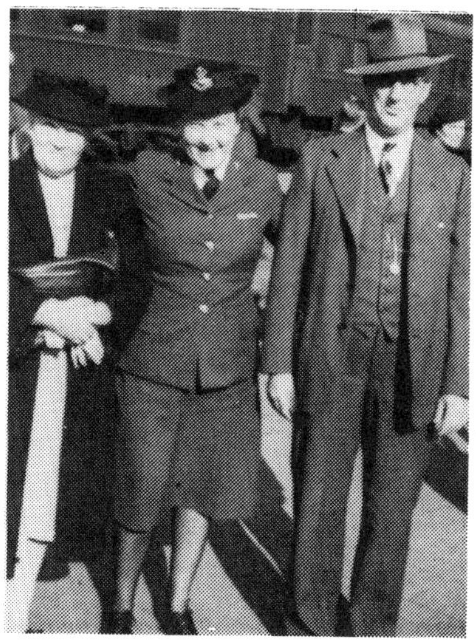

Mary and Alexander Patterson, Marion's parents, 1945. N/S Marion (Patterson) Ferguson on her return from a stint overseas during WW II about two minutes after her arrival and we just about mobbed her.

Accidents were frequent as young, inexperienced pilots trained in old rickety airplanes. British pilots trained at Carberry and other bases in Manitoba during the War because enemy air raids made training too dangerous in Britain.

Marion also served at Saskatoon, Moncton, N.B., and Yarmouth, N.S.

She was posted overseas to Innsworth (Receiving Unit) then to the world famous hospital for burns and plastic surgery, East Grinstead, Sussex, England.

She had a short refresher course for nursing sisters at the University of London and returned to Canada on the *Nieuw Amsterdam.*

Marion was the first lady president of Branch No. 3 Legion at Brandon. She not only was much in demand as a speaker, she also wrote poetry that was recognized by the Legion. The following poem was written in answer to her son's question on Remembrance Day, *"What does it mean, Mum ?"*

Poem by Marion Patterson Ferguson, RCAF
Brandon Branch No. 3
The Royal Canadian Legion.

YOUTH QUESTIONS

"Symbolic of what?"
-the young lad said
As in his hand
He held a poppy red.
"What does it mean?
Why should I care?
You went to war
I wasn't there."
"What's this about the lark,
bravely singing and flying?
What's this about young men
in Flanders fields lying?
It seems to me an awful story
that line about the Flag and Glory."

The old veteran smiled and gently said,
"Son - it's a story about the dead -
Who now in Flanders peacefully sleep
And ask of us - this freedom keep.
A small request for us to do
They gave their lives - for me and you.
I know you're Canadian

I have no doubt -
But the cost of lives
Is what the poppy's about."

"Many stood and were counted
And held high their ideals,
They fought for our rights -
They believed in fair deals,
The right to be free
to worship and speak -
The right to work and play
And keep - A BELIEF
That man must trust and love
Our God on high, in Heaven above."

"Among white crosses, row on row,
This red poppy wildly does grow
To let mankind remember and say
I'm free to live as I wish to-day,
So son, look and care,
Wear a poppy with pride,
For the men who years ago
Marched side by side, and sang
And gave the best they had -
Their very life
for you - m'lad."

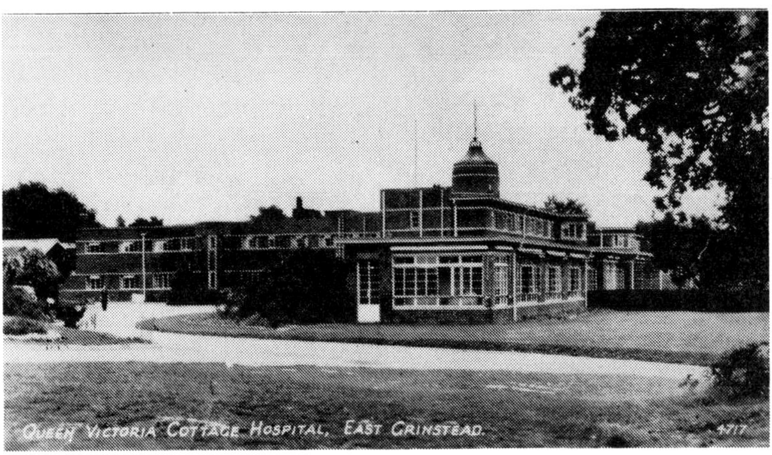

Queen Victoria Hospital, East Grinstead.
Canadian Forces photo 4717

Anna E. Harman

Graduated from: Victoria Hospital School of Nursing, Prince Albert, Saskatchewan. Year: 1944

Military History:

Service: RCAF

Rank: Major

Served: April 1951 to 1977

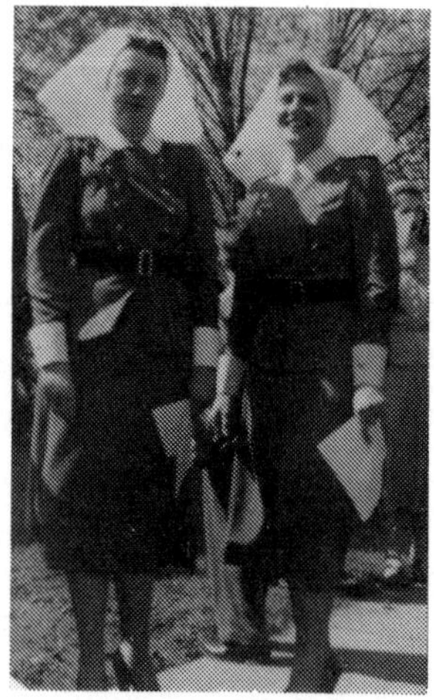

L-R: F/O Ann Harman, F/O Dorothy White Flight nurses graduation April 1954

Two brothers were in the RCAF during WW II. I wanted a change in nursing activity so in April 1951 I became a nursing sister in the RCAF.

I suppose the highlight of my military career was the tour of duty in Europe. Most important, though, were the friends I made and the capable people I worked with.

Nursing in the Service gave me an experience in many fields of health care – surgical, medical, obstetrical, public health, industrial and administrative. There were opportunities to attend many courses and seminars, and to learn new and modern techniques. Postings would find any nurse working in a large hospital or a small hospital, out-patient centres, public health, etc. Each and every tour of duty was interesting.

One interesting posting I had was from Hawaii, Air Evacuation Squadron, to RCAF detachment Fort Nelson. Some thought it was poetic justice – from grass skirts to mukluks in one easy move. We had a well-equipped hospital but only staffed to care for the Army and RCAF personnel and their families. Fort Nelson was situated 300 miles north of Dawson Creek and 600 miles from Whitehorse on the Alaska Highway and had the only hospital facilities. A lot of our patients came from travellers on the Alaska Highway, natives from the Indian reserve or workers in the area.

The Department of Highways had stations about every 50 miles and would inform us of medical problems on the way to us. Some serious ones were not reported accurately, or visa versa. One example was of a car accident involving U.S. soldiers, one with a possible fractured hip and broken jaw. At 3 A.M. the young man in question walked into the hospital carrying his kit bag and chewing gum.

Another time, we received a report that a young girl had been mauled by a bear and had a few lacerations to her face. It took over 100 sutures to her face and ear to close the gashes.

Across the Nelson was an Indian reserve; we saw the occasional patient but the Indian midwife looked after all the obstetrical cases. One night, a young man came to the hospital for help as his wife was having her first baby. The senior medical officer and I, with all our equipment, went back in the boat to the village. After the examination, the doctor decided we would take her back to the hospital. About 50 feet from shore we hit a submerged log and tore a big hole in the bottom of the boat. The doctor and the husband leaped out, and while swimming, pushed us safely to shore. The poor midwife was really upset with our intrusion and went out of business for a few months – we had quite a few extra deliveries in our hospital during that period.

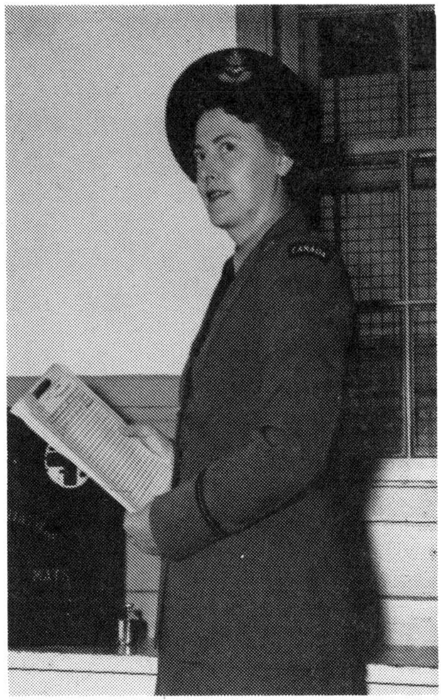

F/O Ann Harman, USAF Hickam, Hawaii 1954
U.S. Defense Department photo

Another incident I'll always remember at Fort Nelson revolves around a little two-year-old girl. The RCMP brought in this little tot who had been physically abused and had a third-degree burn to her hand. The Med/As rigged up a cage-splint for her little hand to protect the dressing. She used this splint as a real weapon. After a period of time she began to trust us and we fell in love with her. Eventually, the social welfare finalized their plans and one of our Nurs/As took her to Vancouver to turn her over to the social welfare people. This little girl just clung to the Nurs/A and the Nurs/A didn't want to turn her over to "strangers." I spent several minutes on the telephone before I convinced my Nurs/A we couldn't keep her.

During the Korean War and post-war, RCAF nurses were

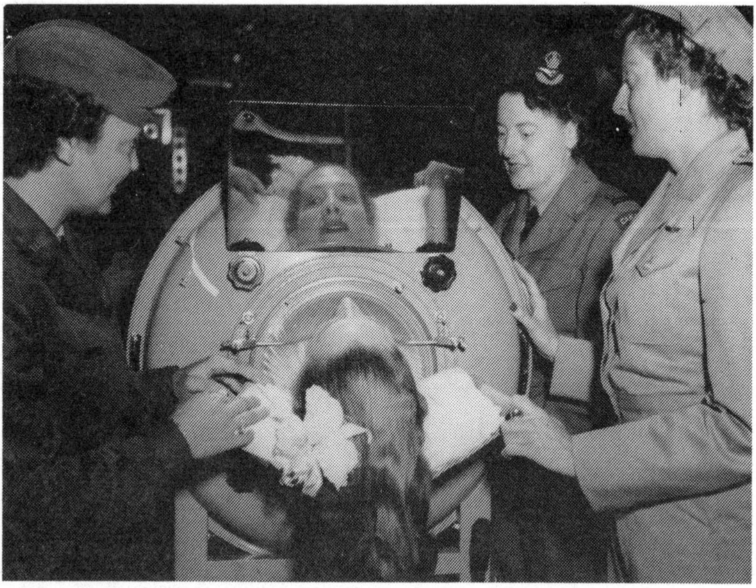

Air evacuation trip to Long Beach, California from Hickam AFB Hawaii 1954. U.S Air Force MATS special mission for a poliomyelitis patient. U.S. Defense Department photo

trained as Flt/Nurses with U.S. Air Force and Navy nurses at the School of Aviation Medicine in Gunter, Alabama. After the 6- to 7-week course in basic theory, the nurses graduated and were presented their Flt/Nurses Wings on a Wings Parade. After graduation they were posted to various bases for air evacuation duties.

The Canadians were posted to 1453rd Air Evacuation Squadron, Hickam Air Force Base, Hawaii, for approximately 3 months to obtain flying experience.

Working with another Flt/Nurse and 2 Med/Techs, the Air Evacuations were from any base in the Pacific such as Japan, Guam, Philippines, back to Hawaii or from Hawaii for onward evacuation to Travis AFB in California. From here, the patients would be transferred by air to hospitals near their homes in the States or Canada.

The Aero-Evac plane was a 4-engine prop cargo plane with a capacity for 60 patients. All treatments, medication, etc., given in the hospital were carried out during transportation. We sometimes had patients on Stryker frames or respirators, etc.

At a later date, the Air Evacuation School was moved to San Antonio, Texas, and after graduation the RCAF Flt/Nurses gained their flying experience at bases Stateside.

A few years later, Armed Forces nurses were given a three-week course in air-evacuation at Trenton, Ontario. They did not receive the coveted Flt/Nurses Wings.

Medical air evacuation in Canada consisted mostly of mercy missions, transporting sick and injured from small hospitals or remote areas to medical centers for care. Now most of the provinces have their own medical evacuation personnel; hence, not much need for service-trained people.

One air evacuation I remember while with the 1453rd Medical Air Evacuation Squadron in Hawaii was a special flight from Honolulu to Long Beach, California. I was a member of the team who took a lady, wife of an airman, with poliomyelitis and required the iron lung to breathe. This was a 14-hour flight. The iron lung was operated off the aircraft power system but we had battery back-up and were prepared to operate the machine by hand, if necessary.

Another interesting mission of which I was one of the team members, was the transportation by helicopter of a 5-year-old boy from Smith Falls, Ontario, to the Montreal Neurological Hospital, Montreal. We landed in Molson Stadium – a football field right beside the hospital. The little lad had a severe head injury and required some kind of helmet to protect his injury. The football team had a complete football outfit, including helmet, made for him. Apparently, he lived in this outfit night and day and only would part with it long enough to bathe.

During my twenty-five years' service, I did many air evacuations – usually the call came after work or in the evening. The nurses often had to improvise and worked under adverse conditions and used all their skills.

Kathleen (Willis) Holl

Graduated from: Kitchener-Waterloo Hospital School of Nursing, Kitchener, Ontario. Year: 1942

Military History:

Service: RCAF

Rank: F/O

Served: January 1944 to 1945

Highlights of my service with the RCAF:

RCAF Station at Trenton, Ontario, with a hospital of 150 beds.

No. 6 Repair Depot, also at Trenton, Ontario.

RCAF Station at St. Thomas, Ontario, with a 300-bed hospital where we cared for many burn cases.

RCAF Station at Rockcliffe, Ontario, with a 200-bed hospital.

I received my discharge from the RCAF in 1945. Since then I served for three years at Westminster DVA Hospital in London, Ontario, and for three years at Shaughnessy DVA Hospital, Vancouver, B.C.

On 19 May 1956 I married Steven Holl. I was widowed in 1989 and now live in Sheffield, Ontario.

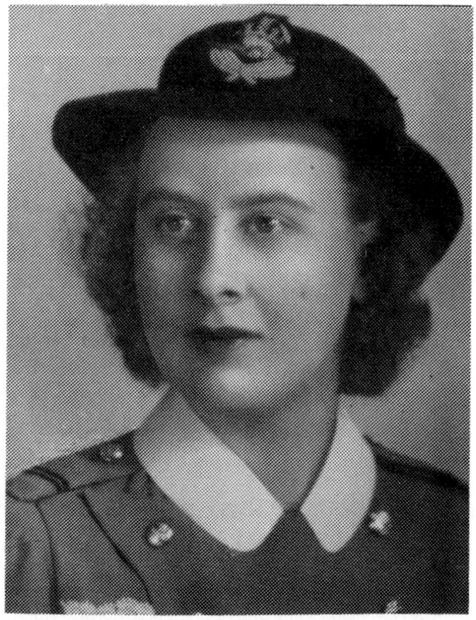

F/O N/S Kathleen (Willis) Holl, 1944

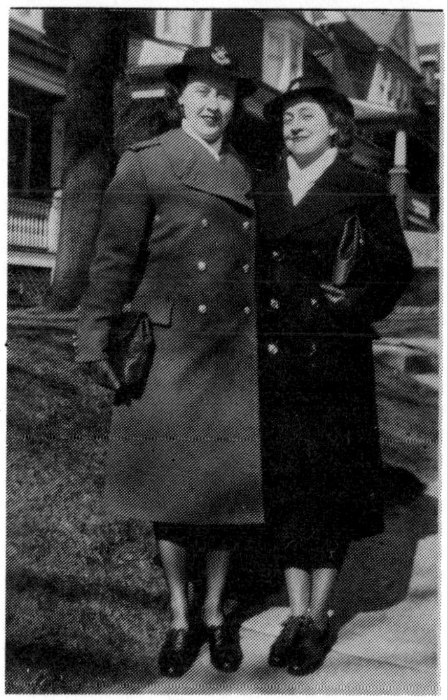

We had just left the staff of Women's College Hospital, Toronto. L: N/S Kathleen (Willis) Holl, R: N/S Bertha (Jones) Rudow. Note how uniform discipline was so important, RCAF coat buttoned same as men.

Marjorie E. Jackson

Graduated from: Brandon General Hospital School of Nursing, Brandon, Manitoba. Year: 1934

Military History:

Service: RCAF

Rank: Flight Lieutenant

Served: 1942 - 1945

I was nursing in Peekskill, New York when Canada declared war. I felt I could contribute, so in 1942 I became a nursing sister in the RCAF.

I was posted to No. 12 Flying Training Station, Brandon, Manitoba. I was there less than a year, and then was posted overseas, August 1942 to East Grinstead, Burns and Plastic Surgery Unit, Sussex, England. At that time we were attached to the East Grinstead Cottage Hospital. There were two Canadian doctors and three Canadian nurses at this hospital.

We used the hospital operating room and patients were housed in Nissen huts. Dr. McIndoe was chief surgeon, Dr. Tilley was a Canadian surgeon. Toronto Burn and Plastic hospital was named in his memory.

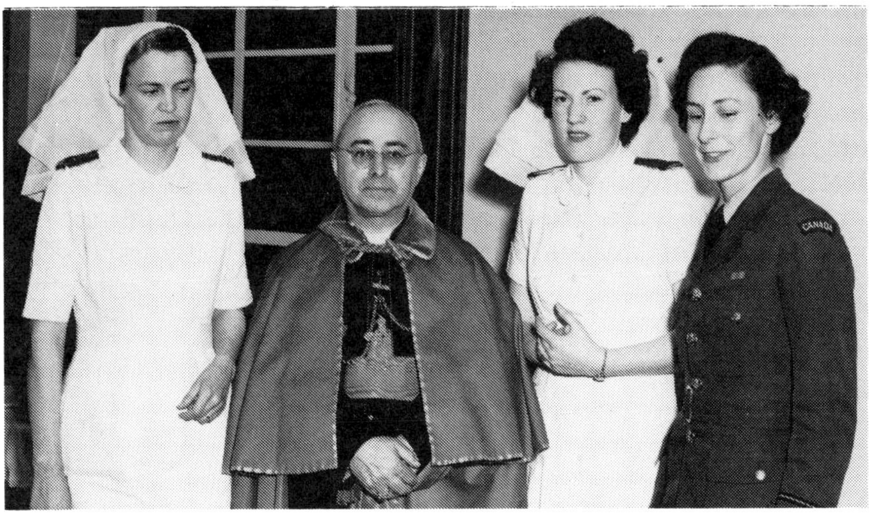

Cardinal Villeneuve with RCAF nurses during a visit to the Queen Victoria Hospital, East Grinstead, Sussex, 20 September 1944. L-R: Matron Marjory Jackson, Cardinal Villeneuve, F/O (N/S) Sally McLellan, F/O (Diet) Elizabeth Rising. Canadian Forces photo PL-32947

In 1944, the Royal Canadian Engineers built a new fully equipped Canadian wing on the hospital property.

I became matron of that wing and then 20 nursing sisters were posted to our hospital.

We had patients referred to us by about 16 different countries. The boys formed a group called Guinea Pigs. This year (1994) in Victoria we will celebrate the Canadian Wings 50th year (now turned over to East Grinstead Hospital).

I came home in 1945 and went to McGill University for hospital administration. I returned to Brandon and was director of nursing there for 25 years. In 1974 I retired and have lived with my sister since then. I enjoyed my service years and have attended many reunions.

EAST GRINSTEAD - RCAF

At East Grinstead, Sussex, World War II was responsible for the growth of one of the world's leading centres of plastic surgery. Surgeons performed a dozen to three dozen operations over a period of a year to two years to repair severe hand and body burns.

Equally important was the restoration of morale and self-assurance. East Grinstead, therefore, handled both highly specialized surgery and the development of a friendly, normal atmosphere to restore mental ease and self-confidence.

Plans to make East Grinstead a centre for advanced plastic surgery began in 1939 when the British Ministry of Health arranged to set up such a centre under the great plastic surgeon Archibald McIndoe, surgeon-in-chief at the 146-bed Queen Victoria Hospital. It was there that a few of the badly burned Battle of Britain pilots formed the Guinea Pig Club in 1941.

Queen Victoria Hospital, East Grinstead's local hospital, allocated use of its plant provided that civilian patients would be accommodated. It is located 30 miles south of London right on "buzz bomb alley." From the beginning, severely burned Canadian airmen were sent there, along with similarly injured airmen of the British and Allied air forces.

In January 1942 Canadian surgeon W/C A. Ross Tilley was posted to the hospital and six months later an anaesthetist and two surgical nurses were also posted to the hospital by the RCAF.

Construction of an all-Canadian wing in the hospital began in late 1943. Construction was done by the Royal Canadian

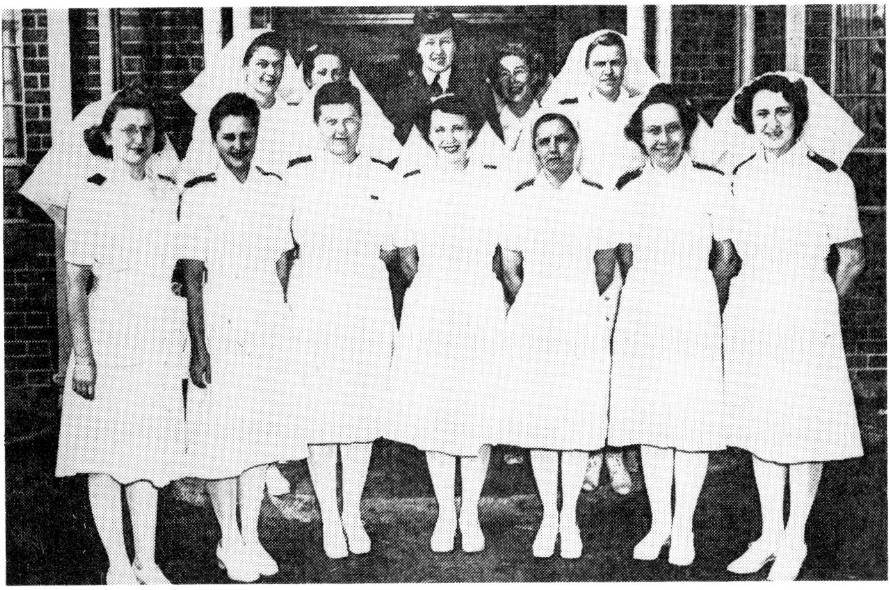

Front Row L-R: F/O (N/S) Mons Stapleford, F/O (N/S) Enid (Faulkner) Matheson, F/O (N/S) Marion (Patterson) Ferguson, F/O (N/S) Hilda (Emke) Moore, F/O (N/S) Frankie Anderson F/O (N/S) E. Matheson, F/O (N/S) Maggie Kaines. Rear L-R: F/O (N/S) Ida (Bishop) Jewsbury, F/O (N/S) Helen Brown, F/O (N/S) Soper, F/O (N/S) Bernie Arnett, Matron Marjory Jackson. Courtesy of the Department of National Defence, Canada, Kardex 181.009(D6391)

Engineers. It came into operation in late July, 1944, with an all-RCAF staff. Accommodation was provided for 50 patients, and when not fully occupied by RCAF casualties, it was filled with burn patients from other services and nations, and civilians.

To care for 50 patients the hospital had a staff of 50 consisting of two surgeons, an anaesthetist, an adjutant, 12 nurses, orderlies, cooks and other general duty personnel. The Canadian medical staff were part of the hospital as a whole, primarily concerned with the Canadian wing, but also working in other parts of the hospital when time permitted and the need arose.

Canadian patients came to East Grinstead from the hospitals where first emergency care was given as quickly as possible after injury. There was a long, slow and painful process of rebuilding. Patients at East Grinstead received much special attention from outside because of the complex nature of their injuries. Part of this was because of the interest in the wonders being performed by the Canadian and British surgeons.

There was a remarkably informal and friendly atmosphere at East Grinstead in which nurses and orderlies, as well as other patients, took an intimate interest in every patient in the place.

The whole staff took a real personal interest in each patient's restoration and recovery.

By the end of the War, East Grinstead had developed into a recognized centre of plastic surgery. Canada's part in this development was the presentation of the war time Canadian wing to the trustees of the Queen Victoria Hospital. This will stand as a memorial, in the words of the dedicatory plaque:

"To the gallant young men of the Royal Canadian
Air Force whose wounds have brought them here and
to the Surgeons, Nurses and Staff who have cared
for them, this building has been erected by the
people of the Dominion Of Canada."
"The Healing of the World
is in its nameless saints." *

*Courtesy of the Department of National Defence, Canada. Kardex 181.099 (D6391).

Ruth M. Laberee

Graduated from: Hotel Dieu School of Nursing, Sherbrooke, Quebec. Year: 1948

Military History:

Service: RCAF

Rank: Captain (Retired)

Served: September 15, 1955 to February 1977

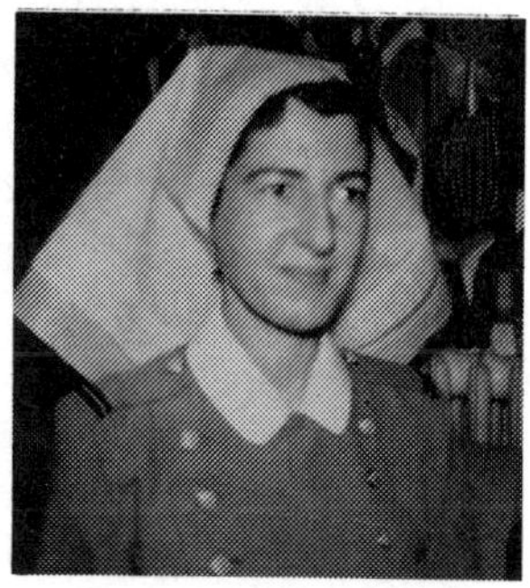

Ruth Laberee 4 (F) Wing, Baden-Soellingen, Germany. NATO Forces 1957-1960. RCAF nursing sister mess kit.

Flight Nursing – RCAF Station Trenton, 1963-65

I completed the Flight Nurse Course on basics at 4 Transport Operational Training Unit, RCAF Stn. Trenton, Ontario, 1 November 1963 following a simulated air medical evacuation flight, aboard a Dakota aircraft.

Fellow students, male and female, alternated as "patients" with simulated fractures, head injuries, etc., while our instructors assessed our nursing care treatments and reports. It was difficult to remain serious, to say the least, in this setting. Our previous classroom experience consisted of lectures, demonstrations, decompression chamber testing sessions, actively participating in simulating ditching exercises in bathing suits at the base indoor swimming pool using a large inflated covered raft. All this hard work would help us become the best possible flight nurses.

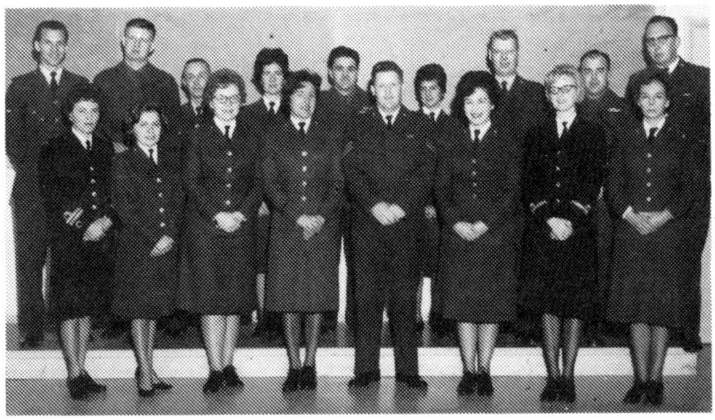

Air Evacuation Course RCAF Station Trenton, 1963. Rear L-R: LAC Thomas; Pte. White; Cpl. Martin; F/L Ruth Laberee; Pte.Gallant; F/O Yvette Gagnon; LAC Wauthier; Sgt. McGilivray; Cpl. Martin L-R: Eve Stymest; Berte Gallant; Janet MacKay; Peggy Corkum; Sgt. Ballantyne; June Parker; Barbara Hudon; Hillary Darlington.

Our destination was McGuire AFB, N.J., where we were to remain overnight. Our U.S. counterparts invited us to join them for a fine dinner. An early bedtime was "suggested" by our flight instructors, due to an early wake-up call for breakfast, followed by preparations for our return-simulated-air evac flight to RCAF St. Hubert, near Montreal.

The roles were reversed on the return trip. Simulated patients of the previous flight had now become the care-givers. Four and one half hours later we arrived at our destination and remained overnight. The following day we returned to our home base Trenton. Flying time – 11 hours and 30 minutes – we had all passed!

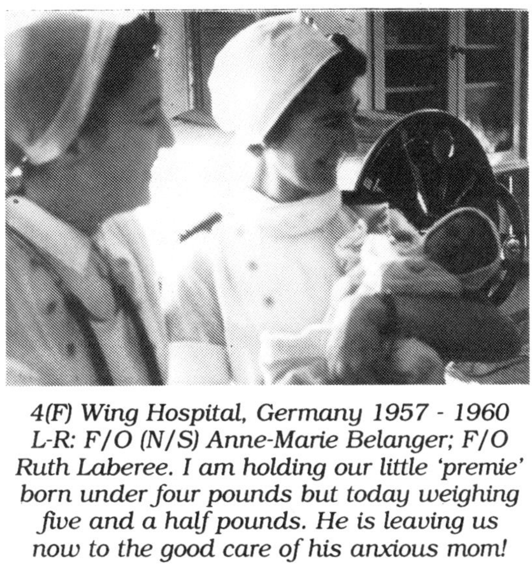

4(F) Wing Hospital, Germany 1957 - 1960 L-R: F/O (N/S) Anne-Marie Belanger; F/O Ruth Laberee. I am holding our little 'premie' born under four pounds but today weighing five and a half pounds. He is leaving us now to the good care of his anxious mom!

Civilian Medical Evacuation by Search and Rescue Squadron.

In the 60s it was not unusual for Search and Rescue Sqn., Trenton, to respond to a civilian request for air-medical evacuation in an isolated area.

From my log book, I remember vividly one cold, windy Saturday morning in March when the duty pilot at Search & Rescue phoned, requesting Flt. Nurse and Med Assistant on call to assist with the transportation of a civilian male patient with head injury, requiring immediate surgery at the Montreal Neurological Hospital.

All was organized quickly: our medical kits, oxygen, stretcher, etc., were placed on board a VERTOL helicopter.

Our destination was Ville Marie, Quebec, with a refuelling stop at RCAF Sta., North Bay, Ontario (a one hour & 35 minute flight).

Weather was worsening after we left North Bay. Strong winds shook the aircraft; visibility was limited due to icing and heavy snowfall preventing the windshield wipers from working effectively. For the pilot, it just seemed like a routine flight.

As we were approaching Ville Marie Hospital, the wind and snow had lessened. A large Red Cross flag appeared into view on the ground below. A group of people had gathered and were waving. The snow had been removed by the fire department crew for safe landing of the helicopter and a path, two feet deep to the hospital entrance had been cleared.

We congratulated the pilot for a job well done and looked forward to a hot cup of coffee.

The patient was safely placed aboard the helicopter. He tolerated the trip well and 2 hours and 25 minutes later the captain had landed his helicopter at Molson Stadium, adjacent to the Montreal Neurological Hospital. There our patient was safely transferred to his final destination.

Ten minutes later we landed at RCAF Stn. St. Hubert for a last refuel stop, then off to home base RCAF Station Trenton... just another routine flight!

Overseas Flights Aboard the Yukon

Regular monthly overseas Air Evac flights usually took place each month from RCAF No.

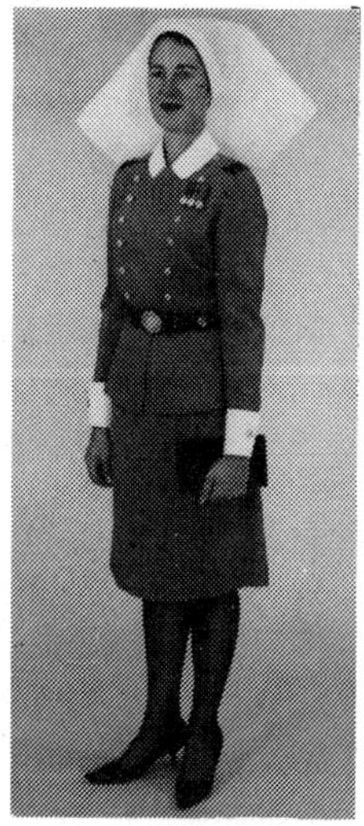

Ruth Laberee 4[F] WING Baden-Soellingen, Germany, NATO Forces. RCAF nursing sister mess kit 1961

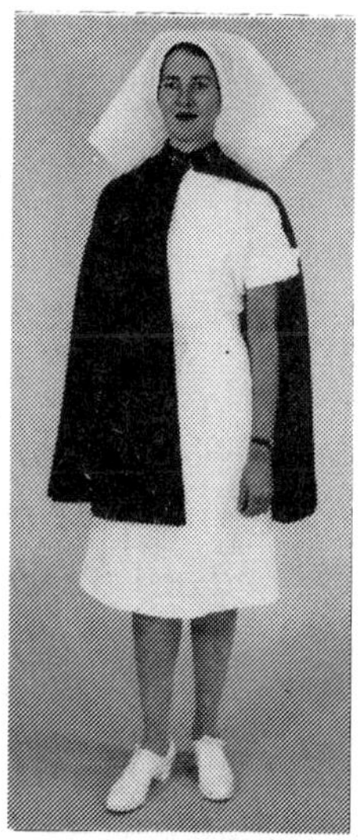

Ruth Laberee RCAF nursing sister, workdress and cape

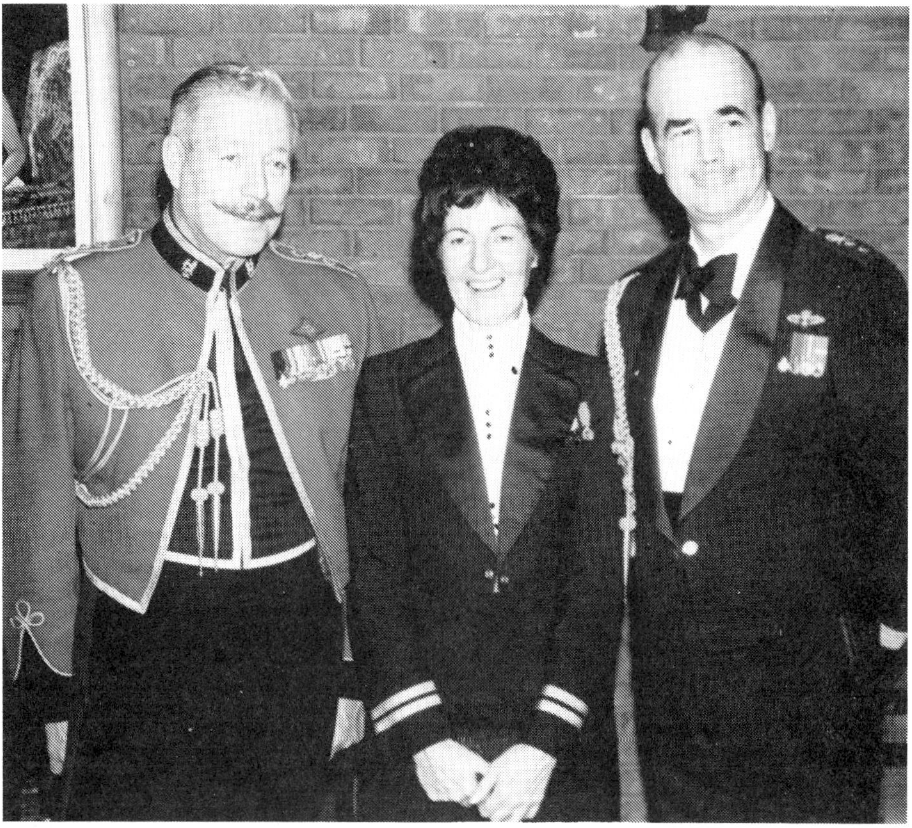

My Retirement Mess Dinner, National Defence Medical Centre CFB Uplands November 1976. L-R: General Cullen, Commandant NDMC, Captain Ruth Laberee, OPD Supervisor, General Leach, Surgeon General.
Canadian Forces photo

1 Wing, Marville, France (flt. time 10 - 11 hours and 30 minutes).

The designated Flt. nurse, Trenton, would fly over on a regular Yukon passenger flight.

The following day, she would then visit patients at the base hospital who had been transferred from different areas of the Canadian NATO bases, and Cyprus, etc., who were destined for Canada the following day.

She was responsible to ensure that all documents were in order, i.e., passports and immunization; confer with the medical officer concerning all patients; receive medication and narcotics if required from pharmacy; check their medical documents, ensuring that no contagious disease was present among travellers – Air evac charts were completed on all patients and sent to designated offices.

Upon arrival at Trenton, all patients and staff were checked through Customs & Immigration (they boarded the aircraft). They then transferred to our base hospital temporarily or "flown" to the National Defence Medical Centre, in Ottawa, usually on a Dakota aircraft, with the same flight nurse. Usually a little party awaited the flight nurse at nurses quarters upon arrival of an o'seas flight. All were anxious to see the PX goodies. The following day, patients destined for the western provinces were boarded on the Cosmopolitan aircraft for onward transfer to their respective bases accompanied by yet another flight nurse.

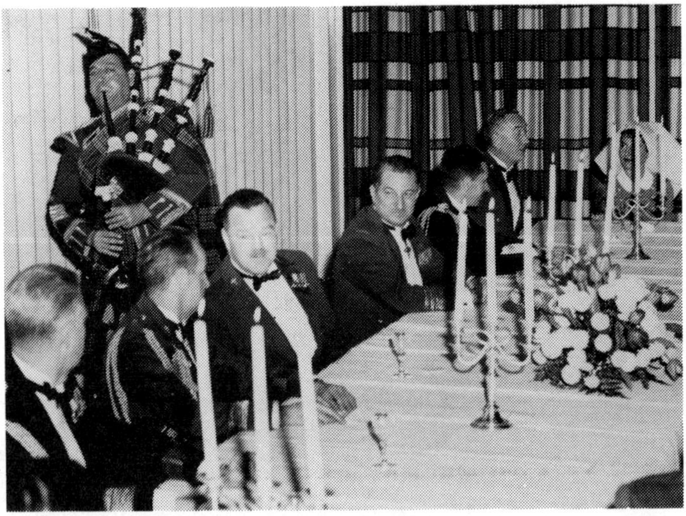

I was chosen Vice President of the Mess Committee. The retirement dinner for Air Commodore A.A.G. Corbet, Deputy Surgeon General Feb., 1961 at RCAF Station Rockcliffe, Ottawa, Ontario. I proposed the toast to the Queen.

Grace (Woodman) MacEachern

Graduated from: Lorraine Hospital School of Nursing at Pembroke, Ontario. Year: 1943

Military History:

Service: RCAF

Rank: Flying Officer.

Served: September 1951 to June 1955

I was training to become a nurse when WW II broke out but didn't finish in time for wartime service. Late 1944 I had a medical and was accepted, but the bomb was dropped in Japan and all medicals, etc., for entrance were cancelled. I was married to an Army veteran, Cranston Scott Woodman, in 1949 and was widowed in 1950. When the Korean War broke out I was accepted into the RCAF. I missed WW II and I didn't want to miss again.

The highlight of my service was being accepted into para-rescue and more so being able to make the course and graduate. In the summer of 1951 the government had decided to train an all-medical rescue team. I was on several searches out of Edmonton and Sea Island.

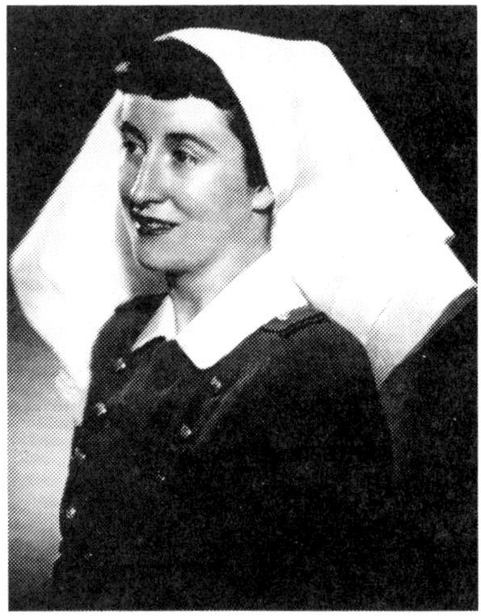

Nursing Sister Grace (Woodman) MacEachern, Edmonton 1955, the year I retired from the RCAF

The RCAF was looking for volunteers for para-rescue and I was fortunate in being chosen. The instructors were fabulous; you had absolute confidence in them. I was in the second para-rescue course that included nursing sisters. We took our outdoor training in the Columbia Icefields in the mountains near Jasper, Alberta, in 1952. We practised how to evacuate a patient on a stretcher while wearing skis. I loved the outdoors and every phase of the training.

My first operational jump was one of the worst jumps I ever made. It was in the mountains where the snow was very deep. We went in as a doctor-nurse rescue team with Sgt. Jamieson as jumpmaster. It was the first combination doctor-nurse jump, the first operational jump for Squadron Leader Dick Wynn and myself, and the first operational jump by a woman in the western world.

The patient we rescued was a geologist doing survey work on Mount Coquitlam when he sustained injuries from a fall. We could not have picked a more unsuitable area for parachuting. Our team was dropped from an RCAF Search and Rescue Squadron Dakota; ordinarily we never jump at night and this was 8:00 P.M. Saturday night. Our information on the possible injuries of Mr. Northcote indicated he had a punctured lung. It was imperative that we get in quickly. A tank of oxygen was parachuted with us. We all landed in the trees.

My parachute became entangled in a tall tree and I was left hanging head down. I worked myself into an upright position, after attaching the 100-foot rope (which all parajumpers wear strapped in their jumpsuits for emergencies such as this) to the bottom straps of the parachute. I had difficulty undoing the snap so I could remove my harness to free myself from the parachute and had to take my gloves off to unfasten the snap link. I slid down part way but I could not hold on to the rope anymore because my hands were burning so much, so I let go and fell the remaining distance to the ground.

The wind was knocked out of me. When I recovered it was too late for me to go in to where the patient was located. I spent a cold night under the trees. At 5:00 A.M. I heard voices. Dr. Wynn and Sgt. Jamieson had located me; they had stayed with the patient. A helicopter was called in and the patient was brought up to snow level. Our helicopter was having mechanical trouble and the U.S. Coastguard came in and evacuated the patient and myself from the snow level. After much persuasion they went back for Dr. Wynne and Sgt. Jamieson but would not go back for any of the ground crew as it was too dicey and risky in the mountains. B.C. Mines recognized us for our rescue work.

I will never forget the look of relief and joy on Mrs. Northcote's face to see her son safe. Her expressed thanks to all involved in the successful rescue made the risk and hard work well worthwhile.

In his post mission report S/L Wynne commended N/S Woodman for her perseverance and determination during the entire mission in spite of her injuries.

To this day, my hands are sensitive from the slide down the rope. After that jump the snap link (the one across the chest) was replaced by a press type release for our parachute harness, similar to the ones used by the Montana Smoke Jumpers.

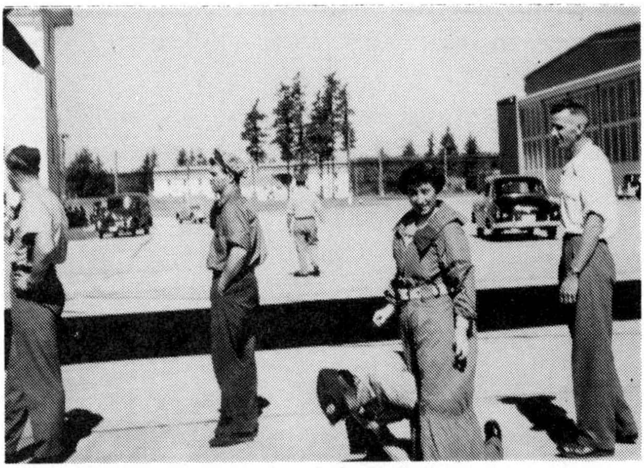

Nursing Sister Grace (Woodman) MacEachern

Summer Camp Abbotsford B.C. July 1952 L-R: Jack Strachan, Grace Woodman, Hank Jenkenson.

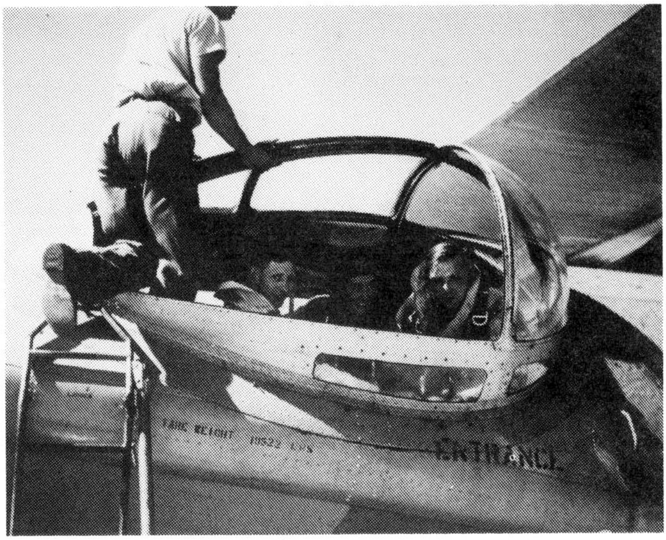

Grace Woodman parachuting at Abbotsford Air Cadets Summer Camp August 1952 This shows landing equipment and the size of the 'chute at Abbotsford, BC, Grace Woodman about 200 feet from the ground coming in for a landing.

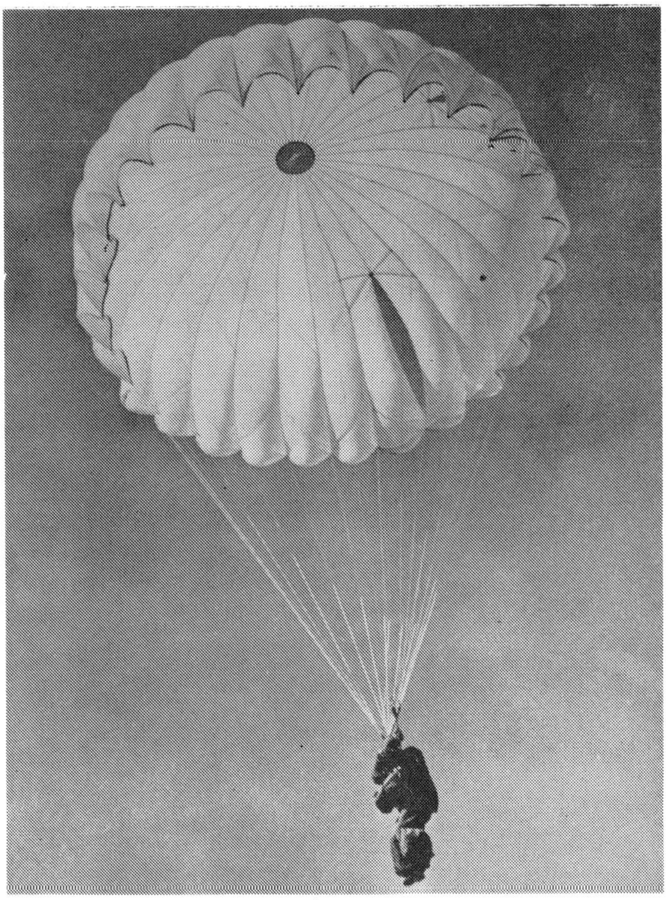

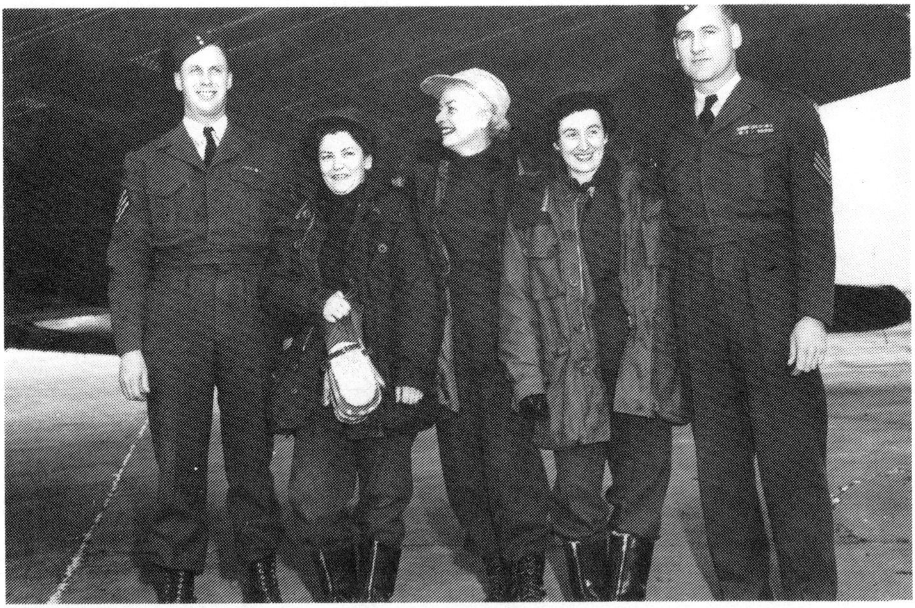

1953, in Edmonton, before simulated search and rescue flight north to Whitehorse for Virginia Kellog, Hollywood script writer who was gathering data for script for "Fox Studio" who were going to make a movie of the para-rescue nurses. I later went up to Jasper with her and Scott Alexander (head of survival school) to show her around survival etc., and the boys did a jump for her. One was also done for her in Whitehorse by the boys.

Taken the night before the operational jump at Sea Island, Vancouver, B.C. We were going to be checked out of a Dakota aircraft but a wind came up and it was put off until the next day and the next day it wasn't a practice but the real thing.

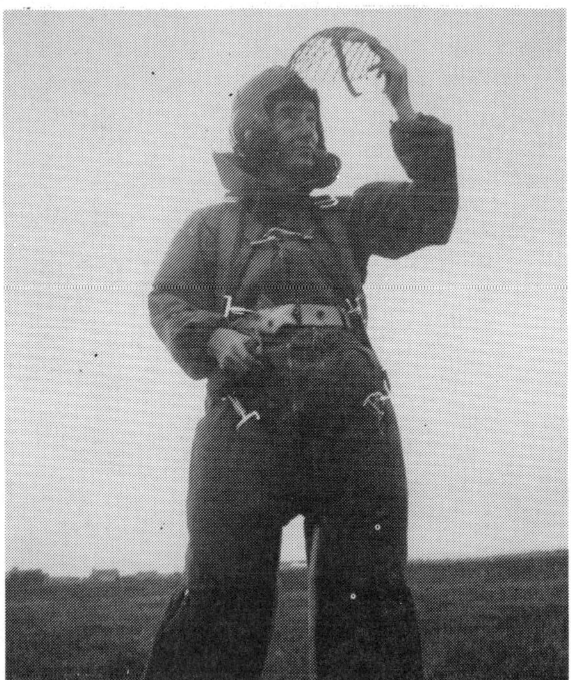

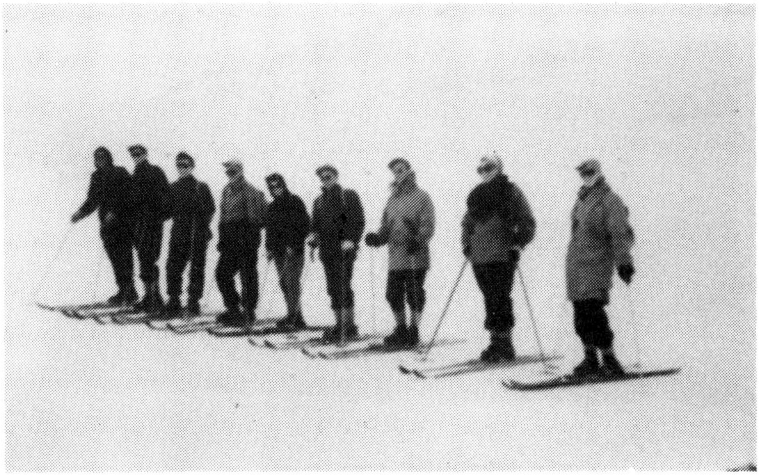

These nine people went to the top of Mount Athabasca around the snowdome. L-R: French ski professional; Don Niven; Larry McNab; Cecil Naughler; N/S Grace Woodman; Tony Chorney; Del Quesnel; Sgt. Ken Clarke; Sgt.Curley Sproat.

In the left corner the other two nurses, Marge Fera and Ruth Kelly and Grace Woodman talking to Dr. Kettles. Out of five nurses Fera, Kelly and Woodman completed the course. Between the first all medical and second all medical course, 10 nurses started and 7 finished

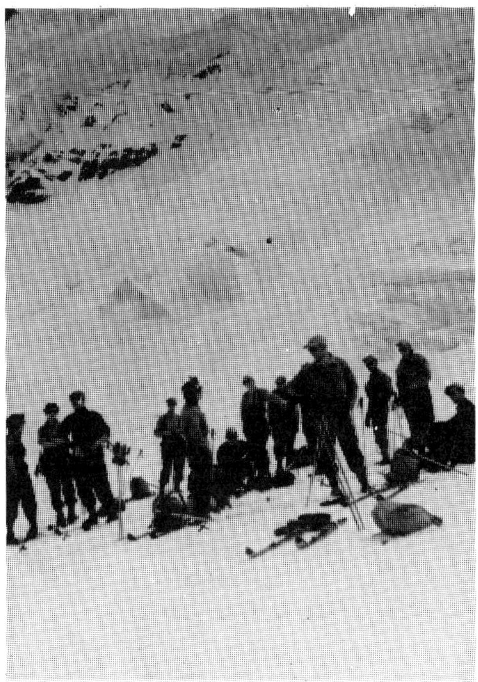

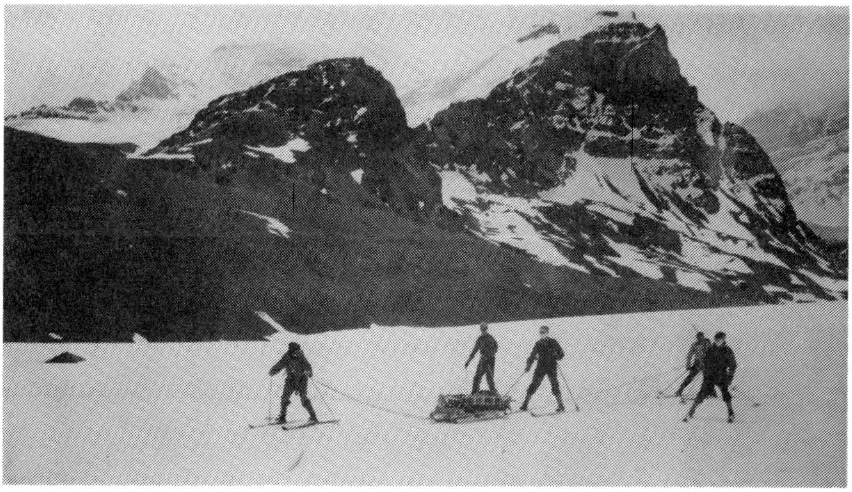

Practicing evacuation in the Icefields. Lead – Grace MacEachern. Ends – Don Niven and Curly Sproat. Dr. Hampson on right side. Behind him, Mr. Weiss, a Swiss fellow who taught us in the Icefields as well as mountain climbing all around Jasper.

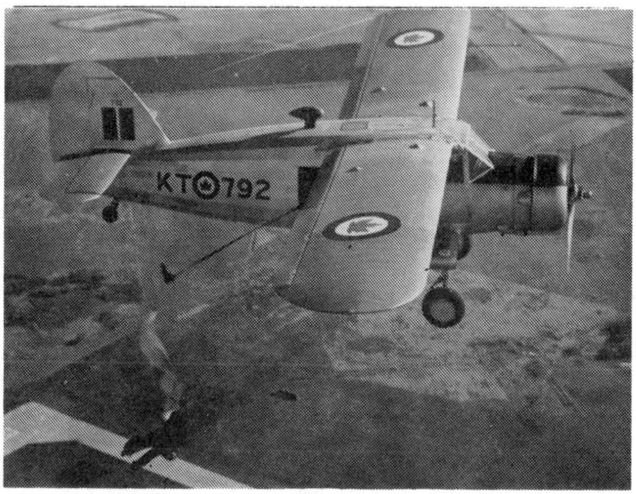

Jump out of a Norseman in 1954 at Namao Airport out of Edmonton by Grace Woodman

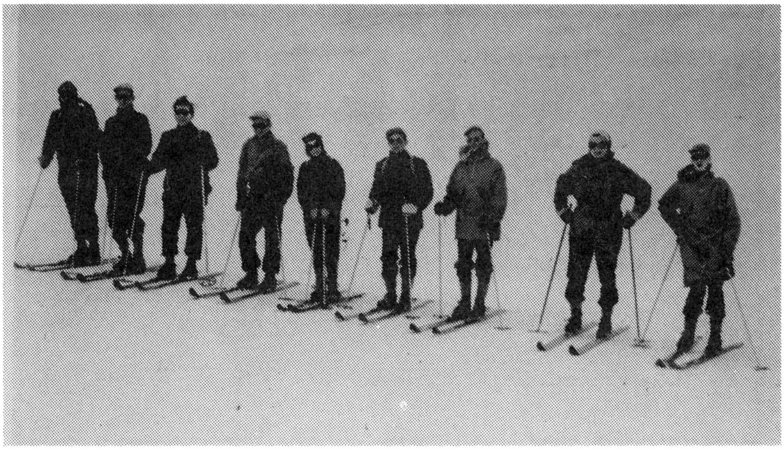

Left - right: Ski pro (French-in French Alps WW ll on patrol for army) Students: Don Nivens; Larry McNab; Cecil Naughler; Grace (Woodman) MacEachern; Tony Chorney; D. Tuechel. Two Instructors: Ken Clarke; Curley Sproat. The second all Medical Course was in winter and this was a first in the Columbia Icefields for anyone to go beyond the ice falls.

The only ones in the course who could ski were the two doctors and Grace Woodman. The doctors didn't want to go which left the ski instructor and myself to get the group up and back down. Quite a trek. The RCAF chose volunteers for an all medical team for para-rescue work. There were only two courses, one in the summer of 1951 and the second one January to June 1952. Ten nurses were selected , but due to injuries only seven completed the course. Our training consisted of six weeks at RCAF Station Edmonton with a view to improve our physical stamina for later training in the Rocky Mountains.

Our day consisted of running, swimming, push, set and chin-ups etc. We then moved into Jasper, Alberta where we were billeted in the town, but spent most of our days at a base camp around Jasper Park airstrip. We learned the art of bush survival, treatment of patients with injuries, rock work and mountain climbing, crossing gorges over rapids with stretchers etc.

Being close to the icefields, we added training in climbing the icefields with three on ropes, cramp-ons (for feet to dig into ice) and ice picks, evacuating a patient in a sled with ropes and on skis. All the time in the outdoors was a real bonus. All of our jumping was done around Jasper, six open jumps on the airstrip and four in the bush. We were a small team but became a very tight one, of helping and caring for each other.

Enid (Faulkner) Matheson

Graduated from: Toronto Western Hospital School of Nursing.
Year: 1940

Military History:

Service: RCAF

Rank: F/O

Served: 1942 to December 1945

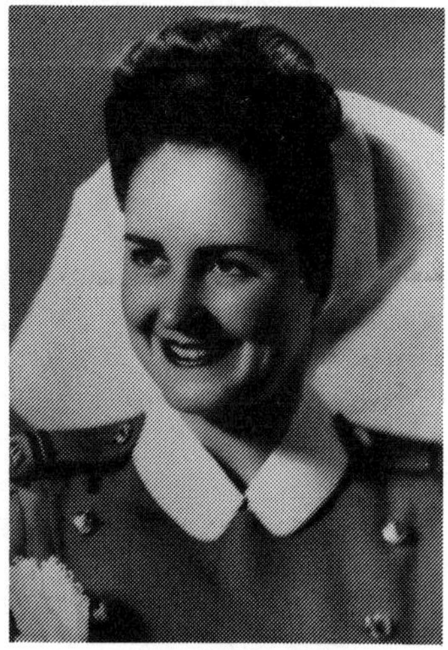

F/O Enid (Faulkner) Matheson

I chose to become a nursing sister in the RCAF first of all for duty to my country. Adventure and travel were also considerations.

My first duty assignment was No. 1 Manning Depot, Toronto, then No. 31 P.D. Moncton, N.B. For my first overseas assignment I was attached to No. 1 Neurological and Plastic Surgery Hospital at Basingstoke. I went for 2 weeks and stayed 6 months. I worked in neurosurgery in the operating room.

From there, I went to East Grinstead in the operating room with Dr. Ross Tilley and the Guinea Pigs.

I returned to Canada in the summer of 1945 to go to the Far East. However, VJ Day came and I was sent to Trenton. There, I worked in the operating room until I was married in December 1945.

Mary J. (Ross) Middlemass

Graduated from: University of Alberta Hospital Faculty of Nursing, Edmonton. Year: 1939

Military History:

Service: RCAF

Rank: Flying Officer

Served: RCAF March 1943 to March 1945 – Captain RCAMC October 1961 to August 1968

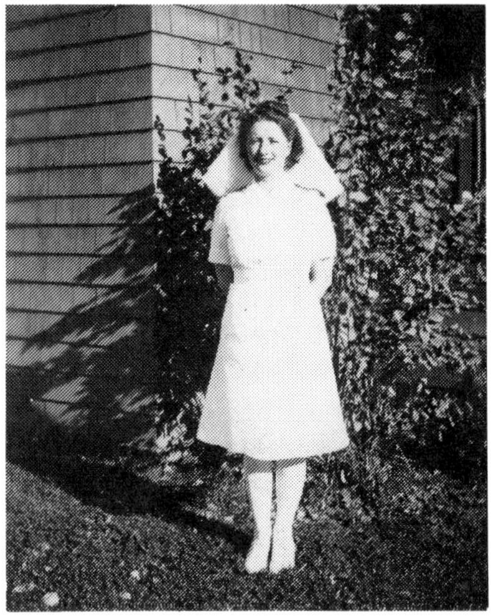

F/O Mary (Ross) Middlemass, 1944

Like many nurses graduating in 1939, a military career was a challenge. It was a different kind of nursing; the opportunity for travel was part of it.

I enlisted in March 1943 and was posted to RCAF Station Patricia Bay, Vancouver Island. My next duty was a course in aviation medicine at Havergel College, Toronto, and was then posted to 2 Air Observers School, Edmonton, until my release in April 1945.

I was called out from the Reserve List by the RCAMC in October 1961 to serve at Camp Wainwright, Alberta, as officer in charge of the Military Hospital.

I retired in August 1968 with rank of Captain, N/S.

Audrey (Adams) Nettleton

Graduated from: Toronto Western Hospital School of Nursing.
Year: 1955

Military History:

Service: RCAF

Rank: Flying Officer

Served: September 1956 to September of 1957

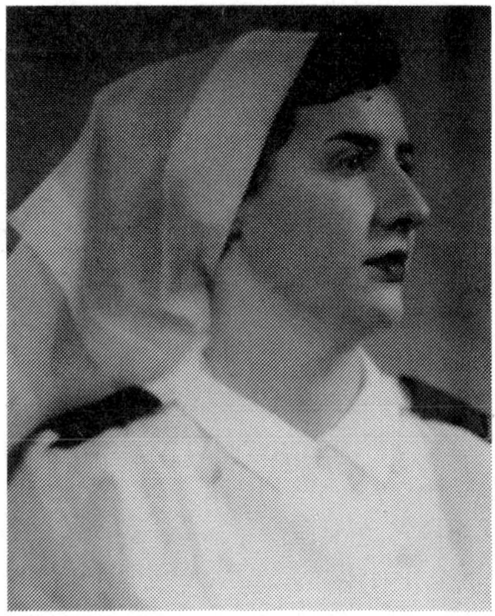

Flying Officer Audrey (Adams) Nettleton RCAF, September 1957, Gravenhurst, Ontario

My service began with three months' indoctrination at the Officers' Training School in London (Crumblin) Ontario, graduating from pilot officer to flying officer on completion. My first assignment was Station Beaverbank (a Dew line site) about 40 miles outside Halifax (now closed). On arrival, there was a medical officer in charge, but he was transferred to Uplands or Rockcliffe soon after I arrived. I was left in charge of a ten-bed hospital to run as a medical inspection room, with several medical assistants, a clerk, a civilian cleaner, and a civilian MO coming in twice a week to do sick parade. The rest of the time I handled sick parade, as well as tend to families who lived on the base. I also had to dispense medications from the well-stocked pharmacy and set up rotation for evening and weekend duties.

Those needing hospitalization were sent to Halifax to the hospital at *Stadacona*, the Infectious Hospital (a case of mumps), or the various civilian hospitals in the case of dependants. I made a point of visiting the hospitals weekly, taking the shift run back to Halifax in the morning and the afternoon run back to Beaverbank. Usually I had coffee at *Stadacona*, in the mess, and lunch in one of the restaurants downtown.

Most of the time there was little to do; play cards with the staff; join the Protestant choir; swim in the pool or play badminton (the latter three during time off, of course).

Twice it was necessary to do some stitching! Once, an airman stood up too fast, and not carefully, from the bottom bunk,

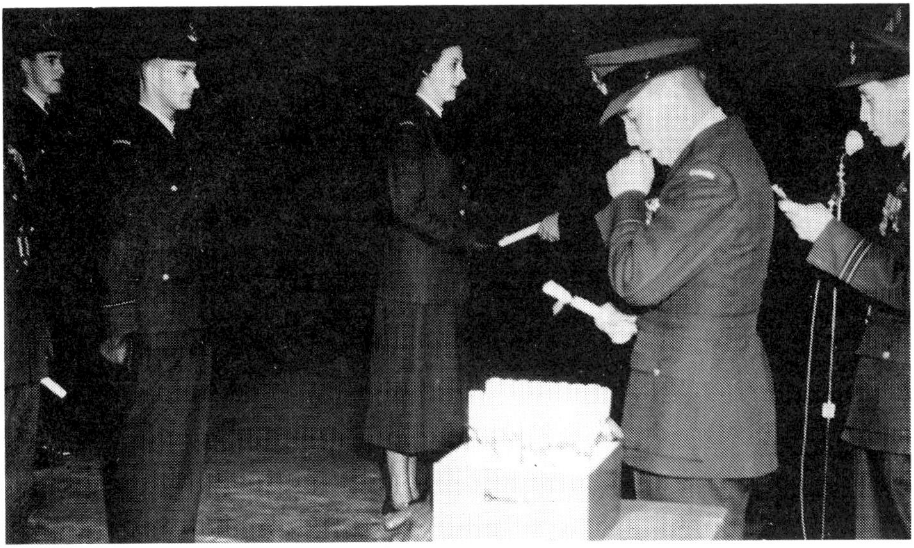

Course 5613 London, Ontario, December 1956. F/O Adams receiving certificate from G/C Guin; F/O V. Devooght; F/L P. Harrow. L-R: F/O Stanley (back); F/O A. Fiske; F/O L. Patrick (back) F/O A. Forget

hitting his head on the top one. The second time it was a Navy officer who lived closer to Beaverbank than *Stadacona* and had already had first aid. There was a third incident where stitches were needed; "the sink came up and hit me on the chin" - but that patient was sent to *Stadacona*! One other time it was necessary to go with the Roman Catholic padre to assist as a widow was consoled following the death of her husband in a car accident.

Since Beaverbank was one of the Dew (Distant Early Warning) stations, there was a period of an exercise called an Alert, during which searches were carried out and security was tighter than usual. It was also necessary for me to inspect the barracks from time to time, with the squadron warrant officer (SWO) present when I entered the men's quarters in case someone was in the washroom or asleep because they were on a later shift.

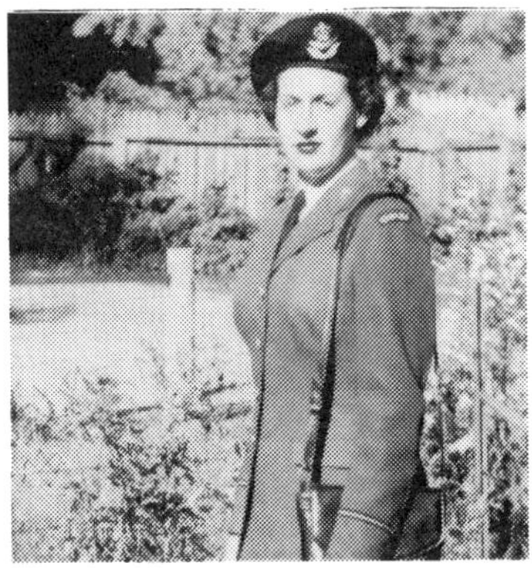

Flying Officer Audrey (Adams) Nettleton RCAF, September 1957, Gravenhurst, Ontario

My military career ended when I requested release to be married in November of 1957. My fiancé (now husband) was leaving to study in England for two years with a view to an overseas posting.

Ruth L. (McTavish) Pearce

Graduated from: St. Joseph's Hospital School of Nursing, Victoria. Year: 1936

Military History:

Service: RCAF

Rank: Flying Officer

Served: 1941 to 1945

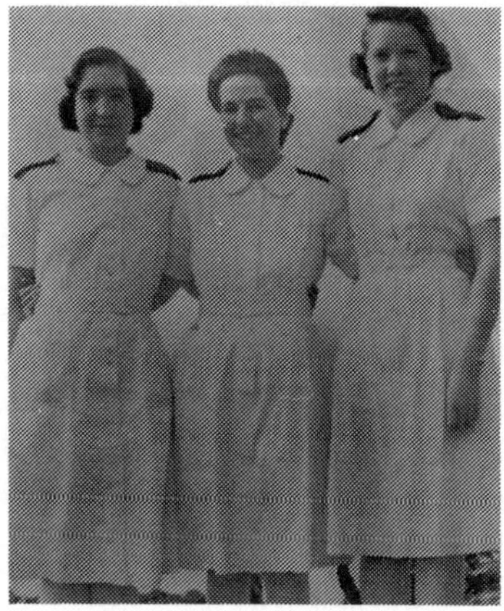

1. Ruth (McTavish) Pearce, Ucelet, BC 1943
2. Natalie Blackwood
3. Evelyn Frostad

Because I wanted a change in my life I chose to become a nursing sister in the RCAF.

It was a great experience and the friends I made were the highlight of my military career.

Shirley Robinson

Graduated from: General and Marine Hospital School of Nursing, Owen Sound, Ontario. Year: 1953

Military History:

Service: RCAF

Rank: Lt. Colonel

Served: 1954 to 1984

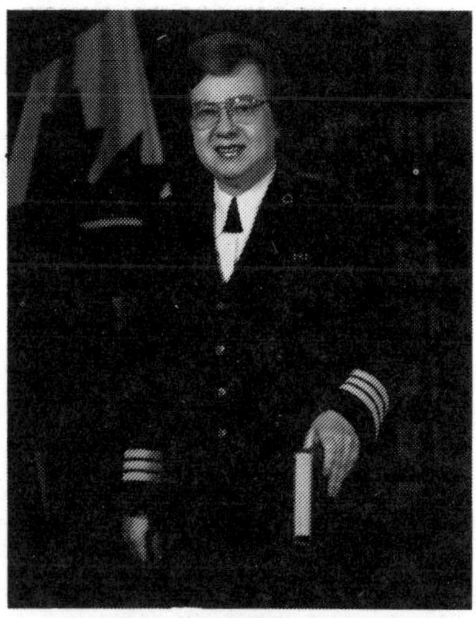

Lt. Colonel Shirley Robinson, retired

I wanted to be in the military for as long as I can remember. I became a registered nurse toward that end, to qualify as an officer. I was interested in adventure and a life with a difference.

I am a native of Lucknow, Ontario, where I received my secondary education. I am a registered nurse by profession having graduated from the General and Marine Hospital School of Nursing, Owen Sound, Ontario, in 1953. I enrolled in the Royal Canadian Air Force as a pilot officer in 1954 and underwent basic officer training in London, Ontario.

I spearheaded efforts to improve and effect progressive change within the CF nursing classification, including renewed emphasis on nurses being good officers as well as good nurses. To this end, I advocated basic training for nursing officers which resulted in the introduction of the Advanced Nursing Officer Course and Nursing Officer Seminars to prepare selected officers for more senior positions.

During my thirty-year career with the Canadian Armed Forces, I served in numerous senior military nursing and administrative positions in Canada and overseas. Including were those of staff officer to the Surgeon General at National Defence Headquarters, Ottawa, and Director of Nursing at the National Defence Medical Centre, Ottawa.

I completed courses in military nursing, medical nursing, nursing unit and nursing service administration; I am a graduate of both junior and senior staff courses from the Canadian Forces Command and Staff College in Toronto, Ontario. Additionally, I completed French language training and Advanced Management courses at St. Jean, Quebec.

Prior to my retirement in 1984, I was deputy director of women personnel at National Defence Headquarters, and as such, was intimately involved with all aspects of women's employment and conditions of service within the Armed Forces. Throughout my career, I endeavoured to improve and advance the military nursing service, and the role and employment opportunities for Canadian Forces women.

Since retirement I have been politically active in efforts to gain career equity for servicewomen by: Co-founding the Association for Women's Equity in the Canadian Forces (AWECF); Presenting written and verbal briefs to federal ministers and other parliamentarians; Acting as consultant to the Canadian Human Rights Commission, and the Status of Women in Canada on the role of military women; Assisting the legal profession in the preparation of discrimination cases against the armed forces; and; Appearing before the media to publicize the importance of equity for military women.

I am a member of: the Council of Canadians; the Human Rights Institute of Canada; the College of Nurses of Ontario.

For devoting a significant part of my life to improving and enhancing the role and opportunities of Canadian Forces women while a member of the armed forces, and since my retirement, I received the Governor General's award in commemoration of the Persons Case in October, 1992.

During my 30-year career as a nursing officer in the Canadian Forces Medical Services, I have served in progressively responsible positions and have gained extensive knowledge and experience in nursing and personnel administration. Throughout my career I have continually endeavoured to improve and enhance the Canadian Forces Nursing Services and the role and employment opportunities for military women.

SHIRLEY ROBINSON RECEIVES GOVERNOR GENERAL'S AWARD IN COMMEMORATION OF THE PERSONS CASE

On October 20, 1992, the Right Honourable Ramon Hnatyshyn, Governor General of Canada, presented Shirley Robinson of Gloucester the Governor General's Award in Commemoration of the Person Case.

The Governor General's Awards are given to individuals who have made an outstanding contribution toward promoting the equality of women in Canada.

The awards commemorate the lengthy legal and political battle for women's constitutional right to be recognized as persons. Led by the efforts of five Alberta women: Emily Murphy,

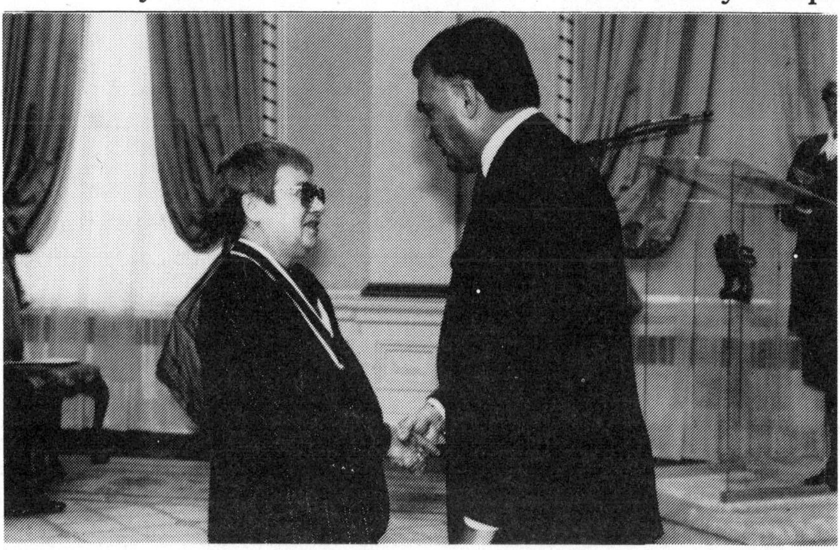

Lt. Colonel Shirley Robinson, retired

Louise McKinney, Nellie McClung, Irene Parlby, and Henrietta Muir Edwards, the Persons Case culminated with the decision rendered by the British Privy Council on October 18, 1929, which declared Canadian women to be persons and thus eligible for appointment to the Senate. The Governor General's Awards in Commemoration of the Persons Case were established in 1979 to celebrate the 50th anniversary of this effort.

Lieutenant-Colonel (Retired) Shirley Robinson has devoted a significant part of her life to improving and enhancing the role and opportunities of women within the Canadian Armed Forces. During her 30-year military career, she was an active advocate of women's equality in employment and conditions of military service. She was appointed Deputy Director of Women Personnel at National Defence Headquarters in 1983. Since retirement in 1984, she has continued her efforts to promote women's equality. Shirley is the co-founder of the Association for Women's Equity in the Canadian Forces, a non-governmental agency which works for women's equal status in the Armed Forces.

Courtesy of: City & Community section of Gloucester Leader, November 1992 page 8.

Margaret (Murray) Rogers

Graduated from: Royal Alexandra Hospital School of Nursing, Edmonton. Year: 1940

Military History:

Service: RCAF

Rank: F.O.

Served: September 1943 to November 1945

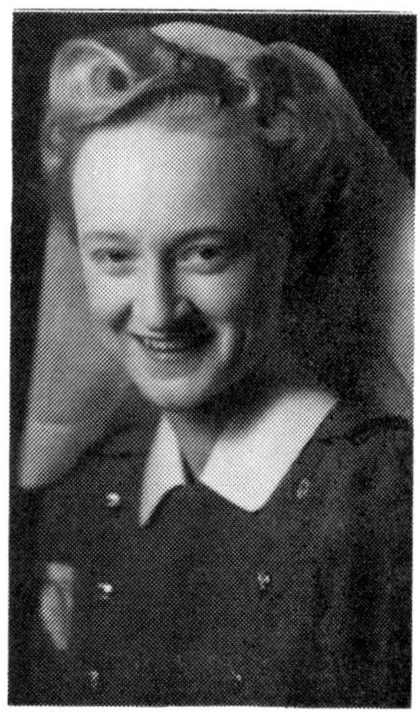

N/S Margaret (Murray) Rogers

As did millions of others, I joined the RCAF to do my part for King and Country

My service time was all west of Winnipeg. I did some air ambulance work; there were no particular highlights.

Rena V. (Mayson) Roskilly

Graduated from: the Royal Alexandra Hospital School of Nursing, Edmonton. Year: 1940

Military History:

Service: RCAF

Rank: F/O (N/S)

Served: 8 October 1943 to 29 September 1945

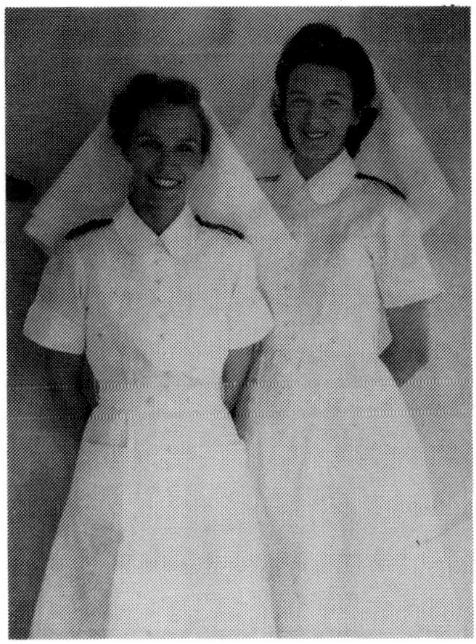

Calgary; L-R: F/O N/S Mary Westway, Senior N/S No. 10 RD, RCAF; F/O N/S Rena (Mayson) Roskilly, RCAF

After working general duty and as operating room nurse in Kimberly and District Hospital and at Banff Mineral Springs Hospital I enlisted in the RCAF in May of 1943. This enlistment took place at Western Air Command, Calgary, Alberta. Working as a civilian, waiting for my commission, my first duty was in an "H" hut isolation hospital at No. 10 Repair Depot, Calgary, Alberta. Here I was confronted and confounded by the many accents of Australian, New Zealand, English, Scottish, Welsh and Irish airmen-in-training in the Air Commonwealth Training Plan. But before long I began to understand all of them. This isolation hospital took care of the many boys infected by what we considered "childhood" diseases, i.e., mumps, chicken pox, measles and many cases of scarlet fever.

When these diseases finally were cured and there were no further new infections, I went up to the new Station Hospital (10 RD) and served there until May 1945. I received my commission in October 1943. During that time I served as ward sister in the operating room. In July 1944 I was posted on temporary duty for one month to the School of Aviation Medicine in Toronto, Ontario, and for the first time saw a part of eastern Canada beyond the Saskatchewan border. It was a very enjoyable and informative course – also giving us time for weekend exploration of surrounding areas including Niagara Falls.

When my fiancè returned following his tour of operations as

a rear air gunner in the Special Duties Squadron, we were married in Calgary in March 1945.

Bill was stationed at RCAF Station, Abbotsford, BC. After asking for and receiving a posting to Pacific Command, I was stationed at RCAF Station, Patricia Bay, BC, one of the most beautiful spots in Canada. There were trees in blossom everywhere; cherry and apple trees and the famous B.C. Dogwood trees all in a misty soft and gentle air.

While I was there, besides the usual nursing duties there were two memorable and hectic duties – days on VE Day and nights on VJ Day – these two I'll never forget.

My husband received his discharge on the 21st of September, 1945 and I on the 29th of September, 1945.

We returned to Kimberly, B.C., to start civilian life and to raise our family (three daughters). Since that time I worked part-time while the girls were small and returned to work full time in the operating room, retiring as head nurse, OR in 1978.

I enjoyed my two years serving as a nursing sister in the RCAF and will always look back with fondness to the memories and people I met in those years.

Maureen Seymour

Graduated from: Royal Jubilee Hospital School of Nursing, Victoria, B.C. Year: 1944

Military History:

Service: RCAF

Rank: F/L

Served: 4 September 1949 to 18 August 1965

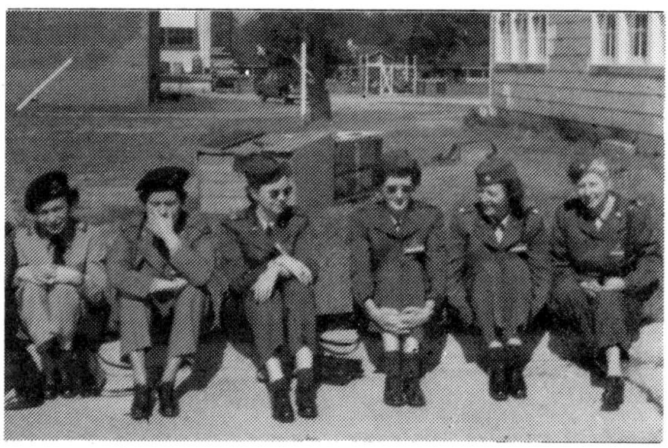

M. Seymour at U.S. School of Aviation Medicine Flight Nurse Course. Gunter Air Force Base. June 1953, second from left - Maureen Seymour

I spent a day aboard a U.S. Navy submarine when based at Hickam AFB. Very cramped quarters and very strict discipline – saluting, etc. We looked through the periscope. One experienced the same sensation when diving or resurfacing as going up in an aircraft and landing.

We took air evacuation training in two phases; the initial phase was six weeks at U.S. Gunter Air Force Base, Alabama, where we set up litters, learned crash procedures, and practised putting on a parachute. We simulated evacuation procedures. We also learned swimming because our flights took us over the ocean.

The second phase was the practical aspect of our training. We spent three months at U.S. Hickam Air Force Base, Hawaii, with Medical Air Evacuation Squadron (MAES), 1453 Squadron. From there we flew to Tokyo with refueling stops at Wake Island or Johnson Island, a man-made island in the Pacific Ocean. During refueling all patients were off-loaded; they were not allowed to remain on the aircraft but were taken by ambulance to a U.S. hospital where personal care and food were provided.

When we flew Hawaii to Tokyo there was an overnight or two-day turnaround. We had breakfast in Tokyo, then breakfast again when we arrived back at Hickam Air Force Base.

Patients were very well screened in Tokyo and Air Force nurses could refuse a patient. Because of this screening process, there were seldom any adverse situations. There were sometimes two or three patients on Stryker frames; we turned them every two hours.

There was the capacity for 120 patients on these pressurized "flying boxcars." They were staffed with two nurses and two technicians. There were four patient categories. On the flight from Hickam to Travis AFB in California, there was usually one nurse and one technician as there were fewer patients.

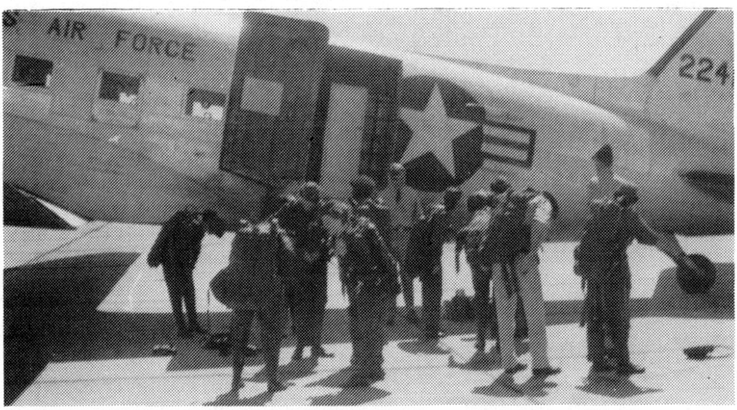

Maureen Seymour at Gunter AFB, USAF

After the three-month practical experience we went back to Canada. I was stationed at RCAF Station Rockcliffe, Ontario, then at Four Wing, Germany.

In 1955 there was a poliomyelitis epidemic at One Wing affecting both military personnel and civilian dependants. We gave 10 cc of gamma globulin, 5 cc in each hip; there were no deaths.

After 16 years in the RCAF I attended the University of Toronto to obtain a B.Sc. in administration.

Signe (Johnson) White

Graduated from: St. Boniface Hospital School of Nursing ,St. Boniface, Manitoba. Year: 1936

Military History:

Service: RCAF

Rank: Flying Officer

Served: March 1942 to October 1945

I filled out a request to volunteer in case of war or disaster. The RCAF responded and I was a nursing sister in the Royal Canadian Air Force.

My military service took me from Saskatchewan to Newfoundland.

March 1942: Posted to RAF Service Station, Weyburn, Saskatchewan

January 1943: Posted to RAF Operational Training Unit, Debert, N.S.

1944 - 1945: Posted to RCAF, Sydney, N.S., Ferry Command,

Coastal Patrol, Gander, Nfld.

In Gander we treated Newfoundland citizens from remote and isolated areas of the province (150-bed hospital).

Isabel Ziegler

Graduated from: Brandon General Hospital School of Nursing, Brandon, Manitoba. Year: 1949

Military History:

Service: RCAF

Rank: Pilot Officer - Flying Officer, Flight Lieutenant.

Served: 1950 to 1964

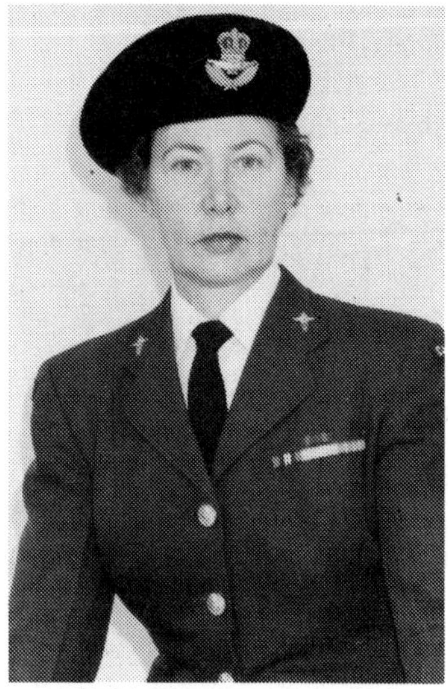

Flight Lieutenant Isabel Ziegler

When I joined the RCAF I really wanted to be a pilot. I was six years old when I first watched a plane fly overhead; I've been fascinated with flying ever since that time. I was in the Women's Division of the RCAF for four years during World War Two and took my discharge in 1945. In 1949 I graduated from Brandon General Hospital School of Nursing.

When I joined in 1950 I became the fiftieth nurse in the RCAF and there were only fifty RCAF nurses in all of Canada. My first assignment was at Station Rockcliffe. That year I was chosen to go for Aeromedical Evacuation Training at Gunter Air Force Base, Alabama, U.S.A. The criteria for acceptance was a commitment to length of service and the ability to cope in a situation when no physician was present. Each nurse had certain preferences; most were hoping to do something where they would move by air, they were quite happy to get in an aircraft to go anywhere as they preferred that mode of travel.

Gunter AFB was the training school for Medical Air Evacuation for all of the U.S.A. although only RCAF nursing sisters went from Canada. After six weeks at Gunter I did three months of practical training with 1453rd Medical Air Evacuation Squadron at Hickam Air Force Base in Hawaii.

This squadron was used to bring the wounded from Korea. From the Korean airfields they all went to Tokyo then to Hickam. We loaded up in Tokyo with patients from the Korean conflict. It was hard on these people when we had to off-load them for aircraft refueling. They were put in an ambulance and taken away from the centre then shuttled back to the aircraft. If they were able to return to the war zone within three months, they stayed at Hickam. For anything longer than that, they were brought back stateside. Canadian patients returned to Canada via RCAF transport. From Travis Air Force Base they were flown to Madigan Army Hospital in Washington State. Canadian nursing sisters accompanied them from Madigan Army Base, Washington State, U.S.A. to the veterans hospital closest to their home in Canada because they were going to have a long hospital stay. The medical staff consisted of one nurse and one medical assistant; there were no physicians on board.

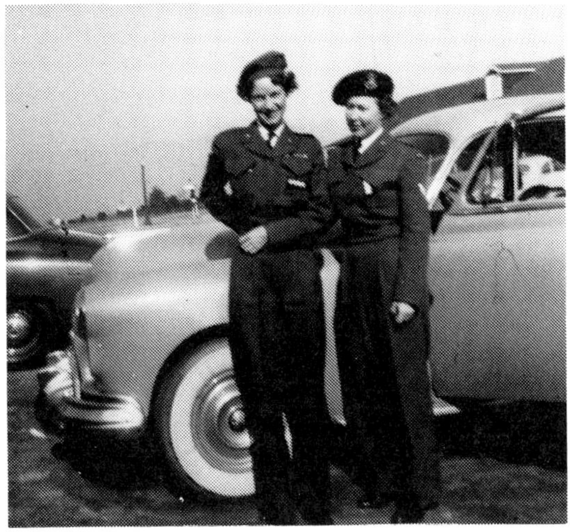

L-R: N/S Jane (Drummond) Beattie, RCAF and N/S Isabel Ziegler, RCAF at U.S. Gunter Air Force Base, January 1951.

When we boarded one of these aircraft to fly to Tokyo to pick up patients we were weighed in as freight. There had to be only a certain number of nurses and medical technicians, then if an aircraft were lost there was not such a great loss of medical personnel. So we were weighed in complete with our medical kit which was a suitcase complete with urinals, bedpans, medication, and, if you were smart, an alarm clock, because all medications had to be given on zebra time. We had two clocks, our wrist watch and one clock in our medical kit which was set on zebra time; that is, Greenwich mean time.

When writing up our notes we had to use local time as well as zebra time to try to keep things in order. A complete record was maintained of the time each patient spent in the air as well as each off-loading and on-loading. When they arrived at U.S.A. Tripler Army Hospital in Hawaii, each patient had a slip of paper listing the miles he had flown, and the time of his medication in zebra time.

Not only were we crossing time zones, we were also crossing the international date line. We had to send a request to the RCAF in Washington, D.C. for remuneration for our expenses. My first request listed the same day twice. I was notified that I'd have to look over my records as I'd made an error and could not have two days with the same date. After much correspondence we reached an agreement, but I'm sure that clerk didn't know anything about crossing the international date line.

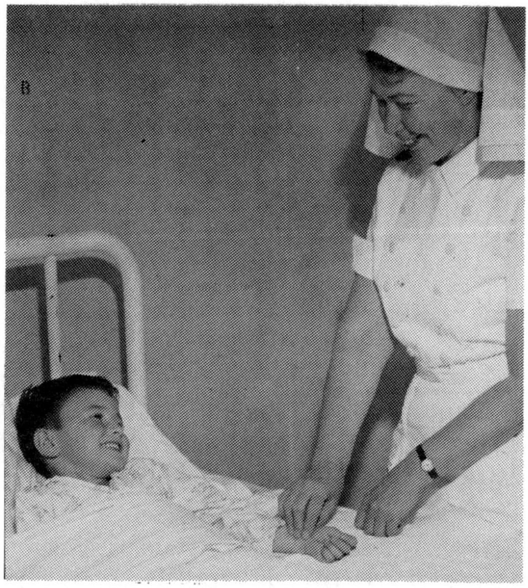

N/S I. Ziegler and a dependant patient at Goose Bay RCAF Hospital, 1951.

We stayed overnight on Wake Island in Quonset huts. Here the bottom bunk was preferable because rats used the top bunks for their own private runway. A sign in the washroom said "Be Careful of Water We Make Water." Ocean water was captured and put through evaporators, therefore, water was very expensive and in short supply.

One time on the way back to Hickam as I was going down the aisle with special diets, a Canadian patient called to me. He got as far as *"Oh Sister"* when my medical technician assistant told him in no uncertain terms that he was speaking to an officer. He was to call her by her rank or say ma'am, definitely not sister. I just caught him by the arm and quietly explained our tradition in the commonwealth countries of referring to us as nursing sisters. Far from it being a derogatory term, we much preferred it to being addressed by our rank. He was very embarrassed, but it did point out one of our differences.

Another time after we started from Hawaii to the Mainland, our captain quietly warned us that we were having a bit of trouble and we might hear an unevenness in the motor. One of our patients, a Canadian paratrooper, noticed it immediately; he had flown enough to know motor sounds. I gave what I hoped was a reassuring answer when the captain called me and said we were at the point of no return and were going to turn back to Hawaii. He was going to do a wide circle and hoped it wouldn't be noticeable. Before long, this same paratrooper called me and told me he could see Search and Rescue aircraft outside the window. We were being paralleled by two Search and Rescue aircraft because of the number of people aboard. They had come from Hickam to catch up to us after the pilot radioed that he was turning back. They had large orange boats slung under their fuselage so they could rescue us if we had to ditch.

As we got closer to Hickam, flying on three engines, we lost a second engine. Fortunately, it was on the opposite side from the other damaged engine so the pilot was able to balance the aircraft. When we touched down on the runway at Hickam, we lost our third engine and came to the end of the runway on one motor. There wasn't a person on board who wasn't relieved as we finally taxied to a stop.

At the end of my three-month practical experience in April 1951, I returned to Canada and was stationed at Goose Bay, Labrador. My friend, Joan Beattie, went to Edmonton as there could not be two nurses with the same qualification at one station. Later, I applied for the Air Force's Para Rescue course when volunteers were requested. I felt I could have contributed much in that field. However, my request was denied as I was already trained in aeromedical evacuation and we could not be dual trained. I did aeromedical evacuation for the year I was at Goose Bay. We cooperated with the Grenfell nurse who was stationed at Happy Valley; a settlement on the outskirts of our military area.

Winnipeg was my next assignment when the poliomyelitis epidemic was at its height. I worked on the isolation ward after having received gamma globulin. The military had one floor of a large civilian isolation hospital in downtown Winnipeg, the King George Hospital. It was part of the Winnipeg Municipal Hospital system. There were five iron lungs to a ward and they were placed head to head in such a way that we could look after two or three patients more easily. The Army brought some large field generators and set them up on our hospital lawn. Only twice while I was on duty did they cut out when there was a power failure due to storms.

This was the first instance in Canada where we had nurses from all three services under one matron, Elizabeth Hodgson, an Army nurse from Shilo Army Base, Manitoba. She was chosen because of her experience during World War Two and she took over one isolation floor. She had to coordinate the Army, Navy and Air Force nurses of this isolation wing and arrange for staffing hours of the medical technicians and nurses. She tried to accommodate Army nurses at Fort Osborne, Navy nurses were split up and Air Force nurses were housed at the RCAF Station. There were so few beds in our quarters that as soon as we got up we rolled up our bed as if we were in a combat area. We put that bedroll in a corner while the next nurse unrolled her bedroll from where she had stored it and climbed into bed. We didn't enter that room once we were up because each nurse had to get a certain number of hours of sleep.

There were technicians, doctors and nurses from all three Services. Unification of the medical services of the Navy, Army and Air Force into one unified medical service didn't take place until January, 1959.

My next assignment was at Comox, B.C. Air Force Base, a Search and Rescue Station. We had a few beds for emergencies but I took most patients by ambulance to HMCS *Naden* in Victoria. I continued search and rescue at Sea Island; from there the patients went to Shaughnessy Veterans hospital. Several times I flew to pick up poliomyelitis patients from Prince George and Prince Rupert. We transported them in an iron lung or in a chestpirator – a plastic appliance taped onto the patient and operated off the aircraft supply system.

We went out when there was a definite patient to be picked up. Civilian small aircraft liked to take any emergency but didn't want anyone with a communicable disease as that required fumigation of their aircraft after the trip. After transporting patients with communicable disease, the RCAF sprayed the plane with a disinfectant and sealed it off for 24 hours.

Several times we picked up premature infants from the interior of B.C. One time, coming back from the B.C. Interior, we had to make an emergency landing on a grass strip in the Fraser Valley when our motor failed. That was my second hair-raising experience with failed motors. Almost as alarming was my experience with JATO or Jet Assisted Take Off.

We went out from Sea Island to a weather ship in the Pacific Ocean in a Grummond Goose, an amphibious aircraft. A young fellow had developed an acute abdomen, and while there was a physician aboard there was no operating room. We landed and got him on the aircraft but the pilot had neglected to tell us he was going to use JATO. It is an electrically operated rocket to put you up in the air; it's like being shot out of a rocket. We left in a cloud of smoke; anyone observing our take off would think we had exploded.

From Sea Island I went to Fort Nelson, then after a short assignment at Winnipeg I was assigned to Three Wing at Zwiebrucken, Germany, from 1959 to 1960. I did only one evacuation there, I took two dependants with tuberculosis to Holland to go on a civilian aircraft on a special flight from Amsterdam to the Vancouver airport. They were noninfectious by this time and thus allowed to fly.

My third assignment at Winnipeg, 1961 to 1964, was my last duty with the RCAF. When U.S. Air Force planes put down here in case of emergency because of bad weather at Fort Nelson, we had to stand by while refueling with high octane took place. Normally USAF planes overshot Winnipeg on their way to Churchill for Arctic testing. A nurse and a medical technician went out with an ambulance and stood by, sometimes for hours while they were on the ground. Then we went back to our regular duties.

At Winnipeg we shared the runway with the civilian airport and were responsible for all civilian emergencies after 4:00 P.M. We used Deer Lodge Veterans Hospital, Winnipeg, Manitoba, for our military patients as our facility was only a Medical Inspection Room.

In 1962 we flew from Winnipeg to Inuvik on a North Star, a four-engine aircraft. We were on an expedition to the Arctic to test the feasibility of a frozen package dinner that could be heated while in flight and served to patients on Aeromedical Evacuation. It was tested on the crew.

I helped to evacuate an airman injured in a helicopter crash during cold weather testing. That was my last Aeromedical Evacuation before my discharge from the RCAF.

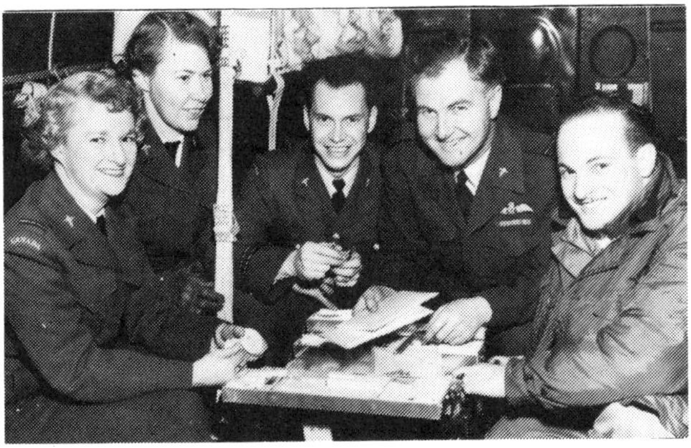

RCAF Sea Island, 2 February 1955 enroute to Sandspit F/O M. Kennedy; F/O I. Ziegler; F/L D. Tanguay; W/C Barclay; LAC G. Barnes aboard Aeromedical Evacuation; planning pickup.

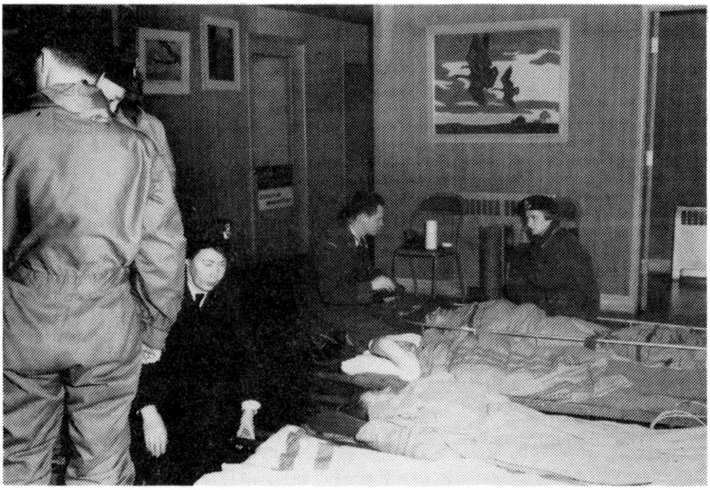

Sandspit Terminal, rescue of 5 survivors of plane crash 1 February 1955. L-R: LAC G. Bierness; F/O Isabel Ziegler; W/C Barclay; F/L B. Tanguay; F/O Margaret Kennedy.

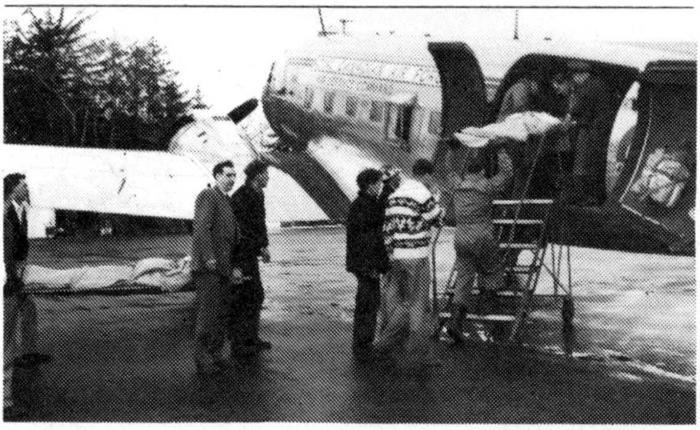

Loading patients at Sandspit, 2 February 1955

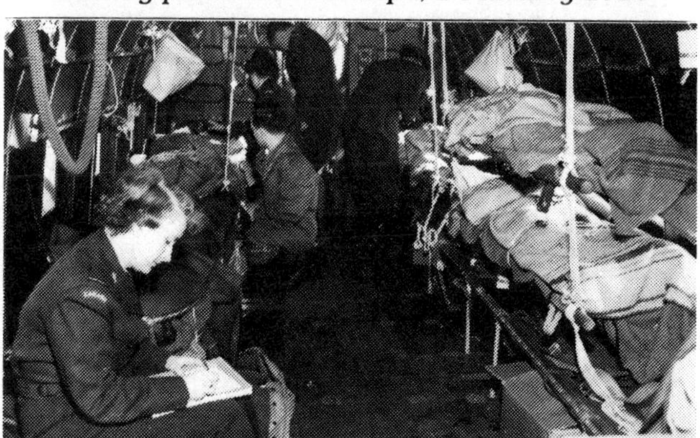

Airborne, Aeromedical Evacuation from Sandspit, returning with patients. L-R: F/O Margaret Kennedy; LAC G. Bierness; F/O Isabel Ziegler; W/C Barclay; F/L B. Tanguay

ABBREVIATIONS

A A	ack-ack/anti-aircraft
ATS	Auxiliary Territorial Service
ADS	Advance Dressing Station
ASU	Advance Surgical Unit
CAMC	Canadian Army Medical Corps
CCS	Casualty Clearing Station
CFMS	Canadian Forces Medical Services
CFMG	Canadian Forces Medical Group
CO	Commanding Officer
Col.	Colonel
C St. J.	Commander Order of St. John
CSR	Central Supply Room
EMS	Emergency Medical Services
ENSA	Entertainments National Services Association
FDS	Field Dressing Station
FSU	Field Surgical Unit
FTU	Field Transfusion Unit
F/O	Flying Officer
F/C	Flight Cadet
IV	Intravenous
LAC	Leading Aircraftsman
LCT	Landing Craft Tank (assault, mechanized, infantry)
LST	Landing Ship Tank
M & V	Meat and vegetables
Med "A"	Medical Assistant
MD	Military District
MO	Medical Officer
NAAFI	Navy, Army and Air Force Institutes, a British organization that provided canteens and/or shops in all their military camps and residential clubs on overseas stations.
NGO	Non-Government Organization
NO	Nursing Officer
OC	Officer Commanding
ORs	Other Ranks
OR	Operating room
OS	Ordinary seaman
P/O	Pilot officer
POW	Prisoner of War
QARANC	Queen Alexandra's Royal Army Nursing Corps
QAIMNS	Queen Alexandra's Imperial Military Nursing Service
RAF	Royal Air Force
RAMC	Royal Army Medical Corps
RCAF	Royal Canadian Air Force
RCAMC	Royal Canadian Army Medical Corps
RCN	Royal Canadian Navy
R & R	Rest and Recreation
SAMNS	South African Military Nursing Service
S/L	Squadron Leader
SMO	Senior Medical Officer
V-1	*Vergeltungswaffe* or Vengeance Force Bomb. Also known as "Buzz Bomb" or "Doodle Bug"
V-2	*Vergeltungswaffe* or Vengeance Force Rocket
VAD	Volunteer Aid Detachment
W/C	Wing Commander
WRCNS	Women's Royal Canadian Naval Service

REFERENCES

Brown, Andrea and Shaffelburg, Diane (1986) *Women in the War Effort.* Board of Education for the City of North York Resource Booklet for Remembrance Day. Produced by: Women's Studies Curriculum and Staff Development Services, North York Schools.

Canadian Military History. Biannual Periodical. Wilfred Laurier University, Waterloo.

Desjardins, Edouard, M.D. (1971) *Heritage: History of the nursing profession in Quebec from the Augustinians and Jeanne Mance to Medicare.* From material researched and supplied by Eileen C. Flanagan & Suzanne Giroux. Published by the Association of Nurses of the Province of Quebec.

Feasby, W.R. (1946 *Official History of the Canadian Medical Services 1939 - 1945. Vol. 1 Organization and Campaigns,* Ottawa, MND.

Gardiner, Juliet (1992) *Overpaid, Oversexed & Over Here: The American GI in World War II Britain.* New York: The Abbeville Press Incorporated.

Gibbon, J.M. & Mathewson, M. (1947). *Three Centuries of Canadian Nursing.* Toronto: The Macmillan Company of Canada Limited.

MacPhail, Sir Andrew (1925*). Official History of the Canadian Forces in the Great War 1914 - 1918. The Medical Services.* Ottawa, MND.

Morton, Desmond (1985). *A Military History of Canada.* Edmonton: Hurtig Publishers.

Nicholson, G.W.L. (1975). *Canada's Nursing Sisters.* Toronto: A.M. Hakkert Ltd.

Richards, Stanley (1994). *Operation Sick Bay.* West Vancouver: Cantaur Publishing.

Stanley, George F.G. (1974) *Canada's Soldiers.* 3rd Edition. Toronto: The Macmillan Company of Canada Ltd.

The New Encyclopaedia Britannica. 1994. 15th Edition. Chicago

War Diaries. All information in the brief history at the beginning of each unit came from the War Diaries at the National Archives of Canada.

INDEX

Only names of those who contributed narratives are included in this index. They are in alphabetical order by maiden name. The married name is listed below.